DOSAGE CALCULATIONS

DOSAGE CALCULATIONS

FOURTH CANADIAN EDITION

Gloria D. Pickar, EdD, RN
Group President and Chief Academic Officer
EmbanetCompass
Orlando, Chicago, Toronto
Former Academic Dean
Seminole State College of Florida
Sanford, Florida

Amy Pickar Abernethy
Associate Professor of Medicine and Nursing
Duke University
Durham, North Carolina

Beth Swart
Ryerson University

NELSON

NELSON

Dosage Calculations, Fourth Canadian Edition
by Gloria D. Pickar, Amy Pickar Abernethy, and Beth Swart

VP, Product and Partnership Solutions:
Anne Williams

Senior Publisher, Digital and Print Content:
Paul Fam

Marketing Manager:
David Groth

Technical Reviewer:
Heather LeBlanc

Content Development Manager:
Suzanne Simpson Millar

Photo and Permissions Researcher:
Natalie Barrington

Production Project Manager:
Jaime Smith

Production Service:
Integra Software Services Pvt. Ltd.

Copy Editor:
Mariko Obokata

Proofreader:
Integra Software Services Pvt. Ltd.

Indexer:
Integra Software Services Pvt. Ltd.

Design Director:
Ken Phipps

Higher Education Design PM:
Pamela Johnston

Interior Design Revisions:
Cenveo Publisher Services

Cover Design:
Trinh Truong

Cover Image:
Tom Merton/Getty Images

Compositor:
Integra Software Services Pvt. Ltd.

Printed and bound in Canada
1 2 3 4 20 19 18 17

For more information contact Nelson Education Ltd., 1120 Birchmount Road, Toronto, Ontario, M1K 5G4. Or you can visit our Internet site at nelson.com

Library and Archives Canada Cataloguing in Publication

Pickar, Gloria D., 1946-, author
Dosage calculations / Gloria D. Pickar, EdD, RN, President and Chief Academic Officer, Compass Knowledge Group, Orlando, Florida, Former Academic Dean, Seminole Community College, Sanford, Florida, Amy Pickar Abernathy, Duke University, Beth Swart, Ryerson University. —Fourth Canadian edition.

Includes index.
ISBN 978-0-17-665715-4 (softcover)

1. Pharmaceutical arithmetic—Textbooks. 2. Textbooks— I. Swart, Beth, author II. Pickar Abernathy, Amy, author III. Title.

RS57.D68 2017 615.1'401513
C2016-907615-6

ISBN-13: 978-0-17-665715-4
ISBN-10: 0-17-665715-0

CONTENTS

PREFACE

Introduction

Dosage Calculations, Fourth Canadian Edition, offers a clear and concise method of calculating drug dosages. The text is directed to students and professionals who want to improve their comfort level with mathematics, and to faculty members who prefer the formula method for calculating dosages. The previous three Canadian and nine U.S. editions have been classroom tested and reviewed by well over 1 million faculty and students, who report that this textbook helped decrease math anxiety and promote confidence in their ability to perform accurate calculations. As one reviewer noted, "I have looked at others [textbooks] and I don't feel they can compare."

The only math prerequisite is the ability to do basic arithmetic. For those who need a review, Chapters 1 and 2 offer an overview of basic arithmetic calculations with extensive exercises for practice.

The text teaches the Three-Step Approach for calculating dosages:

1. Convert measurements to the same unit;
2. Consider what dosage is reasonable; and
3. Calculate using the formula method.

Dosage Calculations, Fourth Canadian Edition, is based on feedback from users of the previous editions and users of other dosage calculation texts. The new edition also responds to changes in the healthcare system by introducing new drugs, replacing outdated drugs, and discussing new or refined ways of administering medications. This revision was designed with the beginning Canadian healthcare provider in mind. The International System (SI) of units is used almost exclusively. The medication dosages and drug labels have been cross-referenced with the current Health Canada drug database so that beginning professionals will be able to recognize names and dosages. The importance of avoiding patient safety incidents, previously referred to as medication errors, is highlighted by the incorporation of applied critical thinking skills in clinical reasoning scenarios based on patient care situations. New to this edition, examples of National Council Licensure Examination (NCLEX) test items are provided at the end of Chapters 5 to 14. These examples will better prepare graduates for their later examinations.

Organization of Content

This text is organized in a natural progression of basic to more complex information. Learners gain self-confidence as they master content in small increments with ample review and reinforcement. Many learners claim that because of using this textbook, they overcame their fear of math for the first time.

Dosage Calculations has 14 chapters, divided into four sections. At the end of each section is a Self-Evaluation, which is a test in workbook format with areas for students to write their answers.

Preceding *Section 1* is a *Mathematics Diagnostic Evaluation*, which allows learners to determine their computational strengths and weaknesses. Section 1 then begins. *Chapters 1* and *2* provide a review of basic arithmetic skills, including fractions, decimals, ratios, percents, and simple equations, with numerous examples and practice problems to ensure that students can apply the skills. *Chapter 3* introduces systems of measurement with a focus on the metric system, which is the standard used in the healthcare field. The household system is included briefly because of its applications for care at home. *Chapter 4* is an overview of the three calculation methods. This overview is accompanied by numerous examples and practice problems to ensure that students can apply the procedures. This section introduces conversion from one unit of measurement to another. The SI system of measurement is emphasized because of its exclusive use in Canada's healthcare sector. However, to challenge students and prepare them for real life, a small number of questions require students to convert imperial values to metric. Even though metric is used in Canada, many individuals still give their weight in pounds and height in feet and inches, which require conversion to metric. Questions using imperial values also emphasize attention to detail. The use of the apothecary and household system is de-emphasized in the chapters, and additional information is provided in the Appendices. The ratio and proportion method of performing conversions is also included; however, in this edition, ratio–proportion is not a major focus because research has shown that using this approach may be more prone to errors in calculations. International, or 24-hour, time is included. Fahrenheit and Celsius temperature conversions are covered in Appendix D.

Section 2 includes Chapters 5 to 7. The information in this section forms the foundation for measuring drug dosages and understanding drug orders and labels.

In *Chapter 5,* users learn to recognize and select appropriate equipment for the administration of medications based on the drug, dosage, and method of administration. Emphasis is placed on interpreting syringe calibrations to ensure that the dosage to be administered is accurate. All photos and drawings have been enhanced to improve clarity, and state-of-the-art technology and information systems have also been updated.

Chapter 6 presents common abbreviations used in healthcare so that learners can become proficient in interpreting medical orders. Generic medication administration records have been used, as appropriate, for examples. In addition, the content on computerized medication administration records has been updated.

It is essential that learners be able to read medication labels to accurately calculate dosages. This skill is developed by having readers interpret the medication labels provided beginning in *Chapter 7.* These labels are from current commonly prescribed medications and are presented in full colour and actual size wherever possible.

In *Section 3,* the reader learns and practises the skill of dosage calculations applied to patients across the life span. *Chapters 8* and *9* guide the reader to apply all the skills mastered to achieve accurate oral and injectable drug dosage calculations. Students learn to think through each problem logically for the right answer and then to apply a simple formula to double-check their thinking. Experience has shown that when this logical but unique system is applied every time to every problem, math anxiety decreases and accuracy increases.

High-alert medications such as insulin and heparin sodium are thoroughly presented. Insulin types, species, and manufacturers have been updated.

Chapter 10 introduces the preparation of therapeutic solutions. Students learn the calculations associated with diluting solutions and reconstituting injectable drugs. This chapter leads to intravenous calculations by fully describing the preparation of solutions. As a result of the expanding role of the nurse and other healthcare providers in the home setting, clinical calculations for home care, such as nutritional feedings, are also discussed.

Chapter 11 covers the calculation of pediatric and adult dosages and concentrates on the body weight method. Emphasis is placed on verifying safe dosages and applying concepts across the life span.

Section 4 presents advanced clinical calculations applicable to both adults and children. Intravenous administration calculations are presented in *Chapters 12* through *14.* Coverage reflects the greater application of IVs in drug therapy. Shortcut calculation methods are presented and explained fully. More infusion devices are included. Heparin and saline locks, types of IV solutions, IV monitoring, IV administration records, and direct IV drugs are presented in *Chapter 12.* Pediatric IV calculations are presented in *Chapter 13,* and obstetric, heparin sodium, insulin, and critical care IV calculations are covered in *Chapter 14.* Ample problems help students master the necessary calculations.

Pedagogy

Each chapter begins with **Objectives** that reflect clear expectations to help students focus on what they are expected to achieve once each chapter is completed. The learning can be readily transferred from the classroom environment to the workplace environment.

Procedures in the text are introduced using **Rule** boxes and **Examples**.

Key concepts are summarized and highlighted in **Quick Review** boxes before each **Review Set,** to allow learners an opportunity to review major concepts prior to working through the problems.

Rationale for Practice boxes identify *why* a specific strategy will help solve a problem.

Math Tips provide memory joggers to assist learners in accurately solving problems.

Learning is reinforced by **Practice Problems** at the conclusion of each chapter.

The importance of calculation accuracy and patient safety is emphasized by patient scenarios that apply critical thinking skills. **Application of Clinical Reasoning** scenarios have also been added to the end-of-chapter problem material, to further emphasize accuracy and safety.

Information to be memorized is identified in **Remember** boxes, and **Caution** boxes alert learners to critical procedures and information.

NEW! New to this edition is the addition of an **Understanding NCLEX Questions** box near the end of Chapters 5 to 14. An example of a standard question used in textbooks is presented with another example of how the question would look as a NCLEX question. The solution is also provided.

NEW! Answers to the Review Sets can be found at the end of each chapter, enabling students to easily check their work as they progress. Solutions to some of the Review Sets are also provided there.

Self-Evaluations at the end of each section provide learners with an opportunity to test their mastery of chapter objectives prior to proceeding to the next section. Two post-tests at the conclusion of the text evaluate the learner's overall skill in dosage calculations. The first test, the *Essential Skills Evaluation*, covers essential skills commonly tested by employers. The second post-test, the *Comprehensive Skills Evaluation*, serves as a comprehensive evaluation of all 14 chapters. Both are presented in a case study format to simulate actual clinical calculations.

An *Answer Key* at the back of the text provides all answers as well as selected solutions to Practice Problems, Self-Evaluations, Essential Skills Evaluation, and the Comprehensive Skills Evaluation.

Appendix B reviews systems of measurement, in particular, the SI system. *Appendix C* describes the apothecary system of measurement. *Appendix D* reviews household units, and *Appendix E* reviews units of measurement for temperature and instructions to convert from one to the other. A general content *index* concludes the text.

Note about the Text

The authors have used the Drug Product Database, Health Canada (www.hc-sc.gc.ca/dhp-mps/prodpharma/databasdon/index-eng.php), for the recommended dosages in this text. There may be some discrepancies among Health Canada, drug monographs, and the *Compendium of Pharmaceuticals and Specialties* (*CPS*) in the dosage range requirements for drugs used as examples in the text. The purpose of this calculations text is to practise calculations. The authors have tried to be as accurate as possible; however, it is the responsibility of the individual administering the drug to ensure that the dosage administered is safe.

Features of the Fourth Canadian Edition

- Content is divided into four main sections to help learners better organize their studies.
- Measurable **Objectives** at the beginning of each chapter emphasize the content to be mastered.
- More than 1200 problems reflecting current drugs and protocols are included for learners to practise their skills and reinforce their learning.
- **Application of Clinical Reasoning** skills apply critical thinking to realistic patient care situations to emphasize the importance of accurate dosage calculations and the avoidance of patient safety incidents.
- Full colour is used to make the text more user-friendly. Chapter elements such as **Rules, Rationale for Practice**, **Math Tips**, **Cautions**, **Remember** boxes, **Quick Reviews**, NCLEX-style test item examples, and **Examples** are colour-coded for easy recognition and use. Colour also highlights **Review Sets** and **Practice Problems.**
- Most syringes and measuring devices are drawn full size to provide accurate scale renderings to help learners master the measurement and reading of dosages.
- Colour has been added to selected syringe drawings throughout the text to *simulate a specific amount of medication,* as indicated in the example or problem. Because the colour used may not correspond to the actual colour of the medication named, *it must not be used as a reference for identifying medications.*
- The math review brings learners up to the required level of basic math competence.
- SI and the conventional metric system notation are used. (The household system of measurement is introduced but not emphasized.)
- **NEW! Understanding NCLEX questions.** An example of a standard question used in textbooks is presented with another example of how the question would look as a National Council Licensure Examination (NCLEX) question. The solution is also be included.
- **Rule** boxes draw the learner's attention to pertinent instructions.
- **Rationale for Practice** boxes provide the reasoning for a specific action or decision when calculating drug dosages.
- **Remember** boxes highlight information to be memorized.
- **Quick Review** boxes summarize critical information throughout the chapters before **Review Sets** are solved.
- **Caution** boxes alert learners to critical information and safety concerns.
- **Math Tips** point out math shortcuts and reminders.
- Content is presented from simple to complex concepts in small increments followed by **Review Sets** and chapter **Practice Problems** for better understanding and to reinforce learning.
- Many problems involving the interpretation of syringe scales are included to ensure that the proper dosage is administered. Once the dosage is calculated, the learner is directed to draw an arrow on a syringe at the proper value.

- Canadian labels of current and commonly prescribed medications are included to help users learn how to select the proper information required to determine the correct dosage. More than 200 labels have been used in this text. The author and publisher have made every effort to include only labels in use today.
- Numerous **Examples** demonstrate the $\frac{D}{H} \times Q = X$ formula method of calculating dosages.
- The dimensional analysis and ratio–proportion methods are included, giving instructors and students a choice of which method to use in calculating dosages.
- Abbreviations, measurements, acronyms, and symbols follow Institution for Safe Medication Practices (ISMP) Canada's "Do Not Use" list.
- Clear instructions are included for calculating IV medications administered in milligram per kilogram per minute.
- Clinical situations are simulated using actual medication labels, syringes, patient care order forms, and medication administration records.
- An **Essential Skills** post-test simulates exams commonly administered by employers for new hires, assesses prior knowledge, and evaluates learning of essential calculation skills. **Comprehensive Skills** evaluates the learner's overall comprehension.
- The general index helps learners and instructors easily find content and skills.

Instructor Resources

The **Nelson Education Teaching Advantage (NETA)** program delivers research-based instructor resources that promote student engagement and higher-order thinking to enable the success of Canadian students and educators. Visit Nelson's **Inspired Instruction** website at nelson.com/inspired/ to find out more about NETA.

The following instructor resources have been created for *Dosage Calculations*, Fourth Canadian Edition. Access these ultimate tools for customizing lectures and presentations at nelson.com/instructor.

NETA Test Bank

This resource was written by Myrna Michelle Davis, Red River College. It includes over 250 multiple-choice questions written according to NETA guidelines for effective construction and development of higher-order questions.

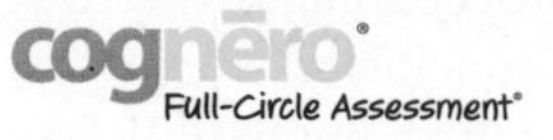

The NETA Test Bank is available in a new, cloud-based platform. **Nelson Testing Powered by Cognero®** is a secure online testing system that allows instructors to author, edit, and manage test bank content from anywhere Internet access is available. No special installations or downloads are needed, and the desktop-inspired interface, with its drop-down menus and familiar, intuitive tools, allows instructors to create and manage tests with ease. Multiple test versions can be created in an instant, and content can be imported or exported into other systems. Tests can be delivered from a learning management system, the classroom, or wherever an instructor chooses. Nelson Testing Powered by Cognero for *Dosage Calculations*, Fourth Canadian Edition, can be accessed through nelson.com/instructor.

NETA PowerPoint

Microsoft® PowerPoint® lecture slides for every chapter have been created by textbook author Beth Swart, Ryerson University. There is an average of 15 slides per chapter, many featuring key figures, labels, tables, and photographs from *Dosage Calculations*, Fourth Canadian Edition. NETA principles of clear design and engaging content have been incorporated throughout, making it simple for instructors to customize the deck for their courses.

Image Library

This resource consists of digital copies of figures, tables, photographs, and drug labels used in the book, in a version with and without labels. Instructors may use these jpegs to customize the NETA PowerPoint or to create their own PowerPoint presentations. An Image Library Key further lists the description and filename of each jpeg.

Instructor's Solutions Manual

This manual, prepared by author Beth Swart, has been independently checked for accuracy by Heather LeBlanc, Oulton College. It contains complete solutions to Review Sets, Practice Problems, Essential Skills Evaluation, and the Comprehensive Skills Evaluation. It also includes suggested answers for the Application of Clinical Reasoning problems.

MindTap

MINDTAP Offering personalized paths of dynamic assignments and applications, **MindTap** is a digital learning solution that turns cookie-cutter into cutting-edge, apathy into engagement, and memorizers into higher-level thinkers. MindTap enables students to analyze and apply chapter concepts within relevant assignments, and allows instructors to measure skills and promote better outcomes with ease. A fully online learning solution, MindTap combines all student learning tools—readings, multimedia, activities, and assessments—into a single Learning Path that guides the student through the curriculum. Instructors personalize the experience by customizing the presentation of these learning tools to their students, even seamlessly introducing their own content into the Learning Path.

Student Ancillaries

MindTap

MINDTAP Stay organized and efficient with ***MindTap***—a single destination with all the course material and study aids you need to succeed. Built-in apps leverage social media and the latest learning technology. For example:

- ReadSpeaker will read the text to you.
- Flashcards are pre-populated to provide you with a jump start for review—or you can create your own.
- You can highlight text and make notes in your MindTap Reader. Your notes will flow into Evernote, the electronic notebook app that you can access anywhere when it's time to study for the exam.
- Quizzes allows you to asses your understanding, and some include a "practice" syringe with a plunger that can be manipulated. Quizzes have been written and checked by Heather LeBlanc, Oulton College.
- Chapter tutorials outline instructions and approaches to safe and accurate dosage calculation. Tutorials have been checked and updated by Heather LeBlanc, Oulton College.

Visit www.nelson.com/student to start using **MindTap**. Enter the Online Access Code from the card included with your text. If a code card is *not* provided, you can purchase instant access at NELSONbrain.com.

ABOUT THE AUTHORS

Gloria D. Pickar, R.N., Ed.D.

Gloria D. Pickar, R.N., Ed.D., is Group President and Chief Academic Officer of EmbanetCompass in Orlando, Florida. She is a former Academic Dean at Seminole State College in Sanford, Florida. She is also the author of nine editions of best-selling *Dosage Calculations*.

Amy Pickar Abernethy, M.D.

Amy Pickar Abernethy, M.D., is Associate Professor of Medicine and Nursing at Duke University in Durham, North Carolina.

Beth Swart, R.N., M.E.S.

Beth Swart, R.N., M.E.S., is a professor at the Daphne Cockwell School of Nursing, Ryerson University, Toronto. She received her diploma of nursing from the Hospital for Sick Children School of Nursing, her B.Sc.N. from the University of Toronto, and her M.E.S. from York University. Beth has taught nursing for more than 40 years, at the diploma level and the baccalaureate level. She is a mentor to students as well as to faculty and instructors. Her areas of expertise are epidemiology and pathophysiology. Beth has also developed innovative online courses using a variety of teaching strategies and technology. Consequently, her major interests are in learning strategies and outcomes. She has been recognized for her teaching excellence. Beth has been an author for Nelson for many years, and has also authored numerous other publications as well.

ACKNOWLEDGMENTS

Reviewers

We wish to thank our many students and colleagues who have provided inspiration and made contributions to the production of the text. We would also like to thank the following reviewers for their insight and suggestions during the development of this edition:

Christine Boyle
Mount Royal University

Lucille Canart
Red River College

Dwayne Pettyjohn
Camosun College

Cindy Skolud
Seneca College of Applied Arts and Technology

Barbara Thompson
Sault College

Diane Valiquette
Bow Valley College

Technical Accuracy Check

Special thanks to Heather LeBlanc, B.Sc. CCPE, RPhT, Lead Instructor, Pharmacy Technician Program, Faculty of Health Science, Oulton College, who checked the accuracy of the dosage calculations and suggested clarifications and corrections wherever applicable in the text and the solutions.

USING THIS BOOK . . .

- Concepts are presented from simple to complex, in small increments, followed by **Quick Review** boxes to reinforce learning.

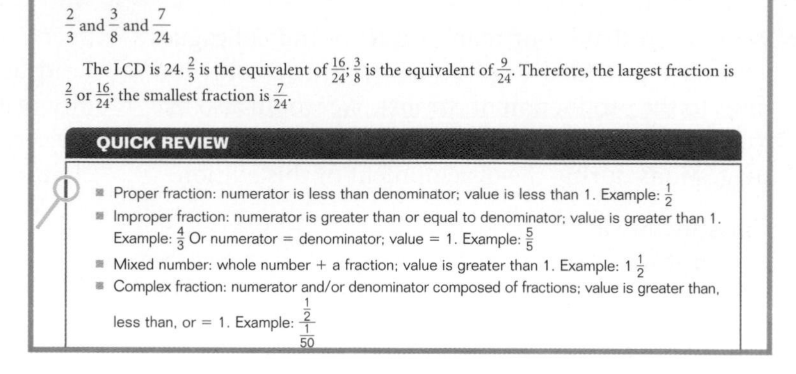

Example:

$\frac{2}{3}$ and $\frac{3}{8}$ and $\frac{7}{24}$

The LCD is 24. $\frac{2}{3}$ is the equivalent of $\frac{16}{24}$; $\frac{3}{8}$ is the equivalent of $\frac{9}{24}$. Therefore, the largest fraction is $\frac{2}{3}$ or $\frac{16}{24}$; the smallest fraction is $\frac{7}{24}$.

QUICK REVIEW

- Proper fraction: numerator is less than denominator; value is less than 1. Example: $\frac{1}{2}$
- Improper fraction: numerator is greater than or equal to denominator; value is greater than 1. Example: $\frac{4}{3}$ Or numerator = denominator; value = 1. Example: $\frac{5}{5}$
- Mixed number: whole number + a fraction; value is greater than 1. Example: $1\frac{1}{2}$
- Complex fraction: numerator and/or denominator composed of fractions; value is greater than, less than, or = 1. Example: $\frac{\frac{1}{2}}{\frac{1}{50}}$

REVIEW SET 12

Use the dimensional analysis method to convert each of the following to the equivalent indicated.

1. 500 mL =	________ L	14. 2 kg = ________ g
2. 0.015 g =	________ mg	15. 5000 mL = ________ L
3. 8 mg =	________ g	16. 1 L = ________ mL
4. 10 mg =	________ g	17. 1 g = ________ mg
5. 60 mg =	________ g	18. 1 mL = ________ L
6. 300 mg =	________ g	19. 23 mcg = ________ mg

- **Review Sets** are inserted after each new topic to encourage learners to stop and check their understanding of the material just presented. Answers to these are available at the end of the chapter. Solutions to selected Review Set items are also available there.

- **Practice Problems** round out each chapter. This is the students' opportunity to put their skills to the test, to identify their areas of strength and the areas in which they need additional study. Answers to these are provided at the end of the book, in the Answers section. Solutions to some Practice Problems are also provided there.

PRACTICE PROBLEMS—CHAPTER 5

1. In the 100-unit insulin syringe, 100 units = ________ mL.
2. The 1-mL syringe is calibrated in ________ of a mL.
3. Can you measure 1.25 mL in a single tuberculin syringe? ________ Explain. ________
4. How would you measure 1.33 mL in a 3-mL syringe? ________

Visuals

- **Photos** and **drug labels** are presented in full colour to help students prepare themselves in practice.

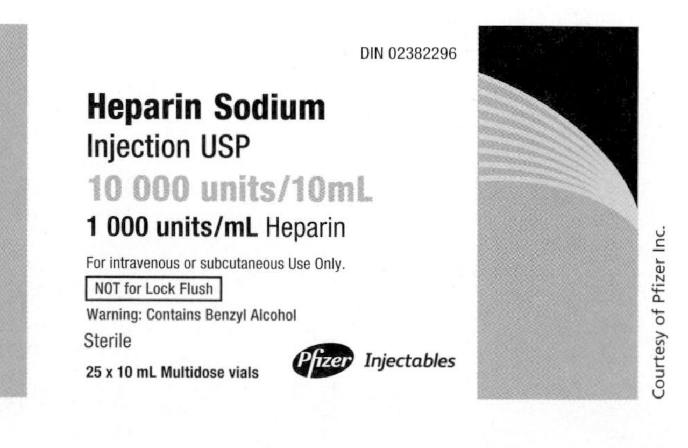

DIN 02382296
Heparin Sodium
Injection USP
10 000 units/10mL
1 000 units/mL Heparin
For intravenous or subcutaneous Use Only.
NOT for Lock Flush
Warning: Contains Benzyl Alcohol
Sterile
25 x 10 mL Multidose vials
Pfizer Injectables

Courtesy of Pfizer Inc.

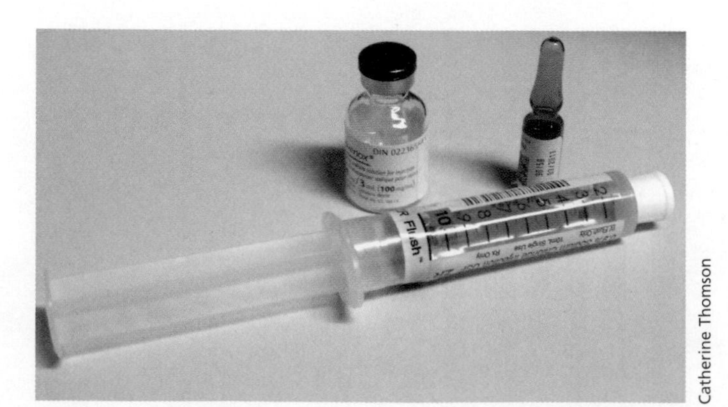

Catherine Thomson

- **Syringes** are drawn full size in most instances, to provide accurate scale renderings to help learners master the reading of injectable dosages.

14. Administer 1.3 mL.

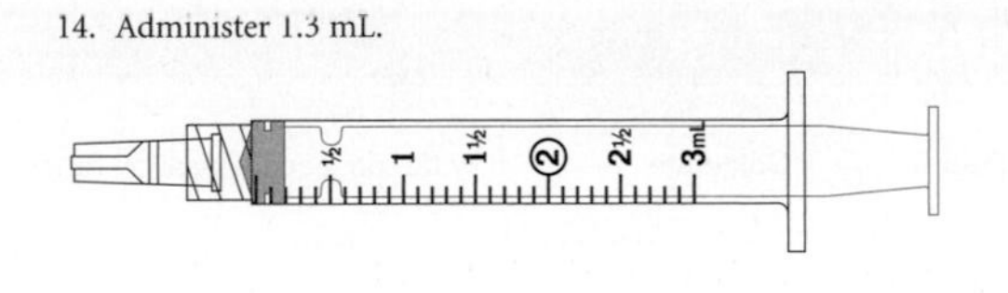

15. Administer 0.33 mL.

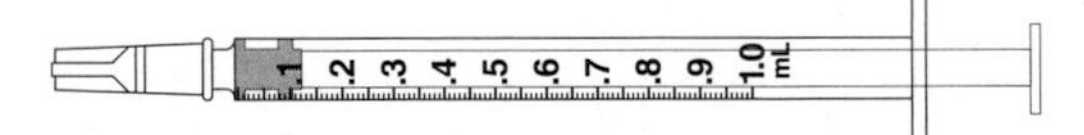

16. Administer 65 units of 100-unit insulin.

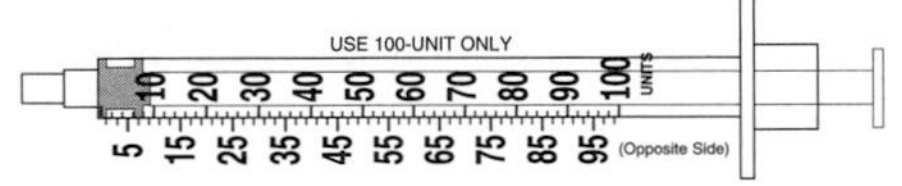

- **Illustrations** simulate critical dosage calculations and dose preparation skills. In particular, colour is used to simulate a specific amount of medication.

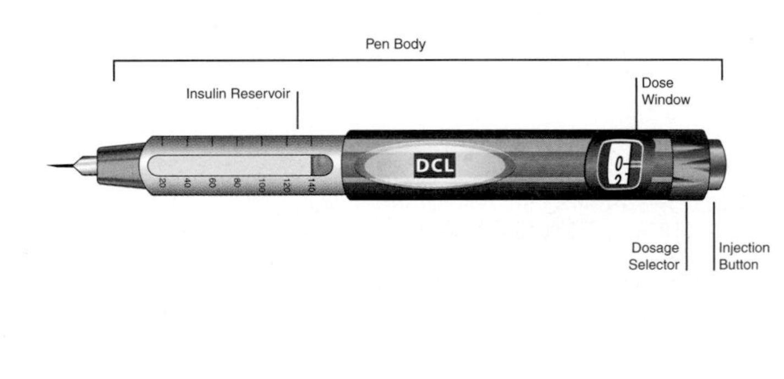

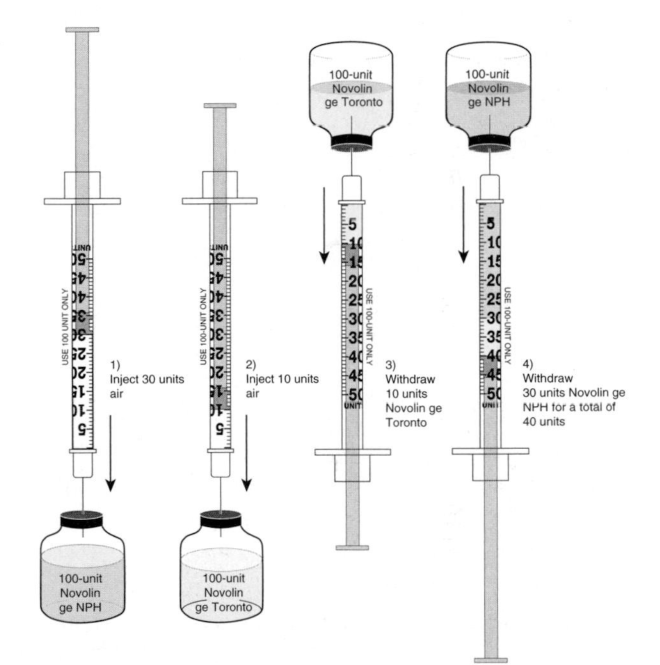

- **Math Tip** boxes provide clues to essential computations, math shortcuts, and reminders throughout the text.

> **MATH TIP**
>
> Incorrect placement of units of measurement can result in an incorrect answer. Even when calculating with dimensional analysis, thinking and reasoning are essential.

- **Caution** boxes alert learners to critical information and safety concerns.

> **CAUTION**
>
> Whenever a decimal fraction (whose value is less than 1) is written in medical notations, the zero MUST precede the decimal point. This practice highlights the decimal point and the fact that the value of the number is less than 1.

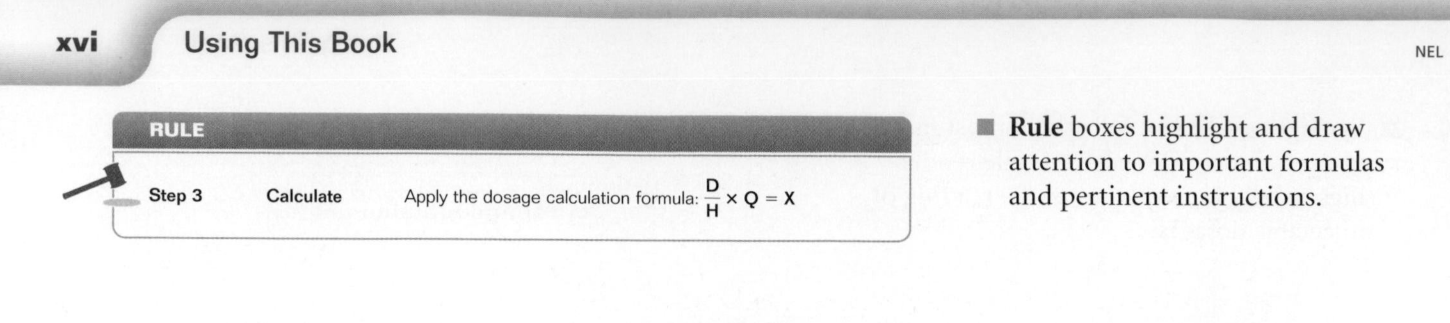

RULE

Step 3 Calculate Apply the dosage calculation formula: $\frac{D}{H} \times Q = X$

- **Rule** boxes highlight and draw attention to important formulas and pertinent instructions.

- **Remember** boxes highlight information that learners should memorize.

REMEMBER

To avoid confusion,

- Always use the capitalized ***L*** to indicate litre. The lower case ***l*** is easily confused with the number one (1);
- Always use ***mcg*** to indicate microgram. The μ symbol is easily misunderstood.

QUICK REVIEW

- Percent (Part) = Percent × Whole Quantity

  Example: What is 15% of 48?

$$15\% \times 48 = \frac{15}{100} \times 48$$

$$= \frac{15}{\cancel{100}_{25}} \times \overset{12}{\cancel{48}} = \frac{\overset{3}{\cancel{15}}}{\cancel{25}_{5}} \times 12 = \frac{3}{5} \times 12 = \frac{36}{5} = 7.2$$

- **Quick Review** boxes summarize critical information that students need to know before the Review Sets are solved.

- **Rationale for Practice** boxes provide the reasoning for a specific action or decision.

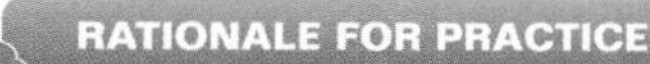

RATIONALE FOR PRACTICE

Some syringes may still be marked in cubic centimetres (cc); however, most drugs are prepared and labelled with the strength given per millilitre (mL). The cubic centimetre and millilitre are equivalent measurements in dosage calculations (1 cc = 1 mL).

UNDERSTANDING NCLEX QUESTIONS

Here's an example of a standard question used in textbooks:

Four-year-old Peter is ordered an oral liquid drug suspension of 4 mL per dose. The best way to administer this medication would be to use a/an:

a. household teaspoon
b. cooking measuring spoon
c. oral syringe
d. graduated medicine cup

Here's how it would look in an NCLEX examination:

The nurse is to discharge a 4-year-old home on an oral liquid drug suspension of 4 mL per dose. Which would the nurse recommend to ensure the highest level of accuracy in home administration of the medication?

a. Using a household teaspoon
b. Using a cooking measuring spoon
c. Using an oral syringe
d. Using a graduated medicine cup

Answer: c. Using an oral syringe

Rationale: The oral syringe would provide the most accurate dose of 4 mL.

- **NEW!** New to this edition is the addition of an **Understanding NCLEX Questions** box near the end of Chapters 5 to 14. An example of a standard question used in textbooks is presented with another example of how the question would look as a NCLEX question. The solution is also provided.

- **Application of Clinical Reasoning skills** are applied to realistic patient care situations to emphasize the importance of accurate dosage calculations and avoiding patient safety incidents. As an added benefit, clinical reasoning scenarios present prevention strategies so that the student can learn how to avoid these patient safety incidents in practice.

APPLICATION OF CLINICAL REASONING

Potential Patient Safety Incident

Incorrect interpretation of order due to misunderstanding of traditional time.

Possible Scenario

A physician prescribed a mild sedative for a patient who is anxious and is scheduled for a sigmoidoscopy in the morning. The order read *diazepam 5 mg orally at 6:00 × 1 dose*. The evening nurse might have assumed that the physician intended this medication to reduce the patient's anxiety and aid him in sleeping the night before the procedure. However, the nurse knew that sleeping aids are usually administered at bedtime, not at the time of evening preparations. The nurse used clinical reasoning and contacted the physician to clarify the order. The physician said she meant for the diazepam to be given at 6 o'clock AM to help the patient relax prior to the actual test.

Potential Outcome

Diazepam would help the patient relax during the sigmoidoscopy and make him drowsy. It is not desirable for the patient to be drowsy or sedated during the evening preparations. Because of the omission of the AM designation, the patient would lose any benefit from the sedative at the intended time if the medication had been administered the evening before the test. The patient would have likely experienced unnecessary anxiety both before and during the test.

Prevention

This scenario emphasizes the benefit of the 24-hour clock. If international time had been in use at this facility, the order would have been written as *diazepam 5 mg orally at 0600 × 1 dose*, clearly indicating the exact time of administration, reducing the risk of a patient safety incident.

Application of Critical Reasoning Additional application problems are provided at the end of the chapter. Answers are provided at the end of the book.

Additional Self-Assessment

Mathematics Diagnostic Evaluation: The *Mathematics Diagnostic Evaluation,* a mini-chapter that precedes Section 1, allows learners to identify their computational strengths and weaknesses.

Self-Evaluation: Self-Evaluations at the end of each section provide learners with an opportunity to test their mastery of chapter objectives prior to proceeding to the next section.

Post-tests: Two tests at the end of the text evaluate the learner's overall skill in dosage calculations. The first test, *Essential Skills Evaluation*, covers essential skills commonly tested by employers. The second test is a *Comprehensive Skills Evaluation.*

Answer Key: At the end of the text is an answer key with selected solutions to Practice Problems, section Self-Evaluations, and post-tests.

DOSAGE CALCULATIONS

FOURTH CANADIAN EDITION

Mathematics Diagnostic Evaluation

To prepare for calculating dosages, it is important to know how to add, subtract, multiply, and divide whole numbers. It is also important to have a working knowledge of fractions, decimals, ratios, percents, and basic problem solving. This text reviews these important mathematical operations, which support all dosage calculations in healthcare.

Set aside $1\frac{1}{2}$ hours in a quiet place to complete the 50 items in the following diagnostic evaluation. Use a notepad and a pencil to work the problems.

Use the results to determine your current computational strengths and weaknesses and to guide your review. A minimum score of 86 is recommended as an indicator of readiness for dosage calculations. If you achieve that score, you may proceed directly to Chapter 3. However, note any problems that are answered incorrectly, and use the related review materials in Chapters 1 and 2 to refresh your arithmetic skills.

This mathematics diagnostic evaluation and the review that follows are provided to enhance confidence and proficiency in arithmetic skills, thereby helping students avoid careless mistakes later when you perform dosage calculations.

Good luck!

Directions:

1. Carry answers to three decimal places and round to two decimal places.

   (Examples: 5.175 = 5.18; 5.174 = 5.17)

2. Express fractions in their lowest terms.

   (Example: $\frac{6}{10} = \frac{3}{5}$)

Mathematics Diagnostic Evaluation

1. 1517 + 0.63 = ________
2. Express the value of 0.7 + 0.035 + 20.006 rounded to two decimal places. ________
3. 9.5 + 17.06 + 32 + 41.11 + 0.99 = ________
4. $19.69 + $304.03 = ________
5. 93.2 − 47.09 = ________
6. 1005 − 250.5 = ________
7. Express the value of 17.156 − 0.25 rounded to two decimal places. ________
8. 509 × 38.3 = ________
9. $4.12 × 42 = ________
10. 17.16 × 23.5 = ________
11. 972 ÷ 27 = ________
12. 2.5 ÷ 0.001 = ________

13. Express the value of $\frac{1}{4} \div \frac{3}{8}$ as a fraction reduced to its lowest terms. ________

14. Express $\frac{1500}{240}$ as a decimal. ________

15. Express 0.8 as a fraction. ________

16. Express $\frac{2}{5}$ as a percent. ________

17. Express 0.004 as a percent. ________

18. Express 5% as a decimal. ________

19. Express $33\frac{1}{3}\%$ as a ratio in lowest terms. ________

20. Express 1:50 as a decimal. ________

21. $\frac{1}{2} + \frac{3}{4} =$ ________

22. $1\frac{2}{3} + 4\frac{7}{8} =$ ________

23. $1\frac{5}{6} - \frac{2}{9} =$ ________

24. Express the value of $\frac{1}{100} \times 60$ as a fraction. ________

25. Express the value of $4\frac{1}{4} \times 3\frac{1}{2}$ as a mixed number. ________

26. Identify the fraction with the greatest value: $\frac{1}{150}, \frac{1}{200}, \frac{1}{100}$ ________

27. Identify the decimal with the least value: 0.009, 0.19, 0.9 ________

28. $\frac{6.4}{0.02} =$ ________

29. $\frac{0.02 + 0.16}{0.4 - 0.34} =$ ________

30. Express the value of $\frac{3}{12 + 3} \times 0.25$ as a decimal. ________

31. 8% of 50 = ________

32. $\frac{1}{2}\%$ of 18 = ________

33. 0.9% of 24 = ________

Find the value of "X." Express your answer as a decimal.

34. $\frac{1:1000}{1:100} \times 250 = X$ ________

35. $\frac{300}{150} \times 2 = X$ ________

36. $\frac{2.5}{5} \times 1.5 = X$ ________

37. $\frac{1\,000\,000}{250\,000} \times X = 12$ ________

38. $\frac{0.51}{1.7} \times X = 150$ ________

39. $X = (82.4 - 52)\frac{3}{5}$ ________

40. $\frac{\frac{1}{150}}{\frac{1}{300}} \times 1.2 = X$ ________

41. Express 2:10 as a fraction in its lowest terms. ________

42. Express 2% as a ratio in its lowest terms. ________

43. If 5 equal medication containers contain 25 tablets in total, how many tablets are in each container? ________

44. A patient is receiving 0.5 milligrams of a medication 4 times a day. What is the total amount of medication in milligrams given each day? ________

45. If 1 kilogram equals 2.2 pounds, how many kilograms does a 66-pound child weigh? ________

46. If 1 kilogram equals 2.2 pounds, how many pounds are in 1.5 kilograms? (Express your answer as a decimal.) ________

47. If 1 centimetre equals $\frac{2}{5}$ inch, how many centimetres are in $2\frac{1}{2}$ inches? (Express your answer as a decimal.) ________

48. If 2.5 centimetres equal 1 inch, how long in centimetres is a 3-inch wound? ________

49. This diagnostic test has a total of 50 problems. If you incorrectly answer 5 problems, what percentage will be answered correctly? ________

50. For every 5 female student nurses in a nursing class, there is 1 male student nurse. What is the ratio of female to male student nurses? ________

Check your work! Answers to these questions are provided next, as well as solutions to some of the questions. Give yourself 2 points for each correct answer.

Perfect score = 100 My score = ________

Readiness score = 86 (43 correct)

Answers to Mathematics Diagnostic Evaluation

1) 1517.63 **2)** 20.74 **3)** 100.66 **4)** $323.72 **5)** 46.11 **6)** 754.5 **7)** 16.91 **8)** 19,494.7 **9)** $173.04 **10)** 403.26 **11)** 36 **12)** 2500 **13)** $\frac{2}{3}$ **14)** 6.25 **15)** $\frac{4}{5}$ **16)** 40% **17)** 0.4% **18)** 0.05 **19)** 1:3 **20)** 0.02 **21)** $1\frac{1}{4}$ **22)** $6\frac{13}{24}$ **23)** $1\frac{11}{18}$ **24)** $\frac{3}{5}$ **25)** $14\frac{7}{8}$ **26)** $\frac{1}{100}$ **27)** 0.009 **28)** 320 **29)** 3 **30)** 0.05 **31)** 4 **32)** 0.09 **33)** 0.22 **34)** 25 **35)** 4 **36)** 0.75 **37)** 3 **38)** 500 **39)** 18.24 **40)** 2.4 **41)** $\frac{1}{5}$ **42)** 1:50 **43)** 5 tablets **44)** 2 milligrams **45)** 30 kilograms **46)** 3.3 pounds **47)** $6\frac{1}{4} = 6.25$ centimetres **48)** 7.5 centimetres **49)** 90% **50)** 5:1

Selected Solutions to Mathematics Diagnostic Evaluation

3)

$$\begin{array}{r} 9.50 \\ 17.06 \\ 32.00 \\ 41.11 \\ 0.99 \\ \hline 100.66 \end{array}$$

6)

$$\begin{array}{r} 1005.0 \\ -250.5 \\ \hline 754.5 \end{array}$$

10)

$$\begin{array}{r} 17.16 \\ 23.5 \\ \hline 8580 \\ 5148 \\ 3432 \\ \hline 403.260 = 403.26 \end{array}$$

12) $0.001\overline{)2.500.} = 2500$ (quotient 2500.)

19) $\dfrac{33\frac{1}{3}}{100} = \dfrac{\frac{100}{3}}{100} = \dfrac{100}{3} \div \dfrac{100}{1} = \dfrac{\cancel{100}}{3} \times \dfrac{1}{\cancel{100}} = \dfrac{1}{3} = 1:3$

23) $1\frac{5}{6} - \frac{2}{9} = \frac{11}{6} - \frac{2}{9} = \frac{66}{36} - \frac{8}{36} = \frac{58}{36} = \frac{29}{18} = 1\frac{11}{18}$

25) $4\frac{1}{4} \times 3\frac{1}{2} = \frac{17}{4} \times \frac{7}{2} = \frac{119}{8} = 14\frac{7}{8}$

29) $\dfrac{0.02 + 0.16}{0.4 - 0.34}$

$$\begin{array}{r} 0.02 \\ +0.16 \\ \hline 0.18 \end{array} \qquad \begin{array}{r} 0.40 \\ -0.34 \\ \hline 0.06 \end{array}$$

$\dfrac{0.18}{0.06} = 0.06.\overline{)0.18.} = 3$ (quotient 3.)

32) $\frac{1}{2}\% = 0.5\% = 0.005$

$$\begin{array}{r} 18 \\ \times\ 0.005 \\ \hline 0.090 = 0.09 \end{array}$$

34) $\dfrac{\frac{1}{1000}}{\frac{1}{100}} \times 250 = \dfrac{1}{\cancel{1000}_{10}} \times \dfrac{\cancel{100}^{1}}{1} \times \dfrac{250}{1} = \dfrac{250}{10} = 25$

45) $66 \text{ pounds} \times \dfrac{1 \text{ kilogram}}{2.2 \text{ pounds}} =$

$$66 \cancel{\text{pounds}} \times \frac{1 \times 10 \text{ kilogram}}{2.2 \times 10 \cancel{\text{pounds}}} =$$

$$\frac{\overset{60}{\cancel{660}}}{\underset{2}{\cancel{22}}} \text{ kilograms} = 30 \text{ kilograms}$$

46)

$$\begin{array}{r} 2.2 \\ \times\ 1.5 \\ \hline 110 \\ 22 \\ \hline 3.30 \end{array}$$

$$1.5 \cancel{\text{kilograms}} \times \frac{2.2 \text{ pounds}}{1 \cancel{\text{kilograms}}}$$

$$= 1.5 \times 2.2 \text{ pounds} = 3.3 \text{ pounds}$$

48) $3 \cancel{\text{inches}} \times \dfrac{2.5 \text{ centimetres}}{1 \cancel{\text{inch}}} = 3 \times 2.5 \text{ centimetres}$

$= 7.5 \text{ centimetres}$

49) $\begin{array}{r} 50 \\ -5 \\ \hline 45 \end{array}$ $\qquad \dfrac{45}{50} = \dfrac{9}{10} = 90\%$

Fractions and Decimals

OBJECTIVES

1. Differentiate between types of fractions.
2. Use fractions in a variety of calculations.
3. Discuss the significance of decimals in calculations.
4. Develop skill in using fractions and decimals in calculations.

Healthcare providers need to understand fractions to be able to interpret and act on medical orders, read prescriptions, and understand patient records and information in healthcare literature. Fractions are also often used in household measures. Proficiency with fractions is essential to success in medication calculations.

FRACTIONS

A *fraction* is a part of a whole number. (See example below.) Fractions are composed of two parts: a *numerator,* the top number, and a *denominator,* the bottom number. The denominator refers to the total number of parts. The larger the number in the denominator, the smaller the value of the pieces (or fraction) of the whole. The numerator refers to a part of the whole that is being considered. The larger the number in the numerator, the more parts of the whole that are being considered. A fraction may also be read as the "numerator divided by the denominator."

Example:

$\frac{1}{4}$ $\frac{\text{numerator}}{\text{denominator}}$

The whole is divided into four equal parts (denominator), and one part (numerator) is considered.

$\frac{1}{4}$ = 1 part of 4 parts, or $\frac{1}{4}$ of the whole.

The fraction $\frac{1}{4}$ may also be read as "1 divided by 4."

MATH TIP

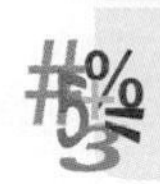

The **d**enominator begins with **d** and is **d**own below the line in a fraction.

Types of Fractions

There are four types of fractions: proper, improper, mixed, and complex. Whole numbers can also be expressed as fractions.

Proper Fractions

Proper fractions are fractions in which the value of the numerator is less than the value of the denominator. The value of a proper fraction is less than 1.

RULE

Whenever the numerator is less than the denominator, the value of the proper fraction must be less than 1.

Example:

$\frac{5}{8}\ \frac{\text{numerator}}{\text{denominator}}$ is less than 1

Improper Fractions

Improper fractions are fractions in which the value of the numerator is greater than or equal to the value of the denominator. The value of an improper fraction is greater than or equal to 1.

RULE

If the numerator is greater than the denominator, the value of the improper fraction must be greater than 1.

Example:

$\frac{8}{5}$ is greater than 1

RULE

If the numerator and the denominator are equal, the value of the improper fraction is always equal to 1.

Example:

$$\frac{5}{5} = 1$$

Mixed Numbers

When a whole number and a proper fraction are combined, the result is called a *mixed number.* The value of a mixed number is always greater than 1.

RULE

If a fraction and a whole number are written together, the fraction value is always greater than 1.

Example:

$1\frac{5}{8} = 1 + \frac{5}{8}$; $1\frac{5}{8}$ is greater than 1

Complex Fractions

Complex fractions are fractions in which the numerator, the denominator, or both may be a proper fraction, an improper fraction, or a mixed number. The value may be less than, greater than, or equal to 1.

Examples:

$\frac{\frac{5}{8}}{\frac{1}{2}}$ is greater than 1 $\frac{\frac{5}{8}}{2}$ is less than 1 $\frac{1\frac{5}{8}}{\frac{1}{5}}$ is greater than 1 $\frac{\frac{1}{2}}{\frac{2}{4}} = 1$

Whole Numbers

Whole numbers have an unexpressed denominator of 1.

Examples:

$1 = \frac{1}{1}$ $3 = \frac{3}{1}$ $6 = \frac{6}{1}$ $100 = \frac{100}{1}$

Fractions at Work

Being able to *convert* is a skill that must be mastered in order to become competent in medication calculation. In this chapter, you will learn to convert between the various types of fractions and to convert fractions to decimals and decimals to fractions. In later chapters, you will learn to convert between units of measurement. Conversion between the different types of fractions simplifies calculations.

Besides conversion, other requisite skills of mastery in fractions for use in medication calculations include comparing fractions, finding *equivalent fractions,* reducing fractions to their *lowest terms,* and finding *lowest common denominators* (LCDs).

Equivalent Fractions

Fractions of equal value can be expressed in several ways. If the numerator and the denominator of a fraction are either multiplied or divided by the same *nonzero* number, the fraction does not change in value. The resulting fraction has the same value as the original fraction and can be called an *equivalent fraction.*

MATH TIP

When changing a fraction, if you want to keep the same equivalent value, you must do the same thing (multiply or divide by the same number) to the numerator and to the denominator.

Examples:

$\frac{2}{4} = \frac{2 \div 2}{4 \div 2} = \frac{1}{2}$ $\frac{1}{3} = \frac{1 \times 3}{3 \times 3} = \frac{3}{9}$

Reducing Fractions to Their Lowest Terms

When calculating dosages, it is usually easier to work with fractions using the smallest numbers possible. Finding these equivalent fractions is called *reducing the fraction to its lowest terms* or *simplifying the fraction.*

RULE

To reduce a fraction to its lowest terms, *divide* both the numerator and the denominator by the *largest nonzero whole number* that will go evenly into both.

Patience is required to reduce a fraction that has large numbers. Sometimes the procedure for reducing a fraction to its lowest terms seems like trial and error. It may need to be reduced several times. Guidelines for reducing fractions are as follows:

- Even numbers are divisible by 2 and sometimes by multiples of 2.
- Numbers ending in 5 or 0 are divisible by 5 and sometimes by multiples of 5.
- Certain numbers are called prime numbers because they cannot be reduced any further. Examples are 2, 3, 7, 11, 13, and 17. See if a prime number will divide evenly into the numerator and denominator.

Example:

Reduce $\frac{7}{28}$ to its lowest terms.

7 can evenly divide into both the numerator (7) and the denominator (28).

$$\frac{7 \div 7}{28 \div 7} = \frac{1}{4}$$

Example:

Reduce $\frac{6}{12}$ to its lowest terms.

6 is the largest number that will divide evenly into both 6 (numerator) and 12 (denominator).

$$\frac{6}{12} = \frac{6 \div 6}{12 \div 6} = \frac{1}{2} \text{ in its lowest terms}$$

MATH TIP

If *both* the numerator and the denominator *cannot* be divided evenly by a nonzero number other than 1, then the fraction is already in its lowest terms.

Finding Common Denominators for Two or More Fractions

To compare, add, or subtract fractions, the denominators must be the same. Such computations are made easier when the LCD is used. The LCD is the smallest whole number that can be divided equally by all denominators within the problem.

To find the LCD, first check to see if the largest denominator in the problem is evenly divisible by each of the other denominators. If so, this largest denominator is the LCD.

Example 1:

$\frac{1}{8}$ and $\frac{1}{4}$

The denominator 8 is evenly divisible by 4. Therefore, 8 is the LCD.

$\frac{2}{7}$ and $\frac{5}{14}$ and $\frac{1}{28}$

The denominator 28 is evenly divided by 7 and 14. Therefore, 28 is the LCD.

If the largest denominator is not evenly divisible, find a common denominator by multiplying all the denominators together. This may not provide the LCD. Then try to reduce the fraction by following the rule described above for **reducing fractions to their lowest terms**.

Example 2:

$\frac{3}{8}$ and $\frac{1}{3}$

The denominator 8 is *not* evenly divisible by 3. Therefore, multiply 8 by 3, which equals 24. The number 24 is a common denominator for these two fractions. In this case, the common denominator is the LCD.

$\frac{2}{3}$ and $\frac{1}{4}$ and $\frac{1}{6}$

The number 6 is evenly divisible by 3 but is not evenly divisible by 4. Multiply 3 by 4 by 6 (which equals 72), and reduce the fraction to its lowest terms, as described earlier. An alternative is to only multiply 4 by 6 (which equals 24) because the largest denominator is evenly divisible by the remaining denominator (3) in the example.

Converting Mixed Numbers to Improper Fractions

When calculating medication dosages, it is important to know how to convert a variety of fractions. Mixed numbers can be converted to improper fractions, and improper fractions can be converted to mixed numbers.

RULE

To change or convert a mixed number to an improper fraction, multiply the whole number by the denominator and add the numerator.

Example:

$$1\frac{5}{8} = \frac{(1 \times 8) + 5}{8} = \frac{13}{8}$$

Converting Improper Fractions to Mixed Numbers

RULE

To change or convert an improper fraction to a mixed number or a whole number, divide the numerator by the denominator.

Examples:

$$\frac{8}{5} = 8 \div 5 = 1\frac{3}{5}$$

$$\frac{10}{4} = 10 \div 4 = 2\frac{2}{4} = 2\frac{1}{2}$$

Comparing Fractions

Once the skills of finding equivalent fractions and LCDs, converting mixed numbers and improper fractions, and reducing fractions to their lowest terms have been mastered, comparing two fractions with the same numerators or the same denominators can be mastered. Fractions with different numerators and different denominators can also be compared.

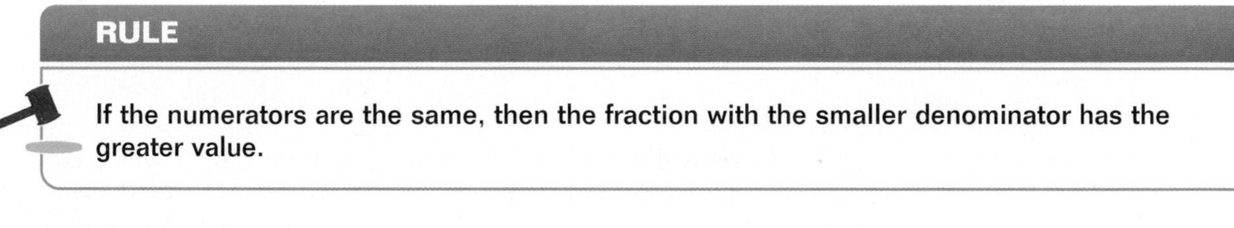

RULE

If the numerators are the same, then the fraction with the smaller denominator has the greater value.

Example:

Compare $\frac{1}{2}$ and $\frac{1}{4}$.

Numerators are both 1.

Denominators: 2 is less than 4.

$\frac{1}{2}$ has a greater value.

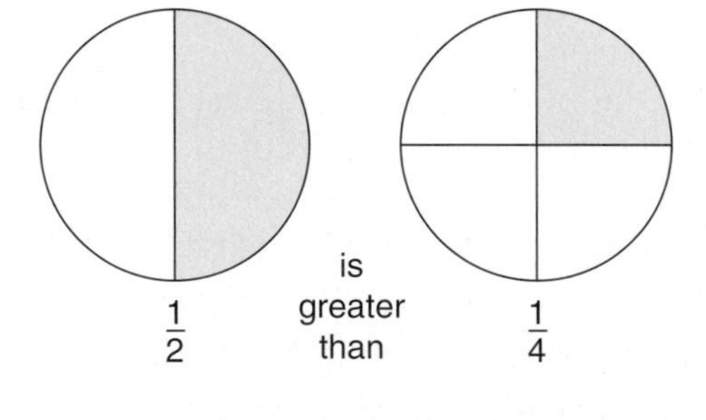
1/2
is
greater
than
1/4

RULE

If the denominators are both the same, then the fraction with the smaller numerator has the lesser value.

Example:

Compare $\frac{2}{5}$ and $\frac{3}{5}$.

Denominators are both 5.

Numerators: 2 is less than 3.

$\frac{2}{5}$ has a lesser value.

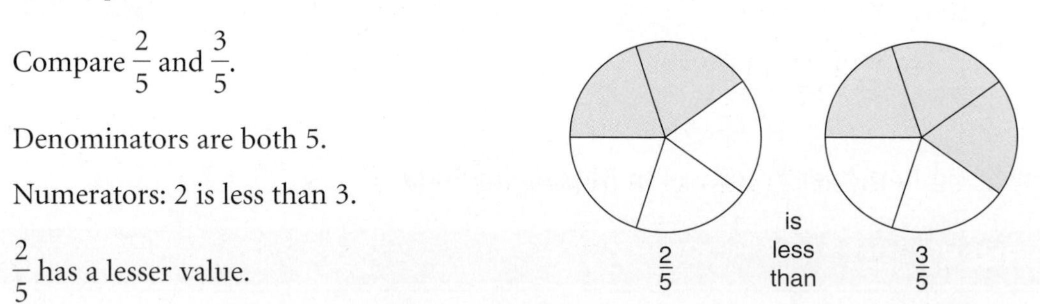
2/5
is
less
than
3/5

If neither the numerators nor the denominators are the same, convert the fractions to equivalent fractions using the LCD. Then compare the numerators as noted in the previous example.

Example:

$\frac{2}{3}$ and $\frac{3}{8}$ and $\frac{7}{24}$

The LCD is 24. $\frac{2}{3}$ is the equivalent of $\frac{16}{24}$; $\frac{3}{8}$ is the equivalent of $\frac{9}{24}$. Therefore, the largest fraction is $\frac{2}{3}$ or $\frac{16}{24}$; the smallest fraction is $\frac{7}{24}$.

QUICK REVIEW

- Proper fraction: numerator is less than denominator; value is less than 1. Example: $\frac{1}{2}$
- Improper fraction: numerator is greater than or equal to denominator; value is greater than 1. Example: $\frac{4}{3}$ Or numerator = denominator; value = 1. Example: $\frac{5}{5}$
- Mixed number: whole number + a fraction; value is greater than 1. Example: $1\frac{1}{2}$
- Complex fraction: numerator and/or denominator composed of fractions; value is greater than, less than, or = 1. Example: $\frac{\frac{1}{2}}{\frac{1}{50}}$
- To change the form of a fraction without changing its value, multiply or divide both the numerator and the denominator by the same nonzero number. Example: $\frac{1}{12} = \frac{1 \times 2}{12 \times 2} = \frac{2}{24}$
- To reduce a fraction to its lowest terms, divide both terms by the largest nonzero whole number that will divide both the numerator and the denominator evenly. Value remains the same. Example: $\frac{6}{10} = \frac{6 \div 2}{10 \div 2} = \frac{3}{5}$
- To convert a mixed number to an improper fraction, multiply the whole number by the denominator and add the numerator; use the original denominator in the fractional part. Example: $1\frac{1}{3} = \frac{4}{3}$
- To convert an improper fraction to a mixed number, divide the numerator by the denominator. Express any remainder as a proper fraction reduced to lowest terms. Example: $\frac{21}{9} = 2\frac{3}{9} = 2\frac{1}{3}$
- When numerators are equal, the fraction with the smaller denominator is greater. Example: $\frac{1}{2}$ is greater than $\frac{1}{3}$
- When denominators are equal, the fraction with the larger numerator is greater. Example: $\frac{2}{3}$ is greater than $\frac{1}{3}$

REVIEW SET 1-1

1. Circle the *improper* fraction(s).

   $\frac{2}{3}$ $1\frac{3}{4}$ $\frac{6}{6}$ $\frac{7}{5}$ $\frac{16}{17}$ $\frac{\frac{1}{9}}{\frac{2}{3}}$

2. Circle the *proper* fraction(s).

   $\frac{1}{4}$ $\frac{1}{14}$ $\frac{14}{1}$ $\frac{14}{14}$ $\frac{144}{14}$

3. Circle the *mixed* number(s) *reduced to their lowest terms.*

   $3\frac{4}{8}$ $\frac{2}{3}$ $1\frac{2}{9}$ $\frac{1}{3}$ $1\frac{1}{4}$ $5\frac{7}{8}$

4. Circle the pair(s) of *equivalent* fractions.

   $\frac{3}{4} = \frac{6}{8}$ $\frac{1}{5} = \frac{2}{10}$ $\frac{3}{9} = \frac{1}{3}$ $\frac{3}{4} = \frac{4}{3}$ $1\frac{4}{9} = 1\frac{2}{3}$

Change the following mixed numbers to improper fractions.

5. $6\frac{1}{2}$ = ________

7. $10\frac{2}{3}$ = ________

6. $1\frac{1}{5}$ = ________

8. $7\frac{5}{6}$ = ________

Change the following improper fractions to whole numbers or mixed numbers; reduce to their lowest terms.

9. $\frac{24}{12}$ = ________

11. $\frac{30}{9}$ = ________

10. $\frac{8}{8}$ = ________

12. $\frac{100}{75}$ = ________

Convert the following fractions to equivalent fractions with the number of parts indicated.

13. $\frac{3}{4}$ to eighths ________

15. $\frac{2}{5}$ to tenths ________

14. $\frac{1}{4}$ to sixteenths ________

16. $\frac{2}{3}$ to ninths ________

Circle the correct answer.

17. Which is larger? $\frac{1}{150}, \frac{1}{100}$

18. Which is smaller? $\frac{1}{1000}, \frac{1}{10\,000}$

19. Which is larger? $\frac{2}{9}, \frac{5}{9}$

20. Which is smaller? $\frac{3}{10}, \frac{5}{10}$

21. A patient is to drink a 300-mL bottle of magnesium citrate prior to his X-ray study. He is able to drink 180 mL. What portion of the bottle remains? (Express your answer as a fraction reduced to its lowest terms.) ________

22. Mrs. Gardiner is 3 days post-colon resection and has positive bowel sounds. She is tolerating ice chips well. Her fluid intake has been changed to 200 mL twice daily and is to be increased by $\frac{1}{2}$ daily for 3 days. What is the total fluid intake for day 2, day 3, and day 4?
Day 2________ Day 3________ Day 4________

23. A class consists of 3 men and 57 women. What fraction of the students in the class are men? (Express your answer as a fraction reduced to its lowest terms.)
____

24. A student answers 18 out of 20 questions correctly on a test. Write a proper fraction (reduced to lowest terms) to represent the portion of the test questions that were answered correctly. ________

25. Mr. Lee is informed that it is safe to reduce his caloric intake by $\frac{1}{8}$, $\frac{1}{6}$, or $\frac{1}{4}$. If Mr. Lee chooses to reduce his caloric intake by the maximum amount, he will choose to reduce his intake by which fraction? ________

Check your work! Answers to all Review Sets are provided at the end of each chapter. Worked solutions for select Review Sets are also provided there.

Addition and Subtraction of Fractions

To add or subtract fractions, all the denominators must be the same. Finding the LCD is the first step in adding or subtracting fractions. Then convert the fractions to equivalent fractions with the LCD. These operations were examined in the previous section.

RULE

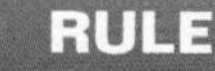

To add or subtract fractions,

1. **Find the LCD, and convert all fractions to equivalent fractions with the LCD; then**
2. **Add or subtract the numerators, place that value in the numerator, and use the LCD as the denominator; and**
3. **Convert to a mixed number or reduce the fraction to its lowest terms.**

MATH TIP

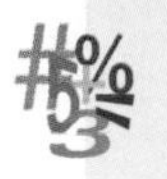

To *add or subtract fractions*, no calculations are performed on the denominators. Once they are all converted to the LCD, perform the mathematical operation (addition or subtraction) on the *numerators* only, and use the LCD as the denominator.

Adding Fractions

Example 1:

$$\frac{3}{4} + \frac{1}{4} + \frac{2}{4}$$

1. Find the LCD. This step is not necessary in this example because the fractions already have the same denominator.

2. Add the numerators: $\frac{3 + 1 + 2}{4} = \frac{6}{4}$

3. Convert to a mixed number, and reduce to its lowest terms: $\frac{6}{4} = 1\frac{2}{4} = 1\frac{1}{2}$

Example 2:

$$\frac{1}{3} + \frac{3}{4} + \frac{1}{6}$$

1. Find the LCD: 12. The number 12 is the LCD that 3, 4, and 6 will all equally divide into.

   Convert to equivalent fractions in twelfths.

   $$\frac{1}{3} = \frac{1 \times 4}{3 \times 4} = \frac{4}{12}$$

   $$\frac{3}{4} = \frac{3 \times 3}{4 \times 3} = \frac{9}{12}$$

   $$\frac{1}{6} = \frac{1 \times 2}{6 \times 2} = \frac{2}{12}$$

2. Add the numerators, and use the common denominator: $\frac{4+9+2}{12} = \frac{15}{12}$

3. Convert to a mixed number, and reduce to its lowest terms: $\frac{15}{12} = 1\frac{3}{12} = 1\frac{1}{4}$

Subtracting Fractions

Example 1:

$\frac{15}{18} - \frac{8}{18}$

1. Find the LCD. This is not necessary in this example because the denominators are the same.
2. Subtract the numerators, and use the common denominator: $\frac{15-8}{18} = \frac{7}{18}$
3. Reduce to its lowest terms: not necessary. No further reduction is possible.

Example 2:

$1\frac{1}{10} - \frac{3}{5}$

1. Find the LCD: 10. The number 10 is the LCD that both 10 and 5 will equally divide into.

   Convert to equivalent fractions in tenths:

   $1\frac{1}{10} = \frac{11}{10}$

   $\frac{3}{5} = \frac{3 \times 2}{5 \times 2} = \frac{6}{10}$

2. Subtract the numerators, and use the common denominator: $\frac{11-6}{10} = \frac{5}{10}$
3. Reduce to its lowest terms: $\frac{5}{10} = \frac{1}{2}$

   Let us review one more time how to add and subtract fractions.

QUICK REVIEW

To add or subtract fractions,

- Convert to equivalent fractions with LCD.
- Add or subtract the numerators; place that value in the numerator. Use the LCD as the denominator.
- Convert the answer to a mixed number or reduce to its lowest terms.

REVIEW SET 1-2

Add, and reduce the answers to their lowest terms.

1. $7\frac{4}{5} + \frac{2}{3} =$ ________

2. $\frac{3}{4} + \frac{2}{3} =$ ________

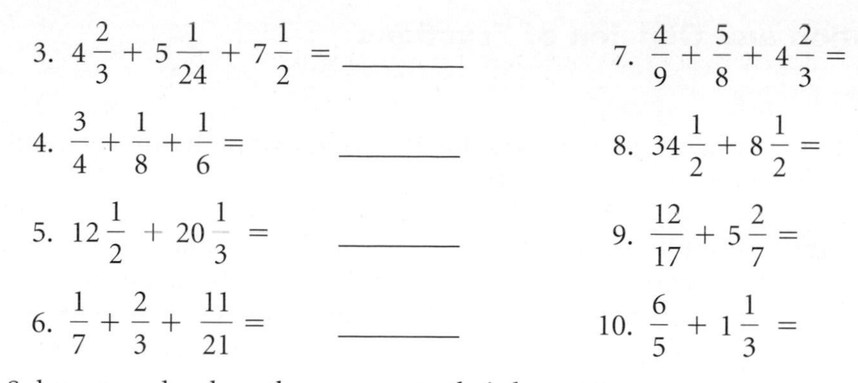

3. $4\frac{2}{3} + 5\frac{1}{24} + 7\frac{1}{2} =$ ________

7. $\frac{4}{9} + \frac{5}{8} + 4\frac{2}{3} =$ ________

4. $\frac{3}{4} + \frac{1}{8} + \frac{1}{6} =$ ________

8. $34\frac{1}{2} + 8\frac{1}{2} =$ ________

5. $12\frac{1}{2} + 20\frac{1}{3} =$ ________

9. $\frac{12}{17} + 5\frac{2}{7} =$ ________

6. $\frac{1}{7} + \frac{2}{3} + \frac{11}{21} =$ ________

10. $\frac{6}{5} + 1\frac{1}{3} =$ ________

Subtract, and reduce the answers to their lowest terms.

11. $\frac{3}{4} - \frac{1}{4} =$ ________

16. $2\frac{3}{5} - 1\frac{1}{5} =$ ________

12. $8\frac{1}{12} - 3\frac{1}{4} =$ ________

17. $14\frac{3}{16} - 7\frac{1}{8} =$ ________

13. $\frac{1}{8} - \frac{1}{12} =$ ________

18. $25 - 17\frac{7}{9} =$ ________

14. $100 - 36\frac{1}{3} =$ ________

19. $4\frac{7}{10} - 3\frac{9}{20} =$ ________

15. $\frac{1}{3} - \frac{1}{6} =$ ________

20. There are $17\frac{1}{2}$ litres of hydrogen peroxide currently in stock in central supply. If central supply usually has 27 litres of hydrogen peroxide in stock, how many litres have been used? ________

21. Ms. Lewenski's medical regime includes fluid restriction. She is to receive $\frac{2}{3}$ of her total day's fluids in the morning and $\frac{1}{4}$ of the fluids in the afternoon. What fraction of the day's fluids does Ms. Lewenski have left to take in the evening? ________

22. Mr. Booth is receiving $\frac{1}{2}$ tablet 3 times daily. How many tablets is he receiving daily?

____

23. Ms. Coady is trying to make sure to drink sufficient fluids daily. She drinks $1\frac{1}{2}$ glasses before breakfast, 1 glass at breakfast, $\frac{2}{3}$ glass in mid-morning, and $1\frac{3}{4}$ glasses at noon. What is the total number of glasses (including fraction of glasses) that Ms. Coady has had to drink by afternoon? ________

24. Mr. Grady is recording walking achievements in a rehabilitation program. His goal is to walk 8 kilometres this week. So far, he has walked $1\frac{1}{4}$ km, $1\frac{1}{3}$ km, $1\frac{1}{2}$ km, and 1 km. How many kilometres are left for him to walk in order to meet his goal for this week?

____

25. As camp nurse, you are encouraging healthy eating. Apples are sectioned and available at meals and snack breaks. In the last 2 days, $54\frac{1}{2}$ and $57\frac{3}{4}$ apples have been consumed. How many apples in total were eaten in the previous 2 days? ________

Check your work! Answers to all Review Sets are provided at the end of each chapter. Worked solutions for select Review Set exercises are also provided there.

Multiplication and Division of Fractions

Multiplying Fractions

To multiply fractions, multiply numerators (for the numerator of the answer), and multiply denominators (for the denominator of the answer).

Simplification of fractions is helpful in reducing math errors. Cancelling fractions is a method of simplifying fraction multiplication by reducing numerators and denominators by a common factor. Cancellation (like reducing to lowest terms) is based on the fact that the division of both the numerator and the denominator by the same whole number does not change the value of the resulting number. In fact, it makes the calculation simpler because smaller numbers are being used.

Example:

$$\frac{1}{3} \times \frac{250}{500}$$

Numerator and denominator of $\frac{250}{500}$ are both divisible by 250.

$$= \frac{1}{3} \times \frac{\overset{1}{\cancel{250}}}{\underset{2}{\cancel{500}}} = \frac{1}{3} \times \frac{1}{2} = \frac{1}{6}$$

Also, a numerator and a denominator of any of the fractions involved in the multiplication may be cancelled when they can be divided by the same whole number. This is called *cross-cancellation.*

Example:

$$\frac{1}{8} \times \frac{8}{9} = \frac{1}{\underset{1}{\cancel{8}}} \times \frac{\overset{1}{\cancel{8}}}{9} = \frac{1}{1} \times \frac{1}{9} = \frac{1}{9}$$

Cultural Note: In some countries, the word *of* is used instead of *times* for multiplication of fractions. It might be simpler to understand multiplication of fractions by substituting *of* for times. For example, $\frac{1}{2}$ of 4 is 2, $\frac{1}{2}$ of $\frac{1}{4}$ is $\frac{1}{8}$, and $\frac{1}{4}$ of $\frac{1}{2}$ is $\frac{1}{8}$.

RULE

To multiply fractions,

1. Reduce and cancel terms, if possible;
2. Multiply numerators for the numerator of the answer, and multiply denominators for the denominator of the answer; and
3. Reduce to lowest terms.

Example 1:

$$\frac{3}{4} \times \frac{2}{6}$$

1. Reduce terms: Divide 2 and 6 by 2

$$\frac{3}{4} \times \frac{\overset{1}{\cancel{2}}}{\underset{3}{\cancel{6}}} = \frac{3}{4} \times \frac{1}{3}$$

Cancel terms: Divide 3 and 3 by 3

$$\frac{\overset{1}{\cancel{3}}}{4} \times \frac{1}{\underset{1}{\cancel{3}}} = \frac{1}{4} \times \frac{1}{1}$$

2. Multiply numerators and denominators:

   $\frac{1}{4} \times \frac{1}{1} = \frac{1}{4}$

3. Reduce to lowest terms: not necessary.

Example 2:

$\frac{15}{30} \times \frac{2}{5}$

1. Reduce terms: Divide 15 and 30 by 15

   $\frac{\overset{1}{\cancel{15}}}{\underset{2}{\cancel{30}}} \times \frac{2}{5} = \frac{1}{2} \times \frac{2}{5}$

   Cancel terms: Divide 2 and 2 by 2

   $\frac{1}{\underset{1}{\cancel{2}}} \times \frac{\overset{1}{\cancel{2}}}{5} = \frac{1}{1} \times \frac{1}{5}$

2. Multiply numerators and denominators:

   $\frac{1}{1} \times \frac{1}{5} = \frac{1}{5}$

3. Reduce to lowest terms: not necessary.

MATH TIP

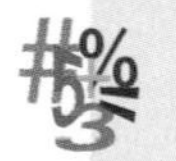

When multiplying a fraction by a nonzero whole number, the same rule applies as for multiplying fractions. First convert the whole number to a fraction with a denominator of 1; the value of the number remains the same.

Example 3:

$\frac{2}{3} \times 4$

1. No terms to cancel. (The numbers 2 and 4 cannot be cancelled because both are numerators. To do so would change the value.) Convert the whole number to a fraction.

   $\frac{2}{3} \times 4 = \frac{2}{3} \times \frac{4}{1}$

2. Multiply numerators and denominators:

   $\frac{2}{3} \times \frac{4}{1} = \frac{8}{3}$

3. Convert to a mixed number.

   $\frac{8}{3} = 8 \div 3 = 2\frac{2}{3}$

MATH TIP

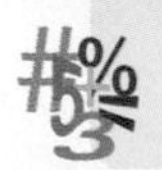

To multiply mixed numbers, first convert them to improper fractions, and then multiply.

Example 4:

$3\frac{1}{2} \times 4\frac{1}{3}$

1. Convert: $3\frac{1}{2} = \frac{7}{2}$

   $4\frac{1}{3} = \frac{13}{3}$

   Therefore, $3\frac{1}{2} \times 4\frac{1}{3} = \frac{7}{2} \times \frac{13}{3}$

2. Reduce and cancel: not necessary. No numbers can be reduced or cancelled.

3. Multiply: $\frac{7}{2} \times \frac{13}{3} = \frac{91}{6}$

4. Convert to a mixed number: $\frac{91}{6} = 15\frac{1}{6}$

Dividing Fractions

The division of fractions uses three terms: *dividend, divisor,* and *quotient.* The *dividend* is the fraction being divided or the first number. The *divisor,* the number to the right of the division sign, is the fraction the dividend is divided by. The *quotient* is the result of the division. To divide fractions, the divisor is inverted, and the operation is changed to multiplication. Once inverted, the calculation is the same as for multiplication of fractions.

Example:

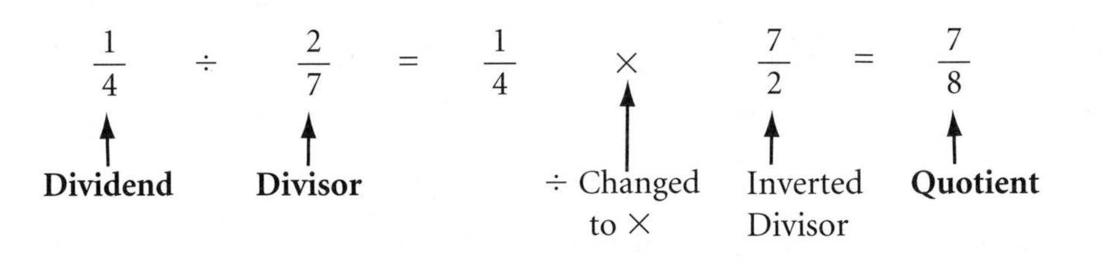

RULE

To divide fractions,

1. **Invert the terms of the divisor, and change ÷ to ×;**
2. **Cancel terms, if possible;**
3. **Multiply the resulting fractions; and**
4. **Convert the result (quotient) to a mixed number, or reduce to its lowest terms.**

Example 1:

$\frac{3}{4} \div \frac{1}{3}$

1. Invert divisor, and change ÷ to ×: $\frac{3}{4} \div \frac{1}{3} = \frac{3}{4} \times \frac{3}{1}$

2. Cancel: not necessary. No numbers can be cancelled.

3. Multiply: $\frac{3}{4} \times \frac{3}{1} = \frac{9}{4}$

4. Convert to mixed number: $\frac{9}{4} = 2\frac{1}{4}$

Example 2:

$\frac{2}{3} \div 4$

1. Invert divisor, and change ÷ to ×: $\frac{2}{3} \div \frac{4}{1} = \frac{2}{3} \times \frac{1}{4}$

2. Cancel terms: $\frac{\overset{1}{\cancel{2}}}{3} \times \frac{1}{\underset{2}{\cancel{4}}} = \frac{1}{3} \times \frac{1}{2}$

3. Multiply: $\frac{1}{3} \times \frac{1}{2} = \frac{1}{6}$

4. Reduce: not necessary; already reduced to its lowest terms.

MATH TIP

To divide mixed numbers, first convert them to improper fractions.

Example 3:

$1\frac{1}{2} \div \frac{3}{4}$

1. Convert: $1\frac{1}{2} = \frac{3}{2}$

2. Invert divisor, and change ÷ to ×: $\frac{3}{2} \times \frac{4}{3}$

3. Cancel: $\frac{\overset{1}{\cancel{3}}}{\underset{1}{\cancel{2}}} \times \frac{\overset{2}{\cancel{4}}}{\underset{1}{\cancel{3}}} = \frac{1}{1} \times \frac{2}{1}$

4. Multiply: $\frac{1}{1} \times \frac{2}{1} = \frac{2}{1}$

5. Reduce: $\frac{2}{1} = 2$

MATH TIP

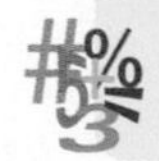

Multiplying complex fractions also involves the division of fractions. Study this carefully.

Example 4:

$$\frac{\frac{1}{150}}{\frac{1}{100}} \times 2$$

1. Convert: Express 2 as a fraction. $\frac{\frac{1}{150}}{\frac{1}{100}} \times \frac{2}{1}$

2. Rewrite complex fraction as division: $\frac{1}{150} \div \frac{1}{100} \times \frac{2}{1}$

3. Invert divisor and change ÷ to ×: $\frac{1}{150} \times \frac{100}{1} \times \frac{2}{1}$

4. Cancel: $\frac{1}{\cancel{150}_{3}} \times \frac{\cancel{100}^{2}}{1} \times \frac{2}{1} = \frac{1}{3} \times \frac{2}{1} \times \frac{2}{1}$

5. Multiply: $\frac{1}{3} \times \frac{2}{1} \times \frac{2}{1} = \frac{4}{3}$

6. Convert to mixed number: $\frac{4}{3} = 1\frac{1}{3}$

This example appears difficult at first, but when solved logically, one step at a time, it is similar to the others.

QUICK REVIEW

- To multiply fractions, cancel terms, multiply numerators, and multiply denominators.
- To divide fractions, invert the divisor, cancel terms, and multiply.
- Convert to a mixed number or reduce to lowest terms.

REVIEW SET 1-3

Multiply, and reduce the answers to their lowest terms.

1. $\frac{3}{10} \times \frac{1}{12} =$ ________
2. $\frac{12}{25} \times \frac{3}{5} =$ ________
3. $\frac{5}{8} \times 1\frac{1}{6} =$ ________
4. $\frac{1}{100} \times 3 =$ ________
5. $\frac{\frac{1}{6}}{\frac{1}{4}} \times \frac{\frac{3}{2}}{3} =$ ________
6. $\frac{\frac{1}{150}}{\frac{1}{100}} \times 2\frac{1}{2} =$ ________
7. $\frac{30}{75} \times 2 =$ ________
8. $9\frac{4}{5} \times \frac{2}{3} =$ ________
9. $\frac{3}{4} \times \frac{2}{3} =$ ________
10. $4\frac{2}{3} \times 5\frac{1}{24} =$ ________
11. $\frac{3}{4} \times \frac{1}{8} =$ ________

Divide, and reduce the answers to their lowest terms.

12. $\frac{3}{4} \div \frac{1}{4} =$ ________

13. $6\frac{1}{12} \div 3\frac{1}{4} =$ ________

14. $\frac{1}{8} \div \frac{7}{12} =$ ________

15. $\frac{1}{33} \div \frac{1}{3} =$ ________

16. $5\frac{1}{4} \div 10\frac{1}{2} =$ ________

17. $\frac{1}{60} \div \frac{1}{2} =$ ________

18. $2\frac{1}{2} \div \frac{3}{4} =$ ________

19. $\dfrac{\frac{1}{20}}{\frac{1}{3}} =$ ________

20. $\dfrac{\frac{3}{5}}{\frac{3}{4}} \div \dfrac{\frac{4}{5}}{1\frac{1}{9}} =$ ________

21. The nurse is maintaining calorie counts (or counting calories) for a patient who is not eating well. The patient ate $\frac{3}{4}$ of an apple. If one large apple contains 80 calories, how many calories did the patient consume? ________

22. How many seconds are there in $9\frac{1}{3}$ minutes? ________

23. A bottle of children's acetaminophen contains 30 tablets. If each dose for a 2-year-old child is $1\frac{1}{2}$ tablets, how many doses are available in this bottle? ________

24. Ms. Flynn needs to take $1\frac{1}{2}$ tablets of medication 3 times per day for 7 days. Over the 7 days, how many tablets will she take? ________

25. Mr. Suzuki's water pitcher is still $\frac{1}{3}$ full. If he drank 850 millilitres of water, how many millilitres does the pitcher hold?________

Check your work! Answers to all Review Sets are provided at the end of each chapter. Worked solutions for select Review Set exercises are also provided there.

DECIMALS

The Arabic system of numeration is positional. This means that the value of any numeral is determined by the position it occupies in a number. Starting at the right and moving to the left, the value assigned to the numerical places is 10 times greater than the value of the place that preceded it. The number 6 724 925 is assigned the places shown in the following example:

6	7	2	4	9	2	5
Millions	Hundred thousands	Ten thousands	Thousands	Hundreds	Tens	Ones

Decimal numbers, commonly called *decimals*, are numeric values that include a whole number, a decimal point, and a decimal fraction. Numbers to the left of a decimal point have a value greater than 1. They are also called *whole numbers.* Numbers to the right of a decimal point have a value less than 1.

Since many medications involve dosages that contain decimals, it is essential that healthcare providers understand decimals, recognize the relative values of decimals, and understand the importance of correct decimal placement to be able to add, subtract, multiply, and divide decimals. Identifying the relative value provides the opportunity to think about the answer to the calculation before doing the math. Being able to think about the answer and evaluate the math is important in administering correct medication dosages. A common error associated with medication administration is improper decimal placement.

RULE

When dealing with decimals, think of the decimal point as the *centre* that separates whole and fractional amounts. The position of the numbers in relation to the decimal point indicates the place value of the numbers.

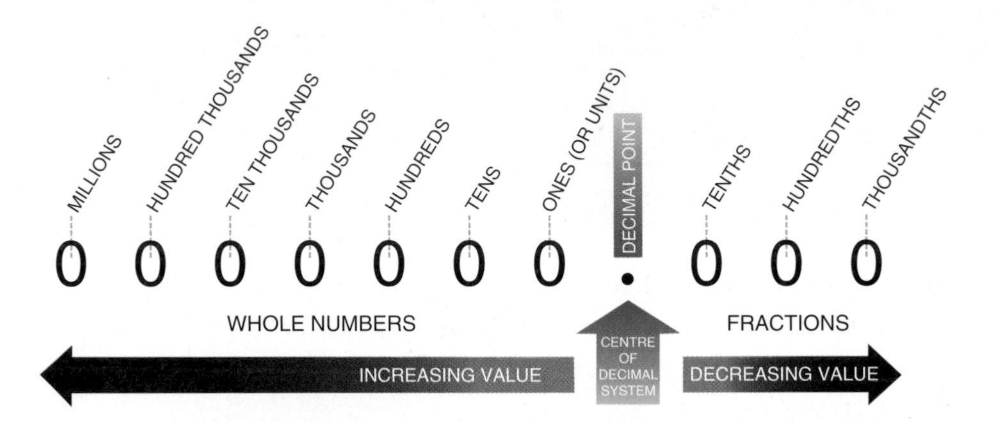

Example 1:

10.1 is higher than 9.15

Example 2:

3.2 is higher than 2.99

Example 3:

7.01 is higher than 6.99

MATH TIP

The decimal portion of the number ends in th(s).

Examples:

0.001 = one thousand*th*

0.02 = two hundred*ths*

0.7 = seven ten*ths*

Decimal fractions are numbers that are less than 1. They are fractions with a denominator of 10, 100, 1000, or any power of 10.

Examples:

Decimal	Fraction
0.1	$= \frac{1}{10}$
0.01	$= \frac{1}{100}$
0.001	$= \frac{1}{1000}$

Decimal numbers are numeric values that include a whole number, a decimal point, and a decimal fraction.

Examples:

Whole number → 4.67

4.67

Decimal point   Fraction numbers

RULE

The decimal number is read by stating the whole number first, the decimal point as *and*, and then the decimal fraction by naming the value of the last decimal place.

Example:

Look carefully at the decimal number 4.125. The last decimal place is thousandths. Therefore, the number is read as "four and one hundred twenty-five thousandths."

5	Thousandths
2	Hundredths
1	Tenths
4 .	Ones

Examples:

The number 6.2 is read as "six and two tenths."

The number 10.03 is read as "ten and three hundredths."

Writing Decimals

The fraction portion of a decimal number indicates an understood denominator of 10 or some power of 10. To eliminate possible confusion and avoid errors when the number is less than 1, always place a zero to the left of the decimal point.

Example:

Decimal Number	Fraction
0.3	$\frac{3}{10}$
0.18	$\frac{18}{100}$
0.175	$\frac{175}{1000}$

CAUTION

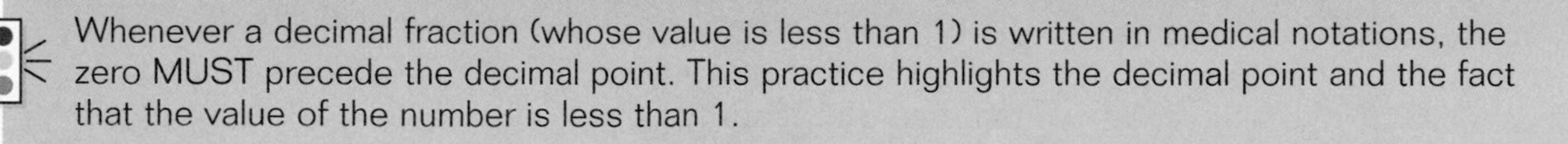

Whenever a decimal fraction (whose value is less than 1) is written in medical notations, the zero MUST precede the decimal point. This practice highlights the decimal point and the fact that the value of the number is less than 1.

CAUTION

There should not be a trailing zero at the end of a decimal.

RULE

Zeros added *after* the last digit of a decimal fraction *do not* change its value. A trailing zero should not be used because it may be misinterpreted and lead to an error.

Reading Decimals

When there is a zero (0) to the left of the decimal, the zero is not read aloud *except* when the nurse is taking a verbal order over the phone from a prescriber. When repeating back an order for a medication involving a decimal, the zero should be read aloud to prevent a patient safety incident.

For example, "zero point three" would be the verbal interpretation of the first example in the above series.

Comparing Decimals

Being able to understand the relative value of decimals and recognizing the high and low values of each decimal number is key to calculating and administering accurate medication dosages. The relative value of a number is determined by the spaces to the left of the decimal point—the more spaces, the higher the value. If the number of spaces in two decimal numbers is the same, then compare the actual numbers. The first place from the left where they differ determines the relative value of each number.

For example, when comparing 23.5 and 25.3, the first place from the left where the two numbers differ is in the ones value; that is, the number 3 is less than the number 5. Therefore, the number 23.5 is less than 25.3. If the numbers to the left of the decimal point do not differ, begin comparing numbers to the right of the decimal point until you find a difference in the numbers. For example, compare 31.53 and 31.64. The numbers to the left of the decimal point are the same (both are 31); in the first space to the right of the decimal point, they differ. Since 5 is less than 6, the number with the lesser value is 31.53.

CAUTION

A common error in comparing decimals is to overlook the decimal place values and misinterpret higher numbers for greater amounts and lower numbers for lesser amounts. This is a common error in medication administration.

MATH TIP

Decimal amounts can be accurately compared by aligning the decimal points and adding zeros, so that the numbers to be compared have the same number of decimal places. Remember that adding zeros at the end of a decimal fraction does not change the original value.

Example 1:

Compare 0.125, 0.05, and 0.2 to find which decimal fraction is largest.

Align decimal points and add zeros.

$0.125 = \frac{125}{1000}$ or one hundred twenty-five thousandths

$0.05\mathbf{0} = \frac{50}{1000}$ or fifty thousandths

$0.2\mathbf{00} = \frac{200}{1000}$ or two hundred thousandths

Now it is easy to see that 0.2 is the greater amount and 0.05 is the least. At first glance, it might be easy to be tricked into thinking that 0.2 is the least amount and 0.125 is the greater amount. This kind of error can have drastic consequences in dosage calculations and patient safety.

Example 2:

Suppose 0.5 micrograms of a drug has been ordered. The recommended maximum dosage of the drug is 0.25 micrograms, and the minimum recommended dosage is 0.125 micrograms. Comparing decimals, you can see that the ordered dosage is not within the allowable range.

0.125 micrograms (recommended minimum dosage)

0.25**0** micrograms (recommended maximum dosage)

0.5**00** micrograms (ordered dosage)

It is now obvious that 0.5 micrograms is outside the allowable limits of the safe dosage range of 0.125 to 0.25 micrograms for this medication. In fact, it is twice the allowable maximum dosage.

Example 3:

0.25 = 0.25**0**

Twenty-five hundredths equals two hundred fifty thousandths.

The last zero does not change the value of the decimal; therefore, it is not necessary. The preferred notation is 0.25 rather than 0.250.

Conversion between Fractions and Decimals

To expedite medication calculations, it is frequently necessary to be able to know equivalency between fractions and decimal numbers and/or to use both fractions and decimal numbers in the required medication calculation.

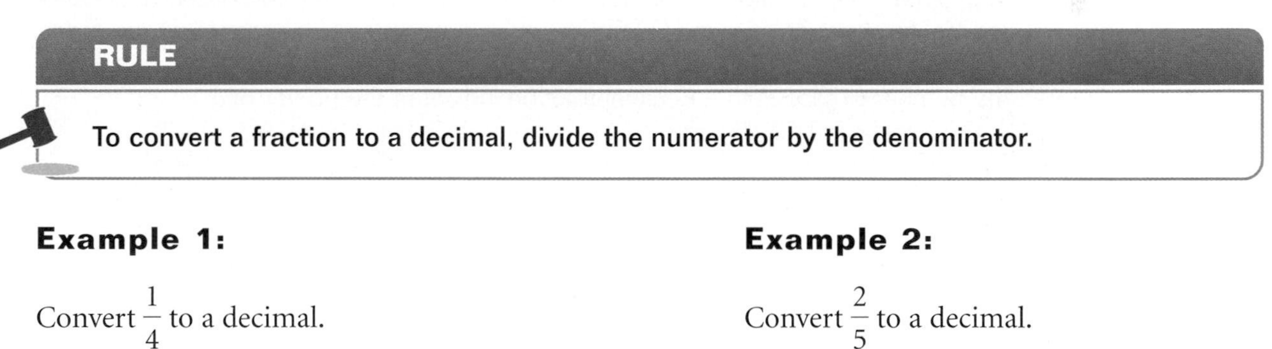

RULE

To convert a fraction to a decimal, divide the numerator by the denominator.

Example 1:

Convert $\frac{1}{4}$ to a decimal.

$$\frac{1}{4} = 4\overline{)1.00} = 0.25$$

(quotient .25; 8, 20, 20)

Example 2:

Convert $\frac{2}{5}$ to a decimal.

$$\frac{2}{5} = 5\overline{)2.0} = 0.4$$

(quotient .4; 20)

RULE

To convert a decimal to a fraction,

1. **Express the decimal number as a whole number in the numerator of the fraction;**
2. **Express the denominator of the fraction as the number 1 followed by as many zeros as there are places to the right of the decimal point; and**
3. **Reduce the resulting fraction to its lowest terms.**

Example 1:

Convert 0.125 to a fraction.

1. Numerator: 125
2. Denominator: 1 followed by 3 zeros = 1000
3. Reduce: $\frac{125}{1000} = \frac{1}{8}$

Example 2:

Convert 0.65 to a fraction.

1. Numerator: 65
2. Denominator: 1 followed by 2 zeros = 100
3. Reduce: $\frac{65}{100} = \frac{13}{20}$

QUICK REVIEW

- In decimal fractions, zeros added before the decimal point or at the end of the decimal fraction *do not* change the value. Example: .5 = **0**.5 = 0.5**0**. However, using the leading zero is the only acceptable notation (i.e., in this case, 0.5).
- In a decimal number, zeros added before and/or after the decimal point may change the value. Example: 1.5 ≠ 1.**0**5 and 1.5 ≠ 1**0**.5
- To avoid a patient safety incident, *always* place a zero to the left of the decimal point in a decimal fraction. *Always* read aloud the zero in a medication order involving a decimal fraction. Example: 0.5 is read as "zero point five."
- The number of places in a decimal fraction indicates the power of 10.

  Examples:
  0.5 = five tenths
  0.05 = five hundredths
  0.005 = five thousandths

- Compare decimals by aligning decimal points and adding zeros.

  Example:
  Compare 0.5, 0.05, and 0.005
  0.500 = five hundred thousandths (greatest)
  0.050 = fifty thousandths
  0.005 = five thousandths (least)

- To convert a fraction to a decimal, divide the numerator by the denominator.
- To convert a decimal to a fraction, express the decimal number as a whole number in the numerator and the denominator as the correct power of 10. Reduce the fraction to its lowest terms.

  Example:

  $$0.04 = \frac{4\text{(numerator is a whole number)}}{100\text{(denominator is 1 followed by 2 zeros)}} = \frac{\overset{1}{\cancel{4}}}{\underset{25}{\cancel{100}}} = \frac{1}{25}$$

REVIEW SET 1-4

Complete the following table of equivalent fractions and decimals. Reduce fractions to their lowest terms.

Fraction	Decimal	The decimal number is read as
1. $\frac{1}{5}$	________	____________________
2. ________	________	eighty-five hundredths
3. ________	1.05	____________________
4. ________	0.006	____________________
5. $10\frac{3}{200}$	________	____________________
6. ________	1.9	____________________
7. ________	________	five and one tenth
8. $\frac{4}{5}$	________	____________________
9. ________	250.5	____________________
10. $33\frac{3}{100}$	________	____________________
11. ________	0.95	____________________
12. $2\frac{3}{4}$	________	____________________

Fraction	Decimal	The decimal number is read as
13. ________	________	seven and five thousandths
14. $1000\frac{1}{200}$	________	____________________
15. ________	________	four thousand eighty-five and seventy-five thousandths

16. Change 0.017 to a four-place decimal. ____________________

17. Change 0.2500 to a two-place decimal. ____________________

18. Convert $\frac{75}{100}$ to a decimal. ____________________

19. Convert 0.045 to a fraction reduced to its lowest terms. ____________________

Circle the correct answer.

20. Which is largest?	0.012	0.120	0.021
21. Which is smallest?	0.635	0.6	0.063

22. 0.375 = 0.0375 (True) (False) ________

23. 2.2 grams = 2.02 grams (True) (False) ________

24. 6.5 ounces = 6.500 ounces (True) (False) ________

25. For a certain medication, the safe dosage should be greater than or equal to 0.5 grams but less than or equal to 2 grams. Circle each dosage that falls within this range.

    0.8 grams   0.25 grams   2.5 grams   1.25 grams

Check your work! Answers to all Review Sets are provided at the end of each chapter. Worked solutions for select Review Set exercises are also provided there.

Addition and Subtraction of Decimals

Addition and subtraction are used in the clinical setting when adding dosages, intake of fluids, and hourly outputs, and when calculating amounts in restricted diets. The addition and subtraction of decimals are similar to the addition and subtraction of whole numbers. There are only two simple but essential rules that are different. Healthcare providers must use these two rules to perform accurate dosage calculations for some medications.

So far, decimals have been compared by aligning the decimal points vertically; now decimals will be aligned to add and subtract decimals. Whenever there is an unequal number of spaces to the right and left of a decimal point, add a zero wherever there is a blank space. (These added zeros do not change the value of the number.) Then add and subtract the numbers the same as you add and subtract whole numbers.

RULE

When adding and subtracting decimals, line up the decimal points.

CAUTION

In final answers, eliminate unnecessary zeros at the end of a decimal to avoid confusion.

Example 1:

$$1.25 + 1.75 = \begin{array}{r} 1.25 \\ +1.75 \\ \hline 3.00 \end{array} = 3$$

Example 2:

$$1.25 - 0.13 = \begin{array}{r} 1.25 \\ -0.13 \\ \hline 1.12 \end{array}$$

Example 3:

$$3.54 + 1.26 = \begin{array}{r} 3.54 \\ +1.26 \\ \hline 4.80 \end{array} = 4.8$$

Example 4:

$$2.54 - 1.04 = \begin{array}{r} 2.54 \\ -1.04 \\ \hline 1.50 \end{array} = 1.5$$

RULE

To add and subtract decimals, add zeros at the end of decimal fractions if necessary to make all decimal numbers of equal length.

Example 1:

$$3.75 - 2.1 = \begin{array}{r} 3.75 \\ -2.10 \\ \hline 1.65 \end{array}$$

Example 2:

Add 0.9, 0.65, 0.27, 4.712

$$\begin{array}{r} 0.900 \\ 0.650 \\ 0.270 \\ +4.712 \\ \hline 6.532 \end{array}$$

Example 3:

$$5.25 - 3.6 = \begin{array}{r} 5.25 \\ -3.60 \\ \hline 1.65 \end{array}$$

Example 4:

$$66.96 + 32 = \begin{array}{r} 66.96 \\ +32.00 \\ \hline 98.96 \end{array}$$

QUICK REVIEW

- When adding and subtracting decimals, align the decimal points and add zeros, making all decimals of equal length. Eliminate unnecessary zeros in the final answer.

Examples:

$$1.5 + 0.05 = \begin{array}{r} 1.50 \\ +0.05 \\ \hline 1.55 \end{array}$$

$$0.725 - 0.5 = \begin{array}{r} 0.725 \\ -0.500 \\ \hline 0.225 \end{array}$$

$$7.8 + 1.12 = \begin{array}{r} 7.80 \\ +1.12 \\ \hline 8.92 \end{array}$$

$$12.5 - 1.5 = \begin{array}{r} 12.5 \\ -1.5 \\ \hline 11.0 \end{array} = 11$$

REVIEW SET 1-5

Find the results of the following problems.

1. 0.16 + 5.375 + 1.05 + 16 = ________
2. 7.517 + 3.2 + 0.16 + 33.3 = ________
3. 13.009 − 0.7 = ________
4. 5.125 + 6.025 + 0.15 = ________
5. 175.1 + 0.099 = ________
6. 25.2 − 0.193 = ________
7. 0.58 − 0.062 = ________
8. $10.10 − $0.62 = ________
9. $19 − $0.09 = ________
10. $5.05 + $0.17 + $17.49 = ________
11. 4 + 1.98 + 0.42 + 0.003 = ________

12. $0.3 - 0.03 =$ ________
13. $16.3 - 12.15 =$ ________
14. $2.5 - 0.99 =$ ________
15. $5 + 2.5 + 0.05 + 0.15 + 2.55 =$ ________
16. $0.03 + 0.16 + 2.327 =$ ________
17. $700 - 325.65 =$ ________
18. $645.32 - 40.9 =$ ________
19. $18 + 2.35 + 7.006 + 0.093 =$ ________
20. $13.529 + 10.09 =$ ________
21. A dietitian calculates the sodium in a patient's breakfast: raisin bran cereal = 0.1 grams, 250 mL 2% milk = 0.125 grams, 180 mL orange juice = 0.001 grams, 1 corn muffin = 0.35 grams, and butter = 0.121 grams. How many grams of sodium did the patient consume? ________
22. A prescription is for 30 mg. The stock supply has one tablet of 7.5 mg and one tablet of 15 mg. How many more milligrams of the medication must the nurse get from the pharmacy? ________
23. Ms. Brisson has a hospital bill for $16 709.43. Her insurance company pays $14 651.37. What is her balance due? ________
24. A pharmacist weighs a tube of antibiotic ointment and discovers it weighs 0.15 kg. How much would 20 tubes weigh? ________
25. A community care nurse accounts for one day of work. If the nurse spent 3 hours and 20 minutes at the office, 40 minutes travelling, $3\frac{1}{2}$ hours caring for patients, 24 minutes for lunch, and took a 12-minute break, what is the total number of hours including the break? Express the answer as a decimal. (HINT: First convert each time to hours and minutes.)

____

Check your work! Answers to all Review Sets are provided at the end of each chapter. Worked solutions for select Review Set exercises are also provided there.

Multiplication and Division of Decimals

Multiplying Decimals

The procedure for multiplication of decimals is similar to that used for whole numbers. The only difference is the decimal point, which must be properly placed in the product or answer. Use the following simple rule.

RULE

To multiply decimals,

1. **Multiply the decimals without concern for decimal point placement;**
2. **Count off the total number of decimal places in the numbers multiplied; and**
3. **Place the decimal point in the product to the left of the total number of places counted. If the product has insufficient numbers for correct placement of the decimal point, add as many zeros as necessary to the left of the product to correct this.**

Example 1:

$1.5 \times 0.5 = 1.5$ 1 decimal place

$\times\ 0.5$ 1 decimal place

0.75 The decimal point is located 2 places to the left because a total of 2 decimal places are counted.

Example 2:

$1.72 \times 0.9 = 1.72$ 2 decimal places

$\times\ 0.9$ 1 decimal place

1.548 The decimal point is located 3 places to the left because a total of 3 decimal places are counted.

Example 3:

$5.06 \times 1.3 = 5.06$ 2 decimal places

$\times\ 1.3$ 1 decimal place

1518

506

6.578 The decimal point is located 3 places to the left because a total of 3 decimal places are counted.

Example 4:

$1.8 \times 0.05 = 1.8$ 1 decimal place

$\times\ 0.05$ 2 decimal places

0.090 The decimal point is located 3 places to the left. Notice that a zero has to be inserted between the decimal point and the 9 to allow for enough decimal places.

$0.090 = 0.09$ Eliminate the unnecessary zero.

RULE

When multiplying a decimal by a power of 10, move the decimal point as many places to the right as there are zeros in the multiplier.

Example 1:

1.25×10

The multiplier 10 has 1 zero; move the decimal point 1 place to the right.

$1.25 \times 10 = 1.2.5 = 12.5$

Example 2:

2.3×100

The multiplier 100 has 2 zeros; move the decimal point 2 places to the right. (**Note:** Add zeros as necessary to complete the operation.)

$2.3 \times 100 = 2.30. = 230$

Example 3:

0.001×1000

The multiplier 1000 has 3 zeros; move the decimal point 3 places to the right.

$0.001 \times 1000 = 0.001. = 1$

Dividing Decimals

Decimal fractions occur frequently in calculations as fractions, which require division. Remember two things we have learned about fractions and decimals:

1. The value of the fraction is not changed when the numerator and the denominator are multiplied by the same number.
2. When multiplying a decimal by a power of 10, move the decimal point as many places to the right as there are zeros in the multiplier.

Now follow the steps in the Rule box below to divide decimals.

RULE

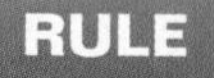

To divide decimals,

1. **Eliminate the decimal point in the divisor (number divided by, or the denominator) by moving the decimal point as many places as necessary to make the divisor a whole number;**
2. **Move the decimal point the same number of places to the right in the numerator (dividend) as you did in the denominator;**
3. **Reduce the fraction to its lowest terms and then divide if necessary;**
4. **Place the decimal point in the *quotient* (answer) above the *new* decimal point place in the *dividend.***

Example 1:

$0.25 \div 0.125$

$= \frac{0.25}{0.125}$

Multiply the numerator and the denominator by 1000, and move the decimal point 3 places to the right.

$= \frac{250}{125}$

In this case, 250 is exactly twice 125. So divide the numerator by the denominator to reduce the fraction to its lowest terms.

$= \frac{250}{125} = 2$

Therefore, $0.25 \div 0.125 = 2$

Example 2:

```
                                40.3   Quotient
100.75  ÷  2.5  =  2.5.)100.7.5  =  40.3
Dividend   Divisor      100
                         07
                         00
                          75
                          75
```

Example 3:

```
                        2825.
56.5 ÷ 0.02 = 0.02.)56.50.  = 2825
                     4
                    16
                    16
                      5
                      4
                     10
                     10
```

MATH TIP

Recall that adding a zero at the end of a decimal number does not change its value (56.5 = 56.50). Adding a zero was necessary in the previous example to complete the operation.

RULE

When dividing a decimal by a power of 10, move the decimal point to the left as many places as there are zeros in the divisor.

Example 1:

0.65 ÷ 10

The divisor 10 has 1 zero; move the decimal point 1 place to the left.

0.65 ÷ 10 = .0.65 = 0.065

(**Note:** Add the zero to the left of the decimal point to avoid confusion and to emphasize that this is a decimal.)

Example 2:

7.3 ÷ 100

The divisor 100 has 2 zeros; move the decimal point 2 places to the left.

7.3 ÷ 100 = .07.3 = 0.073

(**Note:** Add zeros as necessary to complete the operation.)

Example 3:

0.5 ÷ 1000

The divisor 1000 has 3 zeros; move the decimal point 3 places to the left.

0.5 ÷ 1000 = .000.5 = 0.0005

CAUTION

A decimal point placed incorrectly is a major cause of patient safety incidents. It is important to always place the decimal point clearly and correctly.

Rounding Decimals

When dividing, the answer may not "come out even." In some cases it is possible to keep dividing and end up with an answer that is quite long! Sometimes it is convenient and safe to round an answer—that is, to use an approximate answer instead of an exact one.

Rounding Off

Rounding off numbers produces results that can be either larger or smaller than the given number. For many calculations, it is necessary to calculate to thousandths (three decimal places) and round off to hundredths (two places). In this text, instructions will usually specify how many places to carry out your division.

How many places are necessary to carry out the division? The answer depends on the way the medication is dispensed and the equipment needed to administer it. Some tablets can be broken in half. Some liquids are prepared in units of measurement: tenths, hundredths, or thousandths. Some syringes are marked to the nearest tenth, hundredth, or thousandth place. Intravenous rates are usually rounded to the nearest whole number.

RULE

To round off a number,
If the first number to the right of the number to be rounded is greater than or equal to 5, then round up to the next number. If the first number to the right of the number to be rounded is less than 5, then round down.

When rounding for dosage calculations, unnecessary zeros can be dropped. For example, 5.20 rounded to hundredths place should be written as 5.2 because the 0 is not needed to clarify the number.

Examples:

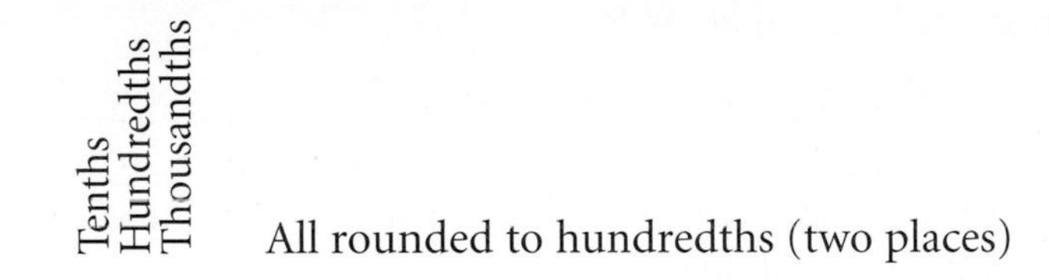

0 . 1 2 3 = 0.12

1 . 7 4 4 = 1.74

5 . 3 2 5 = 5.33

0 . 6 6 6 = 0.67

0 . 3 0 = 0.3 When this is rounded to hundredths, the final zero should be dropped. It is not needed to clarify the number.

RULE

To obtain an answer that is rounded off to the nearest tenth, look at the number in the hundredth place and follow the above rule for rounding off.

Examples:

Tenths
Hundredths

All rounded to tenths (one place)

0 . 1 3 = 0.1

5 . 6 4 = 5.6

0 . 7 5 = 0.8

1 . 6 6 = 1.7

0 . 9 5 = 1.0 = 1 Zero at the end of a decimal is unnecessary.

Rounding Down

The danger of a medication overdose must always be guarded against. Therefore, the amount of medication is often rounded down instead of up. Rounding down is routinely done in pediatrics and when administering high-alert medications to adults.

To round a number down to a particular place, simply drop all the digits after that place. In particular, to round down to the tenths place, simply drop all the digits after the tenths place.

Example:

Round 5.6685 to the nearest hundredth, tenth, and whole number.

5.6685 rounded down to the nearest hundredth = 5.66

5.6685 rounded down to the nearest tenth = 5.6

5.6685 rounded down to the nearest whole number = 5

Note: This is done to avoid medication overdose only. Routinely, in other applications, follow the above rules for rounding off: if the first number to the right of the number to be rounded is equal to or greater than 5, then round up to the next number; if the first number to the right of the number to be rounded is less than 5, then round down.

QUICK REVIEW

- To multiply decimals, place the decimal point in the product to the *left* as many decimal places as there are in the total of the number of places counted in the two decimals multiplied.

  Example:
  $0.25 \times 0.2 = 0.050 = 0.05$ (Zeros at the end of the decimal are unnecessary.)

- To divide decimals, move the decimal point in the divisor and dividend the number of decimal places that will make the divisor a whole number and align it in the quotient.

  Example: $24 \div 1.2$

  $$1.2.\overline{)24.0.} = 20.$$

- To multiply or divide decimals by a power of 10, move the decimal point to the *right* (to *multiply*) or to the *left* (to *divide*) the number of decimal places as there are zeros in the power of 10.

  Examples:
  $5.06 \times 10 = 5.0.6 = 50.6$

  $2.1 \div 100 = .02.1 = 0.021$

- When rounding decimals, add 1 to the place value considered if the next decimal place is 5 or greater.

  Examples:

  Rounded to hundredths: 3.054 = 3.05; 0.566 = 0.57. Rounded to tenths: 3.05 = 3.1; 0.54 = 0.5

REVIEW SET 1-6

Multiply, and round answers to two decimal places.

1. $1.16 \times 5.03 =$ ________
2. $0.314 \times 7 =$ ________
3. $1.71 \times 25 =$ ________
4. $3.002 \times 0.05 =$ ________
5. $75.1 \times 1000.01 =$ ________
6. $16.03 \times 2.05 =$ ________
7. $55.50 \times 0.05 =$ ________
8. $23.2 \times 15.025 =$ ________

Divide, and round answers to two decimal places.

9. $16 \div 0.04 =$ ________
10. $25.3 \div 6.76 =$ ________
11. $0.02 \div 0.004 =$ ________
12. $45.5 \div 15.25 =$ ________
13. $73 \div 13.40 =$ ________
14. $16.36 \div 0.06 =$ ________
15. $0.375 \div 0.25 =$ ________
16. $100.04 \div 0.002 =$ ________

Multiply or divide by the power of 10 indicated. Draw an arrow to demonstrate movement of the decimal point.

17. $562.5 \times 100 =$ ________
18. $16 \times 10 =$ ________
19. $25 \div 1000 =$ ________
20. $32.005 \div 1000 =$ ________
21. $23.25 \times 10 =$ ________
22. $717.717 \div 10 =$ ________
23. $83.16 \times 10 =$ ________
24. $0.33 \times 100 =$ ________
25. $14.106 \times 1000 =$ ________

Check your work! Answers to all Review Sets are provided at the end of each chapter. Worked solutions for select Review Set exercises are also provided there.

PRACTICE PROBLEMS—CHAPTER 1

1. Convert 0.35 to a fraction to its lowest terms. ________

2. Convert $\frac{3}{8}$ to a decimal. ________

Find the least common denominator for the following pairs of fractions.

3. $\frac{5}{7}; \frac{2}{3}$ ________

4. $\frac{1}{5}; \frac{4}{11}$ ________

5. $\frac{4}{9}; \frac{5}{6}$ ________

6. $\frac{1}{3}; \frac{3}{5}$ ________

Perform the indicated operation, and reduce fractions to their lowest terms.

7. $1\frac{2}{3} + \frac{9}{5} =$ ________

8. $4\frac{5}{12} + 3\frac{1}{15} =$ ________

9. $\frac{7}{9} - \frac{5}{18} =$ ________

10. $5\frac{1}{6} - 2\frac{7}{8} =$ ________

11. $\frac{4}{9} \times \frac{7}{12} =$ ________

12. $1\frac{1}{2} \times 6\frac{3}{4} =$ ________

13. $7\frac{1}{5} : 1\frac{7}{10} =$ ________

14. $\dfrac{3}{16} + \dfrac{3}{10} =$ ________

15. $8\dfrac{4}{11}$ divided by $1\dfrac{2}{3} =$ ________

16. $\dfrac{9\frac{1}{2}}{1\frac{4}{5}} =$ ________

17. $\dfrac{13\frac{1}{3}}{4\frac{6}{13}} =$ ________

18. $\dfrac{\frac{1}{10}}{\frac{2}{3}} =$ ________

19. $\dfrac{1}{125} \times \dfrac{1}{25} =$ ________

20. $\dfrac{\frac{7}{8}}{\frac{1}{3}} \div \dfrac{3\frac{1}{2}}{\frac{1}{3}} =$ ________

21. $\dfrac{20}{35} \times 3 =$ ________

22. $2\dfrac{1}{4} \times 7\dfrac{1}{8} =$ ________

Perform the indicated operation, and round the answer to two decimal places.

23. $11.33 + 29.16 + 19.78 =$ ________

24. $93.712 - 26.97 =$ ________

25. $43.69 - 0.7083 =$ ________

26. $66.4 \times 72.8 =$ ________

27. $360 \times 0.53 =$ ________

28. $268.4 \div 14 =$ ________

29. $10.10 - 0.62 =$ ________

30. $5 + 2.5 + 0.05 + 0.15 =$ ________

31. $1.71 \times 25 =$ ________

32. $45 \div 0.15 =$ ________

33. $2974 \div 0.23 =$ ________

34. $51.21 \div 0.016 =$ ________

35. $0.74 \div 0.37 =$ ________

36. $1.5 + 146.73 + 1.9 + 0.832 =$ ________

Multiply or divide by the power of 10 indicated. Draw an arrow to indicate the movement of the decimal point.

37. $9.716 \times 1000 =$ ________

38. $50.25 \div 100 =$ ________

39. $0.25 \times 100 =$ ________

40. $5.75 \times 1000 =$ ________

41. $0.25 \div 10 =$ ________

42. $11.525 \times 10 =$ ________

43. The nurse is to administer 4 tablets with a dosage strength of 0.04 mg each. What total dosage will be given? ________

44. A five-student team completes $\frac{1}{2}$ of an assignment together when one member becomes ill and cannot complete his share. Write a fraction, reduced to its lowest terms, of the remaining portion of the assignment that each student must now do in order to complete the assignment.

____

45. Tablets are labelled 0.1 mg and the nurse is to give $3\frac{1}{2}$ (3.5) tablets. What total dosage is this?

____

46. Last week a nurse earning $17.43 per hour gross pay worked 40 hours plus 6.25 hours of overtime, which is paid at twice the hourly rate. What is the total gross pay for last week for this nurse, including regular and overtime pay? ________

47. The instructional assistant is ordering supplies for the nursing skills laboratory. A single box of 12 urinary catheters costs $98.76. A case of 12 boxes of these catheters costs $975. Calculate the savings per catheter when a case is purchased. ________

48. The nurse is to administer 1.25 mg of a medication. Each tablet of that medication has a strength of 0.5 mg. How many tablets will be administered? ________

49. Mr. Makela is to receive 1200 millilitres of fluid in a 24-hour period. How many millilitres should he drink between the hours of 0700 and 1900 if he is to receive $\frac{2}{3}$ of the total amount during that time? ________

50. A baby weighed 3.7 kilograms at birth. The baby now weighs 6.65 kilograms. How many kilograms did the baby gain? ________

Check your work! Answers to all problems are provided at the end of the book, in the Answers section. Worked solutions for some Practice Problems are also provided there.

ANSWERS TO REVIEW SETS

Review Set 1-1

1) $\frac{6}{6}, \frac{7}{5}$ **2)** $\frac{1}{4}, \frac{1}{14}$ **3)** $1\frac{2}{9}, 1\frac{1}{4}, 5\frac{7}{8}$ **4)** $\frac{3}{4} = \frac{6}{8}, \frac{1}{5} = \frac{2}{10}, \frac{3}{9} = \frac{1}{3}$ **5)** $\frac{13}{2}$ **6)** $\frac{6}{5}$ **7)** $\frac{32}{3}$ **8)** $\frac{47}{6}$ **9)** 2 **10)** 1 **11)** $3\frac{1}{3}$ **12)** $1\frac{1}{3}$ **13)** $\frac{6}{8}$ **14)** $\frac{4}{16}$ **15)** $\frac{4}{10}$ **16)** $\frac{6}{9}$ **17)** $\frac{1}{100}$ **18)** $\frac{1}{10\,000}$ **19)** $\frac{5}{9}$ **20)** $\frac{3}{10}$ **21)** $\frac{2}{5}$ bottle **22)** 600 mL on Day 2; 900 mL on Day 3; 1350 mL on Day 4 **23)** $\frac{1}{20}$ of the class are men **24)** $\frac{9}{10}$ of the questions were answered correctly **25)** $\frac{1}{4}$

Review Set 1-2

1) $8\frac{7}{15}$ **2)** $1\frac{5}{12}$ **3)** $17\frac{5}{24}$ **4)** $1\frac{1}{24}$ **5)** $32\frac{5}{6}$ **6)** $1\frac{1}{3}$ **7)** $5\frac{53}{72}$ **8)** 43 **9)** $5\frac{118}{119}$ **10)** $2\frac{8}{15}$ **11)** $\frac{1}{2}$ **12)** $4\frac{5}{6}$ **13)** $\frac{1}{24}$ **14)** $63\frac{2}{3}$ **15)** $\frac{1}{6}$ **16)** $1\frac{2}{5}$ **17)** $7\frac{1}{16}$ **18)** $7\frac{2}{9}$ **19)** $1\frac{1}{4}$ **20)** $9\frac{1}{2}$ **21)** $\frac{1}{12}$ **22)** $1\frac{1}{2}$ tablets daily **23)** $4\frac{11}{12}$ glasses of fluid **24)** $2\frac{11}{12}$ km left to walk **25)** $112\frac{1}{4}$ apples eaten

Review Set 1-3

1) $\frac{1}{40}$ **2)** $\frac{36}{125}$ **3)** $\frac{35}{48}$ **4)** $\frac{3}{100}$ **5)** 3 **6)** $1\frac{2}{3}$ **7)** $\frac{4}{5}$ **8)** $6\frac{8}{15}$ **9)** $\frac{1}{2}$ **10)** $23\frac{19}{36}$ **11)** $\frac{3}{32}$ **12)** 3 **13)** $1\frac{34}{39}$ **14)** $\frac{3}{14}$ **15)** $\frac{1}{11}$ **16)** $\frac{1}{2}$ **17)** $\frac{1}{30}$ **18)** $3\frac{1}{3}$ **19)** $\frac{3}{20}$ **20)** $1\frac{1}{9}$ **21)** 60 calories **22)** 560 sec **23)** 20 doses **24)** $31\frac{1}{2}$ tablets **25)** 1275 millilitres

Review Set 1-4

1) 0.2, two tenths **2)** $\frac{17}{20}$, 0.85 **3)** $1\frac{1}{20}$, one and five hundredths **4)** $\frac{3}{500}$, six thousandths **5)** 10.015, ten and fifteen thousandths **6)** $1\frac{9}{10}$, one and nine tenths **7)** $5\frac{1}{10}$, 5.1 **8)** 0.8, eight tenths **9)** $250\frac{1}{2}$, two hundred fifty and five tenths **10)** 33.03, thirty-three and three hundredths **11)** $\frac{19}{20}$, ninety-five hundredths **12)** 2.75, two and seventy-five hundredths **13)** $7\frac{1}{200}$, 7.005 **14)** 1000.005, one thousand and five thousandths **15)** $4085\frac{3}{40}$, 4085.075 **16)** 0.0170 **17)** 0.25 **18)** 0.75 **19)** $\frac{9}{200}$ **20)** 0.120 **21)** 0.063 **22)** False **23)** False **24)** True **25)** 0.8 gram and 1.25 grams

Review Set 1-5

1) 22.585 **2)** 44.177 **3)** 12.309 **4)** 11.3 **5)** 175.199 **6)** 25.007 **7)** 0.518 **8)** \$9.48 **9)** \$18.91 **10)** \$22.71 **11)** 6.403 **12)** 0.27 **13)** 4.15 **14)** 1.51 **15)** 10.25 **16)** 2.517 **17)** 374.35 **18)** 604.42 **19)** 27.449 **20)** 23.619 **21)** 0.697 g **22)** 7.5 mg **23)** \$2058.06 **24)** 3 kg **25)** 8.1 h

Review Set 1-6

1) 5.83 **2)** 2.20 **3)** 42.75 **4)** 0.15 **5)** 75 100.75 **6)** 32.86 **7)** 2.78 **8)** 348.58 **9)** 400 **10)** 3.74 **11)** 5 **12)** 2.98 **13)** 5.45 **14)** 272.67 **15)** 1.5 **16)** 50 020 **17)** 562.50. = 56 250 **18)** 16.0. = 160 **19)** .025. = 0.025 **20)** .032.005 = 0.032005 **21)** 23.2.5 = 232.5 **22)** 71.7.717 = 71.7717 **23)** 83.1.6 = 831.6 **24)** 0.33. = 33 **25)** 14.106. = 14 106

SELECTED SOLUTIONS TO REVIEW SETS

Selected Solutions—Review Set 1-1

7) $10\frac{2}{3} = \frac{(3 \times 10) + 2}{3} = \frac{32}{3}$

12) $\frac{100}{75} = 1\frac{25}{75} = 1\frac{1}{3}$

21) 300 mL − 180 mL = 120 mL remaining

$\frac{\cancel{120}^{2}}{\cancel{300}_{5}} = \frac{2}{5}$ bottle remaining

23)
$$\begin{array}{r} 57 \\ +3 \\ \hline 60 \end{array}$$
60 people in class

The men represent $\frac{3}{60}$ or $\frac{1}{20}$ of the class.

25) $\frac{1}{8} = \frac{3}{24}; \frac{1}{6} = \frac{4}{24}; \frac{1}{4} = \frac{6}{24}$

Therefore, $\frac{1}{4}$ is the largest fraction

Selected Solutions—Review Set 1-2

1) $7\frac{4}{5} + \frac{2}{3} = 7\frac{12}{15}$
$$\begin{array}{r} 7\frac{12}{15} \\ +\frac{10}{15} \\ \hline 7\frac{22}{15} \end{array} = 8\frac{7}{15}$$

3) $4\frac{2}{3} + 5\frac{1}{24} + 7\frac{1}{2} = 4\frac{16}{24}$
$$\begin{array}{r} 4\frac{16}{24} \\ 5\frac{1}{24} \\ +7\frac{12}{24} \\ \hline 16\frac{29}{24} \end{array} = 17\frac{5}{24}$$

4) $\frac{3}{4} + \frac{1}{8} + \frac{1}{6} = \frac{18}{24} + \frac{3}{24} + \frac{4}{24} =$

$\frac{18 + 3 + 4}{24} = \frac{25}{24} = 1\frac{1}{24}$

12) $8\frac{1}{12} - 3\frac{1}{4} = 8\frac{1}{12} - 3\frac{3}{12} = 7\frac{13}{12}$

$$\begin{array}{r} 7\frac{13}{12} \\ -3\frac{3}{12} \\ \hline 4\frac{10}{12} = 4\frac{5}{6} \end{array}$$

20) $27 - 17\frac{1}{2} = 26\frac{2}{2}$

$$\begin{array}{r} 26\frac{2}{2} \\ -17\frac{1}{2} \\ \hline 9\frac{1}{2} \text{ litres} \end{array}$$

21) $1 - \left(\frac{2}{3} + \frac{1}{4}\right) - 1 - \left(\frac{8 + 3}{12}\right) = 1 - \frac{11}{12} = \frac{1}{12}$

22) $\frac{1}{2} \times 3 = \frac{3}{2} = 1\frac{1}{2}$ tablets daily

23) $1\frac{1}{2} + 1 + \frac{2}{3} + 1\frac{3}{4} = \frac{3}{2} + 1 + \frac{2}{3} + \frac{7}{4} =$

$\frac{18}{12} + \frac{12}{12} + \frac{8}{12} + \frac{21}{12} = \frac{59}{12} = 4\frac{11}{12}$ cups of fluid

24) $1\frac{1}{4} + 1\frac{1}{3} + 1\frac{1}{2} + 1 = \frac{5}{4} + \frac{4}{3} + \frac{3}{2} + \frac{1}{1} =$

$\frac{15}{12} + \frac{16}{12} + \frac{18}{12} + \frac{12}{12} = \frac{61}{12}$ km walked

$8 \text{ km} - \frac{61}{12} \text{ km} = \frac{96}{12} - \frac{61}{12} = \frac{35}{12} = 2\frac{11}{12}$ km left to walk

25) $54\frac{1}{2} + 57\frac{3}{4} = \frac{218}{4} + \frac{231}{4} = \frac{449}{4} = 112\frac{1}{4}$ apples eaten

Selected Solutions—Review Set 1-3

3) $\frac{5}{8} \times 1\frac{1}{6} = \frac{5}{8} \times \frac{7}{6} = \frac{35}{48}$

5) $\frac{\frac{1}{6}}{\frac{1}{4}} \times \frac{3}{\frac{2}{3}} = \left(\frac{1}{6} \times \frac{4}{1}\right) \times \left(\frac{3}{1} \times \frac{3}{2}\right) = \frac{\overset{2}{\cancel{4}}}{\underset{3}{\cancel{6}}} \times \frac{9}{2} = \frac{\overset{3}{\cancel{18}}}{\underset{1}{\cancel{6}}} = 3$

15) $\frac{1}{33} \div \frac{1}{3} = \frac{1}{33} \times \frac{3}{1} = \frac{3}{33} = \frac{1}{11}$

18) $2\frac{1}{2} \div \frac{3}{4} = \frac{5}{2} \div \frac{3}{4} = \frac{5}{\underset{1}{\cancel{2}}} \times \frac{\overset{2}{\cancel{4}}}{3} = \frac{10}{3} = 3\frac{1}{3}$

24) $3 \times 7 = 21$ doses

$21 \times 1\frac{1}{2} = 21 \times \frac{3}{2} = \frac{63}{2} = 31\frac{1}{2}$ tablets

25) $850 \div \frac{2}{3} = \frac{\overset{425}{\cancel{850}}}{1} \times \frac{3}{\underset{1}{\cancel{2}}} = 1275$ millilitres

Selected Solutions—Review Set 1-4

4) $0.006 = \frac{6}{1000} = \frac{3}{500}$

8) $\frac{4}{5} = 5\overline{)4.0}$ with quotient 0.8, or $\frac{4}{5} = \frac{80}{100} = 0.8$

14) $1000\frac{1}{200} = \frac{2000001}{200} = 200\overline{)2000001.00}$ with quotient 1000.005 or $\frac{1}{200} = \frac{5}{1000} = 0.005$; therefore, 1000.005

$$\begin{array}{r} 200 \\ \hline 0001000 \\ 1000 \\ \hline \end{array}$$

25) 0.8 g is greater than 0.5 g and less than 2 g. Therefore, it is a safe dosage.

0.25 g is less than 0.5 g. Therefore, it is *not* a safe dosage.

2.5 g is greater than 2 g. Therefore, it is *not* a safe dosage.

1.25 g is greater than 0.5 g and less than 2 g. Therefore, it is a safe dosage.

Selected Solutions—Review Set 1-5

2)

$$\begin{array}{r} 7.517 \\ 3.200 \\ 0.160 \\ \underline{33.300} \\ 44.177 \end{array}$$

9)

$$\begin{array}{r} \overset{8\ 9 10}{\$19.00} \\ \underline{-0.09} \\ \$18.91 \end{array}$$

22) 30 mg − (7.5 mg + 15 mg) = 30.0 mg − 22.5 mg = 7.5 mg

$$\begin{array}{r} 30.0 \text{ mg} \\ \underline{-\ 22.5 \text{ mg}} \\ 7.5 \text{ mg} \end{array}$$

25)

$$\begin{array}{r} 3 \text{ h } 20 \text{ min} \\ 40 \text{ min} \\ 3 \text{ h } 30 \text{ min} \\ 24 \text{ min} \\ \underline{12 \text{ min}} \\ 6 \text{ h } 126 \text{ min} \end{array}$$

6 h 126 min = 8 h 6 min (60 minutes/hour)

$$= 8\frac{6}{60} = 8\frac{1}{10} = 8.1 \text{ h}$$

Selected Solutions—Review Set 1-5

8) 23.2 × 15.025 = 348.58

12) 45.5 ÷ 15.25 = 2.9836 = 2.98

CHAPTER

2

Ratios and Percents

OBJECTIVES

1. Interpret values expressed in ratios and percents.
2. Calculate the percent of a quantity.
3. Compare values expressed in fractions, decimals, ratios, and percents.
4. Convert between fractions, decimals, ratios, and percents.

Healthcare providers may use fractions, decimals, percents, and ratios to calculate a variety of medications and treatments. It is important to be able to quickly and accurately convert between them.

RATIOS

A *ratio* is another way of indicating the relationship between two numbers. In other words, it is another way to express a fraction. Ratios can be written as a fraction ($\frac{1}{10}$) or as two numbers separated by a colon (1:10). The latter can be read "one *is to* ten." The colon is a traditional way to write the division sign within a ratio.

Example 1:

3:4 is read "three *is to* four"

Example 2:

On an evening shift, there are 5 nurses and 35 patients. What is the ratio of nurses to patients?
5 nurses to 35 patients = 5 nurses per 35 patients $= \frac{5}{35} = \frac{1}{7}$. This is the same as a ratio of 5:35 or 1:7.

MATH TIP

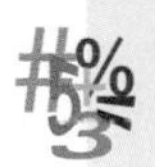

The terms of a ratio are the *numerator* (always to the left of the colon) and the *denominator* (always to the right of the colon) of a fraction. Like fractions, ratios should be stated in their lowest terms.

Example 3:

Epinephrine 1:1000 for injection = 1 part epinephrine to 1000 total parts of solution. The ratio 1:1000 is the same as both $\frac{1}{1000}$ and 0.001.

In some drug solutions such as epinephrine 1:1000, the ratio is used to indicate the drug's concentration. This will be covered in more detail later in this chapter.

The strength of a drug that is diluted can be expressed as a ratio—that is, a numerical relationship between two quantities.

Example 1:

The ratio 1:2 (one to two) means that there is 1 part drug to 2 parts of solution. This solution can also be expressed as $\frac{1}{2}$ strength solution.

Example 2:

The ratio 1:10 (one to ten) means that there is 1 part drug to 10 parts of solution. This solution can also be expressed as $\frac{1}{10}$ strength solution.

Ratio and Proportion

A proportion is an equation that contains two ratios of equal value. Proportions can be used to calculate medication dosages. Although the method is not difficult to learn and use, healthcare providers and researchers who have studied calculation methods used by beginning and seasoned healthcare providers have repeatedly found that using this method seems to result in more patient safety incidents than using dimensional analysis or the "formula method." These latter two methods will be discussed in more detail in Chapter 4.

CAUTION

Although ratios and a medication calculation method called "ratio and proportion" is one way of calculating drug dosages, and is still used successfully by some healthcare providers, evidence is emerging that this methodology holds extra difficulties for the beginning nurse professional who is learning medication calculations (Kohtz & Gowda, 2010; Koohestani & Baghcheghi, 2010; Rice & Bell, 2005). Although the writers acknowledge information about ratios, describe them, and show how to read, write, and convert them in this chapter, for the remainder of this text, it is up to students to decide whether to use ratios in their calculation of medication dosages.

PERCENTS

A percent is a fourth way to show a fractional relationship. Fractions, decimals, ratios, and percents can all be converted from one form to the others. *Percent* comes from the Latin term *per centum,* which means *per hundred.* Conversions of fractions and decimals were discussed in Chapter 1. A percent means a value equal to the number of hundredths—that is, when a percent is written as a fraction, the denominator is always 100.

MATH TIP

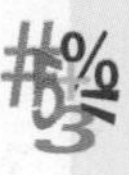

To remember the value of a given percent, replace the % symbol with "/" for *per* and "100" for *cent.* Think: *Percent* (%) means "/100."

Example:

$$3\% = 3 \text{ percent} = 3/100 = \frac{3}{100} = 0.03$$

Converting between Ratios, Percents, Fractions, and Decimals

Understanding the relationship between ratios, percents, fractions, and decimals makes conversion from one to the other quite simple. Now begin by converting a percent to a fraction.

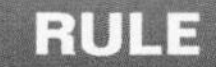

RULE

To convert a percent to a fraction,
1. **Delete the % sign;**
2. **Write the remaining number as the numerator;**
3. **Write "100" as the denominator; and**
4. **Reduce the result to its lowest terms.**

Example:

$$5\% = \frac{5}{100} = \frac{1}{20}$$

It is also easy to express a percent as a ratio.

RULE

To convert a percent to a ratio,
1. **Delete the % sign;**
2. **Write the remaining number as the numerator;**
3. **Write "100" as the denominator;**
4. **Reduce the result to its lowest terms; and**
5. **Express the fraction as a ratio.**

Example:

$$25\% = \frac{25}{100} = \frac{1}{4} = 1{:}4$$

When reading a ratio, the colon is read "*is to.*"

Because the denominator of a percent is always 100, it is easy to find the equivalent decimal. Recall that to divide by 100, the decimal point is moved two places to the left, the number of places equal to the number of zeros in the denominator. This is the hundredths place.

RULE

To convert a percent to a decimal,
1. **Delete the % sign; and**
2. **Divide the remaining number by 100, which is the same as moving the decimal point 2 places to the left.**

Example:

$25\% = \frac{25}{100} = 25 \div 100 = .25. = 0.25$

Conversely, it is easy to change a decimal to a percent.

RULE

To convert a decimal to a percent,
1. **Multiply the decimal number by 100 (move the decimal point 2 places to the right); and**
2. **Add the % sign.**

Example:

$0.25 \times 100 = 0.25. = 25\%$

RULE

To convert a ratio to a percent,
1. **Convert the ratio to a fraction;**
2. **Convert the fraction to a decimal; and**
3. **Convert the decimal to a percent.**

Example:

Convert 1:1000 epinephrine solution to the equivalent concentration expressed as a percent.

1. $1{:}1000 = \frac{1}{1000}$ (ratio converted to fraction)
2. $\frac{1}{1000} = .001. = 0.001$ (fraction converted to decimal)
3. $0.001 = 0.00.1 = 0.1\%$ (decimal converted to percent)

Thus, 1:1000 epinephrine solution = 0.1% epinephrine solution.

Review the preceding example again slowly until it is clear; go over this one step at a time to master these important calculations.

Comparing Percents and Ratios

Healthcare providers frequently administer solutions with the concentration expressed as a percent or ratio. Consider two intravenous solutions given directly into a patient's vein: one is 0.9%; the other is 5%. It is important to be clear that 0.9% is *smaller* than 5%. A 0.9% solution means that there are 0.9 parts of the solid per 100 total parts (0.9 parts is less than one whole part, so it is less than 1%). Compare this to the 5% solution, with 5 parts of the solid (or more than 5 times 0.9 parts) per 100 total parts. Therefore, the 5% solution is much more concentrated, or stronger, than the 0.9% solution. A misunderstanding of these numbers and the quantities they represent can have serious consequences.

Likewise, a solution concentration may be expressed as a fraction percent and as a decimal percent, for example, as $\frac{1}{3}\%$ and 0.45%. Convert these amounts to equivalent decimals to clarify values and compare concentrations.

$$\frac{1}{3}\% = \frac{\frac{1}{3}}{100} = \frac{1}{3} \div \frac{100}{1} = \frac{1}{3} \times \frac{1}{100} = \frac{1}{300} = 0.0033$$

$$0.45\% = \frac{0.45}{100} = 0.0045 \text{ (greater value, stronger concentration)}$$

Example:

Compare solution concentrations expressed as a ratio, such as 1:1000 and 1:100.

$$1{:}1000 = \frac{1}{1000} = 0.001$$

$$1{:}100 = \frac{1}{100} = 0.01 \text{ or } 0.010 \text{ (add zero for comparison); 1:100 is a stronger concentration.}$$

QUICK REVIEW

- Fractions, decimals, ratios, and percents are related equivalents.

  Example: $1{:}2 = \frac{1}{2} = 0.5 = 50\%$
- Like fractions, ratios should be reduced to their lowest terms.

  Example: $2{:}4 = 1{:}2$
- To express a ratio as a fraction, the number to the left of the colon becomes the numerator, and the number to the right of the colon becomes the denominator. The colon in a ratio is equivalent to the division sign in a fraction.

  Example: $2{:}3 = \frac{2}{3}$
- To change a ratio to a decimal, convert the ratio to a fraction, and divide the numerator by the denominator.

  Example: $1{:}4 = \frac{1}{4} = 1 \div 4 = 0.25$
- To change a percent to a fraction, drop the % sign and place the remaining number as the numerator over the denominator 100. Reduce the fraction to its lowest terms.
  Think: per (/) cent (100).

  Example: $75\% = \frac{75}{100} = \frac{3}{4}$
- To change a percent to a ratio, first convert the percent to a fraction in its lowest terms. Then, place the numerator to the left of a colon and the denominator to the right of the colon.

  Example: $35\% = \frac{35}{100} = \frac{7}{20} = 7{:}20$
- To change a percent to a decimal, drop the % sign, and divide the remaining number by 100.

  Example: 4% = .04. = 0.04
- To change a decimal to a percent, multiply by 100, and add the % sign.

  Example: 0.5 = 0.50. = 50%
- To change a ratio to a percent, first convert the ratio to a fraction. Convert the fraction to a decimal and then the decimal to a percent.

  Example: $1{:}2 = \frac{1}{2} = 1 \div 2 = 0.5 = 0.50. = 50\%$

REVIEW SET 2-1

Change the following ratios to fractions that are reduced to their lowest terms.

1. $3:150 =$ ________
2. $6:10 =$ ________
3. $0.05:0.15 =$ ________

Change the following ratios to decimals; round to two decimal places, if needed.

4. $20:40 =$ ________
5. $\frac{1}{1000}:\frac{1}{150} =$ ________
6. $0.3:4.5 =$ ________
7. $1\frac{1}{2}:6\frac{2}{9} =$ ________

Change the following ratios to percents; round to two decimal places, if needed.

8. $12:48 =$ ________
9. $0.08:0.64 =$ ________
10. $7:10 =$ ________
11. $50:100 =$ ________

Change the following percents to fractions that are reduced to their lowest terms.

12. $45\% =$ ________
13. $0.5\% =$ ________
14. $1\% =$ ________
15. $66\frac{2}{3}\% =$ ________

Change the following percents to decimals; round to two decimal places, if needed.

16. $2.94\% =$ ________
17. $33\% =$ ________
18. $0.9\% =$ ________

Change the following percents to ratios that are reduced to their lowest terms.

19. $16\% =$ ________
20. $25\% =$ ________
21. $50\% =$ ________

Which of the following is largest? Circle your answer.

22. 0.9% 0.9 $1:9$ $\frac{1}{90}$
23. 0.05 $\frac{200}{400}$ 0.025 $1:25$
24. 0.0125% 0.25% 0.1% 0.02%
25. $\frac{1}{150}$ $\frac{1}{300}$ 0.5 $\frac{2}{3}\%$

Check your work! Answers to all Review Sets are provided at the end of each chapter. Worked solutions for selected Review Sets are also available there.

PERCENT MEASURES

Percent strengths are used extensively in intravenous solutions and for a variety of other medications, such as eye drops and ointments and other topical (for external use) ointments. Since percent (%) means "parts per hundred," the higher the percent strength, the stronger the solution or ointment. **Note:** Percent notations are made with no space between the quantity and the symbol, for example, 15%.

Another way the healthcare provider uses percents is in calculating an amount. For example, a patient reports that he drank 75% of a 200-mL cup of coffee with breakfast. To record the amount he actually drank in his chart, determine the value of 75% of 200 mL.

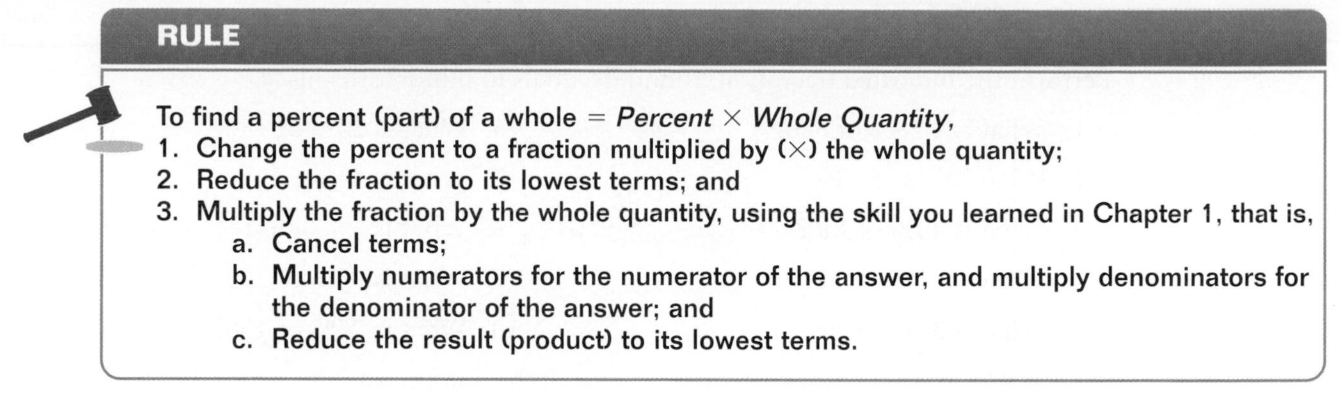

RULE

To find a percent (part) of a whole = *Percent* × *Whole Quantity*,

1. **Change the percent to a fraction multiplied by (×) the whole quantity;**
2. **Reduce the fraction to its lowest terms; and**
3. **Multiply the fraction by the whole quantity, using the skill you learned in Chapter 1, that is,**
   a. **Cancel terms;**
   b. **Multiply numerators for the numerator of the answer, and multiply denominators for the denominator of the answer; and**
   c. **Reduce the result (product) to its lowest terms.**

To continue with the example in the text:

Percent (Part) = Percent × Whole Quantity

1. Change 75% to a fraction and multiply by the whole quantity:

   $\frac{75}{100} \times 200$ mL

2. Reduce the fraction to its lowest terms:

   reduces down by dividing each number by 25; that is, 75 divided by 25 = 3; 100 divided by 25 = 4

   $\frac{\overset{3}{\cancel{75}}}{\underset{4}{\cancel{100}}} \times 200$ mL

3. Multiply $\frac{3}{4} \times 200$:

   a. 4 reduces to 1 and 200 reduces to 50 when each is divided by 4

   $\frac{3}{\underset{1}{\cancel{4}}} \times \overset{50}{\cancel{200}}$ mL

   b. Multiply 3 × 50 mL = 150 mL

   c. Note that the denominator is 1.

4. Therefore, 75% of 200 mL is 150 mL.

MATH TIP

In a mathematical expression, the word *of* means *times* and means that you should multiply.

QUICK REVIEW

- Percent (Part) = Percent × Whole Quantity

  Example: What is 15% of 48?

  $15\% \times 48 = \frac{15}{100} \times 48$

  $= \frac{15}{\underset{25}{\cancel{100}}} \times \overset{12}{\cancel{48}} = \frac{\overset{3}{\cancel{15}}}{\underset{5}{\cancel{25}}} \times 12 = \frac{3}{5} \times 12 = \frac{36}{5} = 7.2$

REVIEW SET 2-2

Perform the indicated operation; round decimals to hundredths place.

1. What is 0.25% of 520? ________
2. What is 5% of 95? ________
3. What is 40% of 140? ________
4. What is 0.7% of 62? ________
5. What is 3% of 889? ________
6. What is 20% of 75? ________
7. What is 4% of 20? ________
8. What is 7% of 34? ________
9. What is 15% of 250? ________
10. What is 75% of 150? ________
11. Mr. Ping is prescribed an anti-infective in the amount of 500 milligrams by mouth twice a day for 10 days to treat pneumonia. He received a bottle of 20 tablets. How many tablets has Mr. Ping taken if he has used 40% of the 20 tablets? ________
12. Ms. Cho is on oral fluid restrictions of 1200 millilitres for a 24-hour period. For breakfast and lunch she has consumed 60% of the total fluid allowance. How many millilitres has she consumed? ________
13. Ms. Little's hospital bill for surgery is $17 651.07. Her insurance company pays 80%. How much will she owe? ________
14. Table salt (sodium chloride) is 40% sodium by weight. If a box of salt weighs 750 grams, how much sodium is in the box of salt? ________
15. Mr. Yoder has an average daily intake of 3500 calories. At breakfast he eats 20% of the total daily caloric allowance. How many calories did he ingest? ________

Check your work! Answers to all Review Sets are provided at the end of each chapter. Worked solutions for selected Review Sets are also available there.

PRACTICE PROBLEMS—CHAPTER 2

Find the equivalent decimal, fraction, percent, and ratio forms. Reduce fractions and ratios to their lowest terms; round decimals to two places.

	Decimal	Fraction	Percent	Ratio
1.	________	$\frac{2}{5}$	________	________
2.	0.05	________	________	________
3.	________	________	17%	________
4.	________	________	________	1:4
5.	________	________	6%	________
6.	________	$\frac{1}{6}$	________	________
7.	________	________	50%	________
8.	________	________	________	1:100
9.	0.09	________	________	________
10.	________	$\frac{3}{8}$	________	________
11.	________	________	________	2:3

12.	________	$\frac{1}{3}$	________	________
13.	0.52	________	________	________
14.	________	________	________	9:20
15.	________	$\frac{6}{7}$	________	________
16.	________	________	________	3:10
17.	________	$\frac{1}{50}$	________	________
18.	0.06	________	________	________
19.	0.04	________	________	________
20.	________	________	10%	________

Convert as indicated.

21. 1:25 to a decimal ________
22. $\frac{10}{400}$ to a ratio ________
23. 0.075 to a percent ________
24. 17:34 to a fraction ________
25. 75% to a ratio ________

Perform the indicated operation. Round decimals to hundredths.

26. What is 35% of 750? ________
27. What is 7% of 52? ________
28. What is 8.3% of 24? ________

Identify the strongest solution in each of the following:

29. 1:40 1:400 1:4 ________
30. 1:10 1:200 1:50 ________

To calculate the following, use your skills of reducing terms, multiplying and dividing fractions, and converting fractions to decimals. Express answers as decimals rounded to the nearest hundredth.

31. $1680 \times \frac{20}{400} =$ ________
32. $\frac{4}{75} \div \frac{1}{300} =$ ________
33. $\frac{3}{15} \times 5 =$ ________
34. $2.2 \times 250 \div 500 =$ ________
35. $0.6 \times \frac{200}{1.2} =$ ________
36. $11\frac{7}{9} \times 3 =$ ________
37. $\frac{1}{8} \div \frac{1}{3} \times 2 =$ ________
38. $\frac{7}{4} \times 12 =$ ________

39. $\frac{9}{0.6} \times 8 =$ ________

40. $\frac{0.4}{0.1} \times 22.5 =$ ________

41. There are 368 people employed at a hospital. If $\frac{3}{8}$ of the employees are nurses, $\frac{1}{8}$ are maintenance/cleaners, $\frac{1}{4}$ are technicians, and $\frac{1}{4}$ are all other employees, calculate the number of employees that each fraction represents. ________

42. A portion of meat totalling 125 grams contains 20% protein and 5% fat. How many grams each of protein and fat does the meat contain? ________ protein ________ fat

43. The total points for a course in a nursing program is 308. A nursing student needs to achieve 75% of the total points to pass the semester. How many points are required to pass? ________

44. To work off 90 calories, Angie must walk for 27 minutes. How many minutes would the patient need to walk to work off 200 calories? ________

45. The prescriber orders a record of a patient's fluid intake and output. The patient drinks 25% of a bowl of broth. How many millilitres of intake will be recorded if the bowl holds 200 millilitres?
____

46. The recommended daily allowance (RDA) of a particular vitamin is 60 milligrams. If a multivitamin tablet claims to provide 45% of the RDA, how many milligrams of the particular vitamin would a patient receive from the multivitamin tablet? ________

47. A patient received an intravenous medication at a rate of 6.75 milligrams per minute. After 42 minutes, how much medication has she received? ________

48. A person weighed 60 kilograms at his last health care provider's office visit. At today's visit the patient has lost 5% of his weight. How many kilograms has the patient lost?
____

49. The cost of a certain medication is expected to decrease by 17% next year. If the cost is $12.56 now, how much would you expect it to cost at this time next year? ________

50. A patient is to be started on 150 milligrams of a medication and then decreased by 10% of the original dose for each dose until he is receiving 75 milligrams. When he takes his 75-milligram dose, how many total doses will he have taken? (HINT: Be sure to count his first (150 milligrams) and last (75 milligrams) doses.) ________

Check your work! Answers to all problems are provided at the end of the book, in the Answers section. Worked solutions for some Practice Problems are also provided there.

ANSWERS TO REVIEW SETS

Review Set 2-1

1) $\frac{1}{50}$ **2)** $\frac{3}{5}$ **3)** $\frac{1}{3}$ **4)** 0.5 **5)** 0.15 **6)** 0.07 **7)** 0.24 **8)** 25% **9)** 12.5% **10)** 70% **11)** 50% **12)** $\frac{9}{20}$ **13)** $\frac{1}{200}$ **14)** $\frac{1}{100}$ **15)** $\frac{2}{3}$ **16)** 0.03 **17)** 0.33 **18)** 0.01 **19)** 4:25 **20)** 1:4 **21)** 1:2 **22)** 0.9 **23)** $\frac{200}{400}$ **24)** 0.25% **25)** 0.5

Review Set 2-2

1) 1.3 **2)** 4.75 **3)** 56 **4)** 0.43 **5)** 26.67 **6)** 15 **7)** 0.8 **8)** 2.38 **9)** 37.5 **10)** 112.5 **11)** 8 tablets **12)** 720 mL **13)** $3530.21 **14)** 300 g **15)** 700 calories

SELECTED SOLUTIONS TO REVIEW SETS

Review Set 2-1

1) $\frac{3}{150} = \frac{\cancel{3}^{1}}{\cancel{150}_{50}} = \frac{1}{50}$

3) $\frac{\cancel{0.05}^{1}}{\cancel{0.15}_{3}} = \frac{1}{3}$

5) $\frac{\frac{1}{1000}}{\frac{1}{150}} = \frac{1}{\cancel{1000}_{100}} \times \frac{\cancel{150}^{15}}{1} = \frac{15}{100} = 0.15. = 0.15$

9) $0.08{:}\ 0.64 = \frac{0.08}{0.64} = \frac{1}{8} = 0.125;$

$0.125 = \frac{125}{1000} = \frac{12.5}{100} = 12.5\%$

13) $0.5\% = \frac{0.5}{100} = 0.5 \div 100 = 0.00.5 = 0.005$

$= \frac{5}{1000} = \frac{1}{200}$

16) $2.94\% = \frac{2.94}{100} = 2.94 \div 100 = 0.02.94 = 0.029 = 0.03$

22) Convert to decimals and compare:

0.9%	= 0.009
0.9	= 0.900 (largest)
1:9	= 0.111
1:90	= 0.011

Review Set 2-2

1) $0.0025 \times 520 = 1.3$

8) $0.07 \times 34 = 2.38$

11) 0.4×20 pills = 8 tablets

13) 80% of $17 651.07 = 0.8 × $17 651.07 = $14 120.86

$17 651.07	total bill
−14 120.86	paid by insurance company
$3530.21	owed by Ms. Little

14) 0.4×750 g = 300 g

15) 0.2×3500 calories = 700 calories

REFERENCES

Kohtz, C. & Gowda, C. (2010). Teaching drug calculation in nursing education. *Nurse Educator, 35*(2), 83–86. doi:10.1097/NNE.0b013e3181ced8a8

Koohestani, H. & Baghcheghi, N. (2010). Comparing the effects of two educational methods of intravenous drug rate calculations on rapid and sustained learning of nursing students: Formula method and dimensional analysis method. *Nurse Education in Practice, 10*(4), 233–237. doi:10.1016/j.nepr.2009.11.011

Rice, J. N., & Bell, M. L. (2005). Using dimensional analysis to improve drug dosage calculation ability. *Journal of Nursing Education, 44*(7), 315–318.

CHAPTER

3

Systems of Measurement

OBJECTIVES

1. Identify the International System of Units (SI).
2. Accurately express the SI units commonly used in the health sector.
3. Accurately interpret the relationship between selected SI prefixes.
4. Recognize common equivalents between the SI and the household systems.
5. Identify and accurately express non-SI units used in the health sector.
6. Convert between traditional and international time.

Measurement systems have been developed and modified by custom and local adaptations throughout history. Three measurement systems for calculating drug dosages have been used in Canada in the past century: the household system, the apothecary system, and the most current, the International System of Units (SI). The SI system will be the focus for this chapter. Information on the apothecary and household systems will be included in the appendices.

Converting between the systems is less common now in the health sector, but there are a few instances in which this may still be necessary, such as a healthcare provider working in the community and/or giving instructions to a patient or family. On a day-to-day basis, Canadians may use a variety of measurement systems. For example, it is not uncommon to measure sugar by the teaspoon, a picture frame in inches, or buy grocery produce by the pound. Similarly, a Canadian-educated healthcare provider may choose to work in a country whose health sector uses a variety of measurement systems. Therefore, it is still relevant for Canadian healthcare providers to understand some approximate conversions between the various systems.

THE INTERNATIONAL SYSTEM OF UNITS

The decimal metric system, based on the metre and kilogram, can be historically traced to the French Revolution (1789–1799). In 1875, the Bureau International des Poids et Mesures (BIPM) was established in France. Its mandate was to provide "the basis for a single, coherent system of measurement to be used throughout the world" (BIPM, 2006, para. 1). Over time, the system evolved and, even today, continues to be refined. In 1960, after a long series of international discussions, the Système International d'Unités was established. In English, the system is known as the *International System of Units.*

It is believed that 98% of the world population uses metric units. The SI is considered the most up-to-date version of the metric system (U.S. Metric Association, 2016). The SI is coherent, logical, and simpler to use than other systems. Its globally uniform descriptions, terms, and symbols enhance international communication. These factors, plus the elimination of the need to convert between various systems, can help ensure safety in healthcare.

Although use of the metric system was legalized in Canada in 1871, it was 100 years before Canada proclaimed a Weights and Measures Act to start the process of ensuring that "all units of measurement used in Canada shall be determined on the basis of [SI]" (Government of Canada, 2016, p. 3). Ten years after this proclamation, with much discussion and planning, the health sector implemented its plan for conversion to SI. Due to government flip-flopping, customer apathy, and administrative stubbornness, Canadian metrication stumbled and stalled. Finally, in 1983, a moratorium on metrication was declared.

Today, even though a hodgepodge of SI and imperial systems is commonly used in Canada, the health sector has maintained the conversion to SI.

One of the features of the SI is the use of seven *base units* (Figure 3-1), compared with the numerous units used in other systems. Five of these units are commonly used in the health sector: length, mass, time, thermodynamic temperature, and amount of substance.

Base Quantity	Base Unit	Symbol
Length	Metre[1]	m
Mass	Kilogram	kg
Time, duration	Second	s
Thermodynamic temperature	Kelvin[2]	K
Amount of substance	Mole[3]	mol

FIGURE 3-1 SI Units Used in the Health Sector[4]

One of the advantages of SI is that it is logical. Since SI is based on the decimal system, prefixes are used to express extremely large and extremely small numbers. Multiples and submultiples commonly used in the health sector and their respective symbols and values are shown in Figure 3-2.

Prefix	Symbol	Numerical Value	Alternative Way of Expressing
kilo	k	1000	10^3
centi	c	0.01	10^{-2}
milli	m	0.001	10^{-3}
micro	mcg[5]	0.000 001	10^{-6}

FIGURE 3-2 SI Prefixes[6]

REMEMBER

Metric Conversion of Grams, Milligrams, and Micrograms
1000 micrograms (mcg) = 1 milligram (mg)
1000 milligrams (mg) = 1 gram (g)
1000 grams (g) = 1 kilogram (kg)

Even where the SI system is officially recognized as the only system of units, some non-SI units, defined in terms of SI units, are still widely used because of historical reasons or because they are deeply embedded in our culture. Two that are commonly used in the health sector are units of time and volume. See Figure 3-3.

---

[1] *Metre* and *meter* are both correct spellings. Most nations use the former, while the latter is commonly used in the United States.

[2] Note: The temperature commonly used in SI is Celsius, a derivative of the base unit, Kelvin. Celsius, Kelvin, and Fahrenheit temperature units are discussed in more detail in Appendix D.

[3] Mole is defined as the number of atoms in exactly 12 g of carbon-12 isotope. Many chemistry reports of blood tests are expressed in molar units. Drug plasma levels are reported in molar units in SI, for example, millimoles per litre (mmol/L).

[4] See Appendix A for the complete list of base units and a reference for additional information to explore the other units.

[5] The official symbol is μ (Greek lower case letter *mu*), but to avoid confusion in expressing medication dosages, *mc* (without the italics) is recommended.

[6] See Appendix A for a list of SI base units and prefixes.

Quantity	Unit	Symbol	Relation to SI
Time	Minute	min	1 min = 60 s
	Hour	h	1 h = 3600 s
	Day	d	1 d = 86 400 s
Volume	Litre[7]	L or l[8]	

FIGURE 3-3 Commonly Used Non-SI Units

RULES

The following 10 rules will help ensure correct writing and interpretation of metric notation:

1. **The unit always follows the amount; for example, 5 g *not* g 5;**
2. **No period is used after the unit abbreviation because it may be mistaken for the number 1 if written poorly; for example, do not write 20 mg.; instead, write 20 mg;**
3. **Do not add an "s" to make the unit plural because it may be misread for another unit; for example, 5 mL *not* 5 mLs;**
4. **Separate the amount from the unit so that the number and unit of measure do not run together because the unit can be mistaken as a zero or zeros, risking a 10-fold to 100-fold overdose; for example, 20 mg *not* 20mg;**
5. **Place a space for amounts with more than 4 digits; for example, 1000 units but 10 000 units *not* 10,000 units and *not* 10000 units;**
6. **Decimals are used to designate fractional amounts; for example, 1.5 mL not $1\frac{1}{2}$ mL;**
7. **Use a leading zero to emphasize the decimal point for fractional amounts less than 1; without the zero, the amount may be interpreted as a whole number, resulting in a serious overdose; for example, 0.5 mg *not* .5 mg;**
8. **Omit unnecessary or trailing zeros that can be misread as part of the amount if the decimal point is not seen; for example, 1.5 mg *not* 1.50 mg;**
9. **Do not use the abbreviation μg for microgram because it might be mistaken for mg, which is 1000 times the intended amount; for example, 150 mcg *not* 150 μg; and**
10. **Do not use the abbreviation cc for mL because the unit can be mistaken for zeros; for example, 500 mL *not* 500 cc.**

Always ask the writer for clarification if unsure about the abbreviation or notation used. Never guess.

REMEMBER

To avoid confusion,

- Always use the capitalized ***L*** to indicate litre. The lower case ***l*** is easily confused with the number one (1);
- Always use ***mcg*** to indicate microgram. The ***μ*** symbol is easily misunderstood.

CAUTION

You may see ***gram*** abbreviated as ***Gm*** or ***gm***, litre as lower case ***l***, or millilitre as ***ml***. These abbreviations should be avoided because they are too easily misinterpreted. You should only use the standardized SI symbols. Use ***g*** for gram, ***L*** for litre, and ***mL*** for millilitre.

[7] *Litre* and *liter* are both correct spellings. Most nations use the former, while the latter is used primarily in the United States.

[8] To avoid confusion with the number one (1), the symbol for the litre should be a capital L.

CAUTION

The SI symbols for milligram (*mg*) and millilitre (*mL*) appear to be similar, but in fact mg is a mass unit and mL is a volume unit. Confusing these two units can have dire consequences in dosage calculations. Learn to clearly differentiate them now.

QUICK REVIEW

In SI,

- The common units are gram, litre, metre, and mole.
- Subunits are designated by the appropriate prefix and the base unit (such as *milli*gram) and standardized symbols (such as *mg*).
- The SI symbol always follows the amount.
- Decimals are used to designate fractional amounts.
- Use a zero to emphasize the decimal point for fractional amounts of less than 1.
- Omit unnecessary zeros.
- Multiply or divide by 1000 to derive most equivalents needed for dosage calculations.
- When in doubt about the exact amount or the symbol used, do not guess. Ask the writer to clarify.

REVIEW SET 3-1

1. The system of measurement most commonly used for prescribing and administering medications is the ________ system.
2. Litre and millilitre are SI units that measure ________.
3. Gram and milligram are SI units that measure ________.
4. Metre and millimetre are SI units that measure ________.
5. 1 mg is ________ of a gram.
6. There are ________ mL in a litre.
7. 10 mL = ________ L
8. Which is largest—kilogram, gram, or milligram? ________
9. Which is smallest—kilogram, gram, or milligram? ________
10. 0.3 litre = ________ mL
11. 1000 mcg = ________ mg
12. 1 kg = ________ g
13. 1 cm = ________ mm

Select the *correct* metric notation.

14. .3 g, 0.3 Gm, 0.3 g, .3 Gm, 0.30 g ________
15. $1\frac{1}{3}$ ml, 1.33 mL, 1.33 ML, $1\frac{1}{3}$ ML, 1.330 mL ________
16. 5 Kg, 5.0 kg, kg 05, 5 kg, 5 kG ________
17. 1.5 mm, $1\frac{1}{2}$ mm, 1.5 Mm, 1.50 MM, $1\frac{1}{2}$ MM ________
18. mg 10, 10 mG, 10.0 mg, 10 mg, 10 MG ________

Interpret these SI abbreviations.

19. mcg ________
20. mL ________
21. mmol ________
22. g ________
23. mm ________
24. kg ________
25. cm ________

Check your work! Answers to all Review Sets are provided at the end of each chapter. Worked solutions for select Review Sets are also provided there.

ALTERNATIVE SYSTEMS OF MEASUREMENT

As noted in the opening of this chapter, Canadians may use a variety of measurement units on a daily basis, even though SI units are the only units used in the healthcare system. Sometimes, Canadian healthcare providers work in the community, so it is appropriate to know equivalent measurement units for common measurements that could be more familiar to the individual patient and/or family. For this purpose, the following table notes five units of volume, one unit of mass, and one unit of length with which Canadian healthcare providers working in a community context should be familiar. The values shown are approximate equivalents. See Appendices B and C (pages 533–535), respectively, for information on an alternative system of measurement called the apothecary system, and more information on the household system of measurement.

REMEMBER

Unit	SI Approximate Equivalent
1 teaspoon (tsp)	5 mL
1 tablespoon (Tbs)	15 mL
1 cup	240 mL
1 quart (qt)	1 L
1 fluid ounce (oz)	30 mL
2.2 pounds (lb or #)	1 kg
1 inch (in or ")	2.54 cm

SPECIAL CLASSES OF UNITS OF MEASUREMENT

Units and milliequivalents are measurements used to indicate the strength or potency of a drug. Neither can be directly converted into any other system of measurement.

Units describe biological effects that cannot yet be known or defined precisely in SI units. Since medications measured this way are important for human health and safety, the World Health Organization takes responsibility to define International Units for these substances. Technically, the *unit* is a measurement of standardized potency versus a mass per volume, as in the majority of medications. Insulin, hormones, vitamins, anticoagulants, and penicillin are common examples of medications measured in units. Some drugs that were once standardized by units may later be synthesized to their chemical composition but still retain units as the indicator of their potency.

Milliequivalents (mEq) compose a measurement of combining or reacting value or power versus mass per volume. Technically, the milliequivalent measures the strength of an ion concentration. It is the expression of the number of grams of a drug contained in 1 mL of a normal solution. Milliequivalents are used to measure a variety of mineral and electrolyte replacements and supplements. Potassium chloride is a common electrolyte replacement that is ordered in milliequivalents.

It is not necessary to learn conversions for the international unit, unit, or milliequivalent because medications prescribed in these measurements are also prepared and administered in the same system.

CAUTION

The abbreviations U (unit) and IU (international unit) are included in the Institute for Safe Medication Practices Canada "Do Not Use" list. Instead, the written words *unit* and *units* should be used because these abbreviations are frequently misinterpreted and often involved in harmful incidents.

Example 1:

Heparin sodium 800 units subcutaneously is prescribed. *Heparin sodium 10 000 units/10 mL (1000 units/mL)* is the available stock drug.

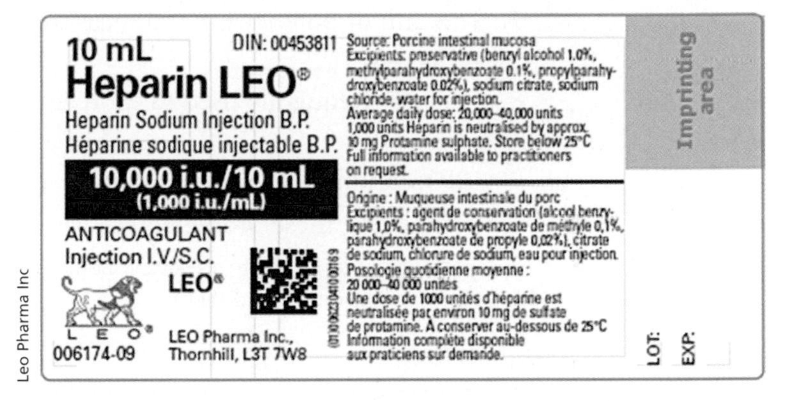

Leo Pharma Inc

Example 2:

Potassium chloride 40 mEq orally is prescribed. *Potassium chloride 20 mEq/tablet* is the stock drug.

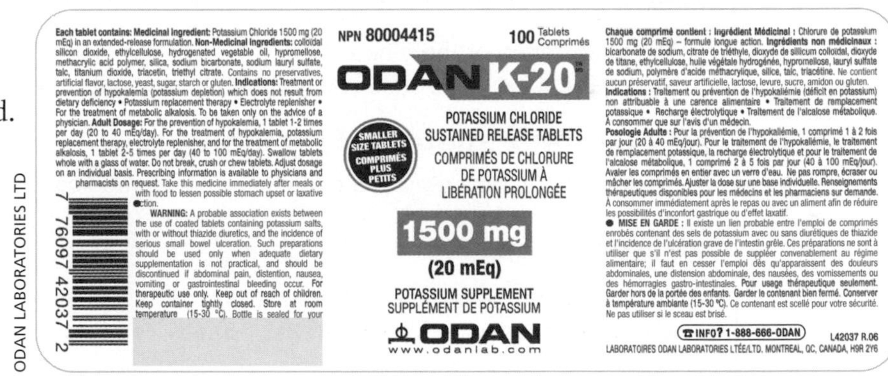

ODAN LABORATORIES LTD

Example 3:

Oxytocin 2 milliunits (0.002 units) intravenous per minute is prescribed. *Oxytocin 10 units/mL* to be added to 1000-mL intravenous solution is available.

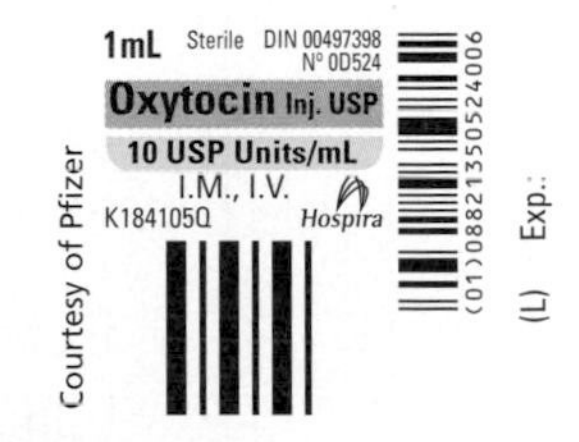

Courtesy of Pfizer

QUICK REVIEW

- Some symbols and abbreviations are obsolete or can lead to patient safety incidents. Do not use U, IU, cc, and μg.
- No conversion is necessary for units, and mEq, because the ordered dosage and supply dosage are in the same system.
- 1 unit = 1000 milliunits

REVIEW SET 3-2

Interpret the following notations.

1. 1000 units ________
2. 10 mEq ________

Express the following using correct notation.

3. 30 milliequivalents ________
4. 1500 units ________
5. The household system of measurement is commonly used in hospital dosage calculations. (True) (False)
6. Drugs such as heparin sodium and insulin are commonly measured in ________, which is abbreviated ________.
7. The unit of potency used to measure vitamins and chemicals is the ________, and is abbreviated ________.
8. The unit frequently used to express the concentration of replacement electrolytes is ________.
9. 100 milliunits = ________ units

After completing these problems, see page 70 in the answer section to check your answers.

Check your work! Answers to all Review Sets are provided at the end of each chapter. Worked solutions for select Review Sets are also provided there.

APPLICATION OF CLINICAL REASONING

The importance of the placement of the decimal point cannot be overemphasized. Now look at some examples of potential patient safety incidents related to placement of the decimal point.

Potential Patient Safety Incident 1

Not placing a zero before a decimal point on medication orders.

Possible Scenario

An emergency room physician wrote an order for the bronchodilator epinephrine for a patient with severe asthma. The order was written as follows:

epinephrine .5 mg subcutaneously now, repeat dose in 20 minutes if no improvement

Suppose the nurse, not noticing the faint decimal point, administered 5 mg of epinephrine subcutaneously instead of 0.5 mg. The patient would receive 10 times the dose intended by the physician.

Potential Outcome

Within minutes of receiving the injection, the patient would likely complain of headache and develop tachycardia, hypertension, nausea, and vomiting. The patient's hospital stay would be lengthened due to the need to recover from the overdose.

Prevention

This type of patient safety incident is avoided by remembering the rule to place a 0 in front of a decimal to avoid confusion regarding the dosage: 0.5 mg. Further, remember to question orders that are unclear or seem unreasonable.

Application of Critical Reasoning Additional application problems are provided at the end of the chapter. Answers are provided at the end of the book.

APPLICATION OF CLINICAL REASONING

Many patient safety incidents occur by confusing mg and mL. Remember that mg is the amount of the medication, and mL is the volume of the medication preparation.

Potential Patient Safety Incident 2

Confusing mg and mL.

Possible Scenario

Suppose a physician ordered morphine hydrochloride syrup (an opioid analgesic) 20 mg by mouth every 3 h for a patient with cancer. Morphine hydrochloride syrup is supplied in a concentration of 20 mg in 1 mL. The pharmacist supplied a bottle of morphine hydrochloride syrup containing a total volume of 250 mL with 20 mg of morphine hydrochloride in every mL. The nurse, in a rush to give her medications on time, misread the order as 20 mL and gave the patient 20 mL of morphine hydrochloride syrup instead of 1 mL. Therefore, the patient received 400 mg of morphine hydrochloride syrup, or 20 times the correct dosage.

Potential Outcome

The patient could develop a number of complications related to a high dosage of opiates such as respiratory depression, hypotension, hallucinations, nausea, and vomiting.

Prevention

The mg is the amount of a medication, and mL is the volume you prepare. Being rushed or distracted can result in confusing milligrams with millilitres. When distracted or stressed, have another nurse double-check the calculation of the dose.

Application of Critical Reasoning Additional application problems are provided at the end of the chapter. Answers are provided at the end of the book.

TIME AND TEMPERATURE CONVERSIONS

Converting between Traditional and International Time

Any discussion on measurement units and medications must include the unit of *time.* As noted earlier in this chapter, the SI base unit of time is the second. However, due to deeply embedded tradition, the use of non-SI units such as minute, hour, and day are still used with the SI.

Time is an important part of a medication regimen. Canada uses the 12-hour traditional clock day-to-day as do the United States and the United Kingdom. Two exceptions in Canada are individuals who speak French and in Ottawa, the national capital, where 24-hour time is commonly used. A third exception in Canada is the healthcare system. Several decades ago, Canada's healthcare system adopted the 24-hour clock as the standard for its system of time. This 24-hour clock system is also known as *international time.*

A variation of the 24-hour clock is seen in Figure 3-4. The figure uses inner and outer circles of numbers. The numbers of the inner circle correlate with traditional AM time (12:00 midnight to 11:59 AM), time periods that are *ante meridian,* or *before noon.* The numbers on the outer circle correlate with traditional PM time (12:00 noon to 11:59 PM), time periods that are *post meridian,* or *after noon.*

Use of the 24-hour clock decreases the possibility of a patient safety incident when administering medications and documenting the time of medication administration because no two times are expressed by the same number. Using the 24-hour clock decreases the risk for misinterpreting time. Two other advantages of the 24-hour clock are its computer compatibility and the greater ease of calculating the duration of time intervals.

In Canadian health institutions that display time, the time is either digitally displayed in the 24-hour clock format or as a traditional 12-hour clock with a second ring of numbers representing the hours between 1 PM (1300) and midnight (2400).

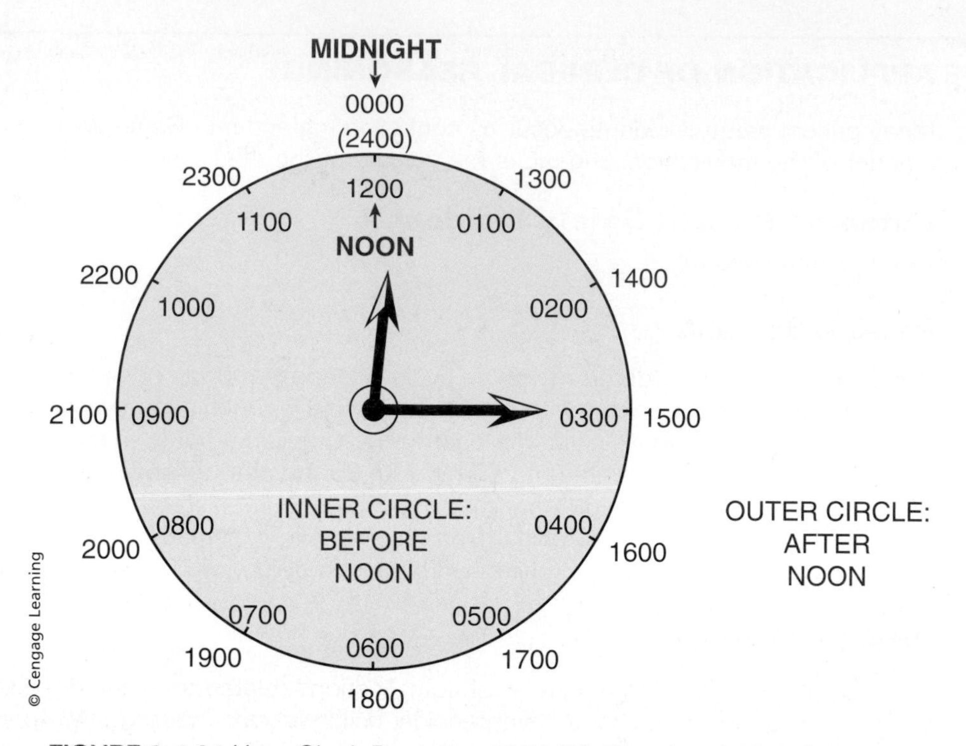

FIGURE 3-4 24-Hour Clock Depicting 0015 (12:15 AM) and 1215 (12:15 PM)

All 24-hour clock times are expressed sequentially with 4 digits without colons and without AM and PM labels. The system starts at midnight. The first 2 digits express the number of hours since midnight. Midnight can be expressed as 2400 or as 0000. It is most frequently written as 2400, but each minute after midnight is written as if midnight were 0000.

RULES

- **For the minutes between 2400 (midnight) and 0100 (1 AM), state each zero before the number of minutes but label it hours.**
- **For hours after 0059, state the number in *hundreds* if the minutes are zero.**
- **For single-digit hours, state the word *zero* before the hours.**
- **To indicate minutes and hours, state the hour (preceded by the *zero* if the hours is single digit) and number of minutes.**

Examples:

0001 (1 minute after midnight) is read "zero zero zero one hour"

0014 (14 minutes after midnight) is read "zero zero fourteen hours"

0100 (1 AM) is read "zero one hundred hours"

0630 (6:30 AM) is read "zero six thirty hours"

1400 (2 PM) is read "fourteen hundred hours"

1840 (6:40 PM) is read "eighteen forty hours"

AM	International Time	PM	International Time
12:00 midnight	2400	12:00 noon	1200
1:00	0100	1:00	1300
2:00	0200	2:00	1400
3:00	0300	3:00	1500
4:00	0400	4:00	1600
5:00	0500	5:00	1700
6:00	0600	6:00	1800
7:00	0700	7:00	1900
8:00	0800	8:00	2000
9:00	0900	9:00	2100
10:00	1000	10:00	2200
11:00	1100	11:00	2300

FIGURE 3-5 Comparison of Traditional and International Time

RULES

1. **International time is designated by a unique 4-digit number.**
2. **No colon is typically used in international time. However, you may see international time represented with a colon, for example, 13:00 for 1300 (for 1:00 PM).**
3. **Minutes after 12:00 AM (midnight) and before 1:00 AM are 0001 through 0059 in international time.**
4. **Traditional time and international time are the same hours starting with 1:00 AM (0100) through 12:59 PM (1259).**
5. **Hours starting with 1:00 PM through 12:00 AM (midnight) are 12:00 hours greater in international time (1300 through 2400).**

MATH TIP

For the hours between 1:00 PM (1300) and 12:00 AM (2400), add 1200 to the traditional time to find the equivalent international time; subtract 1200 from the international time to convert to the equivalent traditional time.

Now apply these rules to convert between the two time systems.

Example 1:

3:00 PM = 3:00 + 12:00 = 1500

Example 2:

2212 = 2212 – 1200 = 10:12 PM

Example 3:

12:45 AM = 0045

Example 4:

0004 = 12:04 AM

Example 5:

0130 = 1:30 AM

Example 6:

11:00 AM = 1100

QUICK REVIEW

- The hours from 1:00 PM through 12:00 midnight are 12:00 hours greater in international time (1300 through 2400).

APPLICATION OF CLINICAL REASONING

Potential Patient Safety Incident

Incorrect interpretation of order due to misunderstanding of traditional time.

Possible Scenario

A physician prescribed a mild sedative for a patient who is anxious and is scheduled for a sigmoidoscopy in the morning. The order read *diazepam 5 mg orally at 6:00 × 1 dose*. The evening nurse might have assumed that the physician intended this medication to reduce the patient's anxiety and aid him in sleeping the night before the procedure. However, the nurse knew that sleeping aids are usually administered at bedtime, not at the time of evening preparations. The nurse used clinical reasoning and contacted the physician to clarify the order. The physician said she meant for the diazepam to be given at 6 o'clock AM to help the patient relax prior to the actual test.

Potential Outcome

Diazepam would help the patient relax during the sigmoidoscopy and make him drowsy. It is not desirable for the patient to be drowsy or sedated during the evening preparations. Because of the omission of the AM designation, the patient would lose any benefit from the sedative at the intended time if the medication had been administered the evening before the test. The patient would have likely experienced unnecessary anxiety both before and during the test.

Prevention

This scenario emphasizes the benefit of the 24-hour clock. If international time had been in use at this facility, the order would have been written as *diazepam 5 mg orally at 0600 × 1 dose*, clearly indicating the exact time of administration, reducing the risk of a patient safety incident.

Application of Critical Reasoning Additional application problems are provided at the end of the chapter. Answers are provided at the end of the book.

REVIEW SET 3-3

Convert the following time equivalents as indicated.

Traditional Time	International Time	Traditional Time	International Time
1. ________	0257	8. ________	1642
2. 3:10 AM	________	9. ________	2356
3. 4:22 PM	________	10. 4:20 AM	________
4. ________	2001	11. 7:31 PM	________
5. ________	1102	12. 12:00 midnight	________
6. 12:33 AM	________	13. 6:45 AM	________
7. 2:16 AM	________	14. ________	0915

15. ________ 2107
16. ________ 1823
17. ________ 0540
18. 11:55 AM ________
19. 10:12 PM ________
20. 9:06 PM ________

Fill in the blanks by writing out the words as indicated.

21. 24-hour time 0623 is stated "________________________________."
22. 24-hour time 0041 is stated "________________________________."
23. 24-hour time 1903 is stated "________________________________."
24. 24-hour time 2311 is stated "________________________________."

Determine the length of each time interval for questions 25 through 33.

25. 0200 to 0600 ________
26. 1100 to 1800 ________
27. 1500 to 2330 ________
28. 0935 to 2150 ________
29. 0003 to 1453 ________
30. 2316 to 0328 ________
31. 8:22 AM to 1:10 PM ________
32. 4:35 PM to 8:16 PM ________
33. 10:05 AM Friday to 2:43 AM Saturday ________

34. The 24-hour clock is imprecise and not suited to healthcare. (True) (False)
35. Indicate whether these international times would be AM or PM when converted to traditional time.
    a. 1030 ________
    b. 1920 ________
    c. 0158 ________
    d. 1230 ________

After completing these problems, see page 70 in the answer section to check your answers.

Check your work! Answers to all Review Sets are provided at the end of each chapter. Worked solutions for select Review Sets are also provided there.

Measurement of Temperature: Converting between the Fahrenheit and Celsius Scales

In Canada, most individuals are familiar with the Celsius scale on a day-to-day basis, as well as in the healthcare setting. Therefore, converting between the Fahrenheit and Celsius scales is considered an academic exercise that does not have to be learned as an additional competency.

For information about these scales and formulas for conversion, please refer to Appendix D, pages 536–538.

PRACTICE PROBLEMS—CHAPTER 3

Give the SI prefix for the following numbers.

1. 0.001 ________
2. 0.000001 ________
3. 0.01 ________
4. 1000 ________

Identify the equivalent unit with a value of 1 that is indicated by the following amounts (e.g., 1000 microunit = 1 unit).

5. 0.001 gram ________
6. 1000 grams ________
7. 0.001 milligram ________
8. 0.01 metre ________

Identify the SI base unit for the following.

9. length ________
10. mass ________
11. volume ________

Interpret the following notations.

12. mg ________
13. mcg ________
14. unit ________
15. mEq ________
16. mL ________
17. km ________
18. mm ________
19. g ________
20. cm ________
21. L ________
22. m ________
23. kg ________
24. mmol ________

Express the following amounts in SI notation.

25. five hundred milligrams ________
26. one-half litre ________
27. five hundredths of a milligram ________

Express the following numeric amounts in words.

28. 375 units ________
29. 2.6 mL ________
30. 20 mEq ________
31. 0.4 L ________
32. 0.17 mg ________
33. If an individual drank 0.25 L, how many mL have been consumed? ________
34. How many mg are in a medication that contains 150 mcg? ________
35. A baby weighs 1.5 kg. What is the equivalent weight in grams? ________
36. A patient is prescribed 0.1 g of a medication. What is the equivalent dose in milligrams? ________
37. A scar measures 15 mm. What is the equivalent length in centimetres? ________
38. A patient is ordered 0.2 mg of a medication. What is the equivalent dose in micrograms? ________
39. How many mL are in a half litre? ________
40. How many g are in 256 000 mcg? ________
41. A patient is prescribed 0.15 g of a medication. What is the equivalent dose in milligrams? ________

Convert the following traditional times to international times.

42. 1:30 PM
43. 12:04 AM
44. 12:00 midnight
45. 6:20 AM

Write out the words to express the following times.

46. 0041 ________

47. 1115 ________

48. 0623 ________

Check your work! Answers to all problems are provided at the end of the book, in the Answers section. Worked solutions for some Practice Problems are also provided there.

APPLICATION OF CLINICAL REASONING

3-1. Describe the clinical reasoning that would prevent a patient safety incident in the following scenario.

Possible Scenario

Suppose a physician prescribed oral warfarin sodium (an anticoagulant) for a patient with a history of phlebitis. The physician wrote an order for 1 mg, but while writing the order placed a decimal point after the 1 and added a 0:

warfarin sodium 1.0 mg orally once per day

Warfarin sodium 1.0 mg was transcribed on the medication record as warfarin sodium 10 mg. The patient received 10 times the correct dosage.

Potential Outcome

The patient could possibly hemorrhage, requiring the antidote, vitamin K, to reverse the effects of the overdose. Remember that not all drugs have antidotes.

Prevention

____

____

3-2. Describe the clinical reasoning that would prevent a patient safety incident or the need to notify the prescribing practitioner.

Possible Scenario

Suppose a physician prescribed oral codeine sulfate (an opioid analgesic) for an adult patient recovering from extensive nasal surgery. The physician wrote the following order for 60 mg of oral solution.

Codeine sulfate solution 60 mg orally every four hours as needed for pain

The surgical unit stocks codeine sulfate solution in two strengths: 10 mg/5 mL and 15 mg/5 mL. The nurse chose the 10 mg/5 mL, confused the mg and mL in calculating, and calculated that the patient needed 12 mL. The nurse was in a rush to help ease the patient's pain yet felt uneasy about the total volume of medication in his original calculation. It seemed that 12 mL of an oral solution usually used for children was a smaller amount than seemed normal. Following the unit's policy of double-checking medication calculations when a stock supply of high-alert medication was being used, a colleague calculated the dosage as 30 mL. They compared their calculation differences, looked back at the original order, and reread the stock medicine label.

Potential Outcome

Because the nurse chose the 10 mg/5 mL strength, the nurse needs 6 times the 5 mL to give the 60 mg ordered (10 mg × 6 = 60 mg). The nurse needs to administer 30 mL (5 mL × 6 = 30 mL) of this medication. Otherwise, the patient will receive only 20% ($\frac{1}{5}$) of the intended amount. The nurse correctly felt uneasy about the amount and followed the surgical unit's protocol, thus avoiding under-medicating his patient for postoperative pain.

Prevention

Check your work! Answers to all Application for Clinical Reasoning problems are provided at the end of the book, in the Answers section.

ANSWERS TO REVIEW SETS

Review Set 3-1

1) metric **2)** volume **3)** weight **4)** length **5)** $\frac{1}{1000}$ or 0.001 **6)** 1000 **7)** 0.01 **8)** kilogram **9)** milligram **10)** 300 **11)** 1 **12)** 1000 **13)** 10 **14)** 0.3 g **15)** 1.33 mL **16)** 5 kg **17)** 1.5 mm **18)** 10 mg **19)** microgram **20)** millilitre **21)** millimole **22)** gram **23)** millimetre **24)** kilogram **25)** centimetre

Review Set 3-2

1) one thousand units **2)** 10 milliequivalents **3)** 30 mEq **4)** 1500 units **5)** False **6)** units, official abbreviation is "u," but its use is *not* recommended; recommended to be written as "units" to reduce errors **7)** international unit, official abbreviation is "IU," but its use is *not* recommended; recommended to be written as "units" to reduce errors **8)** milliequivalents **9)** 0.1

Review Set 3-3

1) 2:57 AM **2)** 0310 **3)** 1622 **4)** 8:01 PM **5)** 11:02 AM **6)** 0033 **7)** 0216 **8)** 4:42 PM **9)** 11:56 PM **10)** 0420 **11)** 1931 **12)** 2400 or 0000 **13)** 0645 **14)** 9:15 AM **15)** 9:07 PM **16)** 6:23 PM **17)** 5:40 AM **18)** 1155 **19)** 2212 **20)** 2106 **21)** "zero-six-twenty-three hours" **22)** "zero-zero-forty-one hours" **23)** "nineteen-zero-three hours" **24)** "twenty-three-eleven hours" **25)** 4 h **26)** 7 h **27)** 8 h 30 min **28)** 12 h 15 min **29)** 14 h 50 min **30)** 4 h 12 min **31)** 4 h 48 min **32)** 3 h 41 min **33)** 16 h 38 min **34)** False **35)** a. AM; b. PM; c. AM; d. PM

SELECTED SOLUTIONS TO REVIEW SETS

Review Set 3-3

28)

$$\begin{array}{r} 2150 \\ -\ 0935 \\ \hline 1215 \end{array} = 12\text{ h }15\text{ min}$$

30) 2316 = 11:16 PM, 0328 = 3:28 AM

11:16 PM → 3:16 AM = 4 h

3:16 AM → 3:28 AM = $\begin{array}{r} 12\text{ min} \\ \hline 4\text{ h }12\text{ min} \end{array}$

32) 4:35 PM → 7:35 PM = 3 h

7:35 PM → 8:16 PM = $\begin{array}{r} 41\text{ min} \\ \hline 3\text{ h }41\text{ min} \end{array}$

REFERENCES

Bureau International des Poids et Mesures (BIPM). (2006). *A concise summary of the International System of Units, the SI*. Retrieved from www.bipm.org/utils/common/pdf/si_summary_en.pdf

Government of Canada. (2016). Weights and Measures Act, R.S.C. 1985. Retrieved from http://laws-lois.justice.gc.ca/PDF/W-6.pdf

Institute for Safe Medication Practices Canada. (2010). ISMP's list of error-prone abbreviations, symbols, and dose designations. Retrieved from www.ismp-canada.org/download/ISMPCanadaListOfDangerousAbbreviations.pdf

United States Metric Association (USMA). (2016). Metric usage and metrication in other countries. Retrieved from www.us-metric.org/metrication-in-other-countries/

CHAPTER

4

Calculation Methods Used in Determining Drug Dosages

OBJECTIVES

1. Apply the dimensional analysis method to solve simple calculation problems.
2. Apply the formula method to solve simple calculation problems.
3. Apply the ratio and proportion method to solve simple calculation problems.
4. Select a method for solving drug dosage problems.

Healthcare providers use different methods to safely calculate medication dosages. The focus of this chapter is on the *dimensional analysis method*. A second method, called the *formula method*, is also introduced in this chapter. The formula method will be applied in Chapter 8 in various calculations. Selecting the method that works the best is an individual choice.

It is important to mention a third method of medication calculation here, the *ratio and proportion method*, as noted in Chapter 2.[1] This method is admittedly useful in many simple medication calculations. However, researchers have reported that students who use the ratio and proportion method for calculating medication dosages are more prone to calculation errors than those who use dimensional analysis. In more complicated calculation problems, it is necessary to complete a series of ratio and proportion calculations to calculate the required medication dosage. In response to this mounting evidence, the emphasis placed on the ratio and proportion method has been reduced.

In summary, according to research, there is a significantly better sustained learning rate among nursing students taught dimensional analysis when compared with those taught the formula method of medication calculation (Koohestani & Baghcheghi, 2010). In earlier research, Rice and Bell (2005) found evidence of the value of teaching dimensional analysis to increase the confidence and accuracy of medication calculation ability among nursing students. Although Kohtz and Gowda (2010) did not find a "significant" difference, they did find that students who used dimensional analysis made fewer mistakes than students who used other methods, even though both groups used calculators.

METHOD 1: DIMENSIONAL ANALYSIS

Dimensional analysis is a centuries-old calculation method known as *units conversion*. It is the method most commonly used in the physical sciences. This method is also known by a variety of other names: *factor labelling, factor analysis,* the *unit factor method,* the *label-factor method,* the *scientific method,* and the *conversion factor method. Dimension* refers to a unit of mass, volume, length, time, and so on. Examples are milligram (mg), litre (L), metre (m), and minute (min).

Dimensional analysis is a practical approach to drug calculations. It is a fast, simple, and organized system for setting up problems. It can be used for all medication problems. Dimensional

[1] See references listed in the Caution box in Chapter 2, page 46.

analysis helps prevent patient safety incidents by allowing you to visualize all parts of the medication problem and to critically think through a problem. It also eliminates the need to memorize formulas because one easy-to-solve equation is needed to determine each answer.

Being able to correctly convert from one unit of measurement to another is a strength of dimensional analysis. This skill is frequently needed in calculating medication dosages when a medication is ordered in one unit but available only in a different unit. In the two examples below, the calculation problem of such conversions is built step by step using dimensional analysis. It is important to master the steps so they can be applied in a variety of medication calculation situations.

Example 1:

Available: 700 mL of liquid
Need to know: how many litres equals 700 mL

Step 1 Establish the "unit path" from the given quantity to the wanted quantity using equivalents as "conversion factors." Make sure that the unit of the desired quantity is in the numerator of either the given quantity or in the unit path.

Remember the information in Chapter 3 about the metric system and SI units: 1 L = 1000 mL. Therefore, when including this information in the problem, the numerator and the denominator are being multiplied by the same value; thus, the value of the equation does not change.

$$700 \text{ mL} \times \frac{1 \text{ L}}{1000 \text{ mL}}$$

Step 2 Cancel terms. In both the numerator and denominator, the unit millilitre (mL) can be cancelled, leaving only the litre (L), which is the desired unit for the answer. This equation is set up correctly to calculate the answer in litres (L).

$$700 \cancel{\text{mL}} \times \frac{1 \text{ L}}{1000 \cancel{\text{mL}}} = 700 \times \frac{1 \text{ L}}{1000}$$

Step 3 Reduce the fraction to its lowest terms. (Divide both the numerator and the denominator by 100.) Multiply the numerators and the denominators (7 × 1L, and 10, respectively). Divide the numerator by the denominator. (Remember how to divide by the power of 10—move the decimal point one place to the left for every power of 10.) Insert zero before the decimal point to emphasize that the quantity is less than 1.

$$\overset{7}{\cancel{700}} \times \frac{1 \text{ L}}{\underset{10}{\cancel{1000}}} = \frac{7 \text{ L}}{\cancel{10}} = .7 \text{ mL} = 0.7 \text{ mL}$$

Therefore, 700 mL = 0.7 L

MATH TIP

When setting up a problem, be sure to always include the units. Carry out the calculations and add the appropriate units to the answer as well. The units that are in the numerator stay above the line, and the units in the denominator stay below the line.

Example 2:

Need to know: how many milligrams (mg) are in 6 grams (g). Use the following format to set up the problem, using the steps discussed above:

Step 1 Establish the "unit path" from the given quantity to the wanted quantity using equivalents as "conversion factors": 1 g = 1000 mg. Make sure that the unit of the desired quantity is in the numerator of either the given quantity or in the unit path.

$$6\text{ g} \times \frac{1000\text{ mg}}{1\text{ g}}$$

Step 2 Cancel terms. In both the numerator and denominator, the unit gram (g) can be cancelled, leaving only the milligram (mg), which is the desired unit for the answer. This equation is set up correctly to calculate the answer in milligrams (mg).

$$6\,\cancel{\text{g}} \times \frac{1000\text{ mg}}{1\,\cancel{\text{g}}}$$

The grams (g) are cancelled in the numerator and denominator. What remains is already reduced to its lowest terms. **Note:** Only milligrams (mg) remain in the answer, which is the desired unit for the answer.

Step 3 Multiply the numerators and denominator, and divide the product of the numerator by the product of the denominator.

$$6\,\cancel{\text{g}} \times \frac{1000\text{ mg}}{1\,\cancel{\text{g}}} = \frac{6000\text{ mg}}{1} = 6000\text{ mg}$$

In this case, the denominator is 1, so the final division result is 6000 mg.

Therefore, 6 g = 6000 mg

RULES

1. **Identify the *desired answer* unit and write it to the left of the equal sign.**
2. **Identify the *given quantity* in the problem and the *desired quantity*, and write them to the right of the equal sign so that the desired quantity is a numerator and the given quantity is written to allow cancellation of units.**
3. **Establish the *unit path* from the given quantity to the wanted quantity using equivalents as "conversion factors." Make sure that the unit of the desired quantity is in the numerator of either the given quantity or in the unit path.**
4. **Carefully check each conversion factor and ensure that it is correctly placed in the numerator or denominator portion of the problem to allow the unwanted units to be cancelled from the problem.**
5. **Cancel the terms as per fraction multiplication described in Chapter 1. The remaining unit(s) should match the unit(s) on the left of the equal sign and be the unit(s) desired. If all the units except the answer unit(s) are not eliminated, recheck the equation.**
6. **Reduce the fractions to their lowest terms; multiply the numerators and denominators; and divide the denominator into the numerator to provide the numerical value of the wanted quantity.**

MATH TIP

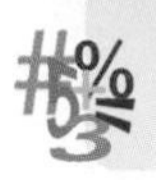

Units can be cancelled the same as numbers and letters in arithmetic and algebra.

MATH TIP

Incorrect placement of units of measurement can result in an incorrect answer. Even when calculating with dimensional analysis, thinking and reasoning are essential.

REVIEW SET 4-1

Use the dimensional analysis method to convert each of the following to the equivalent indicated.

1. 500 mL = ________ L
2. 0.015 g = ________ mg
3. 8 mg = ________ g
4. 10 mg = ________ g
5. 60 mg = ________ g
6. 300 mg = ________ g
7. 0.2 mg = ________ g
8. 1.2 g = ________ mg
9. 0.0025 kg = ________ g
10. 0.065 g = ________ mg
11. 0.005 L = ________ mL
12. 1.5 L = ________ mL
13. 250 mL = ________ L
14. 2 kg = ________ g
15. 5000 mL = ________ L
16. 1 L = ________ mL
17. 1 g = ________ mg
18. 1 mL = ________ L
19. 23 mcg = ________ mg
20. 1.05 g = ________ kg
21. 18 mcg = ________ mg
22. 0.4 mg = ________ mcg
23. 25 g = ________ kg
24. 50 cm = ________ m
25. 10 L = ________ mL

Check your work! Answers to all Review Sets are provided at the end of each chapter. Worked solutions for selected Review Sets are also provided there.

The dimensional analysis method requires three elements: given quantity, desired quantity, and unit path, using equivalent "conversion factors" when necessary to convert from one unit to another. When setting up the calculation problem, set up the conversion factors to permit cancellation of unwanted units. Carefully choose each conversion factor, and ensure that it is correctly placed in the numerator and denominator portion of the problem to allow the unwanted units to be cancelled from the problem. Finally, cancel the units and reduce the numbers to their lowest terms as you learned in Chapter 1, then multiply the numerators, multiply the denominators, and divide the product of the numerators by the product of the denominators to provide the numerical value of the wanted quantity.

CAUTION

Starting the calculation incorrectly will not allow elimination of the undesired units. Knowing when the equation is set up correctly is an essential part of the dimensional analysis method.

...HOD 2: FORMULA

The formula method is a commonly used method for calculating drug dosages.

$$\frac{D}{H} \times Q = \text{Amount to give}$$

D or *desired* dose: drug dose prescribed
H or *have* dose: drug dose available
Q or *quantity:* form and amount in which the drug comes

Example 1:

Prescribed: 500 mg of drug A

Dosage available: 250 mg of drug A in 1 tablet

Use the formula method to calculate the amount of drug A to administer.

$$\frac{\overset{2}{\cancel{500}}\ \cancel{mg}}{\underset{1}{\cancel{250}}\ \cancel{mg}} \times 1 \text{ tablet} = 2 \text{ tablets of drug A}$$

Example 2:

Prescribed: 80 mg of drug B

Dosage available: 100 mg of drug B in 2 mL

Use the formula method to calculate the amount of drug B to administer.

$$\frac{8\cancel{0}\ \cancel{mg}}{\underset{5}{\cancel{10}\cancel{0}}\ \cancel{mg}} \times \cancel{2}\text{ mL} = \frac{8}{5}\text{ mL} = 1.6 \text{ mL}$$

MATH TIP

When putting numbers into a formula, it is important to also include the units. Carry out the calculations and add the appropriate units to the answer as well. The units that are in the numerator stay above the line, and those in the denominator stay below the line.

RULES

To calculate a drug dosage using the formula method,

1. **Memorize the formula, or verify the formula from a resource.**
2. **Place the information from the problem into the formula in the correct position, with all terms in the formula labelled correctly.**
3. **Make sure all measurements are in the same units and systems of measurement, or a conversion must be done *before* calculating the formula.**
4. **Think logically and consider what a reasonable amount to administer would be.**
5. **Calculate the answer.**
6. **Label all answers with the correct units.**
7. **Double-check the math of the calculation.**

REVIEW SET 4-2

Use the formula method to calculate the quantity of drug to administer in the following:

1. A dosage of 0.8 g has been prescribed. The strength available is 1 g in 2.5 mL. ______
2. A dosage strength of 250 mg in 1.5 mL is available. The prescription is for 200 mg. ______
3. The strength available is 1 g in 5 mL. The prescription is for 0.2 g. ______
4. A dosage of 300 mcg is prescribed. The strength available is 500 mcg in 1.2 mL. ______
5. A dosage strength of 1000 units per 1.5 mL is available. Prepare a 1250 unit dose. ______
6. The intravenous solution available has a strength of 200 mEq per 20 mL. Prepare a 50-mEq dosage. ______
7. A dosage of 0.2 mg per 2 mL is available. Prepare a 0.25-mg dosage. ______

Check your work! Answers to all Review Sets are provided at the end of each chapter. Worked solutions for selected Review Sets are also provided there.

If help is required, review the decimal section in Chapter 1 and the SI section in Chapter 3 again for conversions within the SI. Ask for assistance before proceeding further.

METHOD 3: RATIO AND PROPORTION

Ratio and proportion is another method of calculating dosages prescribed by healthcare providers. This method is useful in simple medication calculations. In more complicated calculation providers, a series of ratio and proportion calculations becomes necessary to calculate the required medication dosage.

As noted in Chapter 2, a *ratio* is the numerical relationship between two quantities. When two equal ratios are expressed as an equation, they are said to be a *proportion.*

RULE

In a proportion, the product of the *means* (the two inside numbers) equals the product of the *extremes* (the two outside numbers). Finding the product of the means and the extremes is called *cross-multiplying*.

Example:

Extremes

5:10 = 10:20

Means

$5 \times 20 = 10 \times 10$

$100 = 100$

Because ratios are the same as fractions, the same proportion can be expressed like this: $\frac{5}{10} = \frac{10}{20}$. The fractions are *equivalent,* or equal. The numerator of the first fraction and the denominator of the second fraction are the extremes, and the denominator of the first fraction and the numerator of the second fraction are the means.

Example:

Extreme $\frac{5}{10}$ ⤫ $\frac{10}{20}$ Mean
Mean Extreme

Cross-multiply to find the equal products of the means and extremes.

RULE

If two fractions are *equivalent*, or equal, their cross-products are also equal.

Example:

$\frac{5}{10}$ ⤫ $\frac{10}{20}$

$5 \times 20 = 10 \times 10$

$100 = 100$

When one of the quantities in a proportion is unknown, a letter, such as "X," may be substituted for this unknown quantity. Solve the equation to find the value of "X." In addition to cross-multiplying, there is one more rule to know to solve for "X" in a proportion.

RULE

Dividing or multiplying each side (*member*) of an equation by the same nonzero number produces an equivalent equation.

MATH TIP

Dividing each side of an equation by the same nonzero number is the same as reducing or simplifying the equation. Multiplying each side by the same nonzero number enlarges the equation.

Now examine how to simplify an equation.

Example:

$25X = 100$ (25X means $25 \times X$)

Simplify the equation to find "X." Divide both sides by 25, the number before "X." Reduce to lowest terms.

$$\frac{\overset{1}{\cancel{25}}X}{\underset{1}{\cancel{25}}} = \frac{\overset{4}{\cancel{100}}}{\underset{1}{\cancel{25}}}$$

$\frac{1X}{1} = \frac{4}{1}$ (Dividing or multiplying a number by 1 does not change its value. "1X" is understood to be simply "X.")

$X = 4$

Replace "X" with 4 in the same equation, and you can prove that the calculations are correct.

$25 \times \mathbf{4} = 100$

Now you are ready to apply the concepts of cross-multiplying and simplifying an equation to solve for "X" in a proportion.

Example 1:

$$\frac{90}{2} = \frac{45}{X}$$

You have a proportion with an unknown quantity "X" in the denominator of the second fraction. Find the value of "X."

1. Cross-multiply: $\frac{90}{2} \times \frac{45}{X}$
2. Multiply terms: $90 \times X = 2 \times 45$

   $90X = 90$ (90X means $90 \times X$)
3. Simplify the equation: Divide both sides of the equation by the number before the unknown "X." The terms are being reduced on both sides of the equation.

   $$\frac{\overset{1}{\cancel{90}}X}{\underset{1}{\cancel{90}}} = \frac{\overset{1}{\cancel{90}}}{\underset{1}{\cancel{90}}}$$

   $X = 1$

Try another one. The unknown "X" is a different term.

Example 2:

$$\frac{80}{X} \times 60 = 20$$

1. Convert: Express 60 as a fraction.

   $$\frac{80}{X} \times \frac{60}{1} = 20$$
2. Multiply fractions: $\frac{80}{X} \times \frac{60}{1} = 20$

   $$\frac{4800}{X} = 20$$
3. Convert: Express 20 as a fraction.

   $$\frac{4800}{X} = \frac{20}{1}$$

   This is now a proportion.

4. Cross-multiply: $\frac{4800}{X} \times \frac{20}{1}$

$20X = 4800$

5. Simplify: Divide both sides of the equation by the number before the unknown "X."

$$\frac{\overset{1}{\cancel{20}}X}{\underset{1}{\cancel{20}}} = \frac{\overset{240}{\cancel{4800}}}{\underset{1}{\cancel{20}}}$$

$X = 240$

Example 3:

$$\frac{X}{160} = \frac{2.5}{80}$$

1. Cross-multiply: $\frac{X}{160} \times \frac{2.5}{80}$

$80 \times X = 2.5 \times 160$

$80X = 400$

2. Simplify: $\frac{\overset{1}{\cancel{80}}X}{\underset{1}{\cancel{80}}} = \frac{\overset{5}{\cancel{400}}}{\underset{1}{\cancel{80}}}$

$X = 5$

Example 4:

$$\frac{40}{100} = \frac{X}{2}$$

1. Cross-multiply: $\frac{40}{100} \times \frac{X}{2}$

2. Multiply terms: $100 \times X = 40 \times 2$

$100X = 80$

3. Simplify the equation: $\frac{\overset{1}{\cancel{100}}X}{\underset{1}{\cancel{100}}} = \frac{8\cancel{0}}{10\cancel{0}}$

$X = 0.8$

Calculations that result in an amount less than 1 should be expressed as a decimal. Most medications are ordered and supplied in SI units, and SI is a decimal-based system.

QUICK REVIEW

- A *proportion* is an equation of two equal ratios. The ratios may be expressed as fractions.

  Example: $1:4 = X:8$ or $\frac{1}{4} = \frac{X}{8}$

- In a proportion, the product of the means equals the product of the extremes.

  Example: $1:4 = X:8$ (Extremes: 1 and 8; Means: 4 and X) Therefore, $4 \times X = 1 \times 8$

- If two fractions are equal, their cross-products are equal. This operation is called *cross-multiplying*.

  Example: $\frac{1}{4} \times \frac{X}{8}$ Therefore, $4 \times X = 1 \times 8$, or $4X = 8$

- Dividing each side of an equation by the same number produces an equivalent equation. This operation is called *simplifying the equation*.

  Example: If $4X = 8$, then $\frac{4X}{4} = \frac{8}{4}$, and $X = 2$

REVIEW SET 4-3

Find the value of "X." Express answers as decimals rounded to two places.

1. $\frac{1000}{2} = \frac{125}{X}$ ______
2. $\frac{0.5}{2} = \frac{250}{X}$ ______
3. $\frac{75}{1.5} = \frac{35}{X}$ ______
4. $\frac{1200}{X} \times 12 = 28$ ______
5. $\frac{250}{1} = \frac{750}{X}$ ______
6. $\frac{80}{5} = \frac{10}{X}$ ______
7. $\frac{5}{20} = \frac{X}{40}$ ______
8. $\frac{\frac{1}{100}}{1} = \frac{\frac{1}{150}}{X}$ ______
9. $\frac{2.2}{X} = \frac{8.8}{5}$ ______
10. $\frac{60}{10} = \frac{100}{X}$ ______
11. $\frac{X}{0.5} = \frac{6}{4}$ ______
12. $\frac{25\%}{30\%} = \frac{5}{X}$ ______
13. In any group of 100 nurses, you would expect to find 45 nurses who will specialize in a particular field of nursing. In a class of 240 graduating nurses, how many would you expect to specialize? ______
14. If a patient receives 450 mg of a medication given evenly over 5.5 h, how many milligrams did the patient receive per hour? ______
15. How much salt should be added to 500 mL of water to make a solution that contains 5 g of salt for every 250 mL? ______

Check your work! Answers to all Review Sets are provided at the end of each chapter. Worked solutions for selected Review Sets are also provided there.

Each ratio in a proportion must have the same relationship and follow the same sequence. A proportion compares like things to like things. Be sure the units in the numerators match and the units in the denominators match. Label the units in each ratio.

Example:

How many grams are equivalent to 3.5 kg?

The first ratio of the proportion contains the *known equivalent,* for example, 1 kg : 1000 g. The second ratio contains the *desired unit of measure* and the *unknown equivalent* expressed as "X," for example, 3.5 kg : X g. This proportion in fractional form looks like this:

$$\frac{1 \text{ kg}}{1000 \text{ g}} = \frac{3.5 \text{ kg}}{\text{X g}}$$

CAUTION

Notice that the ratios follow the same sequence. *THIS IS ESSENTIAL.* The proportion is set up so that like units are across from each other. In the above equation, the units in the numerators match (kg), and the units in the denominators match (g).

Cross-multiply to solve the proportion for "X."

$$\frac{1 \text{ kg}}{1000 \text{ g}} \times \frac{3.5 \text{ kg}}{\text{X g}}$$

$\text{X} = 3.5 \times 1000 = 3500 \text{ g}$

The answer is in grams because grams is the unknown equivalent.

$3.5 \text{ kg} = 3500 \text{ g}$

QUICK REVIEW

To use the ratio and proportion method to convert from one unit to another or between systems of measurement,

- Recall the equivalent;
- Set up a proportion: Ratio for known equivalent equals ratio for unknown equivalent;
- Label the units and match the units in the numerators and denominators; and
- Cross-multiply to find the value of the unknown "X" equivalent.

REVIEW SET 4-4

Use the ratio and proportion method to calculate the amount to prepare for each of the following questions.

1. Prescription: 0.2 g of a drug

   Stock dosage: 100 mg/tablet

   How many tablets should be given in one dose? ________

2. Prescription: 600 000 units

   Stock dosage: 400 000 units/mL

   How many mL should be given in one dose? ________

3. Prescription: 160 mg

   Stock dosage: 80 mg/5 mL

   How many mL should be given in one dose? ________

4. Prescription: 7.5 mg

   Stock dosage: 2.5 mg/tablet

   How many tablets should be given in one dose? ________

5. Prescription: 0.125 mg

   Stock dosage: 250 mcg/tablet

   How many tablets should be given in one dose? ________

6. Order: *conjugated estrogens 1.25 mg PO daily*

   Supply: conjugated estrogens 0.625 mg tablets

   Give: ________ tablet(s)

7. Order: *cimetidine hydrochloride 150 mg PO QID with meals & bedtime*

   Supply: cimetidine hydrochloride liquid 300 mg/5 mL

   Give: ________ mL

8. Order: *thiamine hydrochloride 80 mg IM stat*

   Supply: thiamine hydrochloride 100 mg/1 mL

   Give: ________ mL

9. Order: *meperidine hydrochloride 35 mg IM q4h prn for pain*

   Supply: meperidine hydrochloride 50 mg/1 mL

   Give: ________ mL

10. Order: *enoxaparin sodium 3000 units q12h*

    Supply: enoxaparin sodium 40 mg (4000 units)/mL

    Give: ________ mL

11. Order: *lorazepam 2.4 mg IM bedtime prn*

    Supply: lorazepam 4 mg/1 mL

    Give: ________ mL

12. Order: *prednisone 7.5 mg PO daily*

    Supply: prednisone 5 mg (scored) tablets

    Give: ________ tablet(s)

13. Order: *hydrochlorothiazide 30 mg PO BID*

    Supply: hydrochlorothiazide 50 mg/5 mL

    Give: ________ mL

14. Order: *theophylline 160 mg PO q6h*

    Supply: theophylline 80 mg/15 mL

    Give: ________ mL

15. Order: *imipramine hydrochloride 20 mg IM bedtime*

    Supply: imipramine hydrochloride 25 mg/2 mL

    Give: ________ mL

16. Order: *indomethacin 15 mg PO TID*

    Supply: indomethacin suspension 25 mg/5 mL

    Give: ________ mL

17. Order: *lorazepam 2 mg IM 2 h pre-op*

    Supply: lorazepam 4 mg/mL

    Give: ________ mL

18. Order: *phenobarbital 30 mg PO TID*

    Supply: phenobarbital 15 mg tablets

    Give: ________ tablet(s)

19. Order: *glyburide 2.5 mg PO daily*

    Supply: glyburide 1.25 mg

    Give: ________ tablet(s)

20. Order: *chlorpromazine 60 mg IM stat*

    Supply: chlorpromazine 25 mg/mL

    Give: ________ mL

21. Order: *levothyroxine 0.15 mg PO daily*

    Supply: levothyroxine 75 mcg tablets

    Give: ________ tablet(s)

22. Order: *oxtriphylline 160 mg PO q6h*

    Supply: oxtriphylline 100 mg/5 mL

    Give: ________ mL

23. Order: *methylprednisolone sodium succinate 100 mg IV q6h*

    Supply: methylprednisolone sodium succinate 125 mg/2 mL

    Give: ________ mL

24. Order: *fluphenazine hydrochloride 12.5 mg IM STAT*

    Supply: fluphenazine hydrochloride decanoate 25 mg/mL

    Give: ________ mL

25. Order: *amoxicillin 350 mg PO q8h*

    Supply: amoxicillin 250 mg/5 mL

    Give: ________ mL

Check your work! Answers to all Review Sets are provided at the end of each chapter. Worked solutions for selected Review Sets are also available there.

MATH TIP

A proportion is written as two ratios separated by an equal sign, such as 5:10 = 10:20. The two ratios in a proportion may also be separated by a double colon sign, such as 5:10 :: 10:20.

CHECK POINT

At this point, familiarity with a variety of methods to use in calculating medication dosages should be achieved. The ability to recall quickly and accurately from memory the equivalents for conversions should also be achieved. If there is any difficulty understanding the concept of converting from one unit of measurement to another, review the previous chapters and seek additional help from your instructor.

Choose one method that consistently works accurately and most easily for calculating drug dosages. Work the practice problems for Chapter 4. Concentrate on accuracy. One error can be a serious mistake when calculating the dosages of medicines or performing critical measurements of health status.

PRACTICE PROBLEMS—CHAPTER 4

Use dimensional analysis to calculate the amount to prepare for each dose.

1. Order: *lactulose 30 g PO BID*

   Supply: lactulose 667 mg/mL

   Give: ________ mL

2. Order: *penicillin G potassium 500 000 units IM QID*

   Supply: penicillin G potassium 5 000 000 units/20 mL

   Give: ________ mL

3. Order: *cephalexin 100 mg PO QID*

   Supply: cephalexin oral suspension 250 mg/5 mL

   Give: ________ mL

4. Order: *amoxicillin 125 mg PO QID*

   Supply: amoxicillin 250 mg/5 mL

   Give: ________ mL

5. Order: *diphenhydramine hydrochloride 25 mg IM stat*

   Supply: diphenhydramine hydrochloride 50 mg/mL

   Give: ________ mL

6. Order: *diphenhydramine hydrochloride 40 mg PO stat*

   Supply: diphenhydramine hydrochloride 12.5 mg/5 mL

   Give: ________ mL

7. Order: *penicillin G potassium 350 000 units IM BID*

   Supply: penicillin G potassium 500 000 units/2 mL

   Give: ________ mL

8. Order: *diazepam 3.5 mg IM q6h prn*

   Supply: diazepam 5 mg/1 mL

   Give: ________ mL

9. Order: *tobramycin sulfate 90 mg IM q8h*

   Supply: tobramycin sulfate 80 mg/2 mL

   Give: ________ mL

10. Order: *heparin sodium 2500 units subcutaneously BID*

    Supply: heparin sodium 10 000 units/mL

    Give: ________ mL

11. Order: *prochlorperazine maleate 8 mg IM q6h prn*

    Supply: prochlorperazine maleate 5 mg/1 mL

    Give: ________ mL

12. Order: *gentamicin sulfate 60 mg IM q6h*

    Supply: gentamicin sulfate 40 mg/mL

    Give: ________ mL

13. Order: *amikacin sulfate 500 mg IM BID*

    Supply: amikacin sulfate 250 mg/mL

    Give: ________ mL

14. Order: *nystatin oral suspension 250 000 units PO QID*

    Supply: nystatin oral suspension 100 000 unit/per mL

    Give: ________ mL

15. Order: *erythromycin lactobionate 450 mg IV q6h*

    Supply: erythromycin lactobionate 50 mg/mL

    Give: ________ mL

16. Order: *lithium citrate 12 mmol PO TID*

    Supply: lithium citrate 8 mmol/5 mL

    Give: ________ mL

17. Order: *vancomycin 400 mg IV q6h*

    Supply: vancomycin 1 g/20 mL

    Give: ________ mL

18. Order: *levothyroxine sodium 150 mcg PO daily*

    Supply: levothyroxine sodium 0.075 mg tablets

    Give: ________ tablet(s)

19. Order: *amoxicillin 400 mg PO q8h*

    Supply: amoxicillin 250 mg/5 mL

    Give: ________ mL

20. Order: *fosphenytoin 225 mg IV stat*

    Supply: fosphenytoin 150 mg/2 mL

    Give: ________ mL

21. Order: *chlorpromazine hydrochloride 35 mg IM stat*

    Supply: chlorpromazine hydrochloride 25 mg/mL

    Give: ________ mL

22. Order: *Add potassium chloride 30 mEq to 1000 mL D_5W IV*

    Supply: potassium chloride 20 mEq/10 mL

    Add: ________ mL

23. Order: *cefaclor 300 mg PO TID*

    Supply: cefaclor 125 mg/5 mL

    Give: ________ mL

Check your work! Answers to all problems are provided at the end of the book, in the Answers section. Worked solutions for some Practice Problems are also provided there.

APPLICATION OF CLINICAL REASONING

4-1. Describe the clinical reasoning you would implement to prevent this patient safety incident.

Possible Scenario

The order is for *amoxicillin 50 mg PO QID* for a child with an upper respiratory infection. Amoxicillin is supplied in an oral suspension with 125 mg/5 mL. The nurse initially calculated the dose this way:

$$\frac{125\ \cancel{mg}}{50\ \cancel{mg}} \times 5\ mL = \frac{625\ mL}{50} = 12.5\ mL$$

Potential Outcome

The nurse asked a colleague to double-check the dosage, as per institution policy. The scenario became a "near miss"—a "patient safety incident" was averted. The correct amount is 2 mL. If the patient received this large dose, the child would likely develop complications from overdosage of amoxicillin. When the prescriber was notified of the incident, she would likely have ordered the medication discontinued and had extra blood laboratory work done. An incident report would be filed and the family notified of the incident. If you were the colleague asked to double-check the calculation of this medication, what method would you use to set up the calculation problem? Why? Show your calculation of the correct amount of amoxicillin using dimensional analysis.

Prevention

4-2. Describe the clinical reasoning you would implement to prevent this patient safety incident.

Possible Scenario

The order is for *cefotaxime 2 g intravenously immediately* for a patient with a leg abscess. The supply dosage available is 1000 mg/10 mL. The nurse was in a rush to give the medication and calculated the dose this way:

If: $1 \text{ g} = 1000 \text{ mg}$

then: $2 \text{ g} = 1000 \div 2 = 500 \text{ mg}$ (per 5 mL)

When the nurse did a subsequent review of the patient care order, compared it with the dosage available, and considered what was reasonable, the nurse realized that 2 g is equal to 2000 mg, which was twice the amount available in one vial (10 mL). That is, the dosage required would be 2 vials, or $2 \times 10 \text{ mL} = 20 \text{ mL}$ of cefotaxime.

Potential Outcome

If the nurse had administered the 5 mL as originally calculated, the patient would have received only $\frac{1}{4}$ or 25% of the dosage ordered. If this harmful incident had occurred, the leg abscess could have progressed to osteomyelitis (a severe bone infection) because of underdosage.

Prevention

Check your work! Answers to all Application for Clinical Reasoning problems are provided at the end of the book, in the Answers section.

ANSWERS TO REVIEW SETS

Review Set 4-1

1) 0.5 **2)** 15 **3)** 0.008 **4)** 0.01 **5)** 0.06 **6)** 0.3 **7)** 0.0002 **8)** 1200 **9)** 2.5 **10)** 65 **11)** 5 **12)** 1500 **13)** 0.25 **14)** 2000 **15)** 5 **16)** 1000 **17)** 1000 **18)** 0.001 **19)** 0.023 **20)** 0.00105 **21)** 0.018 **22)** 400 **23)** 0.025 **24)** 0.5 **25)** 10 000

Review Set 4-2

1) 2 mL **2)** 1.2 mL **3)** 1 mL **4)** 0.72 mL **5)** 1.9 mL **6)** 5 mL **7)** 2.5 mL

Review Set 4-3

1) 0.25 **2)** 1000 **3)** 0.7 **4)** 514.29 **5)** 3 **6)** 0.63 **7)** 10 **8)** 0.67 **9)** 1.25 **10)** 16.67 **11)** 0.75 **12)** 6 **13)** 108 nurses **14)** 81.82 milligrams/hour **15)** 10 g

Review Set 4-4

1) 2 tablets **2)** 1.5 mL **3)** 10 mL **4)** 3 tablets **5)** 0.5 tablets **6)** 2 **7)** 2.5 **8)** 0.8 **9)** 0.7 **10)** 0.75 **11)** 0.6 **12)** 1.5 **13)** 3 **14)** 30 **15)** 1.6 **16)** 3 **17)** 0.5 **18)** 2 **19)** 2 **20)** 2.4 **21)** 2 **22)** 8 **23)** 1.6 **24)** 16 **25)** 7

SELECTED SOLUTIONS TO REVIEW SETS

Review Set 4-1

2) $\text{mg} = 0.015\,\cancel{\text{g}} \times \frac{1000\text{ mg}}{1\,\cancel{\text{g}}}$

$= 0.015 \times 1000\text{ mg} = 0.015.$

$= 15\text{ mg}$

3) $\text{g} = 8\,\cancel{\text{mg}} \times \frac{1\text{ g}}{1000\,\cancel{\text{mg}}}$

$= \frac{8\text{ g}}{1000} = 0.008.0$

$= 0.008\text{ g}$

7) $\text{g} = 0.2\,\cancel{\text{mg}} \times \frac{1\text{ g}}{1000\,\cancel{\text{mg}}}$

$= \frac{0.2\text{ g}}{1000} = 0.000.2$

$= 0.0002\text{ g}$

9) $\text{g} = 0.0025\,\cancel{\text{kg}} \times \frac{1000\text{ g}}{1\,\cancel{\text{kg}}}$

$= 0.0025 \times 1000\text{ g} = 0.002.5$

$= 2.5\text{ g}$

20) $\text{kg} = 1.05\,\cancel{\text{g}} \times \frac{1\text{ kg}}{1000\,\cancel{\text{g}}}$

$= \frac{1.05\text{ kg}}{1000} = 0.001.05$

$= 0.00105\text{ kg}$

23) $\text{kg} = 25\,\cancel{\text{g}} \times \frac{1\text{ kg}}{1000\,\cancel{\text{g}}}$

$= \frac{25\text{ kg}}{1000} = 0.025.0$

$= 0.025\text{ kg}$

Review Set 4-2

1) $\frac{0.8\,\cancel{\text{g}}}{1\,\cancel{\text{g}}} \times 2.5\text{ mL} = 2\text{ mL}$

2) $\frac{200\,\cancel{\text{mg}}}{250\,\cancel{\text{mg}}} \times 1.5\text{ mL} = 1.2\text{ mL}$

3) $\frac{0.2\,\cancel{\text{g}}}{1\,\cancel{\text{g}}} \times 5\text{ mL} = 1\text{ mL}$

4) $\frac{300\,\cancel{\text{mcg}}}{500\,\cancel{\text{mcg}}} \times 1.2\text{ mL} = 0.72\text{ mL}$

5) $\frac{1250\,\cancel{\text{units}}}{1000\,\cancel{\text{units}}} \times 1.5\text{ mL} = 1.875\text{ mL} = 1.9\text{ mL}$

6) $\frac{50\,\cancel{\text{mEq}}}{200\,\cancel{\text{mEq}}} \times 20\text{ mL} = 5\text{ mL}$

7) $\frac{0.25\,\cancel{\text{mg}}}{0.2\,\cancel{\text{mg}}} \times 2\text{ mL} = 2.5\text{ mL}$

Review Set 4-3

2) $\frac{0.5}{2} = \frac{250}{X}$

$0.5X = 500$

$\frac{\cancel{0.5}X}{\cancel{0.5}} = \frac{500}{0.5}$

$X = 1000$

4) $\frac{1200}{X} \times 12 = 28$

$\frac{1200}{X} \times \frac{12}{1} = 28$

$\frac{14\,400}{X} = \frac{28}{1}$

$28X = 14\,400$

$\frac{\cancel{28}X}{\cancel{28}} = \frac{14\,400}{28}$

$X = 514.285$

$X = 514.29$

5) $\frac{250}{1} = \frac{750}{X}$

$250X = 750$

$\frac{\cancel{250}X}{\cancel{250}} = \frac{750}{250}$

$X = 3$

8) $\frac{\frac{1}{100}}{1} = \frac{\frac{1}{150}}{X}$

$\frac{1}{100}X = \frac{1}{150}$

$\frac{\cancel{\frac{1}{100}}X}{\cancel{\frac{1}{100}}} = \frac{\frac{1}{150}}{\frac{1}{100}}$

$X = \frac{1}{150} \div \frac{1}{100}$

$X = \frac{1}{\underset{3}{\cancel{150}}} \times \frac{\overset{2}{\cancel{100}}}{1}$

$X = \frac{2}{3} = 0.666 = 0.67$

12) $\frac{25\%}{30\%} = \frac{5}{X}$

$\frac{0.25}{0.3} = \frac{5}{X}$

$0.25X = 1.5$

$\frac{\cancel{0.25}X}{\cancel{0.25}} = \frac{1.5}{0.25}$

$X = 6$

13) $\frac{45}{100} = \frac{X}{240}$

$100X = 10\,800$

$\frac{\cancel{100}X}{\cancel{100}} = \frac{10\,800}{100}$

$X = 108$

15) $\frac{X}{500 \text{ mL}} = \frac{5g}{250 \text{ mL}}$

$5 \times 500 = 250X$

$\frac{2500}{250} = \frac{\cancel{250}X}{\cancel{250}}$

$X = 10 \text{ g}$

Review Set 4-4

7) $\frac{300 \text{ mg}}{5 \text{ mL}} = \frac{150 \text{ mg}}{X \text{ mL}}$

$300X = 750$

$\frac{\cancel{300}X}{\cancel{300}} = \frac{750}{300}$

$X = 2.5 \text{ mL}$

10) $\frac{4000 \text{ units}}{1 \text{ mL}} = \frac{3000 \text{ units}}{X \text{ mL}}$

$4000X = 3000$

$X = 0.75 \text{ mL}$

11) $\frac{4 \text{ mg}}{1 \text{ mL}} = \frac{2.4 \text{ mg}}{X \text{ mL}}$

$4X = 2.4$

$\frac{\cancel{4}X}{\cancel{4}} = \frac{2.4}{4}$

$X = 0.6 \text{ mL}$

14) $\frac{80 \text{ mg}}{15 \text{ mL}} = \frac{160 \text{ mg}}{X \text{ mL}}$

$80X = 2400$

$\frac{\cancel{80}X}{\cancel{80}} = \frac{2400}{80}$

$X = 30 \text{ mL}$

18) $\frac{15 \text{ mg}}{1 \text{ tab}} = \frac{30 \text{ mg}}{X \text{ tab}}$

$15X = 30$

$\frac{\cancel{15}X}{\cancel{15}} = \frac{30}{15}$

$X = 2$ tablets

21) $\frac{75 \text{ mcg}}{1 \text{ tab}} = \frac{150 \text{ mcg}}{X}$

$75X = 150$

$\frac{\cancel{75}X}{\cancel{75}} = \frac{150}{75}$

$X = 2$ tablets

23) $\frac{125 \text{ mg}}{2 \text{ mL}} = \frac{100 \text{ mg}}{X \text{ mL}}$

$125X = 200$

$\frac{125\,X}{125} = \frac{200}{125}$

$X = 1.6 \text{ mL}$

24) $\frac{12.5 \text{ mg}}{X} = \frac{25 \text{ mg}}{1 \text{ mL}}$

$25X = 12.5 \times 1$

$\frac{25X}{25} = \frac{12.5}{25}$

$X = 0.5 \text{ mL}$

SECTION 1

Self-Evaluation

Directions:

1. Round decimals to two places, as needed.
2. Express fractions in their lowest terms.

Chapters 1 and 2: Mathematics Review

Multiply or divide by the power of 10 indicated. Draw an arrow to indicate movement of the decimal point.

1. $30.5 \div 10 =$ ________
2. $40.025 \times 100 =$ ________

Identify the lowest common denominator for the following sets of numbers.

3. $\frac{1}{6}, \frac{2}{3}, \frac{3}{4}$ ________
4. $\frac{2}{5}, \frac{3}{10}, \frac{3}{11}$ ________

Complete the operations indicated.

5. $\frac{1}{4} + \frac{2}{3} =$ ________
6. $\frac{6}{7} - \frac{1}{9} =$ ________
7. $1\frac{3}{5} \times \frac{5}{8} =$ ________
8. $\frac{3}{8} \div \frac{3}{4} =$ ________
9. $13.2 + 32.55 + 0.029 =$ ________
10. 20% of $0.09 =$ ________
11. $80.3 - 21.06 =$ ________
12. $0.3 \times 0.3 =$ ________
13. $\frac{1}{150} \div \frac{1}{100} =$ ________
14. $\frac{\frac{1}{120}}{\frac{1}{60}} =$ ________
15. $\frac{16\%}{\frac{1}{4}} =$ ________

Arrange in order from smallest to largest.

16. $\frac{1}{3}, \frac{1}{2}, \frac{1}{6}, \frac{1}{10}, \frac{1}{5}$ ________
17. 0.25, 0.125, 0.3, 0.009, 0.1909 ________
18. Identify the strongest solution of the following: 1:3, 1:60, 1:6 ________

Convert as indicated.

19. 1:100 to a decimal ________
20. $\frac{6}{150}$ to a decimal ________
21. 0.009 to a percent ________
22. $33\frac{1}{3}\%$ to a fraction ________
23. 0.05 to a fraction ________
24. $\frac{1}{2}\%$ to a ratio ________

25. 2:3 to a fraction ________

26. 3:4 to a percent ________

27. $\frac{2}{5}$ to a percent ________

Chapters 3 and 4: Systems of Measurement and Calculation Methods

Find the value of "X" in the following equations. Express your answers as decimals; round to the nearest hundredth.

28. $\frac{0.35}{1.3} \times 4.5 = X$ ________

29. $\frac{0.3}{2.6} = \frac{0.15}{X}$ ________

30. $\frac{0.25}{0.125} \times 2 = X$ ________

31. $\frac{10\%}{\frac{1}{2}\%} \times 1000 = X$ ________

32. $\frac{\frac{1}{100}}{\frac{1}{150}} \times 2.2 = X$ ________

Express the following amount in proper medical notation.

33. one-half millilitre ________

Interpret the following notations.

34. 450 mg ________

35. 0.25 L ________

Choose one of the methods of medication calculation (dimensional analysis, formula method, or ratio and proportion) to solve the following calculation problems. The solutions for the calculation problems focus on the dimensional analysis method. Fill in the missing decimal numbers next to each SI symbol as indicated.

36. 7.13 kg = ________ g = ________ mg = ________ mcg

37. ________ kg = ________ g = ________ mg = 925 mcg

38. ________ kg = ________ g = 125 mg = ________ mcg

39. ________ kg = 16.4 g = ________ mg = ________ mcg

Convert each of the following to the equivalent units indicated.

40. 20 mg = ________ g

41. 56.2 mm = ________ cm

42. 11.59 kg = ________ g

43. Most adults have about 6000 mL of circulating blood volume. This is equivalent to ________ L of blood volume.

Convert the following times as indicated. Designate AM or PM where needed.

Traditional Time	*International Time*
44. 11:35 PM	________
45. ________	1844

46. Tetracycline 250 mg is ordered 4 times daily. The medication label indicates that one capsule contains 0.25 g. How many capsules should be given for one dose? ________

47. Meperidine hydrochloride 60 mg is needed postoperatively for pain. The vial contains 75 mg/mL. How many mL should be given? ________

48. Amoxicillin 500 mg is needed for pneumonia. The suspension is available in 125 mg/5 mL. How many mL need to be prepared? ________

49. Digoxin 125 mcg is needed. The vial label indicates a concentration of 0.5 mg in 2 mL. How many mL are needed? ________

50. A patient needs to receive diphenhydramine hydrochloride 25 mg intravenously. The vial label indicates a concentration of 50 mg/mL. How many mL of diphenhydramine hydrochloride need to be prepared? ________

After completing these problems, see page 503 to check your answers. Give yourself 2 points for each correct answer.

Perfect score = 100 My score = ________

Mastery score = 86 or higher (43 or more correct)

For more practice, go back to the beginning of this section and repeat the Mathematics Diagnostic Evaluation.

Equipment Used in Dosage Measurement

OBJECTIVES

1. Select the appropriate equipment for the medication, dosage, and method of administration ordered.
2. Interpret the calibrations of each device presented.

Now that the system of measurement used in the calculation of dosages has been discussed, the common measuring devices will be examined. In this chapter, the student will learn to recognize and read the calibrations of devices used in both oral and parenteral administration. The oral devices include the medicine cup, the calibrated dropper, and pediatric oral devices. The parenteral devices include the 3-mL syringe, the prefilled syringe, the 1-mL syringe, a variety of insulin syringes, and special safety and intravenous syringes.

ORAL ADMINISTRATION

The Medicine Cup

The 30-mL medicine cup that is used to measure most liquids for oral administration is shown in Figure 5-1. Notice that both the household system and the SI system are calibrated on the cup. Individuals unfamiliar with the metric system may find comparison to the household system helpful in visualizing the amount to be measured. Use of SI is consistent with standards of practice in healthcare and is the most accurate system for measuring medication doses. For volumes less than 10 mL, however, a smaller, more accurate device should be used (see Figures 5-2 and 5-3). Because of differing recommendations for volumes requiring a syringe for accurate measurement, depending on the medication, healthcare providers may sometimes need to make a case-by-case decision regarding whether a syringe or medicine cup is preferable. The institutional policy may also recommend either a syringe or a medicine cup, based on the volume of medication to be administered.

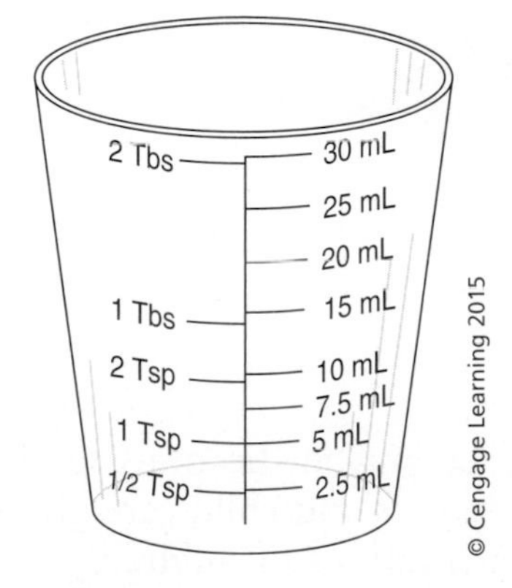

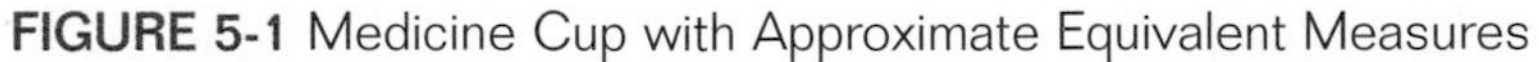
FIGURE 5-1 Medicine Cup with Approximate Equivalent Measures

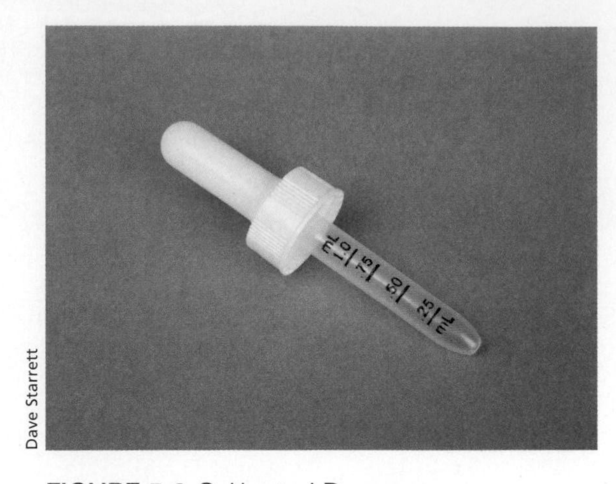

FIGURE 5-2 Calibrated Dropper

The Calibrated Dropper

The calibrated dropper, which is used to administer some small quantities, is shown in Figure 5-2. A dropper is used when giving medicine to children and older adults, and when adding small amounts of liquid to water or juice. Eye and ear medications are also dispensed from a calibrated medicine dropper or squeeze drop bottle.

The amount of the drop varies according to the diameter of the hole at the tip of the dropper. For this reason, a properly calibrated dropper usually accompanies the medicine. It is calibrated according to the way that drug is prescribed. The calibrations are usually given in millilitres, cubic centimetres, or drops.

CAUTION

To be safe, never interchange packaged droppers between medications because drop size varies from one dropper to another.

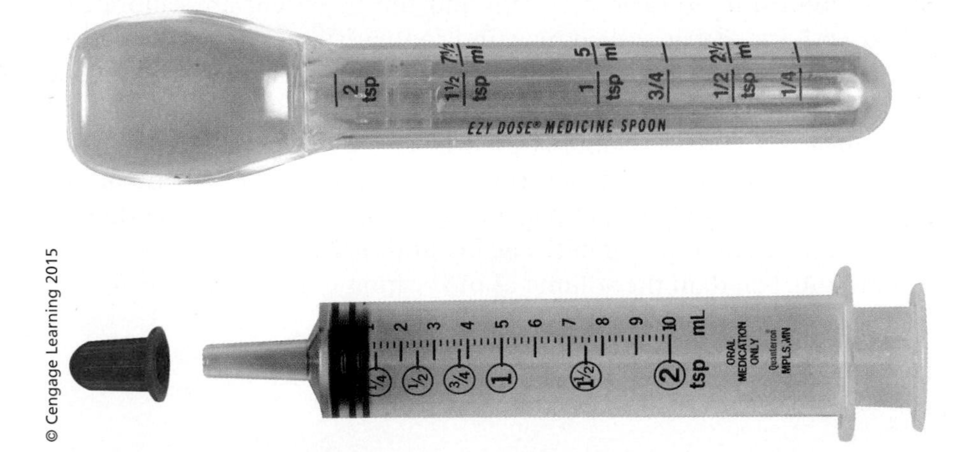

FIGURE 5-3 Devices for Administering Oral Medications to Children

Pediatric Oral Devices

Various types of calibrated devices are available to administer oral medications to children. Two devices intended for oral use only are shown in Figure 5-3. Parents and child care givers should be taught to always use calibrated devices when administering medications to children.

CAUTION

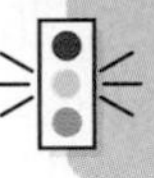

Household spoons vary in size and are not reliable for accurate dosing.

CAUTION

Always prepare and administer small volumes of oral and enteral solutions in oral syringes. This practice avoids placing any non-parenteral products in parenteral syringes. On medication administration record sheets for liquid medications, include the warning "Use oral syringe only."

There are two ways to distinguish oral syringes from parenteral syringes: syringes intended for oral use typically do not have a Luer-Lok hub, and the tip is too large to accommodate a needle. They also usually have a cap on the tip that must be removed before administering the medication. Syringes intended for parenteral use have a Luer-Lok that allows a needle to be secured tightly (see Figure 5-5).

PARENTERAL ADMINISTRATION

The term "parenteral" is used to designate routes of administration other than gastrointestinal. Some examples of parenteral routes of administration are intradermal, subcutaneous, intramuscular, and intravenous routes.

The Three-Millilitre or 3-mL Syringe

A 3-mL syringe assembled with a needle unit is shown in Figure 5-4. The parts of the syringe are identified in Figure 5-5. Notice that the black rubber tip of the suction plunger is visible. The nurse pulls back on the plunger to withdraw the medicine from the storage container. The calibrations are read from the top black ring, not the raised middle section and not the bottom ring. Closely examine the scale in Figure 5-4, which is calibrated in millilitres (mL) and tenths (0.1) of a millilitre. Each 1/2 (or 0.5) millilitre is marked up to the maximum volume of 3 mL.

Dosages are standardized to the syringe calibrations. Standard drug dosages of 1 mL or greater can be rounded to the nearest tenth (0.1) of a mL and measured on the mL scale. Refer to Chapter 1 to review the rules of decimal rounding. For example, 1.45 mL is rounded to 1.5 mL. Notice that the coloured liquid in Figure 5-4 identifies 1.5 mL.

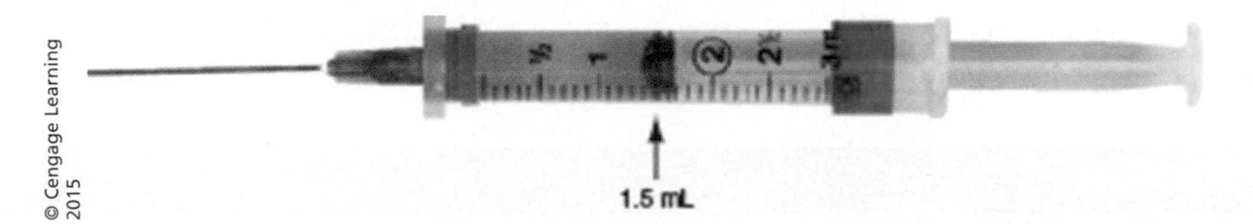

FIGURE 5-4 3-mL Syringe with Needle Unit Measuring 1.5 mL

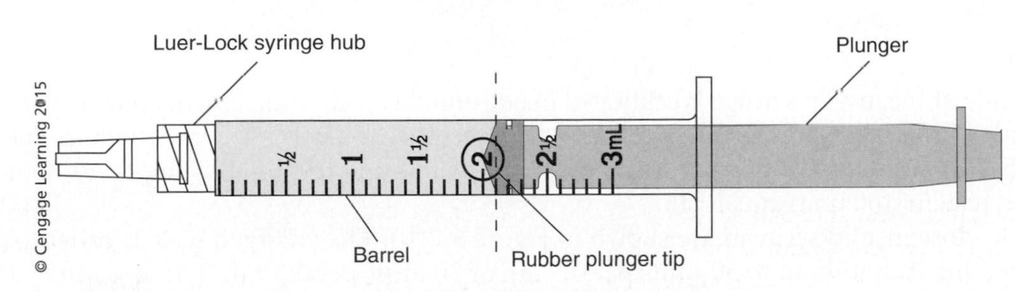

FIGURE 5-5 3-mL Syringe with Needle Unit Measuring 2.1 mL

The Prefilled, Single-Dose Syringe

Figure 5-6 shows two different examples of *prefilled, single-dose syringes.* Such syringes contain the usual single dose of a medication and are to be used only once. The syringe is discarded after the single use. If you are to give *less than the full single dose* of a drug provided in a prefilled, single-dose syringe, you should discard the extra amount *before* injecting the patient.

Example:

The drug order prescribes 7.5 mg of diazepam to be administered to a patient. You have a prefilled, single-dose syringe of diazepam containing 10 mg per 2 mL of solution (as in the first syringe shown in Figure 5-6). You would discard 2.5 mg (0.5 mL) of the drug solution; then 7.5 mg would remain in the syringe. You will learn more about calculating drug dosages beginning in Chapter 8.

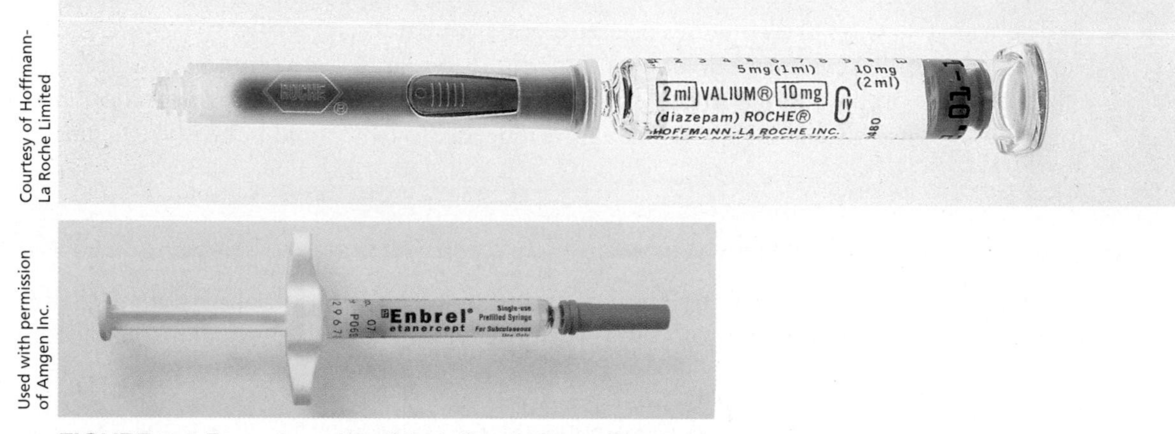

FIGURE 5-6 Examples of Prefilled, Single-Dose Syringes

> **RATIONALE FOR PRACTICE**
>
> **Some syringes may still be marked in cubic centimetres (cc); however, most drugs are prepared and labelled with the strength given per millilitre (mL). The cubic centimetre and millilitre are equivalent measurements in dosage calculations (1 cc = 1 mL).**

The Insulin Syringe

Both sides of a standard 100-unit insulin syringe are shown in Figure 5-7(a). This syringe is to be used for the measurement and administration of 100-unit insulin *only.* The 100 means there are 100 units of insulin in every 1 mL. It must not be used to measure other medications that are measured in units.

> **CAUTION**
>
> One hundred–unit insulin should be measured only in a 100-unit insulin syringe.

One side of the insulin syringe is calibrated in odd-number 2-unit increments (Figure 5-7(a)), and the other side is calibrated in even-number 2-unit increments. The labels are every 10 units. The plunger in Figure 5-8(a) indicates the measurement of 70 units of 100-unit insulin. It is important to note that for 100-unit insulin, 100 units equal 1 mL.

Two lo-dose insulin syringes are shown in Figure 5-7(b). The enlarged scale is easier to read and is calibrated for each unit up to 50 units per 0.5 mL or 30 units per 0.3 mL. The labels are every 5 units. The 30-unit syringe is commonly used for pediatric administration of insulin. The plunger in Figure 5-8(b) indicates the measurement of 19 units of 100-unit insulin.

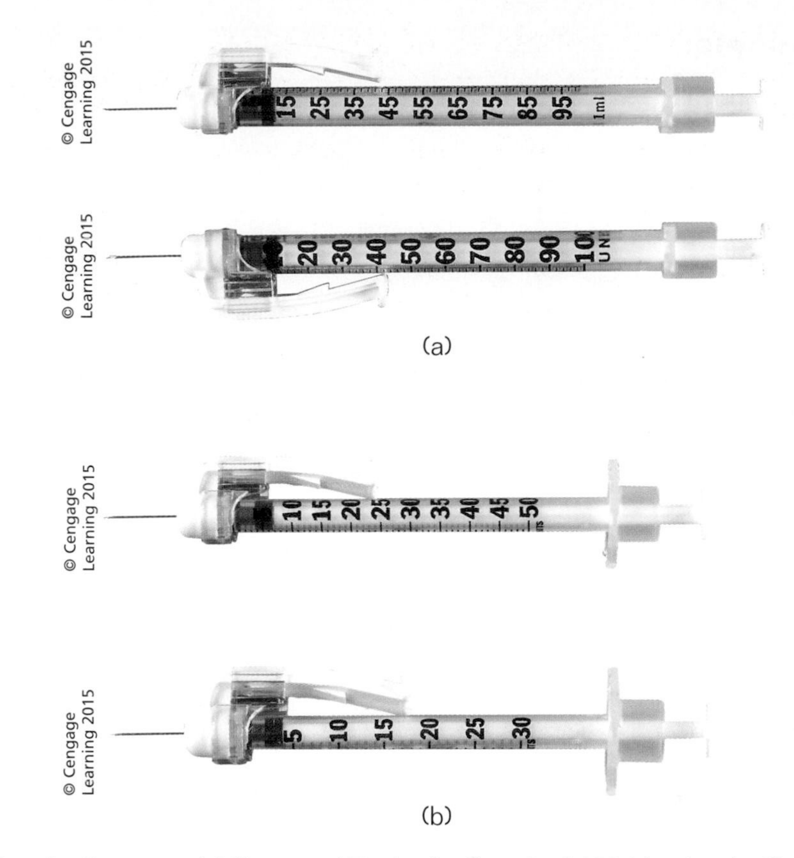

FIGURE 5-7 Insulin Syringes. (a) Front and Back of a Standard 100-Unit Insulin Syringe; (b) Lo-Dose 100-Unit Insulin Syringes, 50 and 30 Units

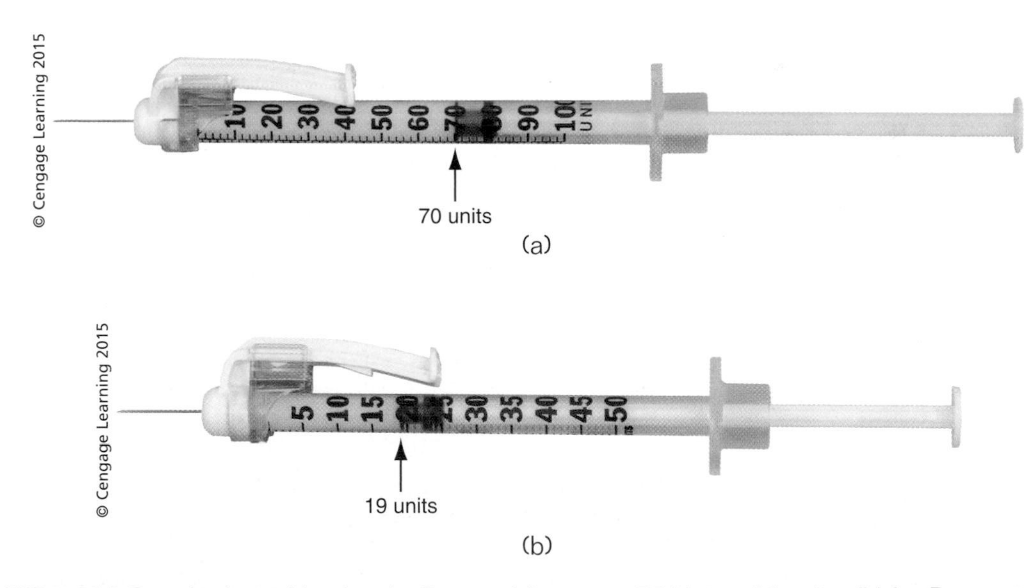

FIGURE 5-8(a) Standard 100-Unit Insulin Syringe Measuring 70 Units of Insulin; (b) Lo-Dose 100-Unit Insulin Syringe Measuring 19 Units of Insulin

The One-Millilitre or 1-mL Syringe

The 1-mL syringe is shown in Figure 5-9. This syringe is also called the tuberculin or TB syringe. It is used when a small dose of a drug must be measured, such as an allergen extract, a vaccine, or a child's medication. Notice that the 1-mL syringe is calibrated in hundredths (0.01) of a millilitre, with each one-tenth (0.1) millilitre labelled on the syringe barrel. Pediatric and critical care doses of less than 1 mL can be rounded to hundredths and measured in the 1-mL syringe. It is preferable to measure all amounts less than 0.5 mL in a 1-mL syringe.

Example:

The amount 0.366 mL is rounded to 0.37 and measured in the 1-mL syringe.

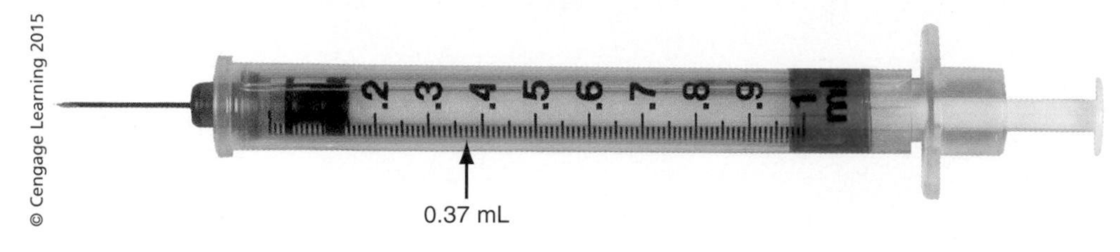

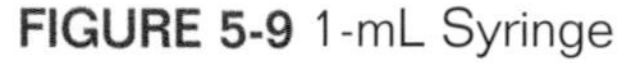

FIGURE 5-9 1-mL Syringe

Safety Syringes

Figure 5-10 shows a 3-mL safety syringe (Figure 5-10(a)), a 1-mL safety syringe (Figure 5-10(b)), and insulin safety syringes (Figures 5-10(c) and (d)). Notice that the needle is protected by a shield to prevent accidental needlestick injury to the nurse after administering an injectable medication.

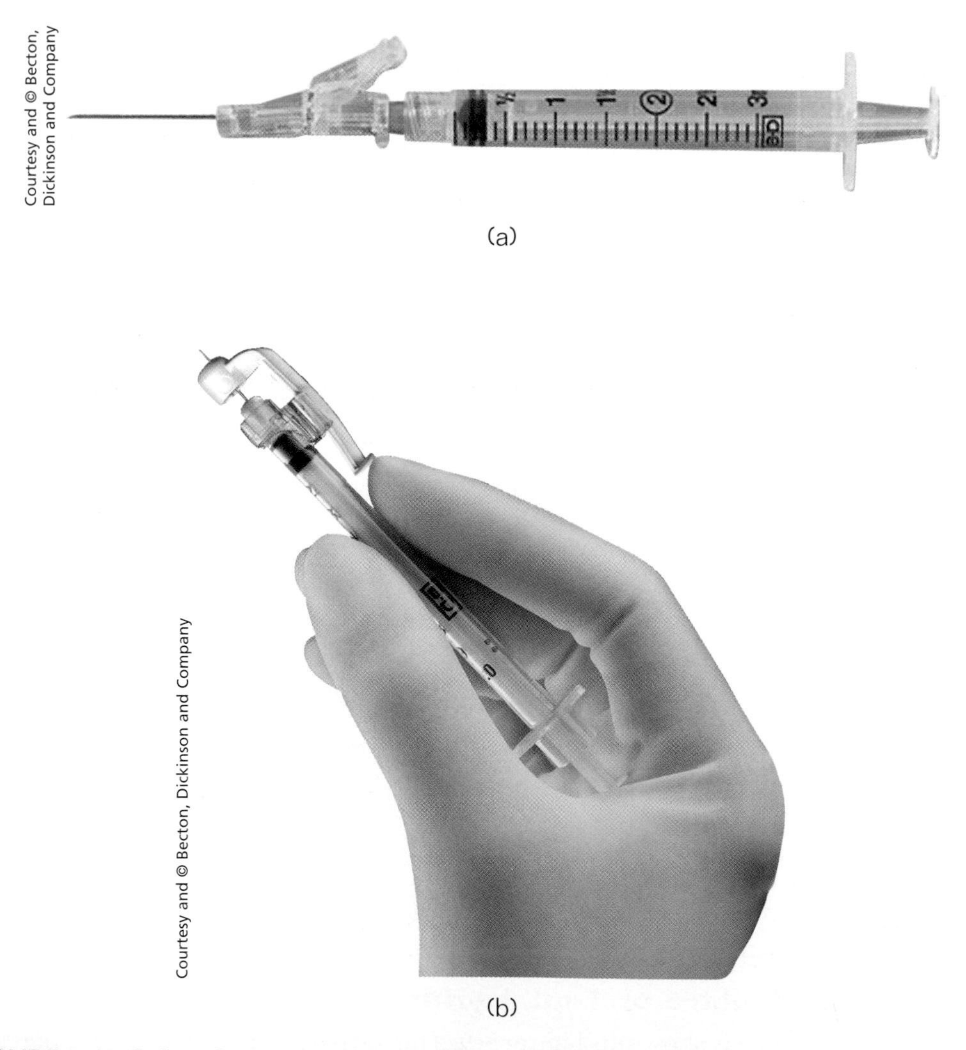

(a)

(b)

FIGURE 5-10 Safety Syringes. (a) 3 mL; (b) 1 mL *(continued)*

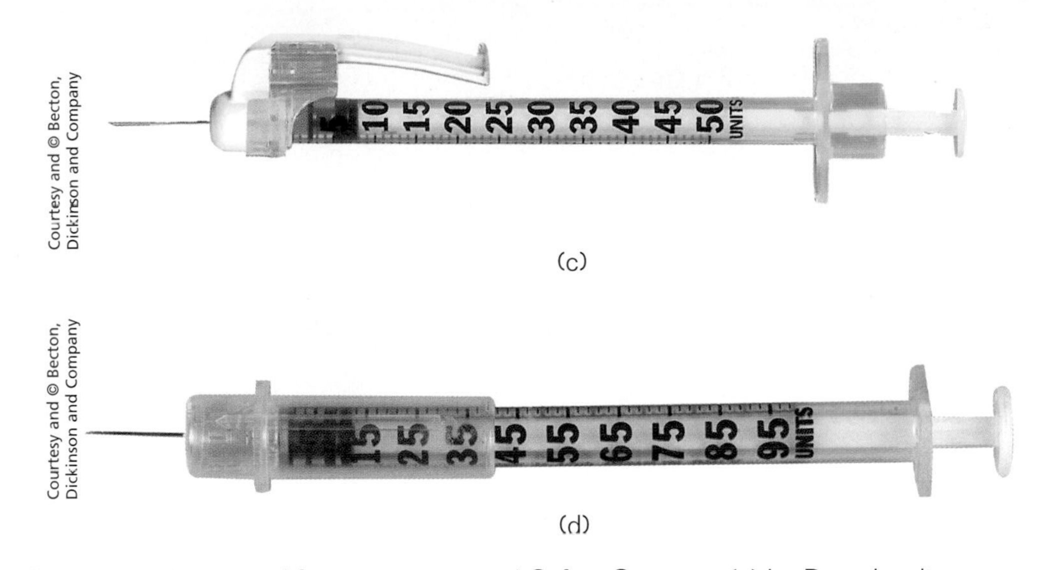

FIGURE 5-10 *(continued from previous page)* Safety Syringes. (c) Lo-Dose Insulin; (d) Standard Insulin

The Intravenous Syringe

Large syringes commonly used to prepare medications for intravenous administration are shown in Figure 5-11. The volume and calibration of these syringes vary. To be safe, examine the calibrations of the syringes, and select the one best suited for the volume to be administered.

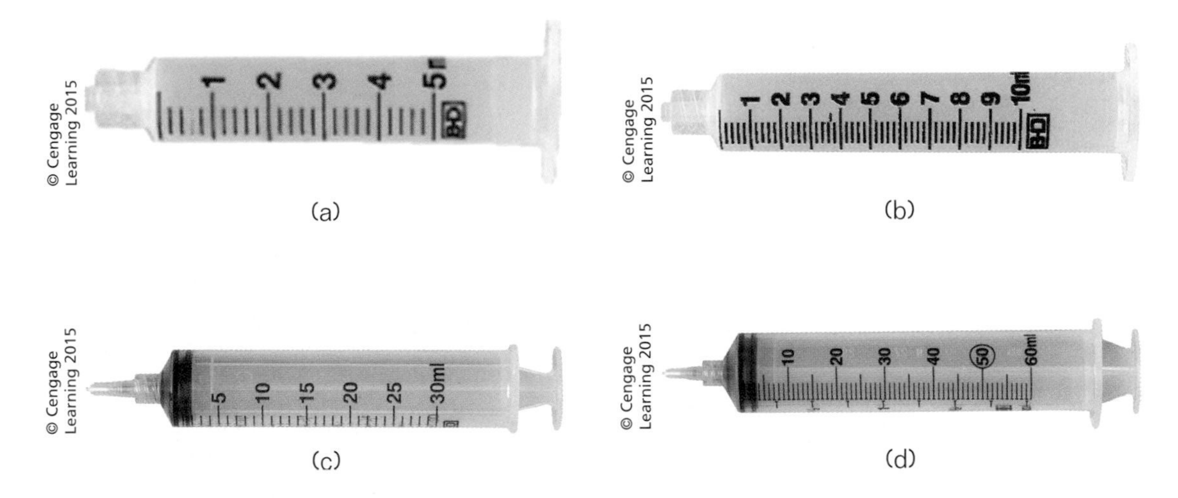

FIGURE 5-11 Intravenous Syringes. (a) 5 mL; (b) 10 mL; (c) 30 mL; (d) 60 mL

The Needle-Free Devices

A needle-free injection system, such as the one in Figure 5-12, is designed to prevent accidental needlesticks during intravenous administration.

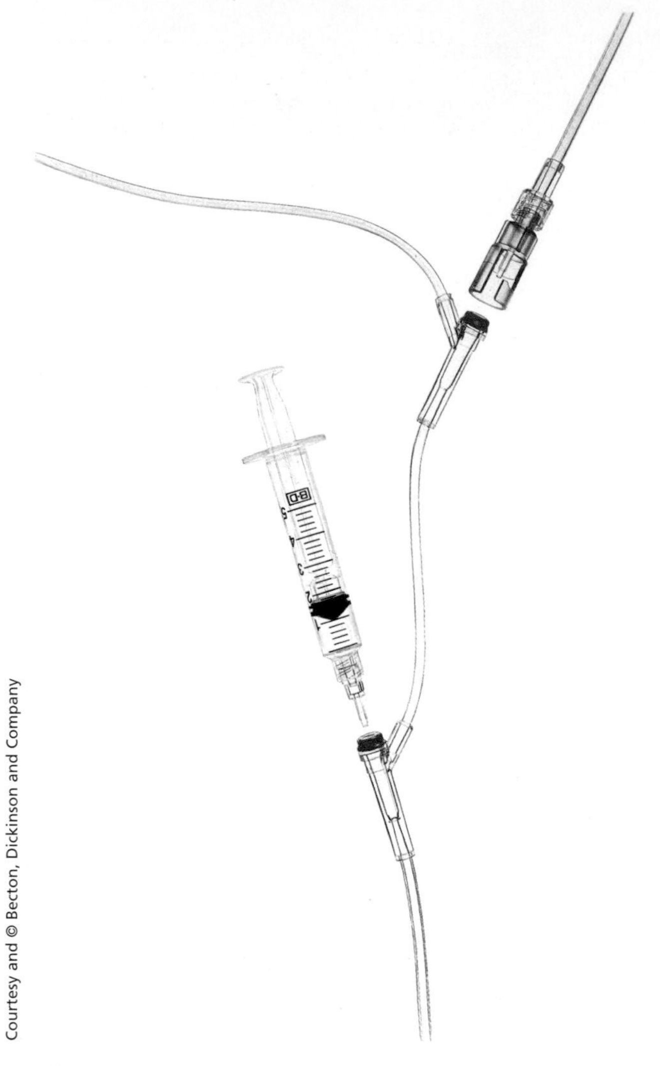

FIGURE 5-12 Needle-Free Injection System

QUICK REVIEW

- The medicine cup has a 30-mL capacity for oral liquids. Amounts less than 10 mL should be measured in a smaller device, such as an oral syringe. It is recommended that the pharmacy dispense all oral liquid medications in patient-specific or unit-of-use oral syringes or in dose medicine cups.
- The calibrated dropper measures small amounts of oral liquids. The size of the drop varies according to the diameter of the tip of the dropper.
- The standard 3-mL syringe is used to measure most injectable drugs. It is calibrated in tenths of a mL.
- The prefilled, single-dose syringe cartridge is to be used once and then discarded.
- The standard 100-unit insulin syringe is used to measure only insulin. It is calibrated for a total of 100 units per 1 mL.
- The lo-dose 100-unit insulin syringe is used for measuring small amounts of insulin. It is calibrated for a total of 50 units per 0.5 mL or 30 units per 0.3 mL. The smaller syringe is commonly used for administering small amounts of insulin.
- The 1-mL syringe is used to measure small or critical amounts of injectable drugs. It is calibrated in hundredths of a mL.
- Syringes intended for injections should never be used to measure or administer oral medications.

REVIEW SET 5-1

1. In which syringe should 0.25 mL of a drug solution be measured? ____________
2. a. Can 1.25 mL be measured in the regular 3-mL syringe? ____________

   b. How? ____________
3. Should insulin be measured in a 1-mL syringe? ____________
4. For the following volumes, select the best measuring device:

   a) 4 mL PO ____________

   b) 20 mL PO ____________

   c) 0.75 mL Subcut ____________

   d) 1.68 mL IV ____________

   e) 5.6 mL IV ____________

   f) 25 units insulin Subcut ____________
5. a. The drop is considered a consistent quantity for comparisons between different droppers. (True) (False)

   b. Why or why not? ____________
6. Can you measure 3 mL in a medicine cup? ____________
7. How would you measure 3 mL of oral liquid to be administered to a child? ____________

   ____
8. The medicine cup indicates that each teaspoon is the equivalent of ________ mL.
9. Describe your action if you are to administer less than the full amount of a drug supplied in a prefilled, single-dose syringe. ____________

   ____
10. What is the primary purpose of safety and needleless syringes? ____________

    ____

Note: The drawings of the syringes in the following questions represent actual sizes.

For questions 11 through 20, draw an arrow to point to the calibration that corresponds to the dose to be administered.

11. Administer 0.75 mL.

12. Administer 1.33 mL.

13. Administer 2.2 mL.

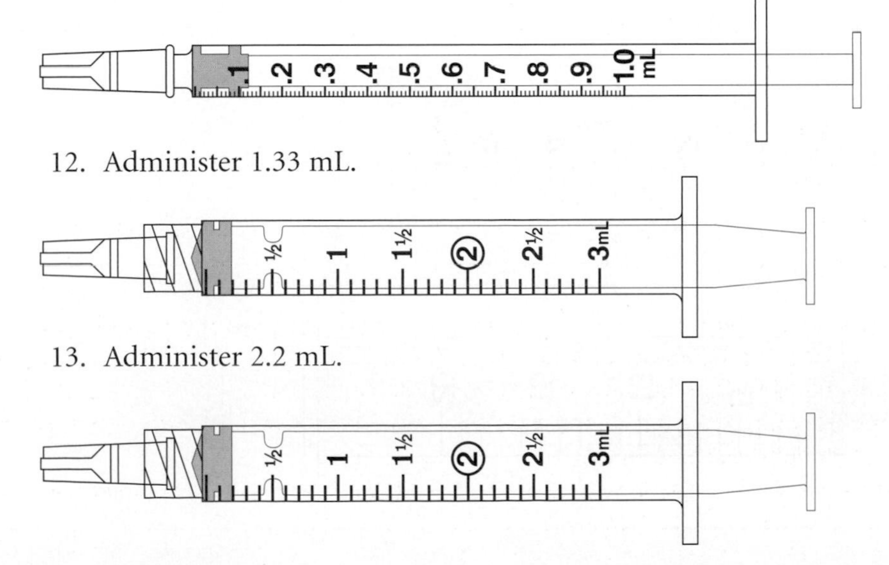

14. Administer 1.3 mL.

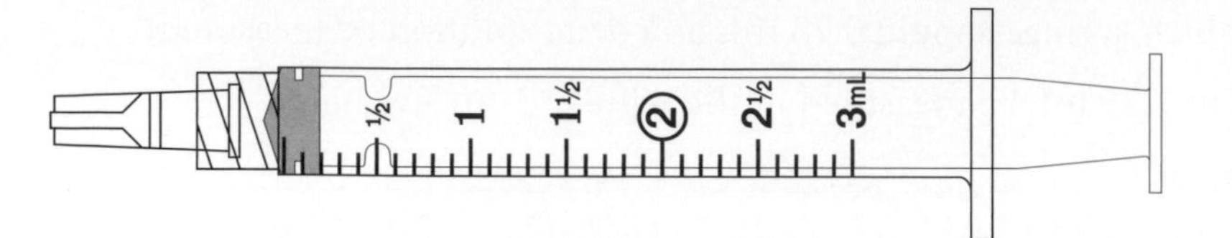

15. Administer 0.33 mL.

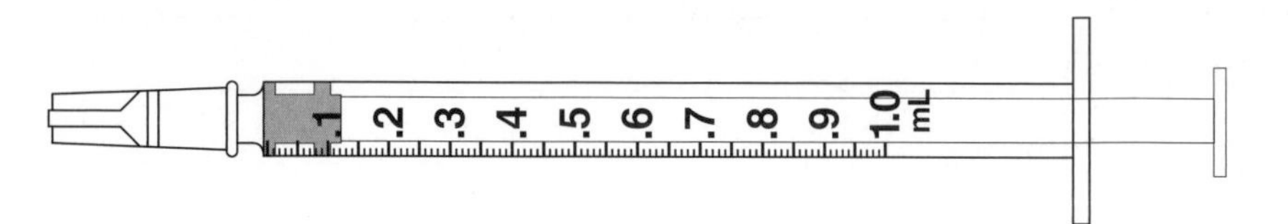

16. Administer 65 units of insulin.

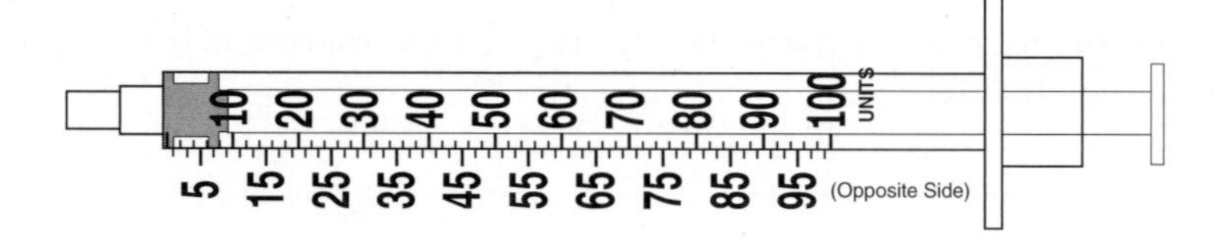

17. Administer 27 units of insulin.

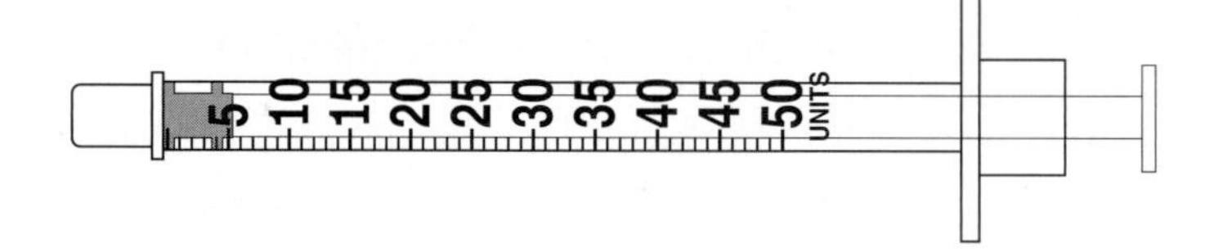

18. Administer 75 units of insulin.

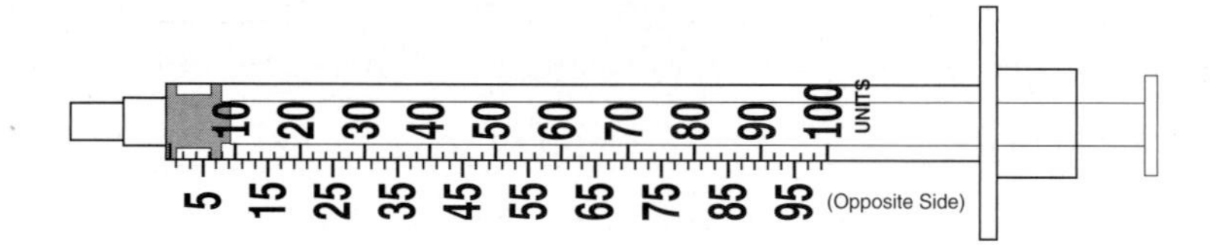

19. Administer 4.4 mL.

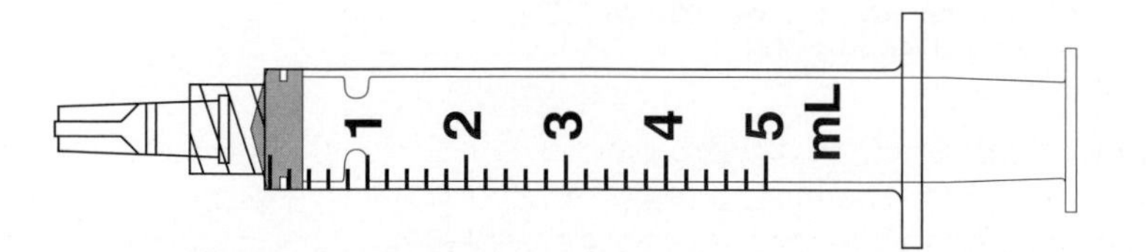

20. Administer 16 mL.

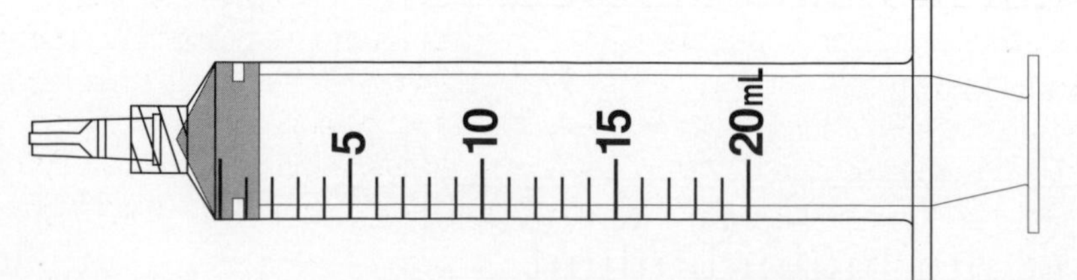

21. On the 5-mL syringe, each calibration is equal to ________. (Express the answer as a decimal.)

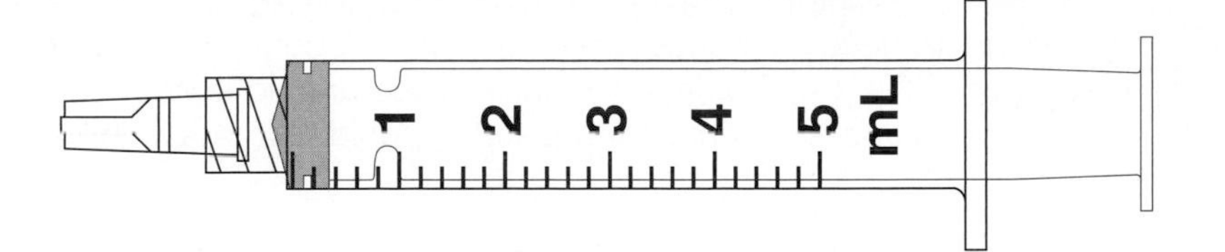

22. On the 20-mL syringe, each calibration is equal to ________.

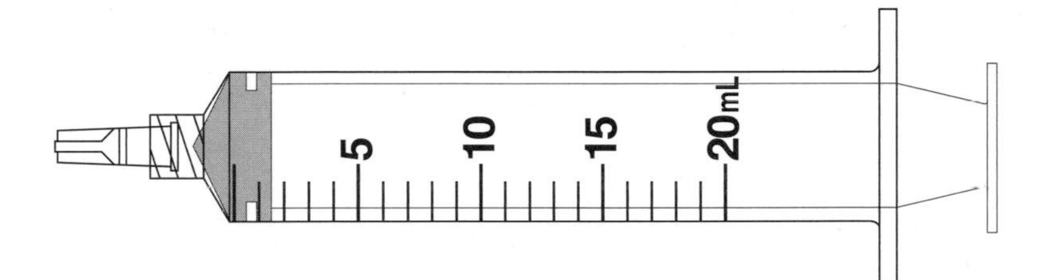

23. On the 10-mL syringe, each calibration is equal to ________. (Express the answer as a decimal.)

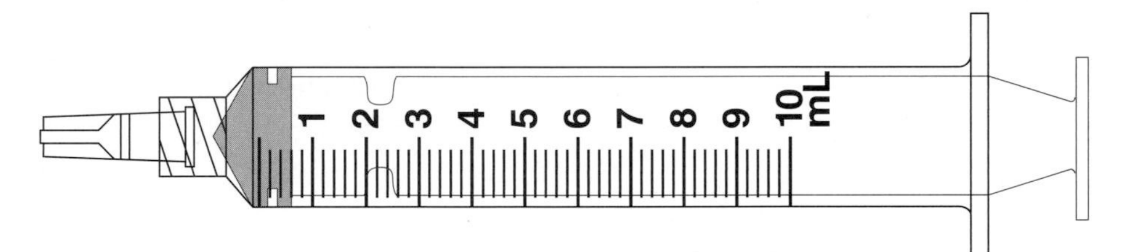

Check your work! Answers to all Review Sets are provided at the end of each chapter. Worked solutions for selected Review Sets are also available there.

APPLICATION OF CLINICAL REASONING

Select the correct equipment to prepare medications. In the following situation, the correct dosage was not given because an incorrect measuring device was used.

Potential Patient Safety Incident

Using an inaccurate measuring device for oral medications.

Possible Scenario

Suppose a pediatrician ordered amoxicillin suspension 250 mg (5 mL or 1 tsp), every 8 hours, to be given to a child. The child should receive the medication for 10 days for otitis media, an ear infection. The pharmacy dispensed the medication in a bottle containing 150 mL, or a 10-day supply. The nurse did not clarify for the mother how to measure and administer the medication. The child returned to the clinic in 10 days for routine follow-up. The nurse asked whether the child had taken all the prescribed amoxicillin. The child's mother stated, "No, we have almost half of the bottle left." When the nurse asked how the medication had been given, the mother showed the bright pink plastic teaspoon she had obtained from the local ice cream parlor. The nurse measured the spoon's capacity and found it to be less than 3 mL. (Remember, 1 tsp = 5 mL.) The child would have received only 3/5, or 60%, of the correct dose.

Potential Outcome

The child did not receive a therapeutic dosage of the medication and was actually underdosed. The child could develop a super infection, which could lead to a more severe illness such as meningitis. Risk of bacterial resistance to the antibiotic could be increased. Inadequate shaking of the suspension prior to measuring could also result in an inaccurate dose of the drug.

Prevention

Teach family members (and patients, as appropriate) to use calibrated measuring spoons or specially designed oral syringes to measure the correct dosage of medication. The volumes of serving spoons may vary considerably, as this situation illustrates. Also teach to adequately shake the medication before measuring and to take all of the medication as ordered to limit the risk of antibiotic resistance.

Application of Critical Reasoning Additional application problems are provided at the end of the chapter. Answers are provided at the end of the book.

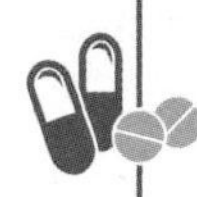

UNDERSTANDING NCLEX QUESTIONS

Here's an example of a standard question used in textbooks:

Four-year-old Peter is ordered an oral liquid drug suspension of 4 mL per dose. The best way to administer this medication would be to use a/an:

a. household teaspoon
b. cooking measuring spoon
c. oral syringe
d. graduated medicine cup

Here's how it would look in an NCLEX examination:

The nurse is to discharge a 4-year-old home on an oral liquid drug suspension of 4 mL per dose. Which would the nurse recommend to ensure the highest level of accuracy in home administration of the medication?

a. Using a household teaspoon
b. Using a cooking measuring spoon
c. Using an oral syringe
d. Using a graduated medicine cup

Answer: c

Rationale: The oral syringe would provide the most accurate dose of 4 mL.

PRACTICE PROBLEMS—CHAPTER 5

1. In the 100-unit insulin syringe, 100 units = ________ mL.
2. The 1-mL syringe is calibrated in ________ of a mL.
3. Can you measure 1.25 mL in a single tuberculin syringe? ________ Explain. ________________

____

____

4. How would you measure 1.33 mL in a 3-mL syringe? ____________________
5. The medicine cup has a ________ mL capacity.
6. To administer exactly 0.52 mL to a child, select a ________ syringe.
7. To administer 5 mL of an oral liquid medication, select ____________________.
8. All droppers are calibrated to deliver standardized drops of equal amounts regardless of the dropper used. (True) (False)
9. The prefilled syringe is a multiple-dose system. (True) (False)
10. Insulin should be measured in an insulin syringe *only*. (True) (False)
11. The purpose of needle-free syringes is ____________________.
12. Medications are measured in syringes by aligning the calibrations with the ________ of the black rubber tip of the plunger. (top ring, raised middle section, or bottom ring)
13. The medicine cup calibrations indicate that 2 tsp are approximately ________ mL.
14. Some syringes are marked in cubic centimetres (cc) instead of millilitres (mL). (True) (False)
15. The ________ syringe is intended to measure a parenteral dose of medication. (standard 3-mL, 1-mL, or insulin)

Draw an arrow to indicate the calibration that corresponds to the dose to be administered.

16. Administer 0.45 mL.

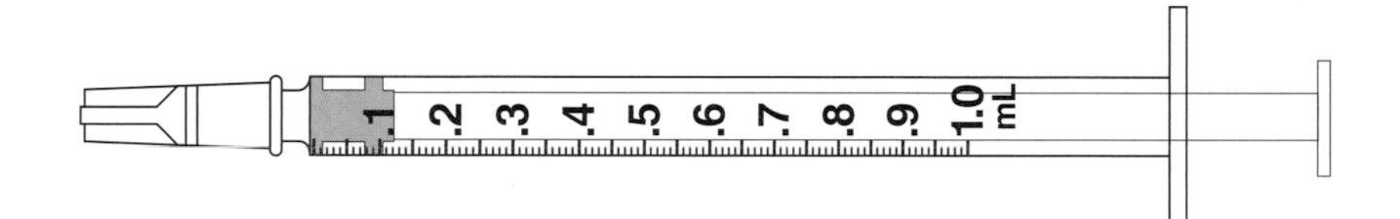

17. Administer 80 units of insulin.

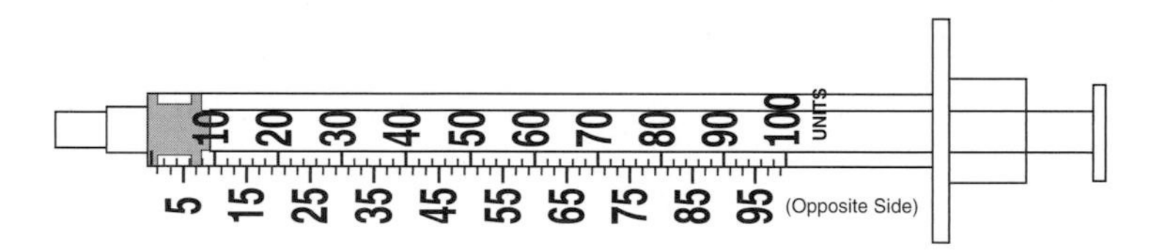

18. Administer 15 mL.

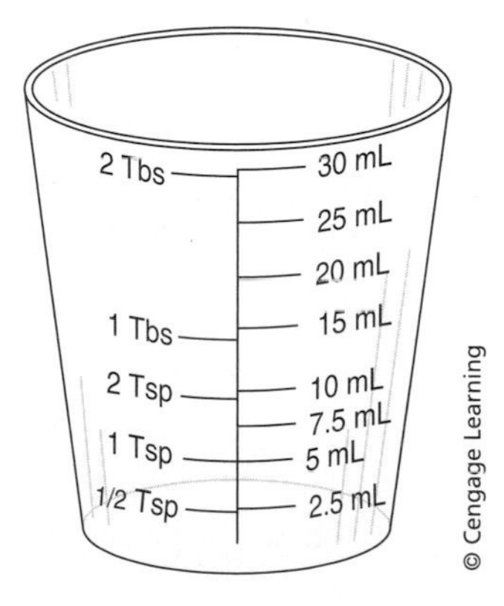

19. Administer 2.4 mL.

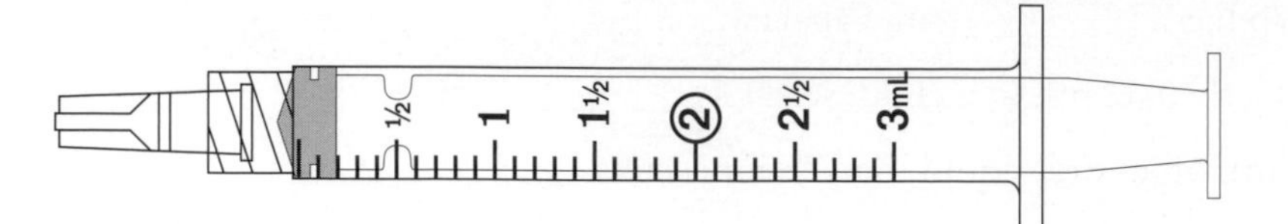

20. Administer 1.1 mL.

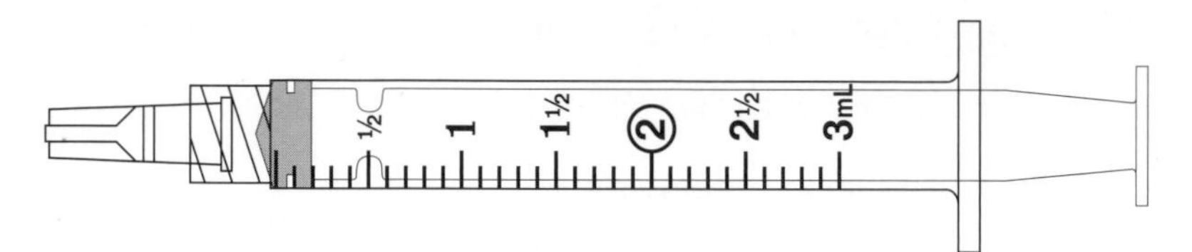

21. Administer 6.2 mL.

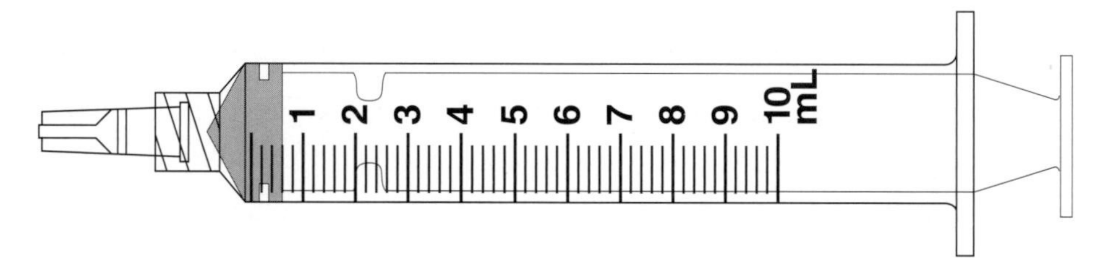

22. Administer 3.6 mL.

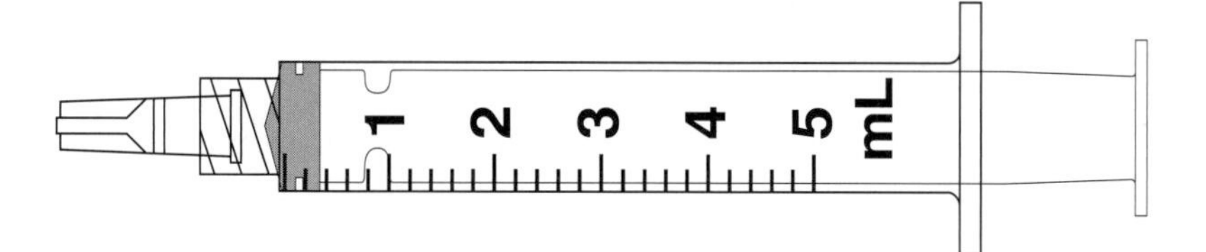

23. Administer 4.8 mL.

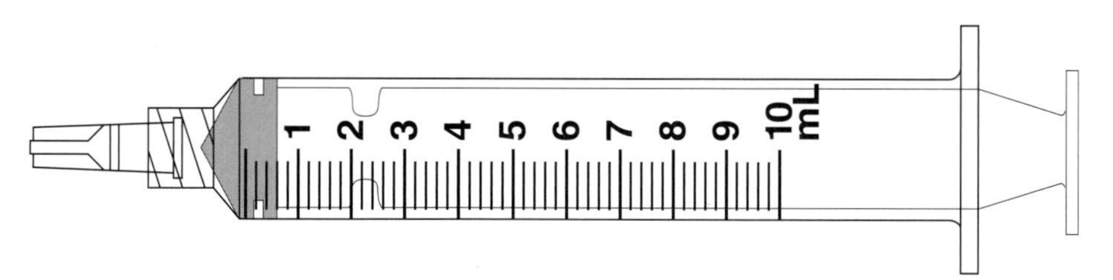

24. Administer 12 mL.

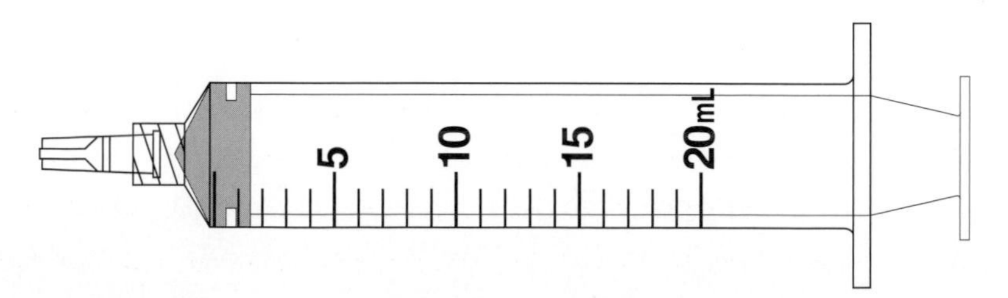

Check your work! Answers to all problems are provided at the end of the book, in the Answers section. Worked solutions for some Practice Problems are also provided there.

APPLICATION OF CLINICAL REASONING

5-1 Describe the clinical reasoning that would prevent this patient safety incident.

Possible Scenario

Suppose a patient with cancer is prescribed oral ondansetron liquid for nausea. Because the patient has had difficulty taking the medication, the nurse decided to draw up the medication in a syringe without a needle to make it easier to give the medication. An unexpected crisis situation disrupted the medication process. Once the crisis was resolved, the nurse attached a needle and injected the oral medication.

Potential Outcome

The medication would be absorbed systemically, and the patient could develop an abscess at the site of injection.

Prevention

____

____

5-2 Describe the clinical reasoning that would prevent this patient safety incident.

Possible Scenario

A child with ear infections is prescribed cefaclor oral liquid as an anti-infective. The medication comes in oral syringes for administration. The nurse fails to remove the cap on the tip of the syringe and attempts to administer the medication.

Potential Outcome

The nurse would exert enough pressure on the syringe plunger that the protective cap could pop off in the child's mouth and possibly cause the child to choke.

Prevention

____

____

Check your work! Answers to all Application of Clinical Reasoning problems are provided at the end of the book, in the Answers section.

ANSWERS TO REVIEW SETS

Review Set 5-1

1) 1-mL syringe (tuberculin) **2)** a. yes; b. Round 1.25 to 1.3 and measure on the mL scale as 1.3 mL. **3)** No **4)** a) 5-mL oral syringe; b) 10-mL oral syringe used twice (most accurate) or a medicine cup; c) 1-mL syringe; d) 2 mL syringe; e) 10-mL syringe; f) 30- or 50-unit lo-dose insulin syringe **5)** a. False; b. The size of the drop varies according to the diameter of the tip of the dropper. **6)** No **7)** Measure the oral liquid in a 3-mL oral syringe, which is not intended for injections. **8)** 5 **9)** Discard the excess prior to injecting the client. **10)** To prevent needlestick injury.

11)

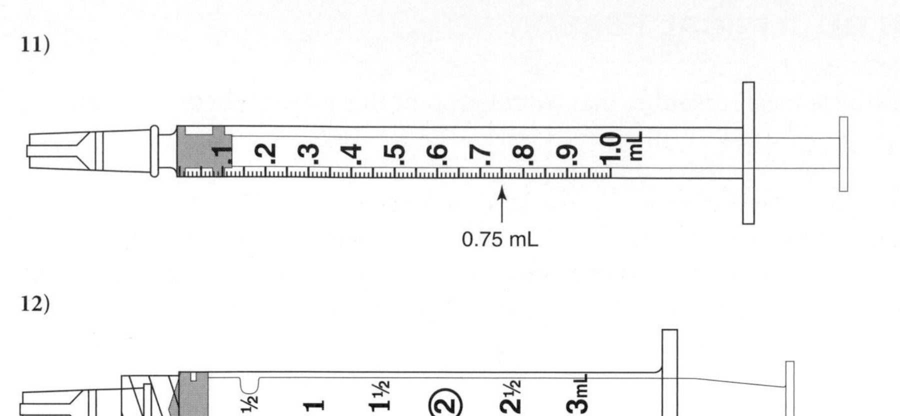

12)

½ 1 1½ 2 2½ 3mL

1.33 mL = 1.3 mL Rounded

13)

½ 1 1½ 2 2½ 3mL

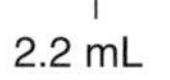

14)

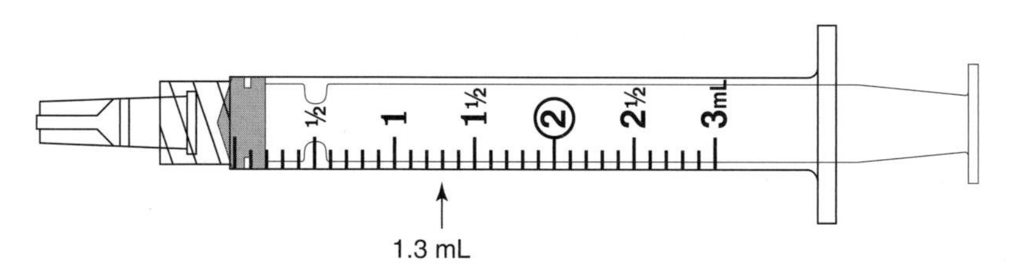

15)

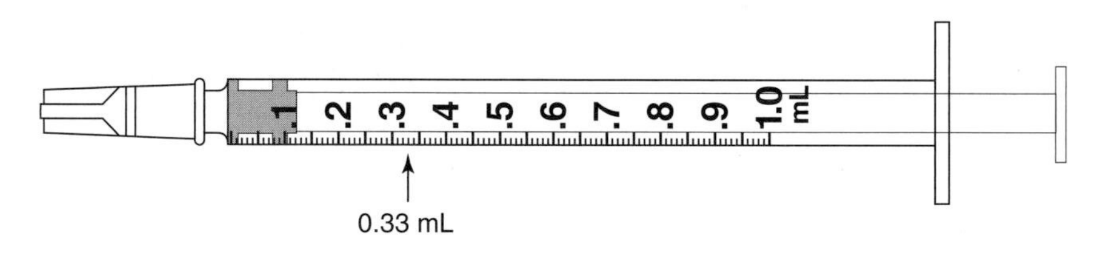

16)

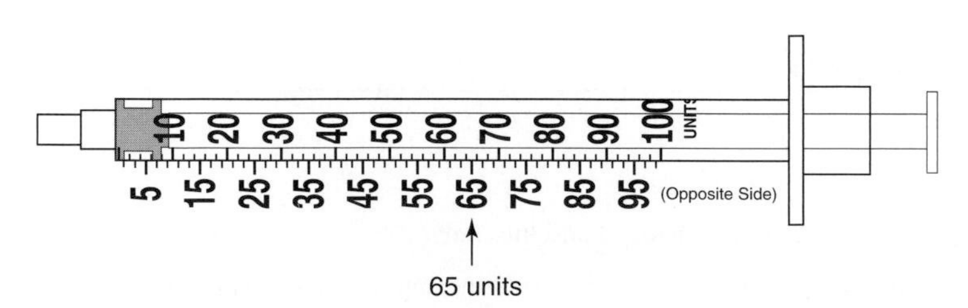

17)

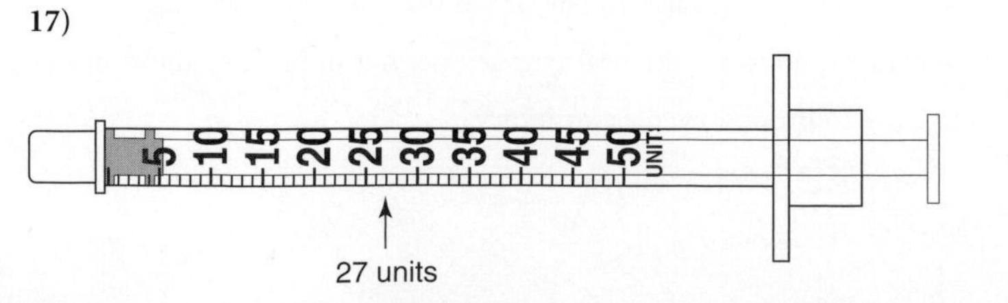

18)

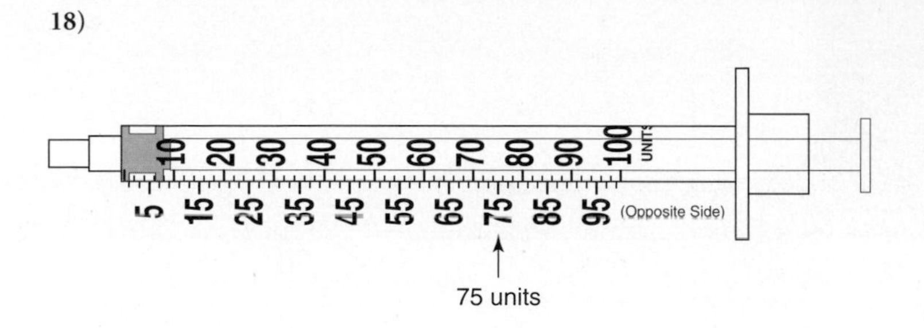

19)

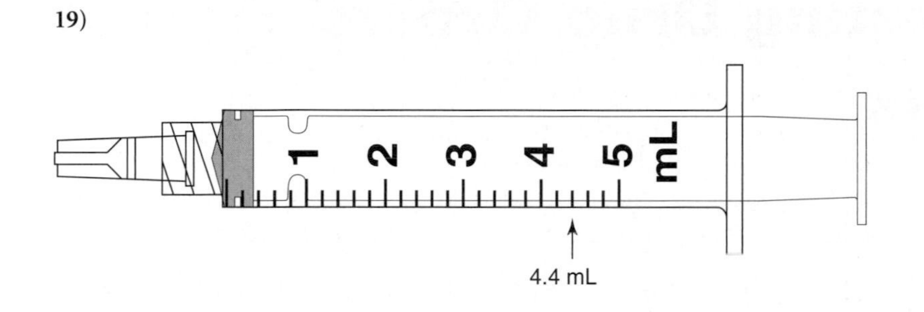

20)

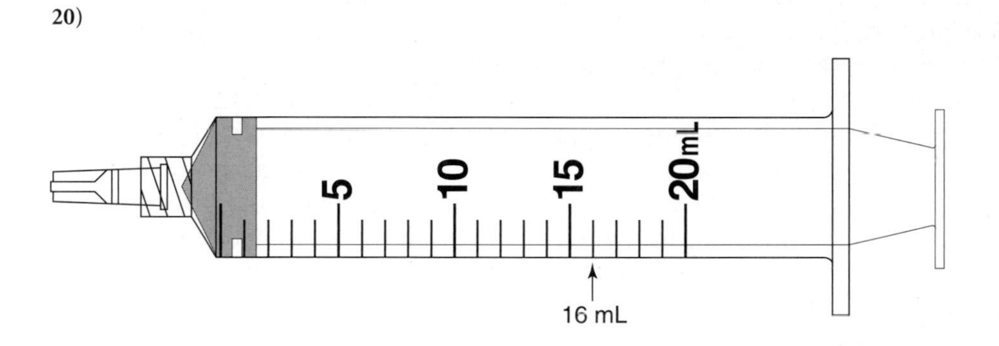

21) 0.2 mL **22)** 1 mL **23)** 0.2 mL

CHAPTER

6

Interpreting Drug Orders

OBJECTIVES

1. Interpret the standard medical abbreviations.
2. Determine notations for the dosage, route, and frequency of the medication to be administered.
3. Interpret medication orders and medication administration records.

The focus in this chapter is on accurate interpretation of a prescription or medication patient care order. However, the goal of ensuring patient safety extends beyond interpretation to adherence to standards and best practices by healthcare providers. In Canada, the provincial/territorial nursing jurisdictions are responsible for ensuring adherence to these standards and best practices. Medication management and administration is continually reviewed and updated to support patient safety. Medication administration requires knowledge, skill, and judgment. Nurses prepare and administer medications according to current evidence-informed rationales and practice-setting policies. Use of sources such as one's specific jurisdictional documents on practice standards, information from the Institute for Safe Medication Practices Canada (ISMP Canada) (www.ismp-canada.org), and current Canadian nursing practice textbooks promotes accurate and effective medication administration practice.

The prescription or medication order conveys the therapeutic drug plan for the patient. It is the responsibility of the nurse to:

- Interpret the order;
- Prepare the exact dosage of the prescribed drug;
- Identify the patient;
- Administer the proper dosage by the prescribed route, at the prescribed time intervals, for the right reason;
- Educate the patient about the medication and allow the right to refuse;
- Record the administration of the prescribed drug; and
- Monitor and document the patient's response for desired (therapeutic) and adverse effects.

Before preparing the correct dosage of the prescribed drug, it is critical to interpret the written patient care order. For brevity and speed, healthcare professions have adopted certain standards and common abbreviations for use in notation. Recognition and interpretation of abbreviations is a skill that develops with practice. However, the use of abbreviations, symbols, and dose designations are potential sources of patient safety incidents. Be sure that the interpretation is always correct; question and check if unsure.

An example of a typical written patient care order is the following:

9/4/XX amoxicillin 500 mg PO QID (pc & bedtime)
J. Prescriber

This order means that the patient should receive 500 milligrams of the antibiotic amoxicillin orally 4 times a day (after meals and at bedtime). The medical notation considerably shortens the written-out order.

MEDICAL ABBREVIATIONS

To ensure patient safety, medication orders must be clear and free from ambiguity, which means minimizing the use of dangerous abbreviations. Nurses, as well as other healthcare providers, must practise to ensure safety in the administration of medications. Misinterpretation of abbreviations contributes to patient safety incidents. The Institute for Safe Medication Practices Canada has identified abbreviations and dose designations that are problematic and has provided recommendations to correct the potential for patient safety incidents. For specific information, see www.ismp.org/newsletters/acutecare/articles/dangerousabbrev.asp.

Medication policies developed by each healthcare facility inform the nurse which abbreviations are acceptable for use in that facility. Accreditation Canada requires that all healthcare agencies implement the "Do Not Use" list of abbreviations, shown on the next page, in all medication-related documentation, both handwritten and entered as free text into a computer, to reduce the potential for medication patient safety incidents. When an abbreviation is not clearly written, it is the responsibility of the nurse to contact the writer of the order containing the abbreviation to obtain clarification and avoid any potential patient safety incidents.

CAUTION

It is critical to know and to adhere to the "Do Not Use" list of medical abbreviations in all medication-related documentation. Only abbreviations acceptable in your nursing practice setting are used in medication documentation.

REMEMBER

Common Medical Abbreviations

Abbreviation	Interpretation	Abbreviation	Interpretation
Route		ad lib	As desired, freely
IM	Intramuscular	prn	When necessary
IV	Intravenous	stat	Immediately, at once
		BID	Twice a day[1]
ID	Intradermal	**Frequency**	
Subcut	Subcutaneously		
GT	Gastrostomy tube	TID	Three times a day[1]
NG	Nasogastric tube	QID	Four times a day[1]
NJ	Nasojejunal tube	min	Minute
PO	By mouth, orally	h/hr	Hour
pr	Per rectum, rectally	qh/qhr	Every hour
Drug Formulations			
		q2h	Every two hours
CR	Controlled release	q3h	Every three hours
ER, XR, XL	Extended release	q4h	Every four hours
EC	Enteric coated	q6h	Every six hours
IR	Immediate release	q8h	Every eight hours
LA	Long acting	q12h	Every twelve hours
SR	Sustained release	**General**	
TR	Timed release	q	Every
Frequency		NPO	Nothing by mouth
ac	Before meals	gtt	Drop
pc	After meals	tab	Tablet

[1] Some healthcare agencies continue to use bid, tid, and qid; some references support avoiding these abbreviations and recommend writing out information in full. BID, TID, and QID appear in ISMP Canada documents and are common in computerized medication administration record sheets (MARS).

Do Not Use

Dangerous Abbreviations, Symbols, and Dose Designations

The abbreviations, symbols, and dose designations found in this table have been reported as being frequently misinterpreted and involved in harmful medication errors. They should NEVER be used when communicating medication information.

Abbreviation	Intended Meaning	Problem	Correction
U	Unit	Mistaken for "0" (zero), "4" (four), or cc.	Use "unit."
IU	International unit	Mistaken for "IV" (intravenous) or "10" (ten).	Use "unit."
Abbreviations for drug names		Misinterpreted because of similar abbreviations for multiple drugs; for example, MS, MSO_4 (morphine sulfate), $MgSO_4$ (magnesium sulfate) may be confused for one another.	Do not abbreviate drug names.
QD QOD	Every day Every other day	QD and QOD have been mistaken for each other, or as 'qid'. The Q has also been misinterpreted as "2" (two).	Use "daily" and "every other day."
OD	Every day	Mistaken for "right eye" (OD = oculus dexter).	Use "daily."
OS, OD, OU	Left eye, right eye, both eyes	May be confused with one another.	Use "left eye," "right eye," or "both eyes."
D/C	Discharge	Interpreted as "discontinue whatever medications follow" (typically discharge medications).	Use "discharge."
cc	Cubic centimetre	Mistaken for "u" (units).	Use "mL" or "millilitre."
μg	Microgram	Mistaken for "mg" (milligram) resulting in one thousand-fold overdose.	Use "mcg."
Symbol	**Intended Meaning**	**Potential Problem**	**Correction**
@	At	Mistaken for "2" (two) or "5" (five).	Use "at."
> <	Greater than Less than	Mistaken for "7" (seven) or the letter "L." Confused with each other.	Use "greater than"/"more than" or "less than"/"lower than."
Dose Designation	**Intended Meaning**	**Potential Problem**	**Correction**
Trailing zero	*X*.0 mg	Decimal point is overlooked resulting in 10-fold dose error.	Never use a zero by itself after a decimal point. Use "***X* mg**."
Lack of leading zero	.*X* mg	Decimal point is overlooked resulting in 10-fold dose error.	Always use a zero before a decimal point. Use "**0.*X*** mg."

Report actual and potential patient safety incidents to ISMP Canada via the Web at www.cmirps-scdpim.ca/

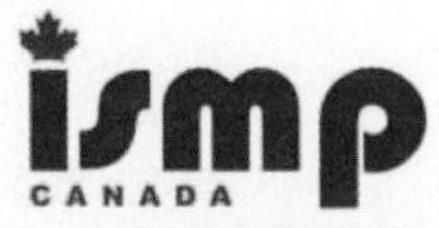

Institute for Safe Medication Practices Canada
Institut pour l'utilisation sécuritaire des médicaments du Canada

The table on previous page lists some common medical abbreviations used in writing drug orders. The abbreviations are grouped according to the route (or method) of administration, the drug formulation, the frequency (time interval), and general terms.

THE DRUG ORDER

The drug order consists of seven parts:

1. Name of the ***patient***
2. Name of the ***drug*** to be administered
3. ***Dose*** of the drug
4. ***Route*** by which the drug is to be administered
5. ***Frequency,*** time, and special instructions related to administration
6. ***Date and time*** when the order was written
7. ***Signature*** of the person writing the order

CAUTION

If any of the seven parts of the drug order is missing or unclear, the order is considered incomplete and is, therefore, not a legal patient care order. The nurse *must obtain* clarification of the order from the writer.

Parts 1 through 5 of the drug order comprise what is considered the original Five Rights of safe medication administration. They are essential, and each one must be routinely checked every time a medication is prepared and administered. Safe administration of medication requires the healthcare provider to accurately document the drug administration. Accurate documentation along with the right reason, the right frequency, and the right site have been added to the Rights of safe medication administration with variance as to how this is expressed across provincial/territorial nursing jurisdictions.

REMEMBER

The Rights of safe and accurate medication administration:

The *right patient* must receive the *right drug* for the *right reason* in the *right amount* by the *right route* in the *right site* at the *right time* and *right frequency*, with the *right to refuse*, followed by the *right documentation.*

Each patient care order follows a specific sequence. The name of the drug is written first, followed by the dosage, route, and frequency. Drugs are identified with generic (non-proprietary) and brand (trade or proprietary) names. The order may be written using generic or brand names, or both. Combination and over-the-counter drugs are often identified by brand name (e.g., Aggrenox contains 200 mg extended-release dipyridamole and 25 mg immediate-release acetylsalicylic acid [ASA or Aspirin]). When correctly written, the trade name of the drug begins with a capital or upper case letter. The generic name begins with a lower case letter.

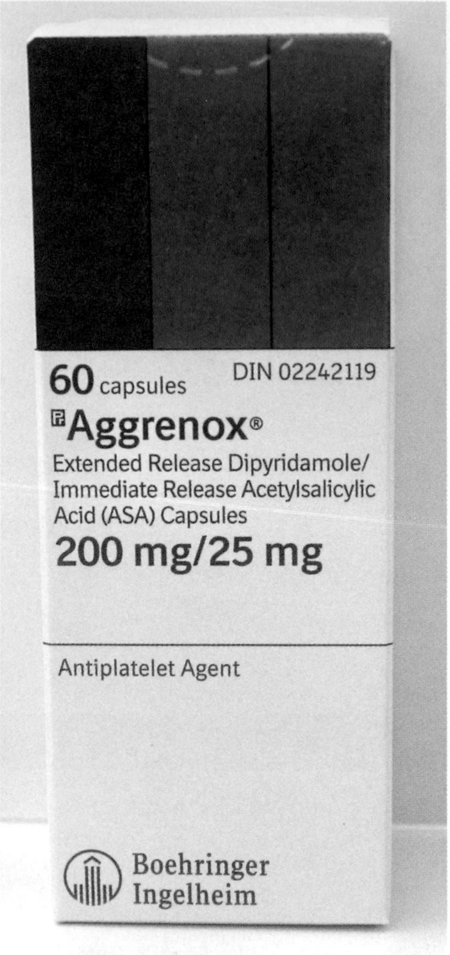

60 capsules DIN 02242119
Aggrenox®
Extended Release Dipyridamole/
Immediate Release Acetylsalicylic
Acid (ASA) Capsules
200 mg/25 mg
Antiplatelet Agent
Boehringer Ingelheim

Courtesy of Boehringer Ingelheim

Aggrenox 25/200 mg ER capsules. Note that the trade name is prominent on the label and begins with an upper case letter, while the generic combination is written below the trade name. Each capsule contains 200 mg dipyridamole ER and 25 mg Aspirin.

CAUTION

The healthcare provider must know current correct information about drugs, whether identified by generic or brand names. Authoritative resources include the Compendium of Pharmaceuticals and Specialties (CPS), Health Canada's Drug Product Database website, drug package enclosures with the manufacturer's information, and licensed pharmacists.

Example:

Pen VK 300 mg PO QID for 10 days

Note: This order could have been written using the generic name (recommended in many jurisdictions). It would look like *penicillin V potassium 300 mg PO QID for 10 days.*

1. *Pen VK* is the brand name of the drug.
2. *300 mg* is the dosage.

3. *PO* is the route.
4. *QID* is the frequency.
5. *For 10 days* indicates that there is a time limit on the use of this medication.

This order means "Give 300 milligrams of penicillin V potassium orally 4 times a day for 10 days."

CAUTION

If the nurse has difficulty interpreting the patient care order, the nurse *must* clarify the order with the prescriber. Usually this person is the physician or another authorized healthcare provider.

The following examples provide the opportunity to practise reading and interpreting patient care orders.

Example 1:

phenytoin 100 mg PO TID

Reads: "Give 100 milligrams of phenytoin orally 3 times a day."

Example 2:

procaine penicillin G 400 000 units IM q6h

Reads: "Give 400 000 units of procaine penicillin G intramuscularly every 6 hours."

Example 3:

meperidine hydrochloride 75 mg IM q4h prn for pain

Reads: "Give 75 milligrams of meperidine hydrochloride intramuscularly every 4 hours when necessary for pain."

CAUTION

The *prn* frequency designates the minimum time allowed between doses. There is no maximum time other than automatic stops as defined by institution policy.

Example 4:

Humulin R insulin 5 units subcutaneously stat

Reads: "Give 5 units of Humulin R insulin subcutaneously immediately."

Example 5:

cephalexin 1 g IV q6h

Reads: "Give 1 gram of cephalexin intravenously every 6 hours."

The administration times are designated by institution policy. For example, TID administration times may be 0900, 1300, and 1700.

QUICK REVIEW

- The *right patient* must receive the *right drug* for the *right reason* in the *right amount* by the *right route* in the *right site* at the *right time, with the right to refuse*, and the *right frequency*, followed by the *right documentation.*
- Understanding patient care orders requires interpreting common medical abbreviations.
- The patient care order must contain the following (in this sequence): drug name, dosage, route, and frequency.
- All parts of the patient care order must be written clearly for accurate, exact interpretation.
- If ever in doubt of the meaning of any part of a patient care order, ask the prescriber to clarify before proceeding.

REVIEW SET 6-1

Interpret the following medication (drug) orders.

1. *naproxen 250 mg PO BID* ______________________________

2. *Humulin R insulin 30 units subcut daily 30 min before breakfast* ______________________________

3. *cefaclor 500 mg PO stat, then 250 mg q8h* ______________________________

4. *levothyroxine 25 mcg PO daily* ______________________________

5. *lorazepam 10 mg IM q4h prn for agitation* ______________________________

6. *cefazolin 500 mg IVPB as per protocol* ______________________________

7. *aluminum hydroxide 10 mL PO hs* ______________________________

8. *atropine sulfate ophthalmic 1% 2 gtt OD q15 min × 4* ______________________________

9. *morphine sulfate 15 mg IM q3–4h prn for pain* ______________________________

10. *digoxin 0.25 mg PO daily* ______________________________

11. *tetracycline 250 mg PO QID* ______________________________

12. *nitroglycerin 0.6 mg SL stat* ______________________________

13. *Sofracort otic suspension 2 gtt AU TID and hs* ______________________________

14. Compare and contrast *TID* and *q8h* administration times. Include sample administration times for each in your explanation. ______________________________

____

15. Describe your action if no method of administration is written. ______________

____

16. Do *QID* and *q4h* have the same meaning? ________ Explain. ______________

____

17. Who determines the medication administration times? ______________

____

18. Name the seven parts of a written medication prescription. ______________

____

19. In Canada, what are the three sources of information on current medication practices?

____

20. Identify the Rights of safe and accurate medication administration as noted in this chapter. ______________________________

____

Check your work! Answers to all Review Sets are provided at the end of each chapter. Worked solutions for selected Review Sets are also available there.

Medication Order and Administration Forms

Hospitals have a special form for recording drug orders. This form may vary across different healthcare settings. All settings require dating on these forms but the date format may vary. Figure 6-1 shows a sample order form. In some jurisdictions and practice areas, orders may be written by healthcare providers other than a physician, and forms may be labelled Patient Care Orders. Find and name each of the seven parts of the patient care orders listed. Notice that the nurse or other healthcare provider

ENTERED	FILLED	CHECKED	VERIFIED
			—

NOTE: A NON-PROPRIETARY DRUG OF EQUAL QUALITY MAY BE DISPENSED - IF THIS COLUMN IS NOT CHECKED!

DATE	TIME WRITTEN	PLEASE USE BALL POINT - PRESS FIRMLY	✓	TIME NOTED	NURSES SIGNATURE
11/3/xx	0815	cephalexin 250 mg PO q6h	✓	0830	B. Swart, RN
		Humulin R Insulin 40 units subcut ac breakfast	✓		
		morphine sulfate 10 mg IV q3 h prn for severe pain	✓		
		codeine phosphate 30 mg PO q4h prn for mild–mod pain	✓		
		acetaminophen 650 mg PO q4h prn for fever greater than 38.3°C	✓		
		furosemide 40 mg IV stat	✓		
		potassium chloride sustained-release tablets 1500 mg PO BID	✓		
		J. Prescriber, MD			
11/3/xx	2200	furosemide 80 mg IV stat	✓		
		J. Prescriber, MD		2210	M. Smith, RN

AUTO STOP ORDERS: UNLESS REORDERED, FOLLOWING WILL BE D/C'D AT 0800 ON:

DATE	ORDER		PHYSICIAN SIGNATURE
		☐ CONT ☐ D/C	PHYSICIAN SIGNATURE
		☐ CONT ☐ D/C	PHYSICIAN SIGNATURE
		☐ CONT ☐ D/C	PHYSICIAN SIGNATURE

CHECK WHEN ANTIBIOTICS ORDERED ☐ Prophylactic ☐ Empiric ☐ Therapeutic

Allergies: None Known

CLIENT DIAGNOSIS Type 1 Diabetes

HEIGHT 166 cm WEIGHT 59 kg

Patient, Mary Q.
#3-11316-7

FORM 959-708 (8-XX) PHYSICIANS ORDER Reynolds + Reynolds LITHO IN U.S.A. K41814 (7-XX) D339360

1

FIGURE 6-1 Prescriber's Order

must verify and initiate each order, ensuring that each of the seven parts is accurate. In some places, the pharmacist may be responsible for verifying the order as part of the computerized record.

The drug orders from the prescriber's order form are transcribed to a medication administration record (MAR), such as the one shown in Figure 6-2. This form may vary across different healthcare settings. The nurse or other healthcare provider uses this record as a guide to

- Check the patient care order;
- Prepare the correct dosage; and
- Record the drug administered.

These three checkpoints help ensure accurate medication administration.

PAGE ____ of ____

MEDICATION ADMINISTRATION RECORD

ORIGINAL ORDER DATE	DATE STARTED / RENEWED	MEDICATION - DOSAGE	ROUTE	SCHEDULE 23-07	SCHEDULE 07-15	SCHEDULE 15-23	DATE 11/3/xx 23-07	11/3/xx 07-15	11/3/xx 15-23	DATE 11/4/xx 23-07	11/4/xx 07-15	11/4/xx 15-23	DATE 11/5/xx 23-07	11/5/xx 07-15	11/5/xx 15-23	DATE 11/6/xx 23-07	11/6/xx 07-15	11/6/xx 15-23
11/3/xx	11/3/xx	cephalexin 250 mg q6h	PO	24 06	12	18		GP 12	MS 18	24JJ 06JJ	GP 12	MS 18						
11/4/xx	11/4/xx	Humulin R insulin 40 units before breakfast	sub-cut		0730						GP 0730Ⓑ							
11/3/xx	11/3/xx	furosemide 40 mg daily	PO		09			GP 09			GP 09							
11/3/xx	11/3/xx	potassium chloride SR 1500 mg BID	PO		09	21			MS 21		GP 09	MS 21						
		PRN																
11/3/xx	11/3/xx	morphine sulfate 10 mg q3h	IV	severe pain				GP 12Ⓛ	MS 18Ⓜ-		10Ⓙ							
11/3/xx	11/4/xx	codeine phosphate 30 mg q4h	PO	mild–mod pain						JJ 06	GP 14							
11/3/xx	11/3/xx	acetaminophen 650 mg q4h	PO	fever greater than 38.3°C				GP 12	MS 16–20	JJ 24–04	GP 08–12							

INJECTION SITES: B - RIGHT ARM; C - RIGHT ABDOMEN; D - RIGHT ANTERIOR THIGH; G - LEFT ARM; H - LEFT ABDOMEN; J - LEFT ANTERIOR THIGH; L - LEFT BUTTOCKS; M - RIGHT BUTTOCKS

DATE GIVEN	TIME	INT.	ONE - TIME MEDICATION - DOSAGE	RT.
11/3/xx	2200	ms	furosemide	IV

SIGNATURE OF NURSE ADMINISTERING MEDICATIONS	DATE 11/3/xx	DATE 11/4/xx	DATE	DATE
23-07		JJ J. Jones, LPN		
07-15	BS B. Swart, RN GP G. Pinar, RN	BS B. Swart, RN GP G. Pinar, RN		
15-23	MS M. Smith, RN	MS M. Smith, RN		

DATE GIVEN	TIME	INT.	MEDICATION-DOSAGE-CONT.	RT.

RECOPIED BY:

CHECKED BY:

ALLERGIES: None Known

Patient, Mary Q.

#3-11316-7

ORIGINAL COPY

602-31 (7-XX) (MPC# 1355)

LITHO IN U.S.A. K6508 (7-92) D39553

PRINTED BY STANDARD REGISTER U.S.A. ZIPSET ®

FIGURE 6-2 Medication Administration Record

COMPUTERIZED MEDICATION ADMINISTRATION SYSTEMS

Most healthcare facilities now use computers to process patient care orders. Patient care orders are either electronically transmitted or manually entered into the computer from an order form, such as the one shown in Figure 6-3. Through the computer, the healthcare provider can transmit the order within seconds to the pharmacy for filling. The computer can keep track of drug stock and usage patterns. Most importantly, it can scan for information previously entered, such as drug incompatibilities, drug allergies,

ENTERED	FILLED	CHECKED	VERIFIED
			—

NOTE: A NON-PROPRIETARY DRUG OF EQUAL QUALITY MAY BE DISPENSED - IF THIS COLUMN IS NOT CHECKED!

DATE	TIME WRITTEN	PLEASE USE BALL POINT - PRESS FIRMLY	✓	TIME NOTED	NURSES SIGNATURE
8/31/XX	1500	procainamide hydrochloride 500 mg PO q6h	✓		
		J. Prescriber, MD		1515	M. Smith, RN
9/3/XX	0830	digoxin 0.125 mg PO daily	✓	0715	B. Swart, RN
		furosemide 40 mg PO daily	✓		
		metoclopramide hydrochloride 10 mg PO stat & ac & at bedtime	✓		
		potassium chloride sustained-release tablets 1500 mg PO BID start 9/4/XX	✓		
		nitroglycerin 0.4 mg SL prn	✓		
		Percocet tab 1 PO q4h prn for mild-moderate pain	✓		
		morphine sulfate 10 mg IV q43h prn for severe pain	✓		
		promethazine hydrochloride 50 mg IV q4h prn for nausea.	✓		
		Administer with morphine sulfate			
		J. Prescriber, MD			

AUTO STOP ORDERS: UNLESS REORDERED, FOLLOWING WILL BE D/C'D AT 0800 ON:

DATE	ORDER		
		☐ CONT ☐ D/C	PHYSICIAN SIGNATURE
		☐ CONT ☐ D/C	PHYSICIAN SIGNATURE
		☐ CONT ☐ D/C	PHYSICIAN SIGNATURE

CHECK WHEN ANTIBIOTICS ORDERED ☐ Prophylactic ☐ Empiric ☐ Therapeutic

Allergies: No known allergies

CLIENT DIAGNOSIS: heart failure

HEIGHT 177.8 cm WEIGHT 74.5 kg

Patient, John D.
#3-81512-3

FORM 959-708 (8-XX) **PHYSICIANS ORDER** Reynolds + Reynolds LITHO IN U.S.A. K41814 (7-XX) D339360

1

FIGURE 6-3 Physician's Order

safe dosage ranges, doses already given, and recommended administration times. The healthcare staff can be readily alerted to potential problems and inconsistencies. The corresponding MAR may also be printed directly from the computer (Figure 6-4).

The computerized MAR may be viewed at the computer or from a printed copy (Figure 6-4). The healthcare provider may be able to look back at the patient's cumulative MARS, document administration times, and comments at the computer terminal and then keep a printed copy of the information obtained and entered. The data analysis, storage, and retrieval abilities of computers make them essential tools for safe and accurate medication administration.

Note that in Figures 6-1, 6-2, 6-3, and 6-4, there is no range for intervals to repeat medication. While this practice of including a range for intervals of medications may still occur in practice, there is a shift to indicate only the minimal interval for repeat. Also, although the generic name is the preferred name when writing an order, brand or trade names still do appear, especially with combination medications, for example, Percocet, a combination of 325 mg acetaminophen and 5 mg oxycodone hydrochloride.

REMEMBER

It is important to be aware and comply with practice in one's specific area of practice.

PHARMACY MAR

START	STOP	MEDICATION	SCHEDULED TIMES	OK'D BY	0001 TO 1200	1201 TO 2400
08/31/xx 1800 SCH		PROCAINAMIDE HCL 500 MG TAB-SR 500 mg Q6H PO	0600 1200 1800 2400	JD	0600 BS 1200 BS	1800 MS 2400 JD
09/03/xx 0900 SCH		DIGOXIN 0.125 MG TAB 1 TAB daily PO	0900	JD	0900 BS	
09/03/xx 0900 SCH		FUROSEMIDE 40 MG TAB 1 TAB daily PO	0900	JD	0900 BS	
09/03/xx 0845 SCH		METOCLOPRAMIDE 10 MG TAB 10 mg AC&HS PO GIVE ONE NOW	0730 1130 1630 2100	JD	0730 BS 1130 BS	1630 MS 2100 MS
09/04/xx 0900 SCH		POTASSIUM CHLORIDE 20 mEq MEQ (equivalent to 1500 mg potassium chloride) SR TAB 2 TAB BID PO START 9-4	0900 1700	JD	0900 BS	2100 BS
09/03/xx 1507 PRN		NITROGLYCERIN 0.4 mg TAB-SL 1 TABLET PRN SL PRN CHEST PAIN		JD		
09/03/xx 1700 PRN		OXYCODONE 5 mg and ACETAMINOPHEN 325 mg Percocet 1 TAB Q4H PO PRN MILD–MODERATE PAIN		JD		
09/03/xx 2100 PRN		MORPHINE SULFATE INJ 10 mg Q3H IV PRN SEVERE PAIN W PHENERGAN		JD		2200 (H) MS
09/03/xx 2100 PRN		PROMETHAZINE (PHENERGAN) INJ 50 mg Q4H IV PRN NAUSEA W morphine sulfate		JD		2200 (H) MS

Gluteus	Thigh
A. Right	H. Right
B. Left	I. Left
Ventro Gluteal	
C. Right	J. Right
D. Left	K. Left
E. Abdomen 1 2 / 3 4	

730-13 (12/xx)

	NURSE'S SIGNATURE	INITIAL
7–3	B. Swart, RN	BS
3–11	M. Smith, RN	MS
11–7	J. Doe, RN	JD

ALLERGIES: NKA

DIAGNOSIS: CHF

Patient: Patient, John D.
Patient# 3-81512-3
Admitted: 08/31/xx
Physician: J. Prescriber, MD
Room: PCU-14 PCU

FIGURE 6-4 Computerized Medication Administration Record

QUICK REVIEW

- Drug orders are prescribed on the Physician's Orders form or similar forms, such as a Patient Care Orders form.
- The person who administers a drug records it on the MAR. This record may be handwritten or computerized.
- All parts of the patient care order must be written clearly for accurate, exact interpretation. If ever in doubt about the meaning of any part of a patient care order, ask the prescriber to clarify.

REVIEW SET 6-2

Refer to the MAR (Figure 6-2) on page 119 to answer questions 1 through 10.

1. What is the route of administration for the insulin? ____________
2. How many times in a 24-hour period will furosemide be administered? ____________
3. What is the only medication ordered to be given routinely at noon? ____________
4. What time of day is the insulin to be administered? ____________
5. A dosage of 1500 mg of potassium chloride sustained-release tablets is ordered. This is equivalent to 20 mEq of potassium. What does *mEq* mean?

   ____
6. The patient requests that the potassium chloride be crushed as the pill is too large to be swallowed. Should the nurse follow the patient's request? Explain.

   ____

   ____
7. The nurse works 1500 to 2300 on November 5. Which routine medications will the nurse administer to Mary Q. Patient during the shift?

   ____
8. Mary Q. Patient has a temperature of 38.9°C. What medication should be administered?

   ____
9. How many times in a 24-hour period will potassium chloride sustained-release tablets be administered? ____________
10. Identify the place on the MAR where the stat IV furosemide was charted. ____________

Refer to the computerized MAR (Figure 6-4) on page 121 to answer questions 11 through 20. Identify the scheduled international time.

11. Scheduled times for administering procainamide hydrochloride ____________
12. Scheduled times for administering digoxin and furosemide ____________
13. Scheduled times for administering metoclopramide ____________
14. Scheduled times for administering potassium chloride sustained-release tablets ____________
15. How often can the morphine sulfate be given? ____________
16. If the digoxin was last given on 09/07/xx at 0900 what are the next time and date it will be given? ____________
17. What is the ordered route of administration for the nitroglycerin? ____________
18. How many times a day is furosemide ordered? ____________
19. The equivalent dosage of digoxin is ________ mcg.
20. Which drugs are ordered to be administered "as necessary"? ____________

Check your work! Answers to all Review Sets are provided at the end of each chapter. Worked solutions for selected Review Sets are also available there.

APPLICATION OF CLINICAL REASONING

It is the responsibility of the nurse to clarify any patient care order that is incomplete, that is, an order that does not contain the essential seven parts discussed in this chapter. Now look at an example in which this type of patient safety incident occurred.

Potential Patient Safety Incident

Failing to clarify incomplete orders.

Possible Scenario

Suppose a prescriber ordered *famotidine tablet PO at bedtime* for a patient with an active duodenal ulcer. Nurse 2 notes there is no dosage listed. Nurse 1 thought the medication came in only one dosage strength, added 20 mg to the order, and sent it to the pharmacy. The pharmacist prepared the dosage written on the prescriber's order sheet. Two days later, during rounds, the prescriber noted that the patient had not responded well to the famotidine. When asked about the famotidine, the nurse explained that the patient had received 20 mg at bedtime. The prescriber informed the nurse that the patient should have received the 40-mg tablet.

Potential Outcome

Potentially, the delay in correct dosage could result in gastrointestinal bleeding or delayed healing of the ulcer.

Prevention

This patient safety incident could have been avoided simply by the prescriber writing the strength of the medication. Since this was omitted, the nurse should have checked the dosage before sending the order to the pharmacy. When the nurse fills in an incomplete order, the nurse is prescribing a medicine that is not within the scope of practice. As well the patient is being exposed to potential harm.

Application of Critical Reasoning Additional application problems are provided at the end of the chapter. Answers are provided at the end of the book.

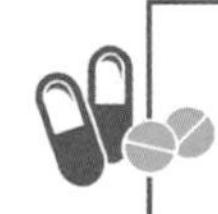

UNDERSTANDING NCLEX QUESTIONS

Here's an example of a standard question used in textbooks:

The following orders were written by a prescriber. Which order is written correctly?

a. Aspirin 2 tablets prn
b. haloperidol ½ tablet at bedtime
c. zolpidem 5 mg PO at bedtime prn
d. levothyroxine (Synthroid) 0.05 mg 1 tablet

Here's how the question would look in an NCLEX examination:

The nurse is checking the following orders written by a prescriber. Which order would the nurse consider to be clear and correct?

a. Aspirin 2 tablets prn
b. haloperidol ½ tablet at bedtime
c. zolpidem 5 mg PO at bedtime prn
d. levothyroxine (Synthroid) 0.05 mg 1 tablet

Answer: c

Rationale: The order has the drug, dosage, route, time, and frequency.

PRACTICE PROBLEMS—CHAPTER 6

Interpret the following abbreviations and symbols without consulting another source.

1. NG ________
2. pr ________
3. ac ________
4. SL ________
5. TID ________
6. q4h ________
7. prn ________
8. PO ________
9. tab ________
10. stat ________
11. ad lib ________
12. IM ________
13. pc ________

Give the abbreviation or symbol for the following terms without consulting another source.

14. nothing by mouth ________
15. drop ________
16. millilitre ________
17. at bedtime ________
18. gram ________
19. 4 times a day ________
20. every hour ________
21. subcutaneous ________
22. intravenous ________
23. twice daily ________
24. every 3 hours ________
25. every 12 hours ________
26. capsule ________
27. kilogram ________

Interpret the following prescriber drug orders without consulting another source.

28. *sustained release* ________________
29. *enteric coated* ________________
30. *long acting* ________________
31. *immediate release* ________________
32. *keterolac tromethamine 60 mg IM stat and q6h* ________________
33. *procaine penicillin G 300 000 units IM QID* ________________
34. *Mylanta tab 1 PO 1 h ac, 1 h pc, at bedtime and q2h during the night prn for gastric upset* ________________
35. *chlordiazepoxide 25 mg PO q6h prn for agitation* ________________
36. *heparin sodium 5000 units subcutaneously stat* ________________
37. *codeine sulfate 150 mg CR tablet q12h for pain* ________________
38. *digoxin 0.25 mg PO daily* ________________
39. *Optimyxin Plus ophthalmic 2 gtt left eye QID* ________________
40. *furosemide 40 mg IM stat* ________________
41. *betamethasone 4 mg IV BID* ________________

Refer to the MAR in Figure 6-5 on page 126 to answer questions 42 through 45.

42. How many units of heparin sodium will the patient receive at 2200? ________________

43. What route is ordered for the Humulin R insulin? ______________________

44. Interpret the order for ciprofloxacin hydrochloride. ______________________

45. If the administration times for the sliding scale insulin are accurate (30 minutes before meals), what times will meals be served? ______________________

Refer to the Computerized Pharmacy MAR in Figure 6-6 on page 127 to answer questions 46 through 49.

46. The prescriber visited at 1700 on 08/08/xx. What order did the prescriber write? ______________________

____

47. Interpret the order for ranitidine hydrochloride. ______________________

48. Which of the routine medication(s) is(are) ordered for 1800? ______________________

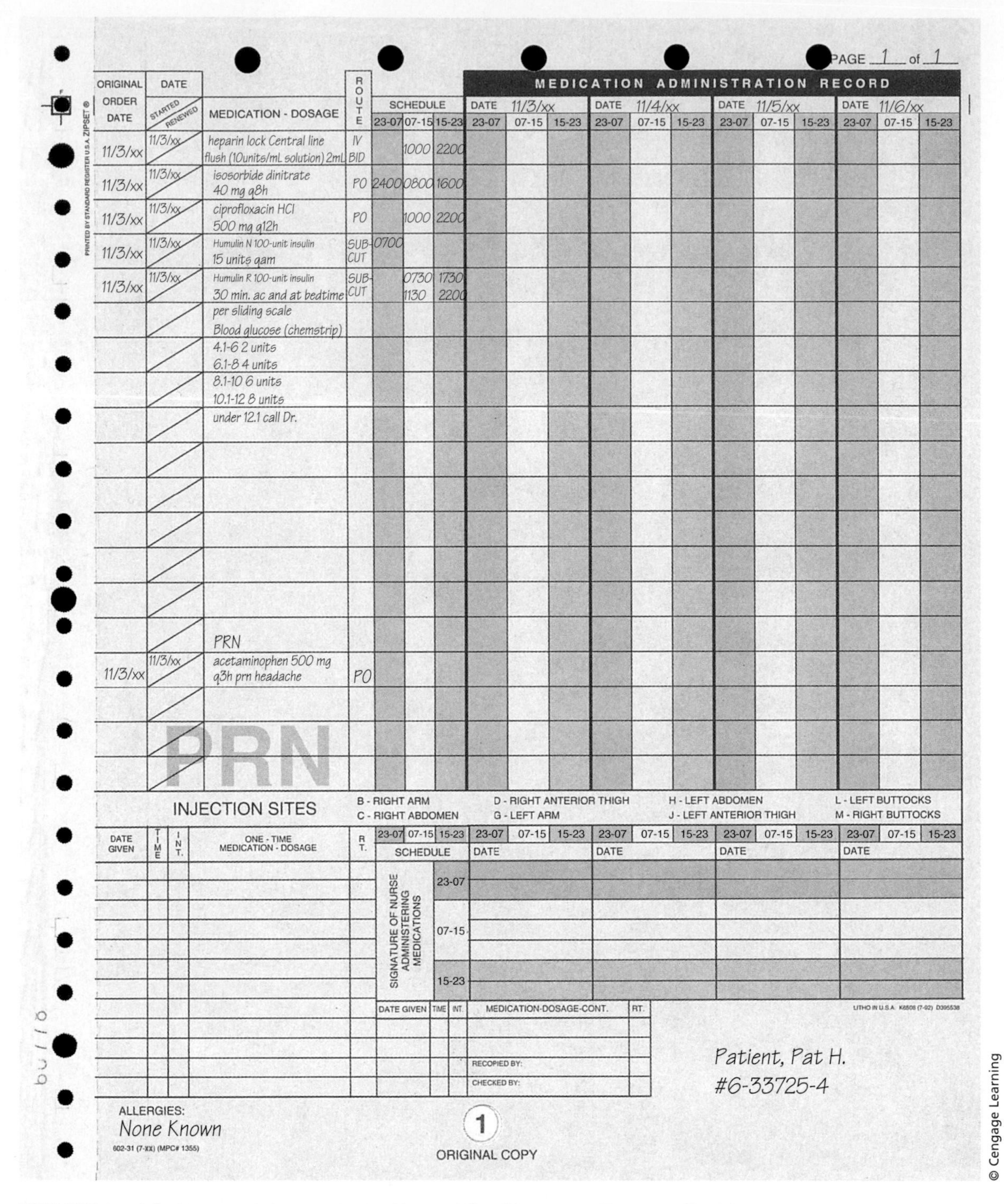

PAGE 1 of 1

MEDICATION ADMINISTRATION RECORD

ORIGINAL ORDER DATE	DATE STARTED / RENEWED	MEDICATION - DOSAGE	ROUTE	SCHEDULE 23-07	SCHEDULE 07-15	SCHEDULE 15-23
11/3/xx	11/3/xx	heparin lock Central line flush (10units/mL solution) 2mL	IV BID		1000	2200
11/3/xx	11/3/xx	isosorbide dinitrate 40 mg q8h	PO	2400	0800	1600
11/3/xx	11/3/xx	ciprofloxacin HCl 500 mg q12h	PO		1000	2200
11/3/xx	11/3/xx	Humulin N 100-unit insulin 15 units qam	SUB-CUT	0700		
11/3/xx	11/3/xx	Humulin R 100-unit insulin 30 min. ac and at bedtime per sliding scale Blood glucose (chemstrip) 4.1-6 2 units 6.1-8 4 units 8.1-10 6 units 10.1-12 8 units under 12.1 call Dr.	SUB-CUT		0730 1130	1730 2200
		PRN				
11/3/xx	11/3/xx	acetaminophen 500 mg q3h prn headache	PO			

DATE 11/3/xx: 23-07 | 07-15 | 15-23
DATE 11/4/xx: 23-07 | 07-15 | 15-23
DATE 11/5/xx: 23-07 | 07-15 | 15-23
DATE 11/6/xx: 23-07 | 07-15 | 15-23

PRN

INJECTION SITES

B - RIGHT ARM
C - RIGHT ABDOMEN
D - RIGHT ANTERIOR THIGH
G - LEFT ARM
H - LEFT ABDOMEN
J - LEFT ANTERIOR THIGH
L - LEFT BUTTOCKS
M - RIGHT BUTTOCKS

DATE GIVEN	TIME	INT.	ONE - TIME MEDICATION - DOSAGE	RT.

SIGNATURE OF NURSE ADMINISTERING MEDICATIONS: 23-07 | 07-15 | 15-23

DATE GIVEN	TIME	INT.	MEDICATION-DOSAGE-CONT.	RT.

RECOPIED BY:

CHECKED BY:

Patient, Pat H.
#6-33725-4

ALLERGIES:
None Known

602-31 (7-XX) (MPC# 1355)

PRINTED BY STANDARD REGISTER U.S.A. ZIPSET ®

1

ORIGINAL COPY

LITHO IN U.S.A.

FIGURE 6-5 Medication Administration Record for Chapter 6 Practice Problems (Questions 42 through 45)

PHARMACY MAR

START	STOP	MEDICATION	SCHEDULED TIMES	OK'D BY	0701 TO 1500	1501 TO 2300	2301 TO 0700
21:00 8/17/xx SCH		MEGESTROL ACETATE (APO-MEGESTROL) 40 mg TAB 2 TABS PO BID	0900 2100				
12:00 8/17/xx SCH		VANCOMYCIN 250 mg CAP 1 CAPSULE PO QID	0800 1200 1800 2200				
9:00 8/13/xx SCH		FLUCONAZOLE (DIFLUCAN) 100 mg TAB 100 MG PO QD	0900				
21:00 8/11/xx SCH		PERIDEX ORAL RINSE 480 mL 30 mL ORAL RINSE BID SWISH & SPIT	0900 2100				
17:00 8/10/xx SCH		RANITIDINE (ZANTAC-C) 150 mg TAB 1 TABLET PO BID WITH BREAK.&SUPPER	0800 1700				
17:00 8/08/xx SCH		DIGOXIN (LANOXIN) 0.125 mg TAB 1 TAB PO daily 1700	1700				
0:01 8/27/xx PRN		LIDOCAINE 5% UNG 35 g TUBE APPLY TOPICAL PRN* TO RECTAL AREA					
14:00 8/22/xx PRN		SODIUM CHLORIDE INJ 10 mL AS DIR IV TID DILUENT FOR ATIVAN IV					
14:00 8/22/xx PRN		LORAZEPAM (ATIVAN)*2 mg INJ 1 MG IV TID PRN ANXIETY					
9:30 8/21/xx PRN		TUCKS 40 PADS APPLY APPLY TOPICAL Q4-6H TO RECTUM PRN					
9:30 8/21/xx PRN		ANUSOL SUPP 1 SUPP 1 SUPP PR Q4-6H					
16:00 8/18/xx PRN		MEPERIDINE* (DEMEROL) INJ 25 mg 10 MG IV Q1H PRN PAIN IN ADDITION TO PCA					

Gluteus — A. Right, B. Left
Thigh — H. Right, I. Left
Ventro Gluteal — C. Right, D. Left
Deltoid — J. Right, K. Left
E. Abdomen — 1 | 2 / 3 | 4 QD
Page 1 of 2

STANDARD TIMES
daily = 0900
BID = Q12H = 0900 & 2100
TID = 0800, 1400, 2200
Q8H = 0800, 1600, 2400
QID = 0800, 1200, 1800, 2200
Q6H = 0600, 1200, 1800, 2400
Q4H = 0400, 0800, 1200. . .
QD DIGOXIN = 1700
QD WARFARIN = 1600

NURSE'S SIGNATURE INITIAL
0701-1500 ______
1501-2300 ______
2301-0700 ______
Ok'd by ______

ALLERGIES: NAFCILLIN
Sulfamethoxazole/Trimethoprim DS
SULFA
TRIMETHOPRIM
CIPROFLOXACIN HCL

Patient: Smith, John
Patient #: 3-90301-4
Physician: J. Physician, M.D.
Room: 407-4 South

FROM: 08/30/xx 0701 TO: 08/31/xx 0700

FIGURE 6-6 Computerized Pharmacy Medication Administration Record for Chapter 6 Practice Problems (Questions 46 through 49)

49. How many hours are between the scheduled administration times for megesterol acetate?

____

Check your work! Answers to all problems are provided at the end of the book, in the Answers section. Worked solutions from some Practice Problems are also provided there.

APPLICATION OF CLINICAL REASONING

6–1 Describe the clinical reasoning that would prevent this patient safety incident.

Possible Scenario

Suppose a prescriber wrote an order for *gentamicin sulfate 100 mg to be given IV q8h* to a patient hospitalized with meningitis. The unit secretary transcribed the order as

gentamicin sulfate 100 mg IV q8h

(0600, 1200, 1800, 2400)

The medication nurse checked the order without noticing the discrepancy in the administration times. Suppose the patient received the medication every 6 hours for 3 days before the patient safety incident was noticed.

Potential Outcome

The patient would have received one extra dose each day, which is equivalent to one-third more medication daily. Most likely, the prescriber would be notified of the patient safety incident, and the medication would be discontinued and serum gentamicin sulfate levels drawn. The levels would likely be in the toxic range, and the patient's gentamicin sulfate levels would be monitored until the levels returned to normal. This patient could be at risk of developing ototoxicity or nephrotoxicity from the overdose of gentamicin.

Prevention

____

____

Check your work! Answers to all Application of Clinical Reasoning Problems are provided at the end of each chapter.

ANSWERS TO REVIEW SETS

Review Set 6-1

1) Give 250 milligrams of naproxen orally 2 times a day. **2)** Give 30 units of Humulin R insulin subcutaneously every day 30 minutes before breakfast. **3)** Give 500 milligrams of cefaclor orally immediately, and then give 250 milligrams orally every 8 hours. **4)** Give 25 micrograms of levothyroxine orally once a day. **5)** Give 10 milligrams of lorazepam intramuscularly every 4 hours as necessary for agitation. **6)** Give 500 milligrams of cefazolin intravenously per piggyback as per protocol. **7)** Give 10 millilitres of aluminum hydroxide orally at bedtime. **8)** Give two drops of 1% atropine sulfate ophthalmic in the right eye every 15 minutes for four applications. **9)** Give 15 mg of morphine sulfate intramuscularly every 3 to 4 hours as needed for pain. **10)** Give 0.25 milligram of digoxin orally once a day. **11)** Give 250 milligrams of tetracycline orally 4 times a day.

12) Give 0.6 mg of nitroglycerin sublingually immediately. **13)** Give two drops of Sofracort otic suspension in both ears 3 times a day and at bedtime. **14)** The abbreviation TID means 3 times a day with no specific interval between times. An attempt is made to give the three doses during waking hours. The abbreviation q8h means every 8 hours. These doses would be given around the clock at 8-hour intervals. For example, administration times for TID might be 0800, 1200, 1700; administration times for q8h could be 0800, 1600, 2400. **15)** Contact the prescriber for clarification. **16)** No, QID orders are given 4 times in 24 hours with no specific interval between times indicated in order, typically during waking hours, whereas q4h orders are given 6 times in 24 hours at 4-hour intervals. **17)** Determined by hospital or institution policy. **18)** Patient, drug, dosage, route, frequency, date and time written, signature of prescriber. **19)** Specific jurisdictional documents on practice standards, information from the Institute for Safe Medication Practices (ISMP), and current Canadian nursing practice textbooks. **20)** The *right patient* must receive the *right drug* for the *right reason* in the *right amount* by the *right route* in the *right site* at the *right time* and the *right frequency*, with the *right to refuse*, followed by the *right documentation*.

Review Set 6-2

1) subcutaneous injection **2)** once **3)** cephalexin **4)** 0730 (before breakfast) **5)** milliequivalent **6)** The potassium chloride tablet is a sustained-release tablet. It should not be crushed, chewed, or sucked; the drug should be swallowed whole because the drug is released at a predetermined rate in order to maintain a constant drug concentration for a specific period of time with minimum adverse effects. **7)** cephalexin and potassium chloride **8)** acetaminophen **9)** twice **10)** in the "One-Time Medication Dosage" section, lower left corner **11)** 0600, 1200, 1800, 2400 **12)** 0900 **13)** 0730, 1130, 1630, 2100 **14)** 0900, 1700 on the 4th of September **15)** every 3 hours, as needed for severe pain **16)** 09/09/xx at 0900 or 9 AM **17)** sublingual, under the tongue **18)** once a day **19)** 125 mcg **20)** nitroglycerin, oxycodone and acetaminophen (Percocet), morphine sulfate, promethazine hydrochloride

CHAPTER

7

Drug Labels

OBJECTIVES

1. Differentiate between the trade and generic names of drugs.
2. Interpret the significant components of a drug label.
3. Recognize the significance of reading and following label instructions.
4. Interpret product label directions.

The prescriber provides the information needed for the drug: the dosage, strength, route, time, and the frequency the drug is to be administered. The nurse prepares the order from the drugs available. The drug label is an important source of information about the drug; in particular, the label provides the formulation of the drug.

TRADE AND GENERIC NAMES

Every pharmaceutical product has three names: a chemical name, a trade or brand name, and a generic name. The chemical name describes the drug's molecular structure. The trade or brand name is the manufacturer's name for a drug. The trade name is usually the most prominent word on the drug label—it is in large type and boldly visible to promote the product. The trade name is followed by the sign ®, meaning that both the name and formulation are registered by the company producing it. The generic name is determined by an international body; however, the trade name is determined by the manufacturer so that a drug may be sold under many trade names but

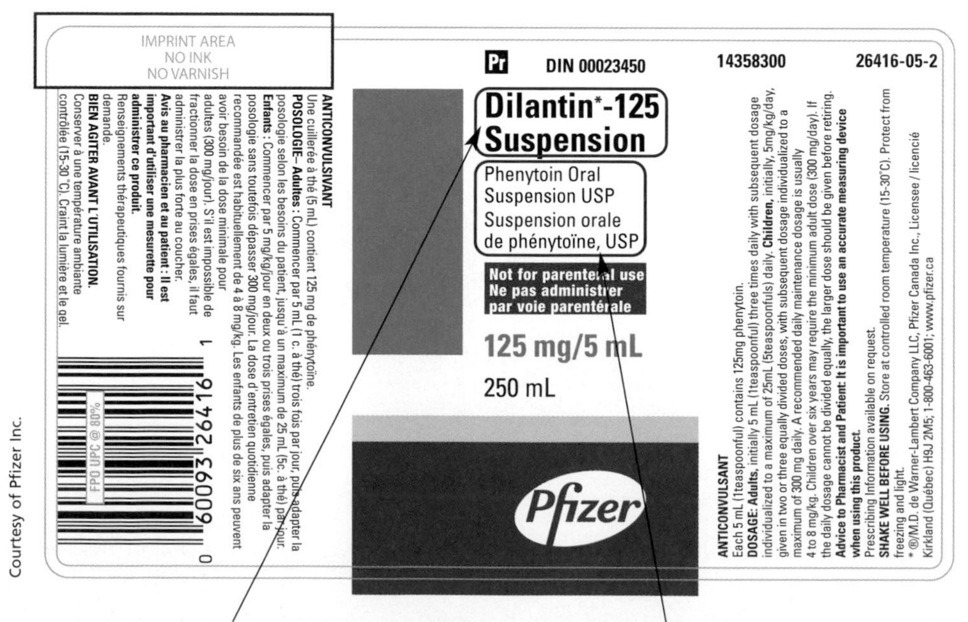

Courtesy of Pfizer Inc.

Trade Name (Dilantin) and Generic Name (phenytoin oral suspension)

the same generic name. The generic name appears directly under the trade name. Sometimes the generic name is also placed inside parentheses. By law, the generic name must be identified on all drug labels. All drugs sold in Canada, whether generic or brand name, must be approved by Health Canada's Therapeutic Products Directorate (TPD) or the Natural and Non-prescription Health Products Directorate (NNHPD) and meet strict guidelines established by Health Canada's Food and Drug Act and Regulations.

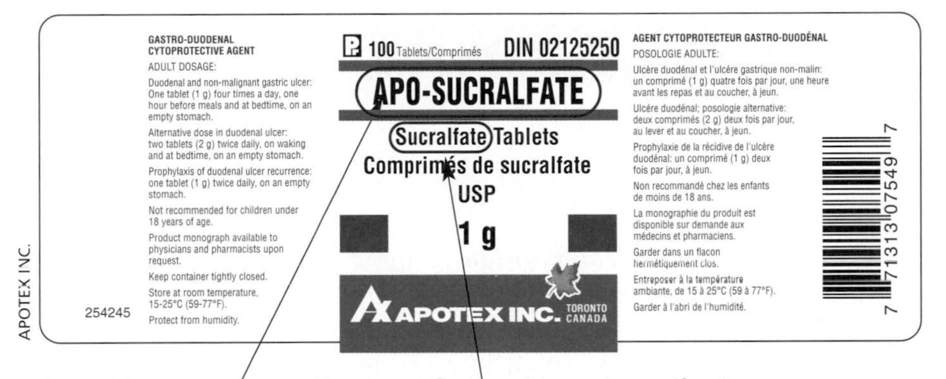

Trade Name (Apo-sucralfate) and Generic Name (sucralfate)

Generic equivalents of many trade-name drugs are ordered as substitutes according to the prescriber's preference or pharmacy policy. Because only the generic name appears on these labels, nurses need to carefully cross-check all medications. Failure to do so could cause inaccurate drug identification. Generic drugs must have the same amount of active ingredient as in the trade-name drug. Non-medicinal ingredients (e.g., fillers and preservatives) in generic drugs may differ from the non-medicinal ingredients in brand-name products, but they are also regulated and subject to a similar review process.

DOSAGE STRENGTH

The dosage strength refers to the dosage *weight* or active portion of drug provided in a specific unit of measurement. The dosage strength of the gemfibrozil tablets in the label below, for example, is

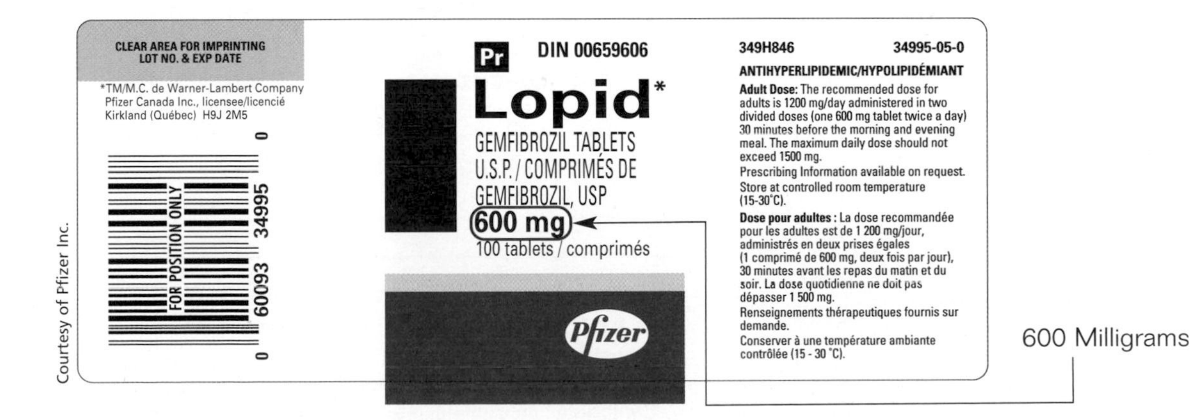

600 milligrams (the weight and specific unit of measurement) per tablet. Some drugs will have two different but equivalent dosage strengths. In the example label below, penicillin V has a dosage strength of 300 mg per 5 mL of liquid solution. This is equivalent to 480 000 units (per 5 mL). The label may or may not include both units of measurements, and in this example, it does. This information allows prescribers to order the drug using either unit of measurement.

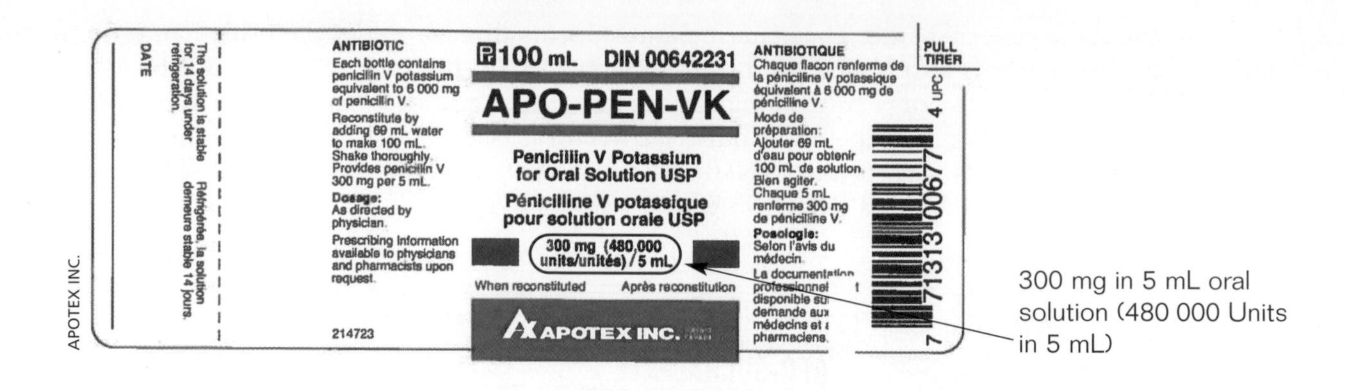

300 mg in 5 mL oral solution (480 000 Units in 5 mL)

FORM

The form identifies the ***structure*** and ***composition*** of the drug. Solid dosage forms for oral use include tablets and capsules. Some powdered or granular medications that are not manufactured in tablet or capsule form can be directly combined with food or beverages and administered. Others must be reconstituted (liquefied) and measured in a precise liquid volume, such as millilitres or drops. They may be a crystalloid (clear solution) or a suspension (solid particles in liquid that separate when held in a container).

Injectable medications may be supplied in solution or dry powdered form to be reconstituted. Once reconstituted, they are measured in millilitres.

Medications are also supplied in a variety of other forms, such as suppositories, inhalers, creams, and patches.

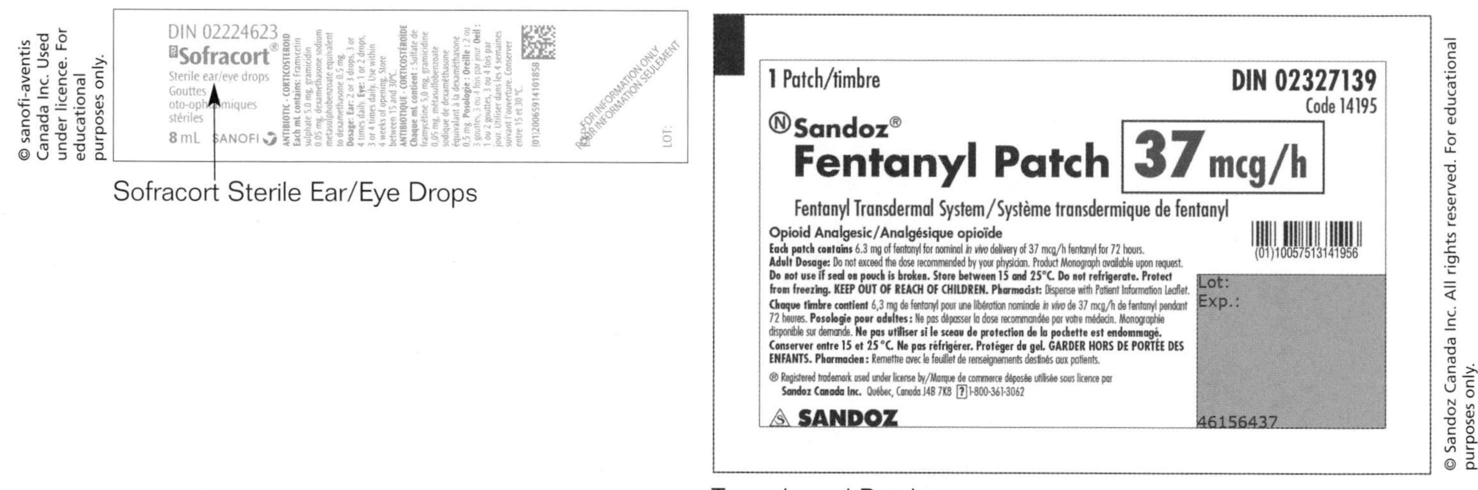

Sofracort Sterile Ear/Eye Drops

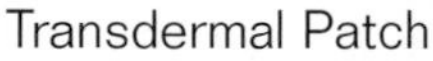

Transdermal Patch

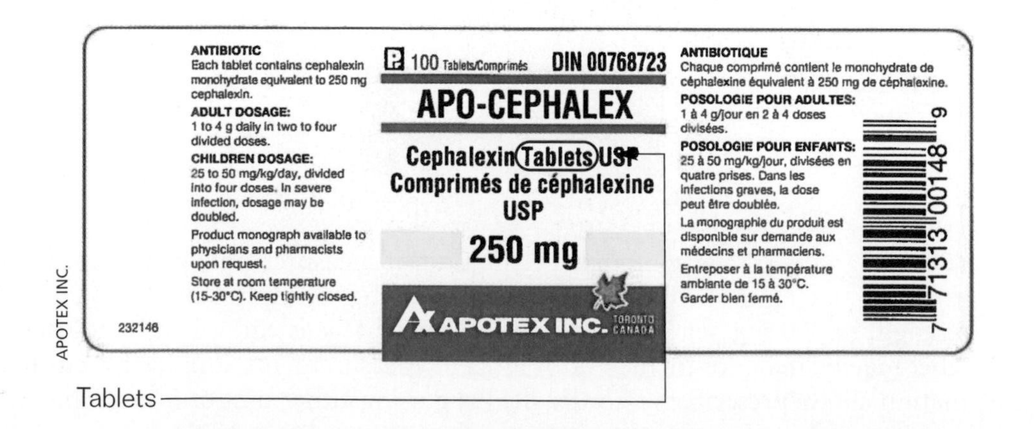

Tablets

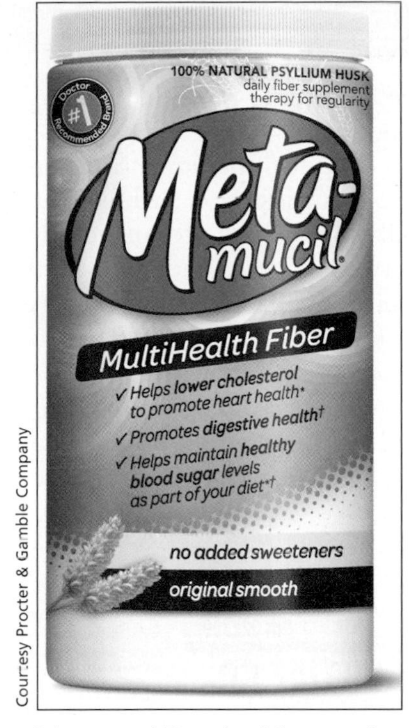

Metamucil Powder Measured in Tablespoons

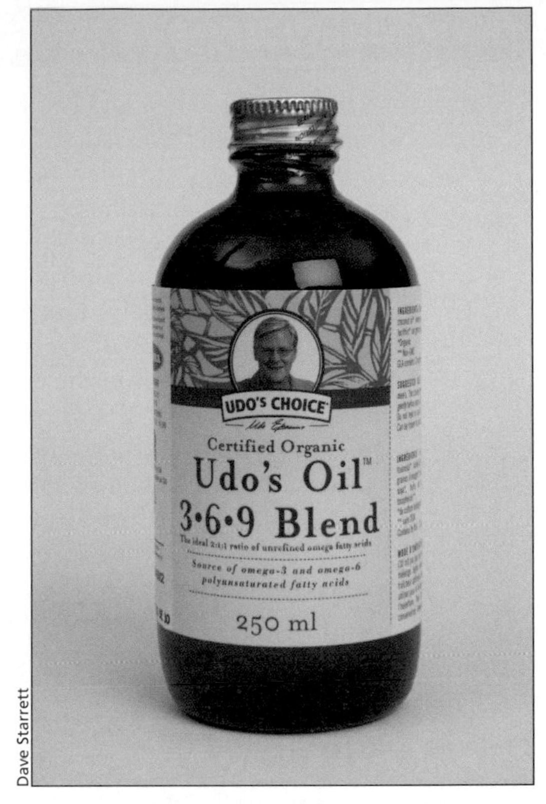

Certified Organic Udo's Oil 3-6-9 Blend

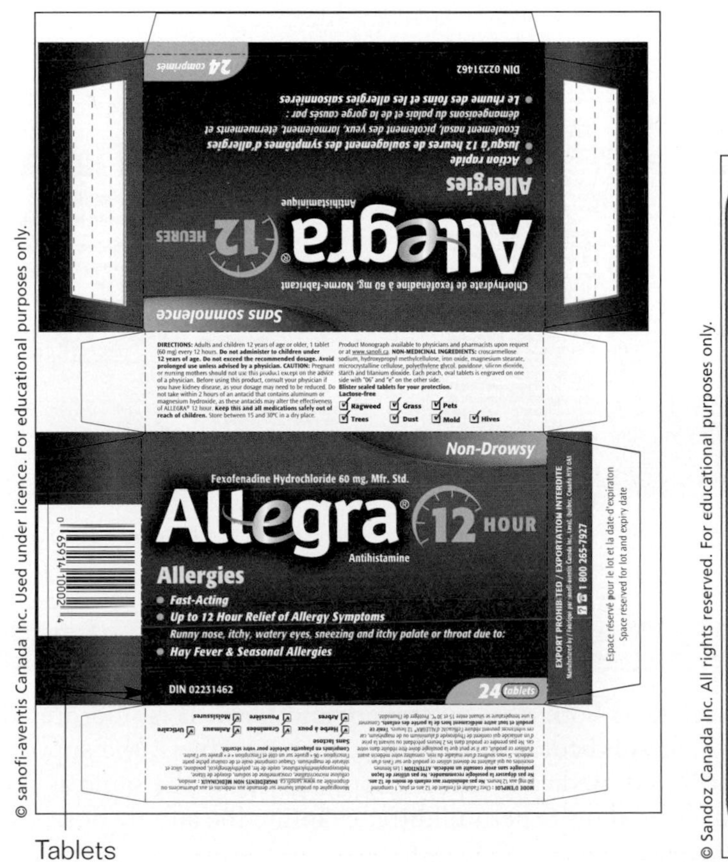

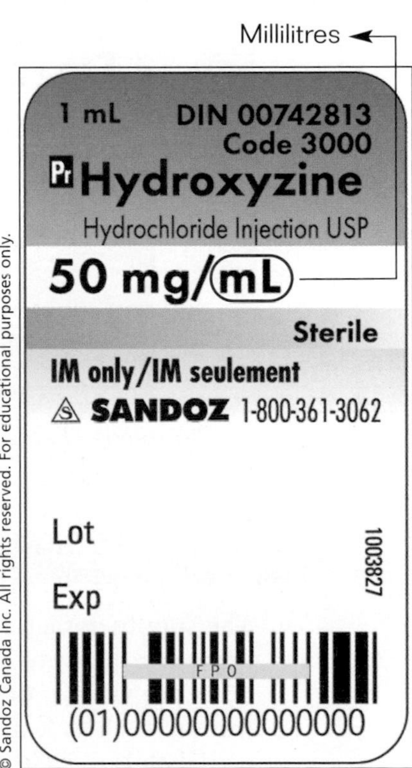

DRUG DELIVERY SYSTEMS

There are newer modes of drug delivery systems and time-release technology that control the rate at which a drug is released or the location in the body where it is released, or both. Usually this methodology refers to time-dependent release in oral drug formulations as opposed to immediate-release (IR) formulations. There are many variations of timed release, such as sustained-release (SR), long-acting (LA), and extended-release (ER) formulations, where prolonged release is intended to maintain the therapeutic window for prolonged periods of time. Another variation, delayed release (e.g., enteric-coated tablets) targets different sites of the gastrointestinal tract (e.g., the small intestine). Controlled-release (CR) or controlled-delivery (CD) drugs prolong the action of the drugs and maintain drug levels within the therapeutic window in an attempt to both avoid peaks in drug concentration and maximize therapeutic efficiency (i.e., to control both the rate of drug release and the site of release). Time-release medications must never be cut, chewed, crushed, or dissolved. In doing so, the timed-release mechanism of the medication is damaged, which results in the immediate release of the drug and the potential for overdose.

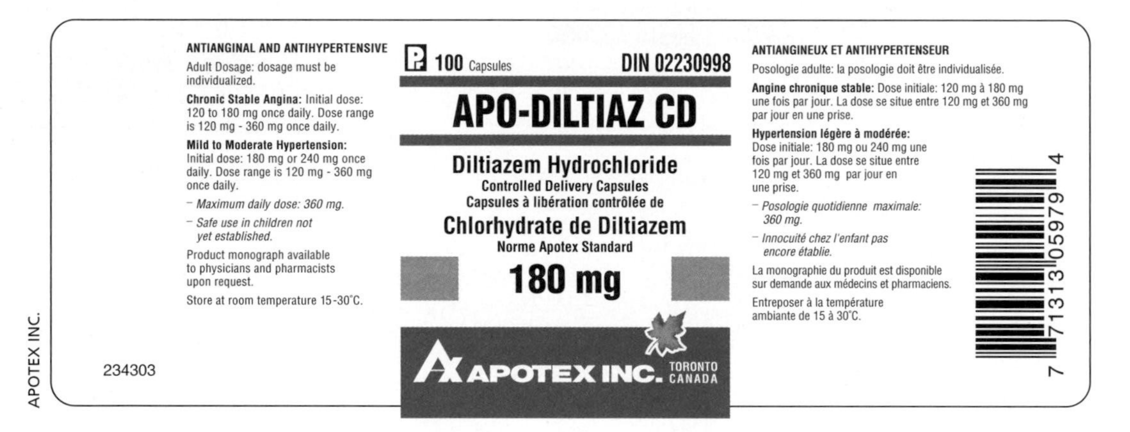

Diltiazem HCl Controlled Delivery Capsule

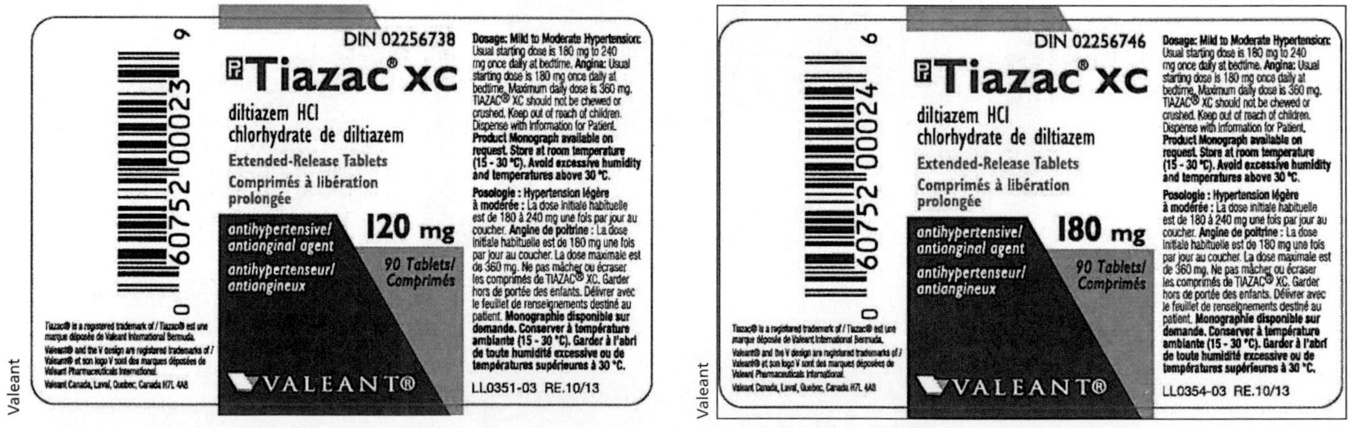

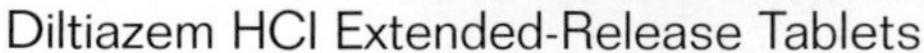
Diltiazem HCl Extended-Release Tablets

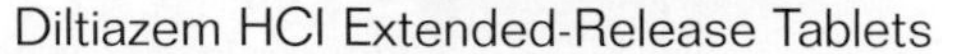
Diltiazem HCl Extended-Release Tablets

SUPPLY DOSAGE

The supply dosage refers to both ***dosage strength*** and ***form.*** It is interpreted as "X measured units per some quantity." For solid-form medications, such as tablets, the supply dosage is X measured units per tablet. For liquid medications, the supply dosage is the same as the medication's concentration, such as X measured units per millilitre. Examine the supply dosages printed on the following labels.

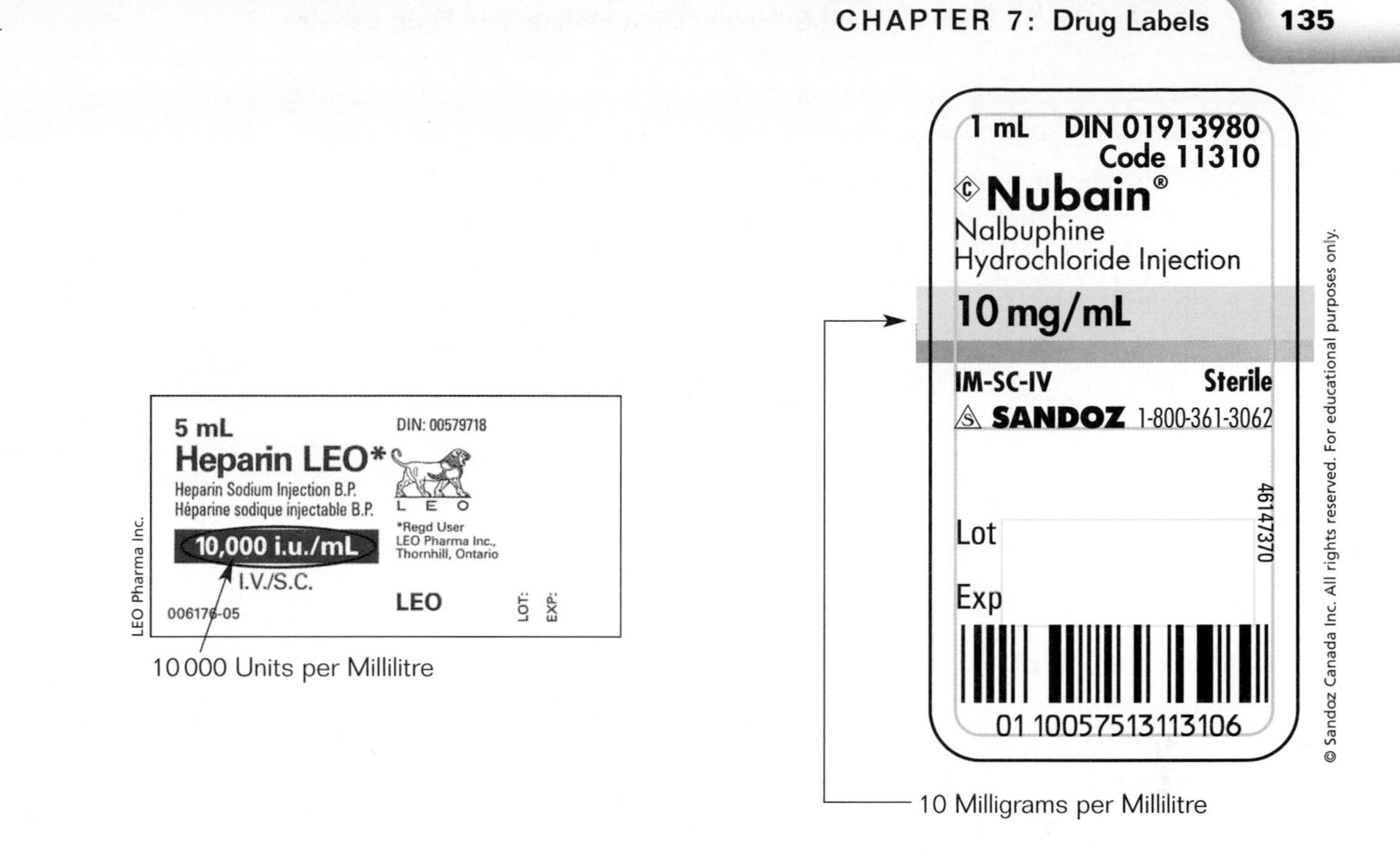

TOTAL VOLUME

The total volume refers to the ***full quantity*** contained in a package, bottle, or vial. For tablets and other solid medications, it is the total number of individual items. For liquids, it is the total fluid volume.

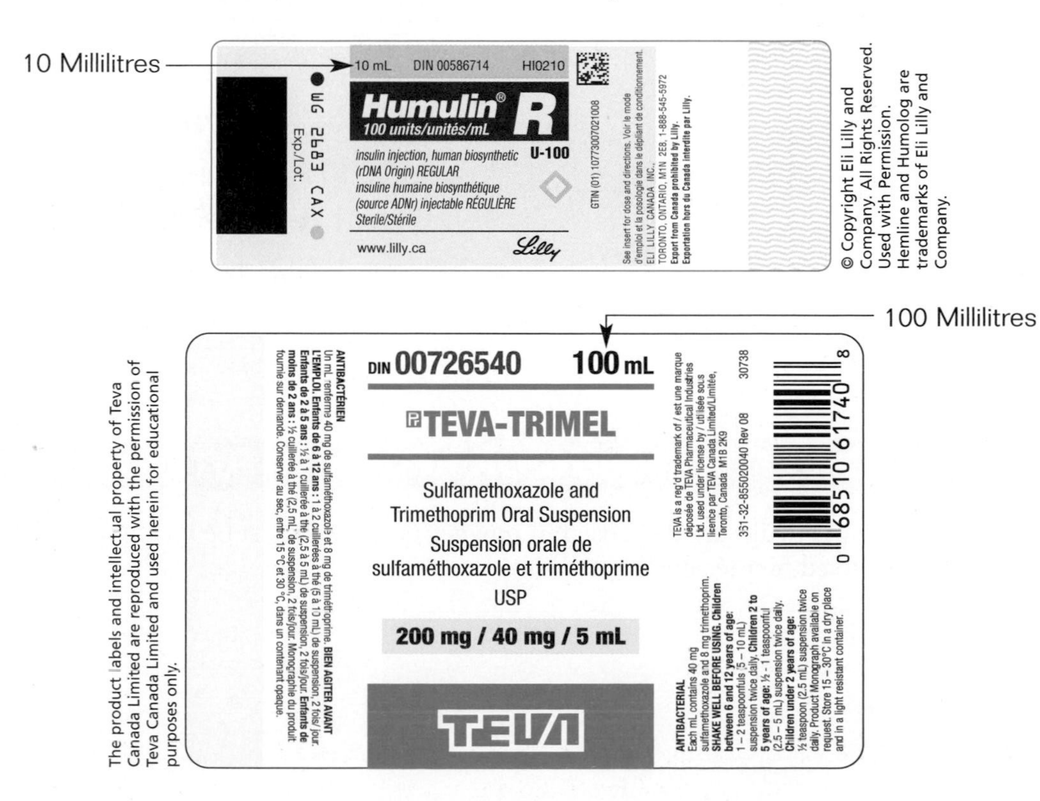

ADMINISTRATION ROUTE

The administration route refers to the ***site*** of the body or ***method of drug delivery*** into the patient. Examples of routes of administration are oral, enteral (into the gastrointestinal tract through a tube), sublingual, injection (IV, IM, subcut), otic, optic, topical, rectal, vaginal, and others. Unless specified otherwise, tablets, capsules, and caplets are intended for oral use.

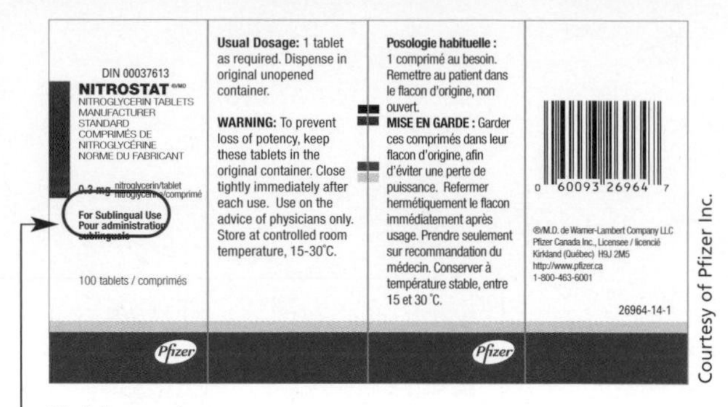

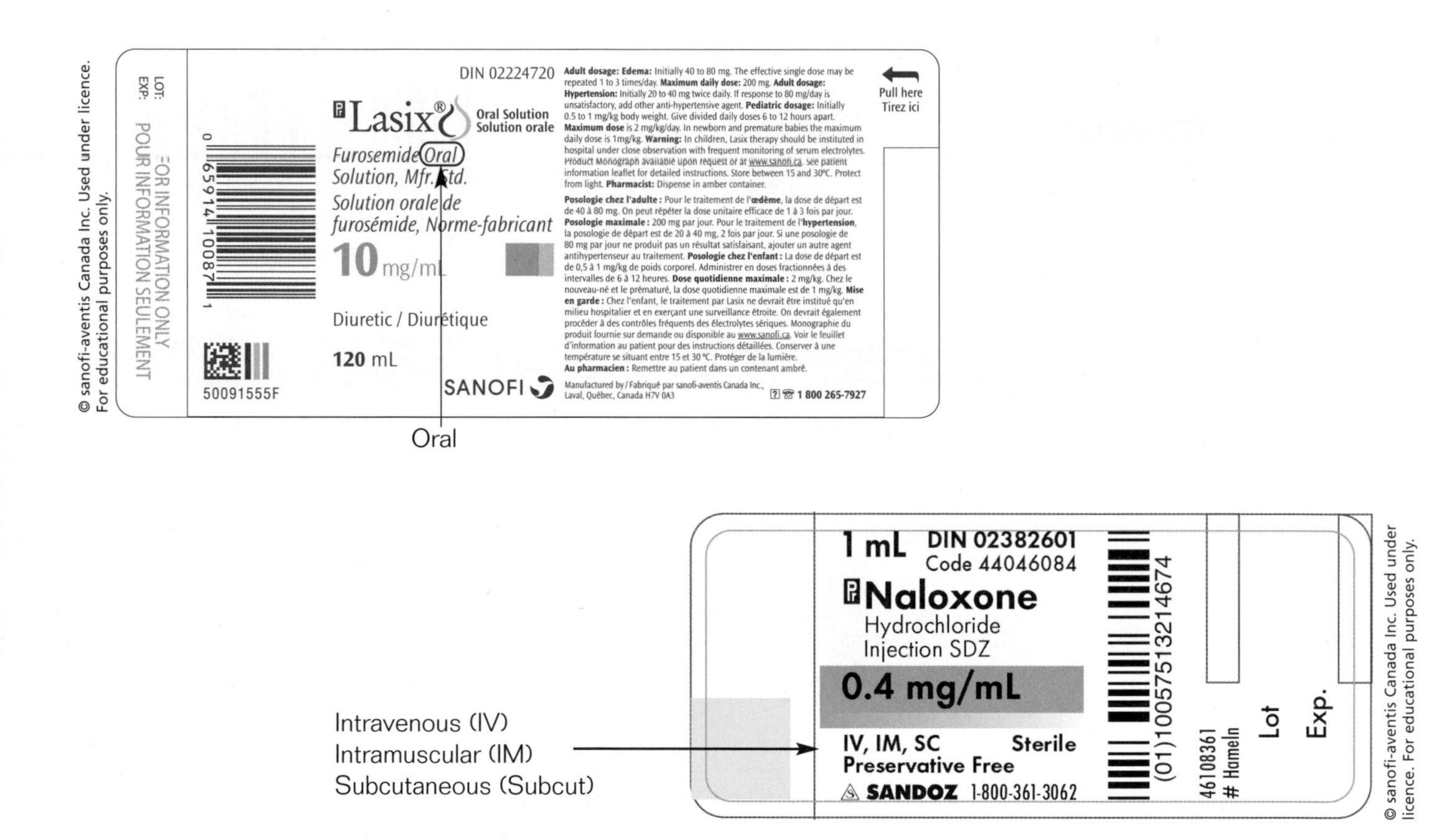

DIRECTIONS FOR MIXING OR RECONSTITUTING

Some drugs are dispensed in ***powder form*** and must be ***reconstituted for use.*** (Reconstitution is discussed further in Chapter 10.)

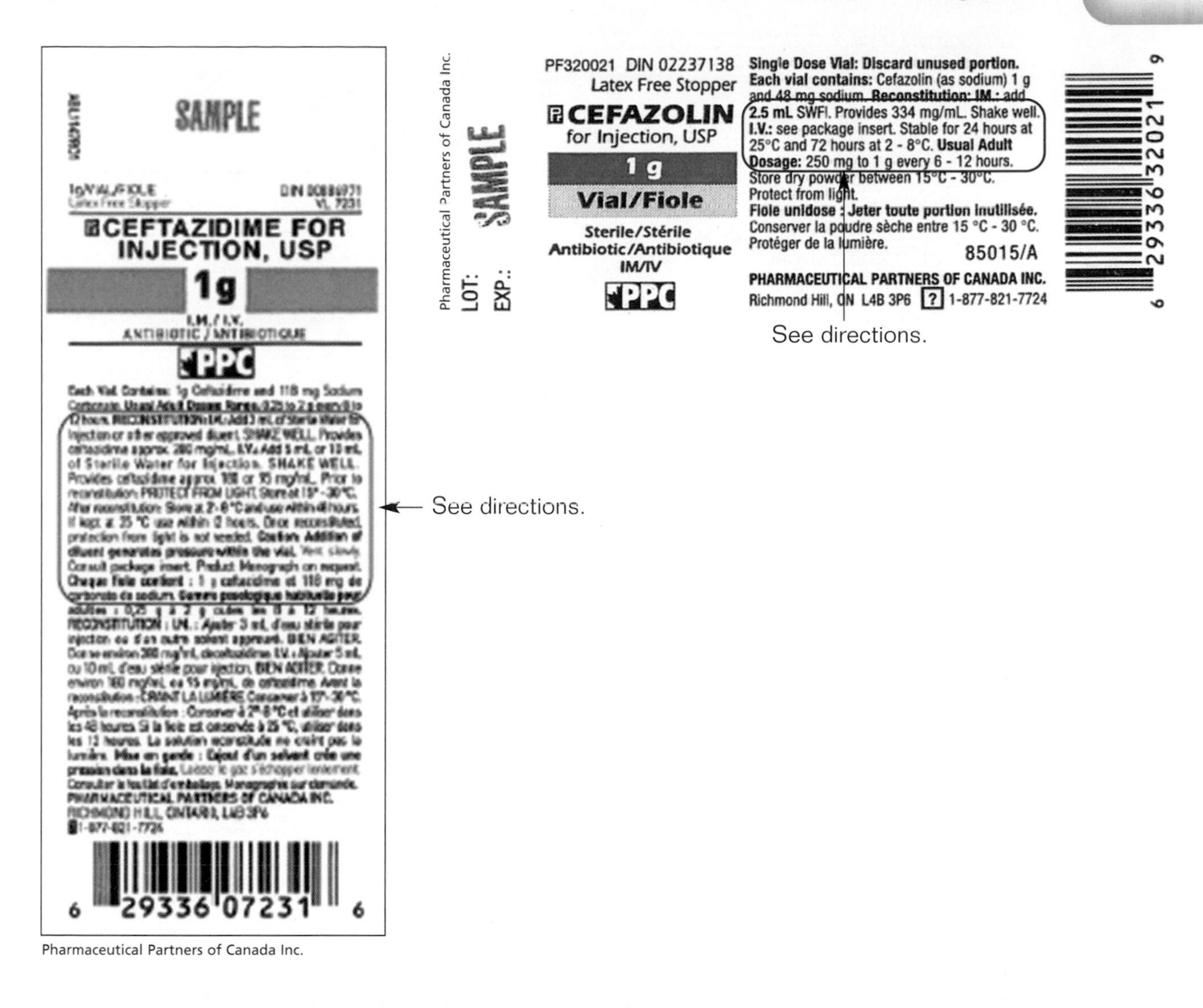

Pharmaceutical Partners of Canada Inc.

SPECIAL INSTRUCTIONS

Manufacturers may print special instructions on the packaging, or specific alerts may be added by the pharmacy before dispensing. Storage instructions such as "refrigerate at all times," "keep in a dry place," "replace cap and close tightly before storing," or "protect from light" may be found on a label. Reconstituted suspensions may be dispensed already prepared for use, and directions may instruct the healthcare provider to "shake well before using" as a reminder to remix the components. Read and follow all label instructions carefully.

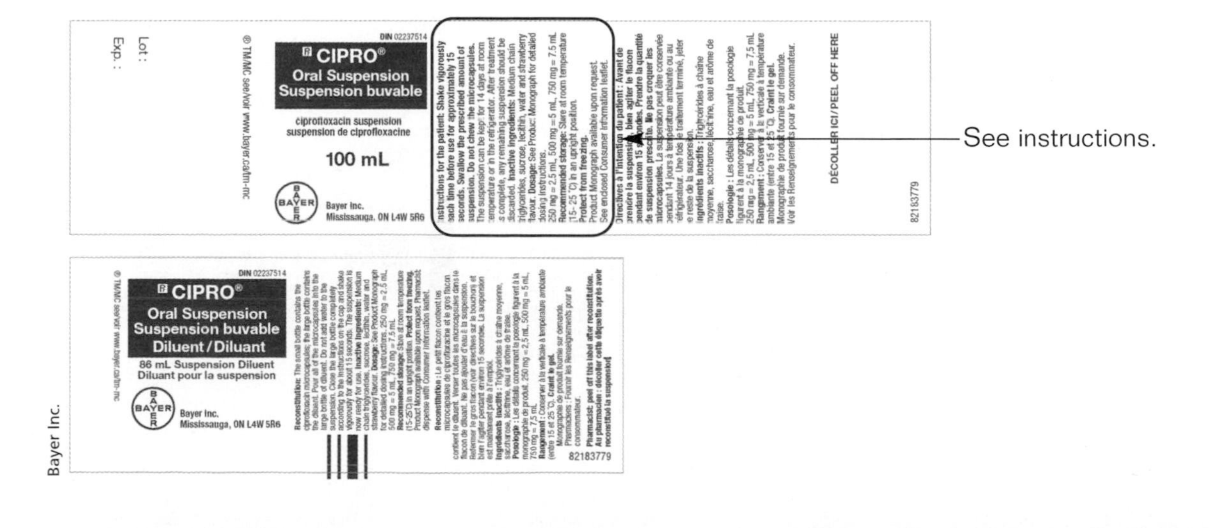

Bayer Inc.

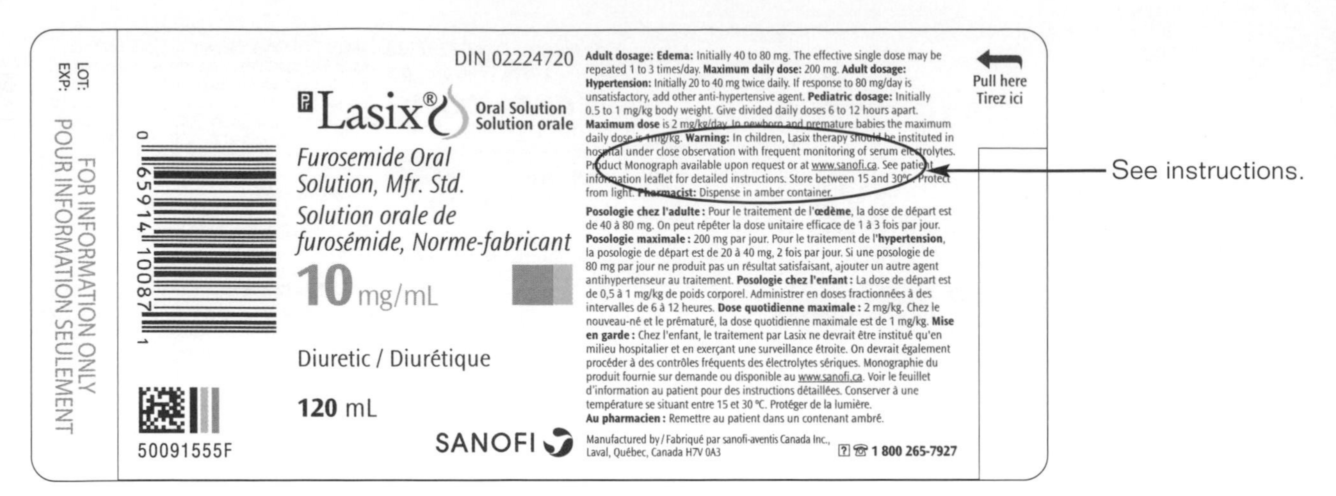
LOT:
EXP:
FOR INFORMATION ONLY
POUR INFORMATION SEULEMENT
0 65914 10087 1
50091555F
DIN 02224720
Lasix®
Oral Solution
Solution orale
Furosemide Oral Solution, Mfr. Std.
Solution orale de furosémide, Norme-fabricant
10 mg/mL
Diuretic / Diurétique
120 mL
SANOFI
Adult dosage: Edema: Initially 40 to 80 mg. The effective single dose may be repeated 1 to 3 times/day. Maximum daily dose: 200 mg. Adult dosage: Hypertension: Initially 20 to 40 mg twice daily. If response to 80 mg/day is unsatisfactory, add other anti-hypertensive agent. Pediatric dosage: Initially 0.5 to 1 mg/kg body weight. Give divided daily doses 6 to 12 hours apart. Maximum dose is 2 mg/kg/day. In newborn and premature babies the maximum daily dose is 1 mg/kg. Warning: In children, Lasix therapy should be instituted in hospital under close observation with frequent monitoring of serum electrolytes. Product Monograph available upon request or at www.sanofi.ca. See patient information leaflet for detailed instructions. Store between 15 and 30°C. Protect from light. Pharmacist: Dispense in amber container.
Posologie chez l'adulte : Pour le traitement de l'œdème, la dose de départ est de 40 à 80 mg. On peut répéter la dose unitaire efficace de 1 à 3 fois par jour. Posologie maximale : 200 mg par jour. Pour le traitement de l'hypertension, la posologie de départ est de 20 à 40 mg, 2 fois par jour. Si une posologie de 80 mg par jour ne produit pas un résultat satisfaisant, ajouter un autre agent antihypertenseur au traitement. Posologie chez l'enfant : La dose de départ est de 0,5 à 1 mg/kg de poids corporel. Administrer en doses fractionnées à des intervalles de 6 à 12 heures. Dose quotidienne maximale : 2 mg/kg. Chez le nouveau-né et le prématuré, la dose quotidienne maximale est de 1 mg/kg. Mise en garde : Chez l'enfant, le traitement par Lasix ne devrait être institué qu'en milieu hospitalier et en exerçant une surveillance étroite. On devrait également procéder à des contrôles fréquents des électrolytes sériques. Monographie du produit fournie sur demande ou disponible au www.sanofi.ca. Voir le feuillet d'information au patient pour des instructions détaillées. Conserver à une température se situant entre 15 et 30 °C. Protéger de la lumière.
Au pharmacien : Remettre au patient dans un contenant ambré.
Manufactured by / Fabriqué par sanofi-aventis Canada Inc., Laval, Québec, Canada H7V 0A3
1 800 265-7927
Pull here
Tirez ici
See instructions.

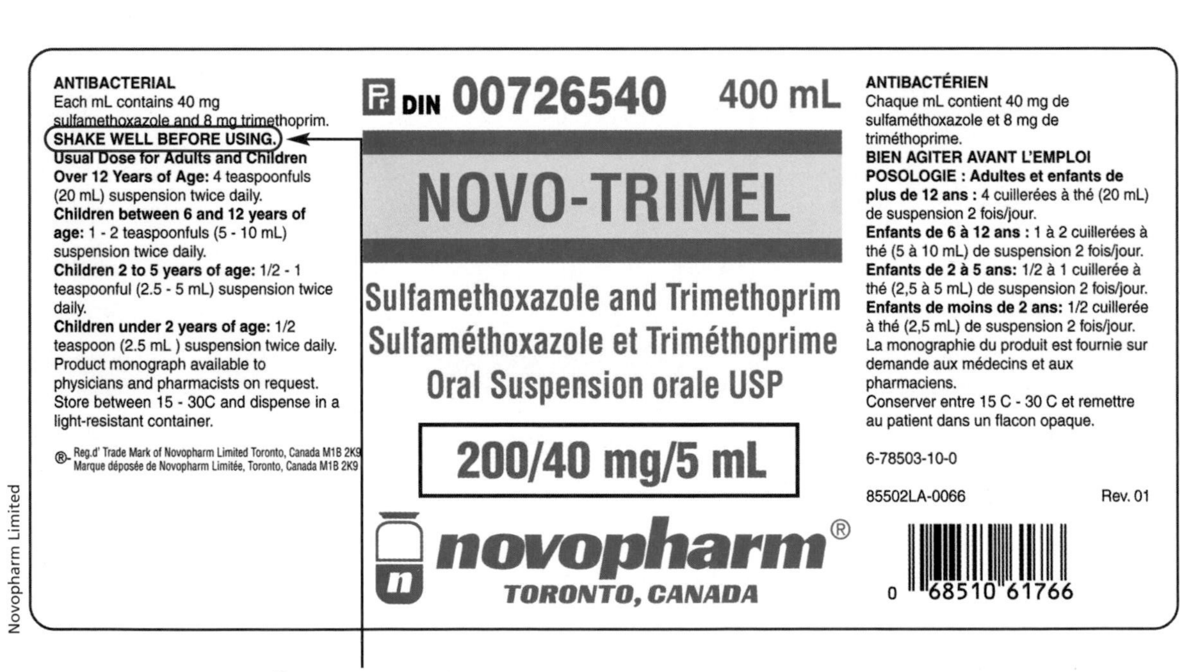
ANTIBACTERIAL
Each mL contains 40 mg sulfamethoxazole and 8 mg trimethoprim.
SHAKE WELL BEFORE USING.
Usual Dose for Adults and Children Over 12 Years of Age: 4 teaspoonfuls (20 mL) suspension twice daily.
Children between 6 and 12 years of age: 1 - 2 teaspoonfuls (5 - 10 mL) suspension twice daily.
Children 2 to 5 years of age: 1/2 - 1 teaspoonful (2.5 - 5 mL) suspension twice daily.
Children under 2 years of age: 1/2 teaspoon (2.5 mL) suspension twice daily.
Product monograph available to physicians and pharmacists on request.
Store between 15 - 30C and dispense in a light-resistant container.
® Reg.d' Trade Mark of Novopharm Limited Toronto, Canada M1B 2K9
Marque déposée de Novopharm Limitée, Toronto, Canada M1B 2K9
DIN 00726540
400 mL
NOVO-TRIMEL
Sulfamethoxazole and Trimethoprim
Sulfaméthoxazole et Triméthoprime
Oral Suspension orale USP
200/40 mg/5 mL
novopharm®
TORONTO, CANADA
ANTIBACTÉRIEN
Chaque mL contient 40 mg de sulfaméthoxazole et 8 mg de triméthoprime.
BIEN AGITER AVANT L'EMPLOI
POSOLOGIE : Adultes et enfants de plus de 12 ans : 4 cuillerées à thé (20 mL) de suspension 2 fois/jour.
Enfants de 6 à 12 ans : 1 à 2 cuillerées à thé (5 à 10 mL) de suspension 2 fois/jour.
Enfants de 2 à 5 ans: 1/2 à 1 cuillerée à thé (2,5 à 5 mL) de suspension 2 fois/jour.
Enfants de moins de 2 ans: 1/2 cuillerée à thé (2,5 mL) de suspension 2 fois/jour.
La monographie du produit est fournie sur demande aux médecins et aux pharmaciens.
Conserver entre 15 C - 30 C et remettre au patient dans un flacon opaque.
6-78503-10-0
85502LA-0066
Rev. 01
0 68510 61766
See instructions.

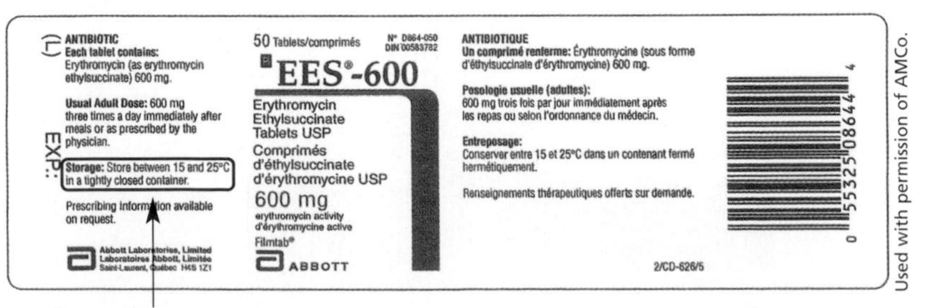
ANTIBIOTIC
Each tablet contains:
Erythromycin (as erythromycin ethylsuccinate) 600 mg.
Usual Adult Dose: 600 mg three times a day immediately after meals or as prescribed by the physician.
Storage: Store between 15 and 25°C in a tightly closed container.
Prescribing Information available on request.
EXP.:
50 Tablets/comprimés
EES®-600
Erythromycin Ethylsuccinate Tablets USP
Comprimés d'éthylsuccinate d'érythromycine USP
600 mg
Filmtab®
ABBOTT
ANTIBIOTIQUE
Un comprimé renferme: Érythromycine (sous forme d'éthylsuccinate d'érythromycine) 600 mg.
Posologie usuelle (adultes):
600 mg trois fois par jour immédiatement après les repas ou selon l'ordonnance du médecin.
Entreposage:
Conserver entre 15 et 25°C dans un contenant fermé hermétiquement.
Renseignements thérapeutiques offerts sur demande.
2/CD-626/5
0 55325 08644 4
See instructions.

NAME OF THE MANUFACTURER

The name of the manufacturer is circled on the following labels.

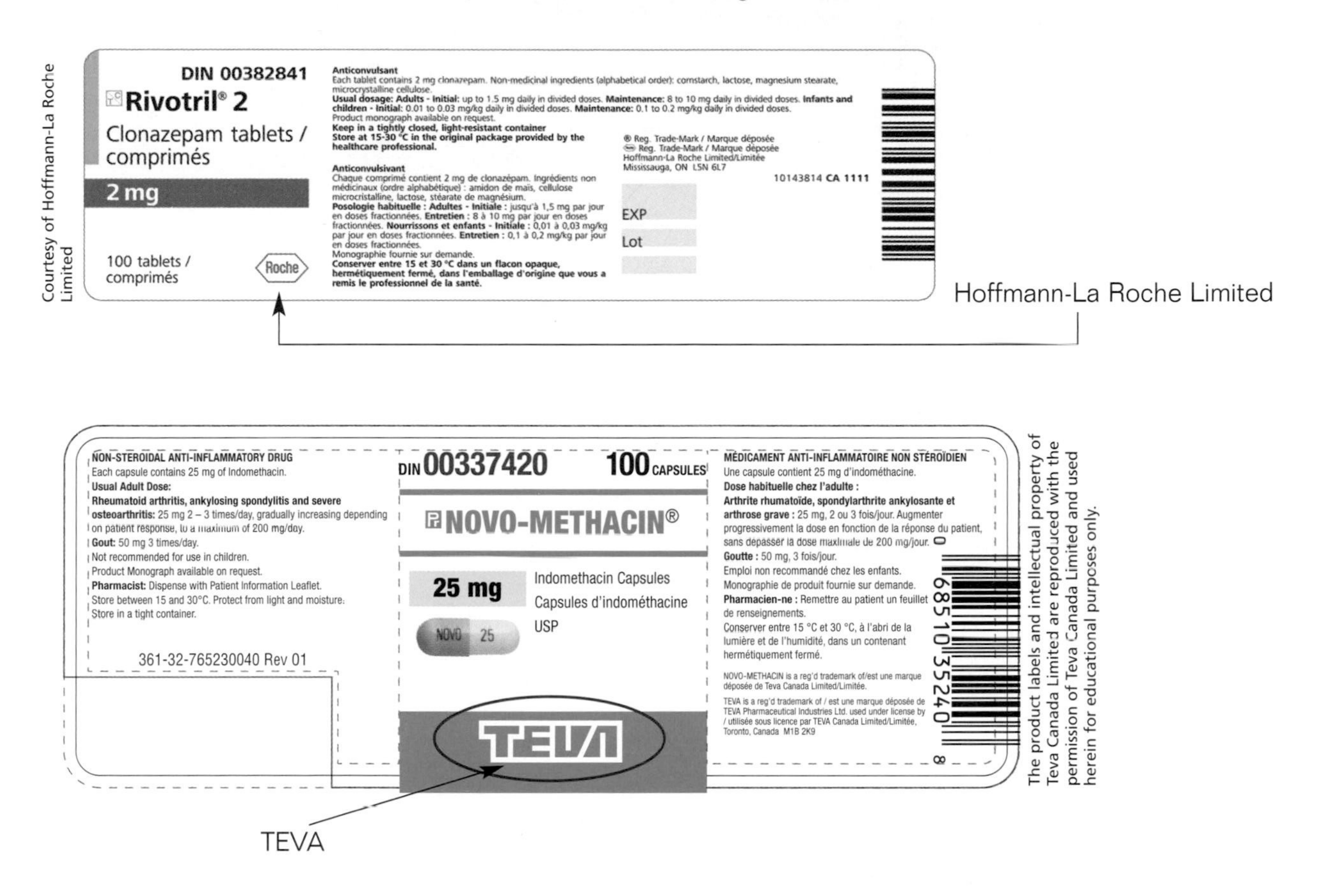
DIN 00382841
Rivotril® 2
Clonazepam tablets / comprimés
2 mg
100 tablets / comprimés
Roche
EXP
Lot
10143814 CA 1111
Hoffmann-La Roche Limited
NON-STEROIDAL ANTI-INFLAMMATORY DRUG
Each capsule contains 25 mg of Indomethacin.
Usual Adult Dose:
Rheumatoid arthritis, ankylosing spondylitis and severe osteoarthritis: 25 mg 2 – 3 times/day, gradually increasing depending on patient response, to a maximum of 200 mg/day.
Gout: 50 mg 3 times/day.
Not recommended for use in children.
Product Monograph available on request.
Pharmacist: Dispense with Patient Information Leaflet.
Store between 15 and 30°C. Protect from light and moisture.
Store in a tight container.
361-32-765230040 Rev 01
DIN 00337420
100 CAPSULES
NOVO-METHACIN®
25 mg
Indomethacin Capsules
Capsules d'indométhacine
USP
NOVO 25
TEVA
MÉDICAMENT ANTI-INFLAMMATOIRE NON STÉROÏDIEN
Une capsule contient 25 mg d'indométhacine.
Dose habituelle chez l'adulte :
Arthrite rhumatoïde, spondylarthrite ankylosante et arthrose grave : 25 mg, 2 ou 3 fois/jour. Augmenter progressivement la dose en fonction de la réponse du patient, sans dépasser la dose maximale de 200 mg/jour.
Goutte : 50 mg, 3 fois/jour.
Emploi non recommandé chez les enfants.
Monographie de produit fournie sur demande.
Pharmacien-ne : Remettre au patient un feuillet de renseignements.
Conserver entre 15 °C et 30 °C, à l'abri de la lumière et de l'humidité, dans un contenant hermétiquement fermé.
0 68510 35240 8
TEVA

EXPIRY DATE

The medication should be used, discarded, or returned to the pharmacy by the expiry date. Further, observe the special instructions about the expiry dates given on labels for reconstituted medications. **Note:** If the day is not indicated on the expiry date, the product expires on the last day of the month indicated. For example, for the haloperidol label on the right, if the expiry date is 7/18, it means July 31, 2018.

LOT OR CONTROL NUMBERS

The Health Canada Food and Drug Regulations require all medication packages to be identified with a lot or control number. The lot or control number is an internal number assigned by the company that will allow it to identify the exact time and date the batch was made. If a drug is recalled, for example, because of damage or tampering, the particular group of medication packages can be quickly identified by the lot number and it can be removed from shelves. This number has been invaluable for recalls of vaccines and over-the-counter medications.

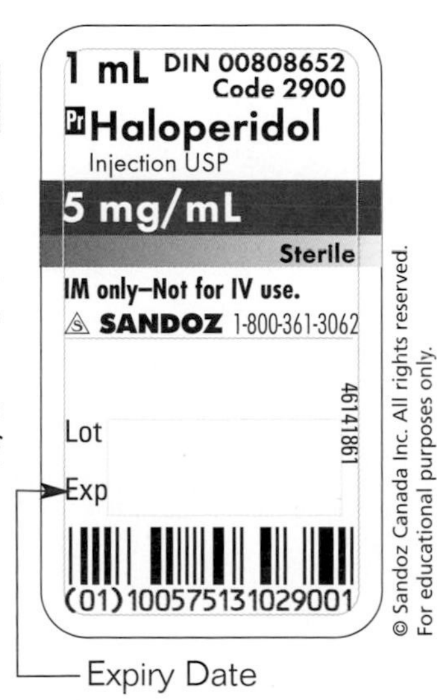
1 mL DIN 00808652
Code 2900
Haloperidol
Injection USP
5 mg/mL
Sterile
IM only–Not for IV use.
SANDOZ 1-800-361-3062
46141861
Lot
Exp
(01)100575131029001
Expiry Date

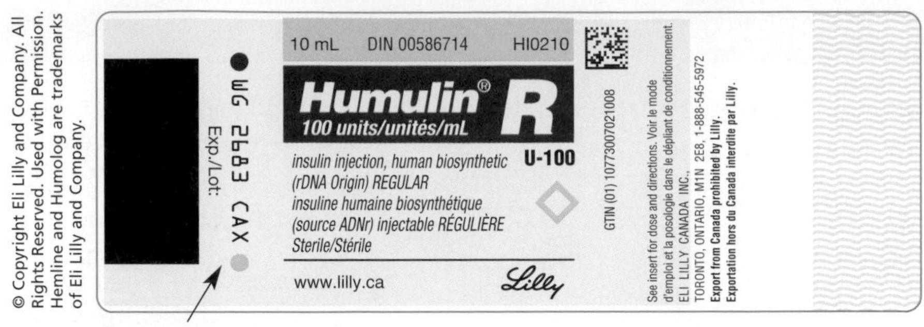

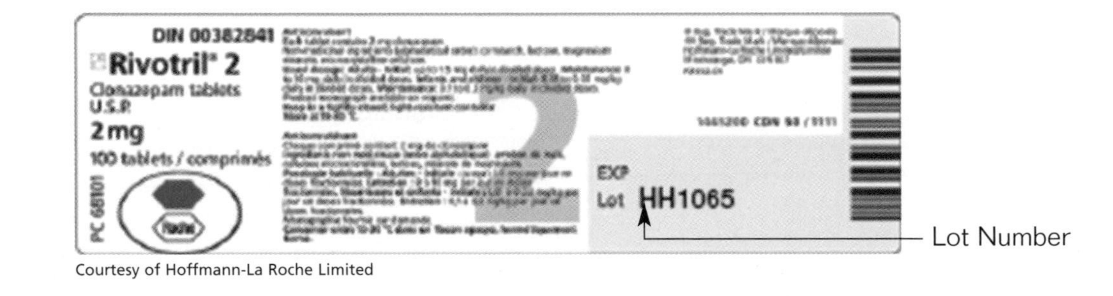

Courtesy of Hoffmann-La Roche Limited

DRUG IDENTIFICATION NUMBER

The Drug Identification Number (DIN) is an 8-digit computer-generated number assigned by the TPD of Health Canada. The DIN indicates to healthcare providers and consumers that this product has been evaluated and meets safety and health benefit expectations. Prescription and over-the-counter drug products assigned a DIN are approved for sale in Canada. The DIN identifies the manufacturer, product name, active ingredient(s), strength(s) of active ingredient(s), pharmaceutical form, and route of administration. For Sandoz-Lisinopril 5 mg, the DIN is 02289199. Related information can be found at www.hc-sc.gc.ca/dhp-mps/prodpharma/activit/fs-fi/dinfs_fd-eng.php.

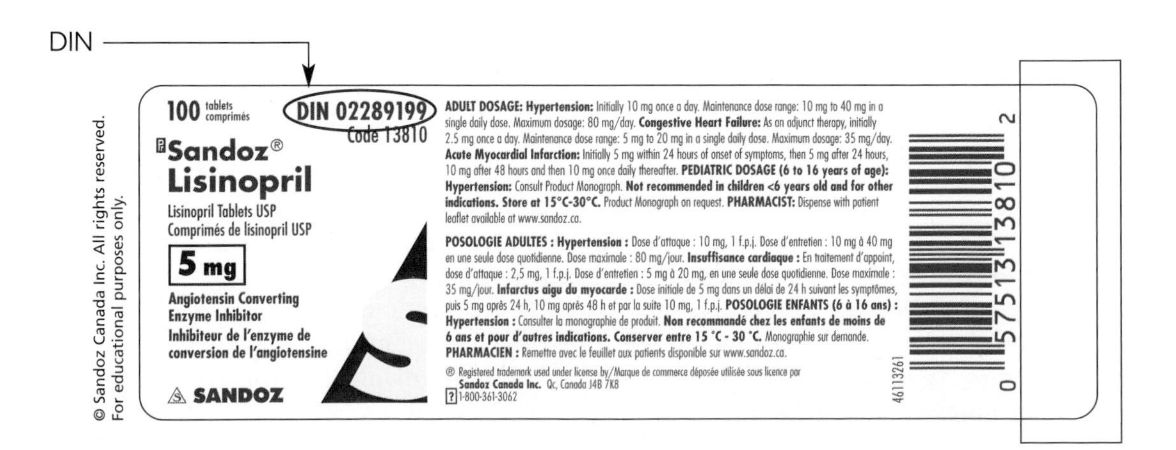

NATURAL PRODUCT NUMBER

Similarly, manufacturers of products considered to be alternative medicines must obtain approval and be licensed to market their products in Canada. Review and assignment of Natural Product Numbers (NPNs) is done by the Natural and Non-prescription Health Products Directorate (NNHPD) of Health Canada, which promotes consumer safety and awareness. The NNHPD ensures that the natural health products (NHPs) are safe, effective, and of high quality. All NHPs must have a product licence and meet requirements for labelling. In the label for Jamieson calcium given below, this number is NPN 80000248. Related information can be found at http://www.hc-sc.gc.ca/dhp-mps/prodnatur/index-eng.php.

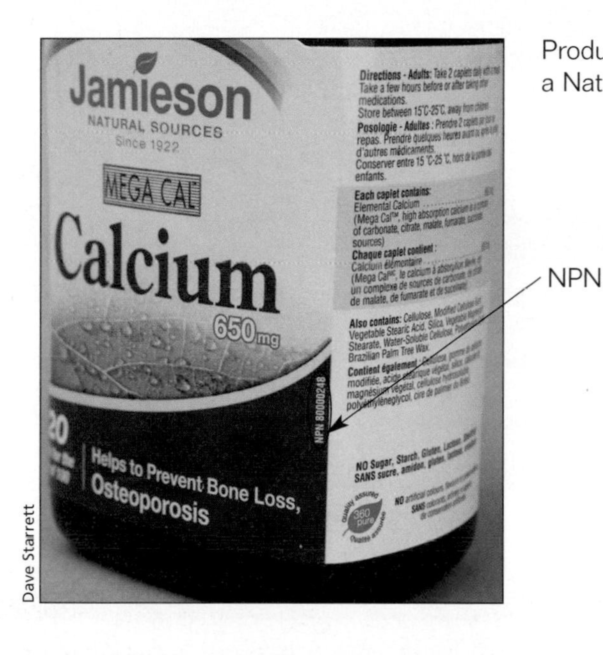

Products considered to be alternative medicines carry a Natural Product Number (NPN).

BAR CODE SYMBOLS

Bar code symbols are commonly used in retail sales. Health Canada has adopted a global bar code standard for pharmaceutical products that have been approved for use in Canada. Machine-readable bar codes ensure accurate medication verification and documentation accuracy. Such a standard is intended to increase medication safety and reduce errors.

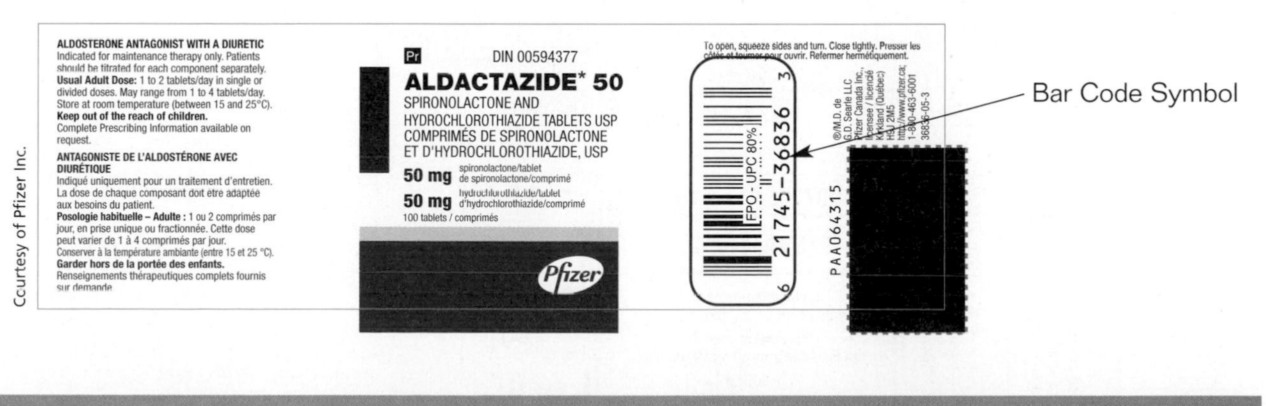

UNIT- OR SINGLE-DOSE LABELS

Most oral medications administered in the hospital setting are available in unit dosages, such as a single capsule or tablet packaged separately in a typical blister pack. The pharmacy provides a 24-hour supply of each drug for the patient. The only major difference in this form of labelling is that the total volume of the container is usually omitted because the volume is ***one*** tablet or capsule. Likewise, the dosage strength is understood as ***per one.*** Injectable medicines are also packaged in single-dose preparations.

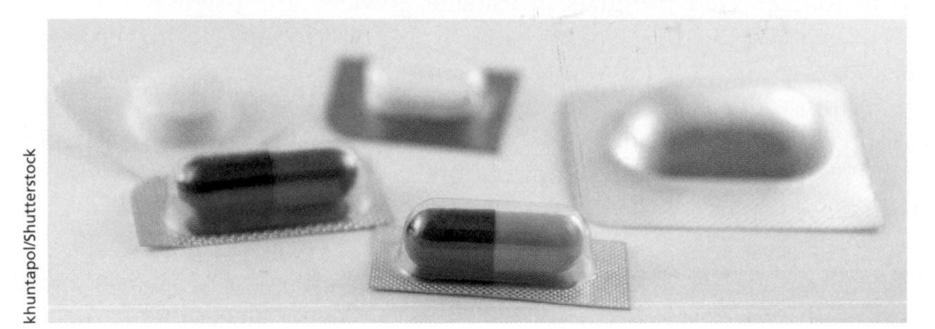

Sample Blister Pack

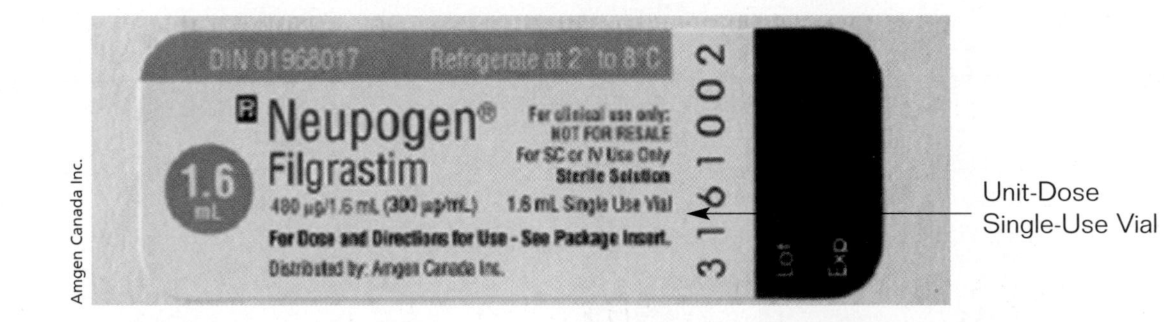

COMBINATION DRUGS

Some medications are a combination of two or more drugs in one form. Examine the labels for acetaminophen/oxycodone hydrochloride and sulfamethoxazole/trimethoprim below and notice the different substances that are combined in each tablet. Combination drugs are usually prescribed by the

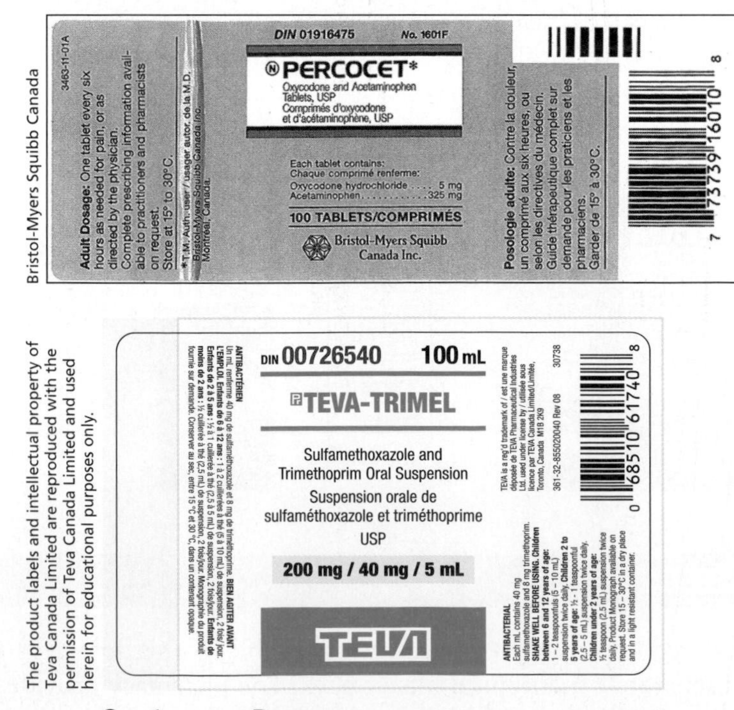

Combination Drugs

number of tablets, capsules, or millilitres to be given, rather than by the dosage strength. The combination medication represents the strength of each component. For example, Percocet contains 5 mg of oxycodone hydrochloride and 325 mg of acetaminophen; Teva-Trimel contains 200 mg of sulfamethoxazole and 40 mg of trimethoprim in every 5 mL of the suspension.

SUPPLY DOSAGE EXPRESSED AS A RATIO OR PERCENTAGE

Occasionally, solutions will be ordered and/or manufactured in a supply dosage expressed as a ratio or percentage.

RULE

Ratio solutions express the *number of grams* of the drug *per total millilitres of solution*.

Example:

Epinephrine 1:1000 contains 1 g pure drug per 1000 mL solution, 1 g:1000 mL = 1000 mg:1000 mL = 1 mg:1 mL.

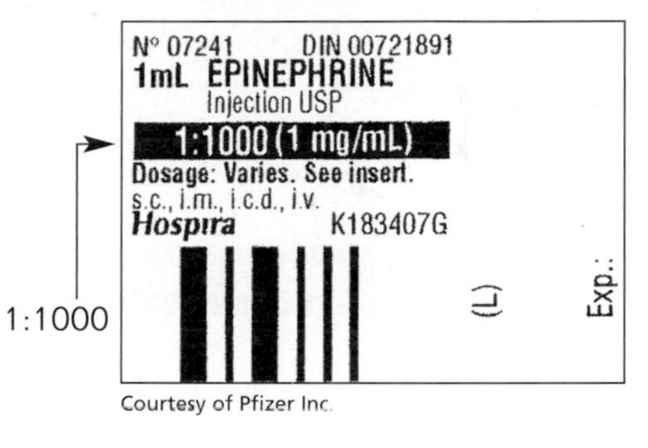

Courtesy of Pfizer Inc.

RULE

Percentage (%) solutions express the *number of grams* of the drug *per 100 millilitres of solution*.

Example:

Lidocaine hydrochloride 2% contains 2 g pure drug per 100 mL solution, 2 g/100 mL = 2000 mg/100 mL = 100 mg/5 mL = 20 mg/mL.

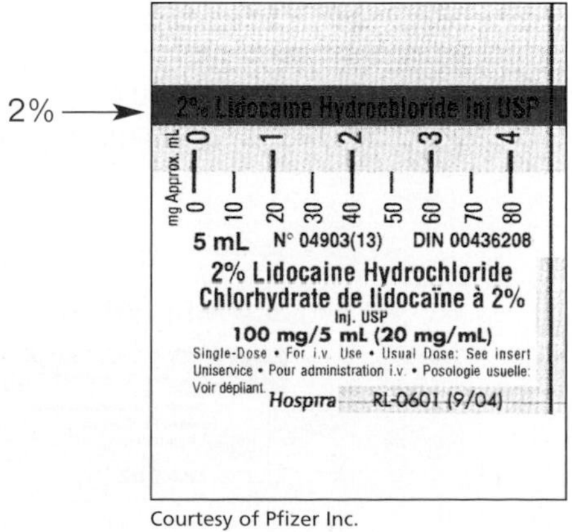

Courtesy of Pfizer Inc.

Although these labels look different from many of the other labels, it is important to recognize that the supply dosage can still be determined. Many times the label will have a more commonly identified supply dosage and not just the ratio or percentage. Examine the epinephrine and lidocaine hydrochloride labels above. On the epinephrine label, the ratio is 1:1000; the supply dosage can also be identified as 1 mg/mL. On the lidocaine hydrochloride label, the percentage is 2%; the supply dosage can also be identified as 20 mg/mL.

CHECKING LABELS

Recall the Rights of Medication Administration: The *right patient* must receive the *right drug* for the *right reason* in the *right amount* by the *right route* in the *right site* at the *right time* and *right frequency*, followed by the *right documentation*. To be absolutely sure the patient receives the right drug, check the label three times.

CAUTION

Before administering a medication to a patient, check the drug label 3 times:

1. Against the patient care order (or medication administration record, MAR)
2. Before preparing the medication
3. After preparing the medication and before administering it

QUICK REVIEW

Read labels carefully to

- Identify the drug and the manufacturer;
- Differentiate between dosage strength, form, supply dosage, total container volume, and administration route;
- Recognize that the drug's supply dosage similarly refers to a drug's weight per unit of measure or *concentration*;
- Find the directions for reconstitution, as needed;
- Note the expiry date;
- Describe the lot or control number;
- Identify the supply dosage on labels with ratios and percents;
- Be sure the right drug is administered.

REVIEW SET 7-1

Use the drug labels A through G to find the information requested in questions 1 through 12. Indicate your answer by letter (A through G).

A

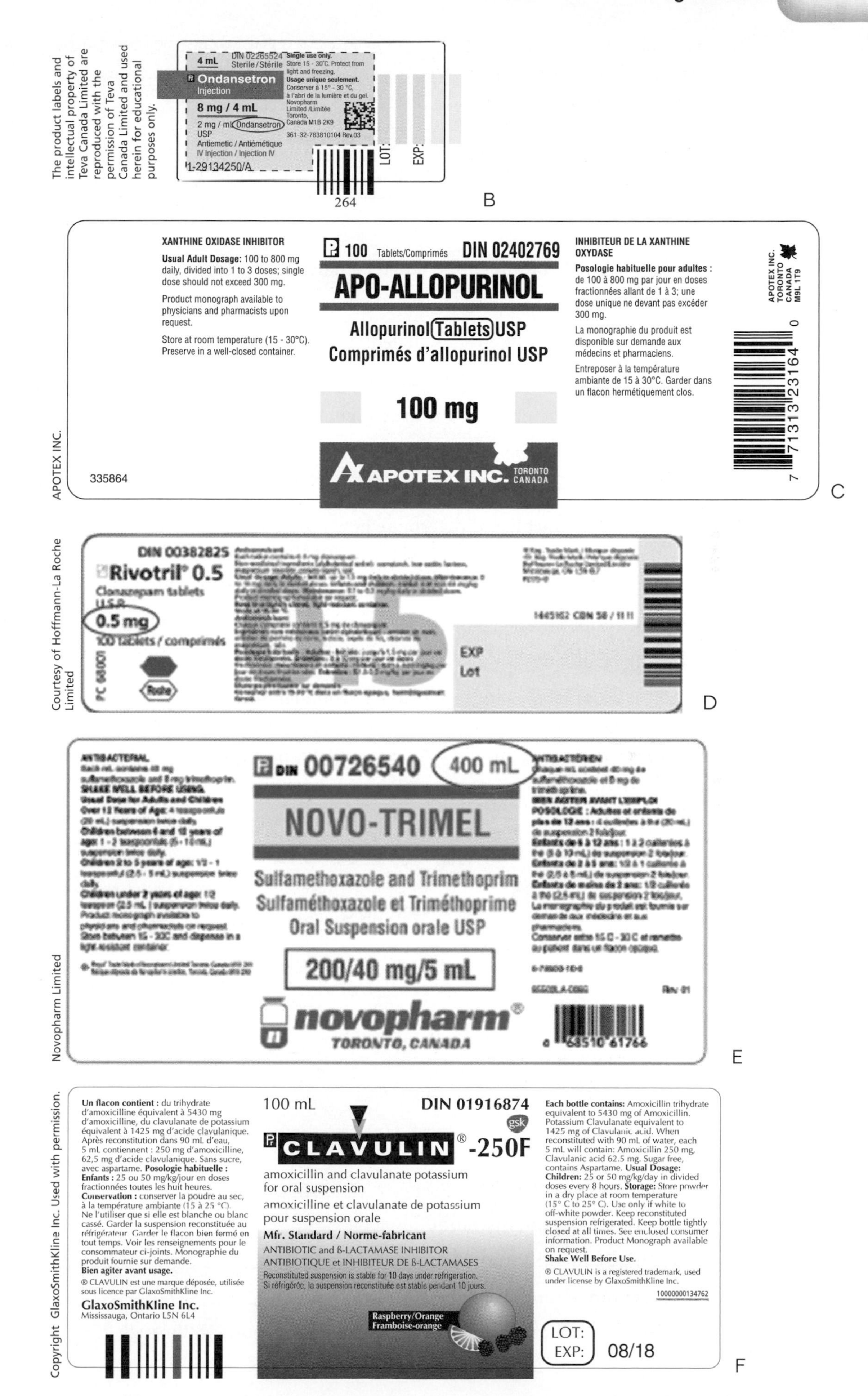
The product labels and intellectual property of Teva Canada Limited are reproduced with the permission of Teva Canada Limited and used herein for educational purposes only.
4 mL
DIN 02265524
Sterile/Stérile
Ondansetron
Injection
8 mg / 4 mL
2 mg / mL Ondansetron
USP
Antiemetic / Antiémétique
IV Injection / Injection IV
Single use only.
Store 15 - 30°C. Protect from light and freezing.
Usage unique seulement.
Conserver à 15° - 30 °C, à l'abri de la lumière et du gel.
Novopharm Limited /Limitée Toronto, Canada M1B 2K9
361-32-783810104 Rev.03
1-29134250/A
LOT:
EXP:
264
B
APOTEX INC.
XANTHINE OXIDASE INHIBITOR
Usual Adult Dosage: 100 to 800 mg daily, divided into 1 to 3 doses; single dose should not exceed 300 mg.
Product monograph available to physicians and pharmacists upon request.
Store at room temperature (15 - 30°C). Preserve in a well-closed container.
335864
100 Tablets/Comprimés
DIN 02402769
APO-ALLOPURINOL
Allopurinol Tablets USP
Comprimés d'allopurinol USP
100 mg
APOTEX INC. TORONTO CANADA
INHIBITEUR DE LA XANTHINE OXYDASE
Posologie habituelle pour adultes : de 100 à 800 mg par jour en doses fractionnées allant de 1 à 3; une dose unique ne devant pas excéder 300 mg.
La monographie du produit est disponible sur demande aux médecins et pharmaciens.
Entreposer à la température ambiante de 15 à 30°C. Garder dans un flacon hermétiquement clos.
APOTEX INC. TORONTO CANADA M9L 1T9
7 71313 23164 0
C
Courtesy of Hoffmann-La Roche Limited
DIN 00382825
Rivotril® 0.5
Clonazepam tablets U.S.P.
0.5 mg
100 tablets / comprimés
PC 68001
Roche
EXP
Lot
D
Novopharm Limited
DIN 00726540
400 mL
NOVO-TRIMEL
Sulfamethoxazole and Trimethoprim
Sulfaméthoxazole et Triméthoprime
Oral Suspension orale USP
200/40 mg/5 mL
novopharm®
TORONTO, CANADA
Rev 01
E
Copyright GlaxoSmithKline Inc. Used with permission.
Un flacon contient : du trihydrate d'amoxicilline équivalent à 5430 mg d'amoxicilline, du clavulanate de potassium équivalent à 1425 mg d'acide clavulanique. Après reconstitution dans 90 mL d'eau, 5 mL contiennent : 250 mg d'amoxicilline, 62,5 mg d'acide clavulanique. Sans sucre, avec aspartame. Posologie habituelle : Enfants : 25 ou 50 mg/kg/jour en doses fractionnées toutes les huit heures. Conservation : conserver la poudre au sec, à la température ambiante (15 à 25 °C). Ne l'utiliser que si elle est blanche ou blanc cassé. Garder la suspension reconstituée au réfrigérateur. Garder le flacon bien fermé en tout temps. Voir les renseignements pour le consommateur ci-joints. Monographie du produit fournie sur demande.
Bien agiter avant usage.
® CLAVULIN est une marque déposée, utilisée sous licence par GlaxoSmithKline Inc.
GlaxoSmithKline Inc.
Mississauga, Ontario L5N 6L4
100 mL
DIN 01916874
gsk
CLAVULIN® -250F
amoxicillin and clavulanate potassium for oral suspension
amoxicilline et clavulanate de potassium pour suspension orale
Mfr. Standard / Norme-fabricant
ANTIBIOTIC and ß-LACTAMASE INHIBITOR
ANTIBIOTIQUE et INHIBITEUR DE ß-LACTAMASES
Reconstituted suspension is stable for 10 days under refrigeration.
Si réfrigérée, la suspension reconstituée est stable pendant 10 jours.
Raspberry/Orange
Framboise-orange
Each bottle contains: Amoxicillin trihydrate equivalent to 5430 mg of Amoxicillin. Potassium Clavulanate equivalent to 1425 mg of Clavulanic acid. When reconstituted with 90 mL of water, each 5 mL will contain: Amoxicillin 250 mg, Clavulanic acid 62.5 mg. Sugar free, contains Aspartame. Usual Dosage: Children: 25 or 50 mg/kg/day in divided doses every 8 hours. Storage: Store powder in a dry place at room temperature (15° C to 25° C). Use only if white to off-white powder. Keep reconstituted suspension refrigerated. Keep bottle tightly closed at all times. See enclosed consumer information. Product Monograph available on request.
Shake Well Before Use.
® CLAVULIN is a registered trademark, used under license by GlaxoSmithKline Inc.
10000000134762
LOT:
EXP: 08/18
F

PHARMACODE

RECONSTITUTION: I.M.: Add 5 mL of sterile water for injection, gives 330 mg cefotaxime/mL. I.V.: Add 10 mL of sterile water for injection, gives 180 mg cefotaxime/mL. I.V. INFUSION: Reconstitute as above, further dilute with 50 to 1000 mL of a recommended infusion solution, see package insert. Use reconstituted solutions within 24 hours if kept between 15 and 25°C or within 48 hours if refrigerated between 2 and 8°C. ECL12B

DIN 02225107
Claforan®
Sterile cefotaxime sodium
Céfotaxime sodique stérile
i.m./i.v.
2 g per vial / par flacon
Antibiotic / Antibiotique
sanofi aventis

RECONSTITUTION : I.M. : Ajouter 5 mL d'eau stérile pour injection. Donne 330 mg de céfotaxime/mL. I.V. : Ajouter 10 mL d'eau stérile pour injection. Donne 180 mg de céfotaxime/mL. PERFUSION I.V. : Reconstituer comme indiqué ci-dessus et diluer avec 50 à 1000 mL d'une solution recommandée pour perfusion intraveineuse, voir la notice ci-incluse. Utiliser les solutions reconstituées dans les 24 heures si elles sont conservées entre 15 et 25 °C et dans les 48 heures si elles le sont à une température se situant entre 2 et 8 °C.

Lot: D1895F2

Exp:

G

1. The total volume of the liquid container is circled. ________
2. The dosage strength is circled. ________
3. The form of the drug is circled. ________
4. The trade name of the drug is circled. ________
5. The generic name of the drug is circled. ________
6. The expiry date is circled. ________
7. The lot number is circled. ________
8. Look at label E and determine how much of the supply drug you will administer to the patient per dose for the order *sulfamethoxazole 100/20 mg.* ________
9. Look at label A and identify the route of administration. ________
10. Identify the labels that have an imprinted bar code symbol. ________
11. Look at label B and identify the supply dosage. ________
12. Look at label F and determine how much of the drug supplied you will administer to the patient per dose for the order *clavulin 100 mg PO q8h x 10 days.* ________

Refer to the following drug label to provide the specific drug information requested in questions 13 through 17.

LOT : 302081

EXP. : 2005 F

SAMPLE

15 mL DIN 02220288
PF370070

PENICILLIN G
Sodium for Injection USP

5 million IU
per Vial/par fiole

IM/IV
Sterile/Stérile
Antibiotic / Antibiotique

Usual adult dose:
1,000,000 to 5,000,000 IU every 4 to 6 hours.
For full prescribing information, see package insert.
Reconstitution: Use Sterile Water for Injection, USP or other recommended diluent.

Volume of diluent	Approximate Concentration /mL	Withdrawable Volume
3.1 mL	1,000,000 IU	5 mL
8.2 mL	500,000 IU	10 mL

Reconstituted solution is stable for 5 days refrigerated or 24 hours room temperature.

Pharmaceutical Partners of Canada Inc.
Richmond Hill, Ontario L4C 9S6
1-877-821-7724

Dose habituelle pour adultes :
1 000 000 à 5 000 000 UI toutes les 4 à 6 heures.
Pour les renseignements posologiques complets, consulter le feuillet d'emballage.
Reconstitution : Utiliser de l'eau stérile pour préparations injectables USP ou un autre diluant recommandé.

Volume de diluant	Concentration approximative/mL	Volume obtenu
3,1 mL	1 000 000 UI	5 mL
8,2 mL	500 000 UI	10 mL

La solution reconstituée est stable pendant 5 jours au réfrigérateur ou pendant 24 heures à la température ambiante.

85009/A

6 29336 37070 2

13. Generic name ____________________
14. Dosage strength ____________________
15. Route of administration ____________________
16. Drug Identification Number ____________________
17. Manufacturer ____________________

Refer to the following drug label to answer questions 18 through 20.

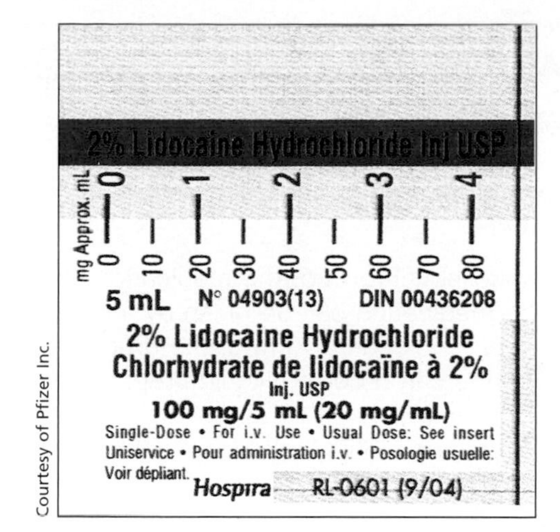

Courtesy of Pfizer Inc.

18. The supply dosage of the drug is ________ %.
19. The supply dosage of the drug is ________ g per 100 mL.
20. The supply dosage of the drug is ________ mg per mL.

Check your work! Answers to all Review Sets are provided at the end of each chapter. Worked solutions for selected Review Sets are also available there.

APPLICATION OF CLINICAL REASONING

Reading the medication labels is critical. Make sure that the drug you want is what you have on hand before you prepare it. Here is an example of a patient safety incident related to reading the label incorrectly.

Potential Patient Safety Incident

Not checking the label for correct dosage.

Possible Scenario

A nurse flushed a triple central venous catheter (an IV with three ports). According to hospital policy, the nurse was to flush each port with 10 mL of normal saline followed by 2 mL of heparin flush solution in the concentration of 100 units/mL. The nurse mistakenly picked up a vial of heparin sodium containing heparin sodium 10 000 units/mL. Without checking the label, she prepared the solution for all three ports. The patient received 60 000 units of heparin sodium instead of 600 units.

Potential Outcome

The patient in this case would be at great risk for hemorrhage, leading to shock and possibly death. Protamine sulfate would be ordered to counteract the action of the heparin sodium.

Prevention

There is no substitute for checking the label before administering a medication. The nurse in this case had three opportunities to catch the patient safety incident, having drawn three different syringes of medication for the three ports.

Application of Critical Reasoning Additional application problems are provided at the end of the chapter. Answers are provided at the end of the book.

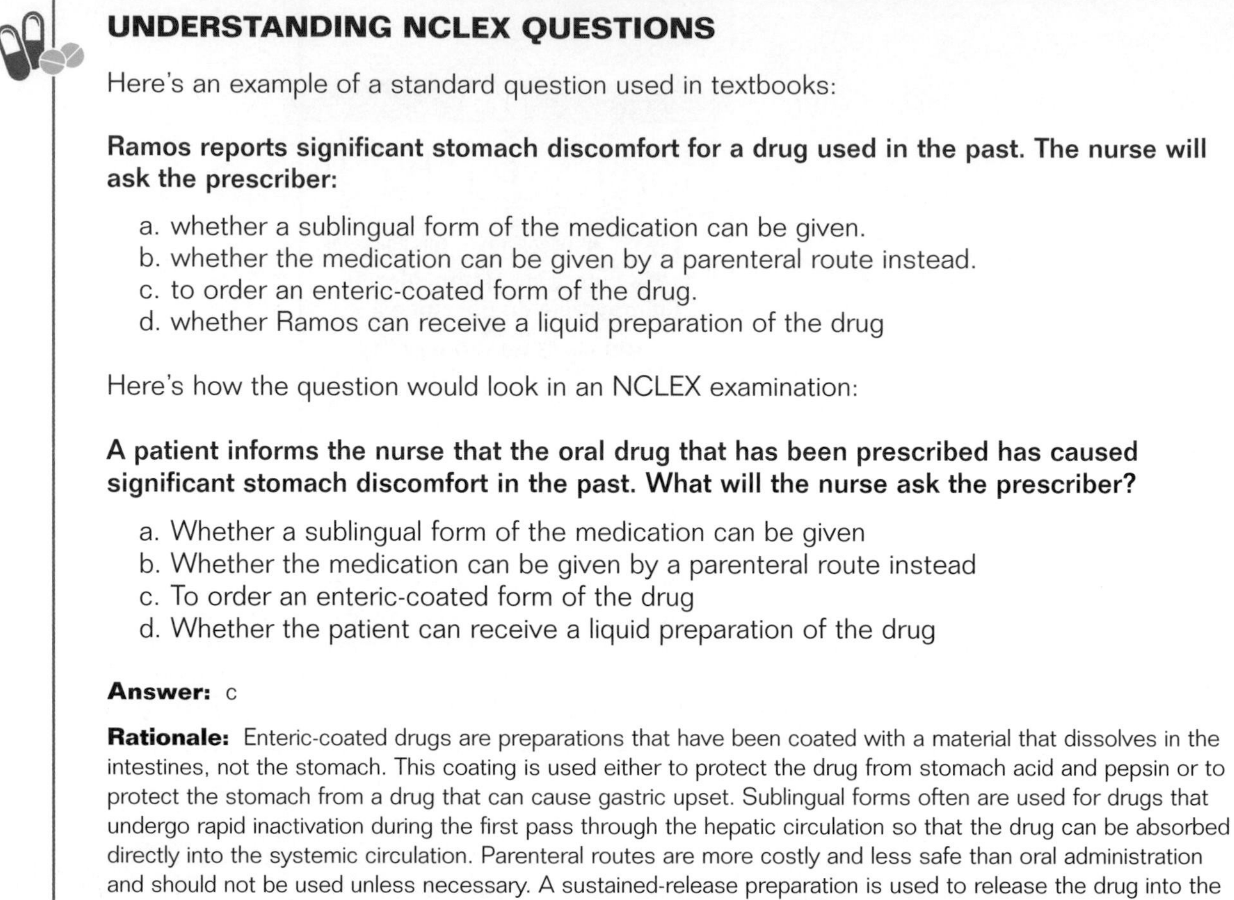

UNDERSTANDING NCLEX QUESTIONS

Here's an example of a standard question used in textbooks:

Ramos reports significant stomach discomfort for a drug used in the past. The nurse will ask the prescriber:

a. whether a sublingual form of the medication can be given.
b. whether the medication can be given by a parenteral route instead.
c. to order an enteric-coated form of the drug.
d. whether Ramos can receive a liquid preparation of the drug

Here's how the question would look in an NCLEX examination:

A patient informs the nurse that the oral drug that has been prescribed has caused significant stomach discomfort in the past. What will the nurse ask the prescriber?

a. Whether a sublingual form of the medication can be given
b. Whether the medication can be given by a parenteral route instead
c. To order an enteric-coated form of the drug
d. Whether the patient can receive a liquid preparation of the drug

Answer: c

Rationale: Enteric-coated drugs are preparations that have been coated with a material that dissolves in the intestines, not the stomach. This coating is used either to protect the drug from stomach acid and pepsin or to protect the stomach from a drug that can cause gastric upset. Sublingual forms often are used for drugs that undergo rapid inactivation during the first pass through the hepatic circulation so that the drug can be absorbed directly into the systemic circulation. Parenteral routes are more costly and less safe than oral administration and should not be used unless necessary. A sustained-release preparation is used to release the drug into the body over a specific period to reduce the number of daily doses required to sustain therapeutic drug levels.

PRACTICE PROBLEMS—CHAPTER 7

Look at the drug labels A through G, and supply the information requested.

Label A:

1. The supply dosage of the drug is ______________________________.
2. The Drug Identification Number is ______________________________.
3. The total volume of drug available is ______________________________.

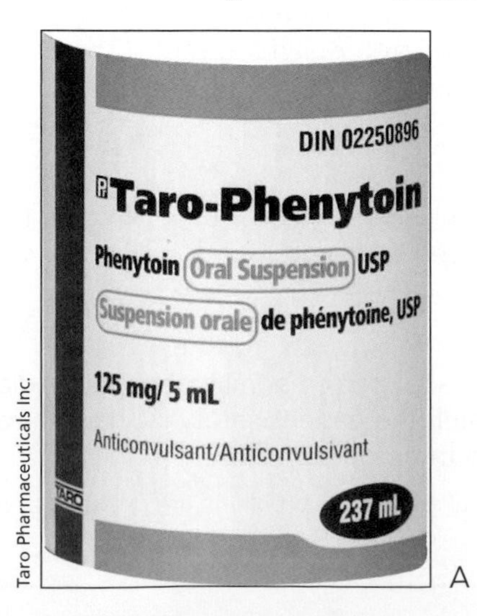

Taro Pharmaceuticals Inc.

A

Label B:

4. The generic name of the drug is____________________.
5. The reconstitution instruction to mix a supply dosage of 100 mg/5 mL for oral suspension is ____________________.
6. The manufacturer of thc drug is____________________.

BIEN AGITER AVANT L'EMPLOI.
Le flacon contient de la céfixime sous forme de trihydrate correspondant à 1 g de céfixime anhydre.
POSOLOGIE – ADULTE : 400 mg, 1 fois par jour. Si nécessaire, 200 mg, 2 fois par jour.
Infections urinaires : 400 mg, 1 fois par jour.
ENFANT : 8 mg/kg/jour, 1 fois par jour. Si nécessaire, 4 mg/kg, 2 fois par jour.
Infections urinaires : 8 mg/kg/jour, 1 fois par jour.
RECONSTITUTION : Secouer légèrement le flacon plusieurs fois pour ameublir la poudre avant la reconstitution. Ajouter un volume total de 33 mL d'eau divisé en DEUX PORTIONS. Bien mélanger après chaque addition. Donne 20 mg/mL. La suspension peut être conservée pendant 14 jours à la température ambiante ou réfrigérée. **Jeter la portion non utilisée.**
Monographie du produit fournie sur demande ou disponible au www.sanofi.ca. Conserver la poudre à une température ambiante contrôlée se situant entre 15 et 30 °C.

(01)20065914106686

DIN 00868965
Suprax®
Cefixime for oral suspension, Mfr. Std. /
Céfixime pour suspension orale, Norme-fabricant
100 mg / **5** ml *
Antibiotic / Antibiotique
50 mL
*when reconstituted / lorsque reconstitué
SANOFI

SHAKE WELL BEFORE USE.
The bottle contains cefixime as trihydrate, corresponding to 1 g cefixime anhydrous.
DOSAGE – ADULTS: 400 mg once daily. If necessary, 200 mg twice daily. **Urinary tract infections:** 400 mg once daily.
CHILDREN: 8 mg/kg/day once daily. If necessary, 4 mg/kg twice daily. **Urinary tract infections:** 8 mg/kg/day once daily.
RECONSTITUTION: Tap the bottle several times to loosen powder contents prior to reconstitution. Add a total volume of 33 mL of water split in TWO PORTIONS. Mix well after each addition. Provides 20 mg/mL. Suspension may be kept for 14 days at room temperature or under refrigeration. **Discard unused portion.** 1230421-E
Product Monograph available upon request or at www.sanofi.ca. Store powder at controlled room temperature between 15 and 30°C.
® Registered trade-mark of / Marque déposée de Astellas Pharma Inc., Osaka, Japan (Japon).
Mfd by / Fabr. par sanofi-aventis Canada Inc., Laval, Québec, Canada H7V 0A3
1 800 265-7927
Lot
Exp.
E50069005E

B

Label C:

7. The total volume of the medication container is____________________.
8. The supply dosage is____________________.
9. How much will you administer to the patient per dose for the order *Methotrexate sodium 25 mg IV stat?*____________________

C

STERILE/ STÉRILE
DIN 02099705
2 mL
METHOTREXATE
Sodium Injection
sodique injectable
50 mg / 2 mL
USP
25 mg / mL
methotrexate per vial
de méthotrexate par fiole
For IM, IV, intra-arterial, intraventricular or intrathecal use. Single use only. Discard unused portion.
Usage IM, IV, intra-artériel, intraventriculaire ou intrathécal. Usage unique seulement. Jeter toute portion inutilisée.
ANTIMETABOLITE
For complete information on dosage and administration and directions for use, see package insert. Store at room temperature protected from light.
PRESERVATIVE FREE
ANTIMÉTABOLITE
Pour les renseignements complets sur la posologie et l'administration, consulter le dépliant de conditionnement. Garder à l'abri de la lumière, à la température ambiante.
SANS AGENT DE CONSERVATION
novopharm®
®-Reg'd Trademark of Novopharm Limited
Marque déposée de Novopharm Limitée
Toronto, Canada M1B 2K9
C
Cytotoxic
Cytotoxique
93.148.375-C
76723LA-0002 Rev. 01
Lot:
Exp:

Novopharm Limited

Label D:

10. The number of doses supplied by this vial is ____________________.
11. The generic name is ____________________.
12. The Drug Identification Number of the drug is ____________________.

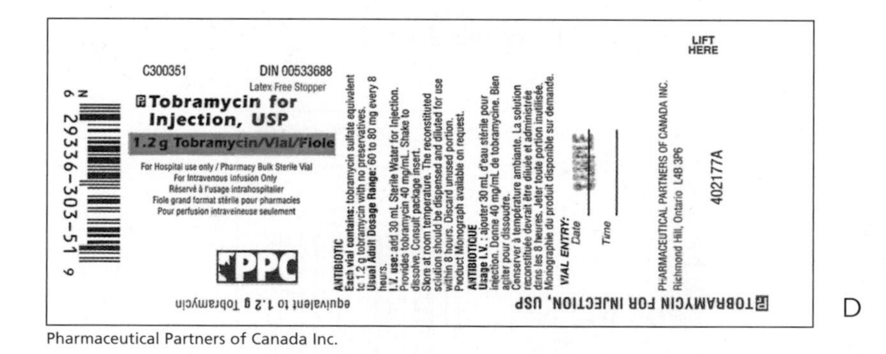

D

Pharmaceutical Partners of Canada Inc.

Label E:

13. The form of the drug is____________________.
14. The total volume of the drug container is____________________.
15. The administration route is____________________.

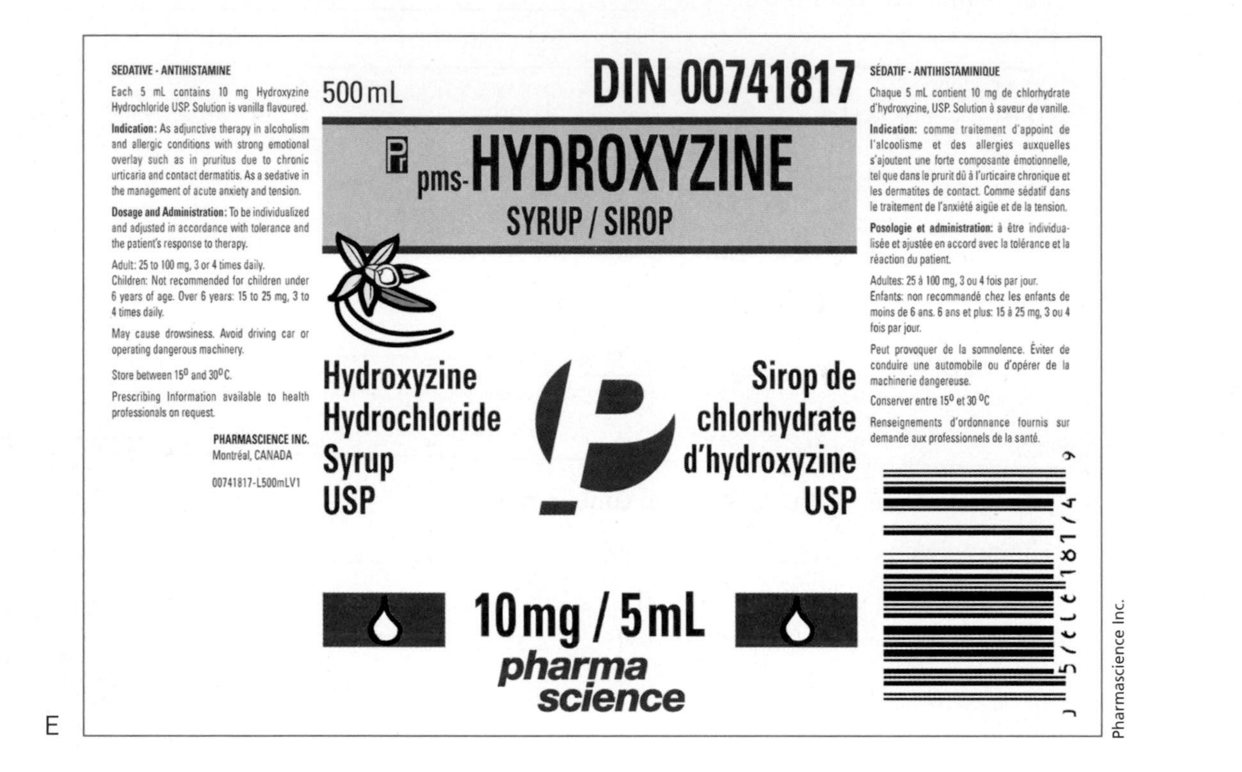
SEDATIVE - ANTIHISTAMINE
Each 5 mL contains 10 mg Hydroxyzine Hydrochloride USP. Solution is vanilla flavoured.
Indication: As adjunctive therapy in alcoholism and allergic conditions with strong emotional overlay such as in pruritus due to chronic urticaria and contact dermatitis. As a sedative in the management of acute anxiety and tension.
Dosage and Administration: To be individualized and adjusted in accordance with tolerance and the patient's response to therapy.
Adult: 25 to 100 mg, 3 or 4 times daily.
Children: Not recommended for children under 6 years of age. Over 6 years: 15 to 25 mg, 3 to 4 times daily.
May cause drowsiness. Avoid driving car or operating dangerous machinery.
Store between 15⁰ and 30⁰C.
Prescribing Information available to health professionals on request.
PHARMASCIENCE INC.
Montréal, CANADA
00741817-L500mLV1
500 mL
DIN 00741817
pms-HYDROXYZINE
SYRUP / SIROP
Hydroxyzine Hydrochloride Syrup USP
Sirop de chlorhydrate d'hydroxyzine USP
10 mg / 5 mL
pharma science
SÉDATIF - ANTIHISTAMINIQUE
Chaque 5 mL contient 10 mg de chlorhydrate d'hydroxyzine, USP. Solution à saveur de vanille.
Indication: comme traitement d'appoint de l'alcoolisme et des allergies auxquelles s'ajoutent une forte composante émotionnelle, tel que dans le prurit dû à l'urticaire chronique et les dermatites de contact. Comme sédatif dans le traitement de l'anxiété aigüe et de la tension.
Posologie et administration: à être individualisée et ajustée en accord avec la tolérance et la réaction du patient.
Adultes: 25 à 100 mg, 3 ou 4 fois par jour.
Enfants: non recommandé chez les enfants de moins de 6 ans. 6 ans et plus: 15 à 25 mg, 3 ou 4 fois par jour.
Peut provoquer de la somnolence. Éviter de conduire une automobile ou d'opérer de la machinerie dangereuse.
Conserver entre 15⁰ et 30 ⁰C
Renseignements d'ordonnance fournis sur demande aux professionnels de la santé.
Pharmascience Inc.

E

Label F:

16. The name of the drug manufacturer is____________________.
17. The form of the drug is____________________.
18. The appropriate temperature for storage of this drug is____________________.

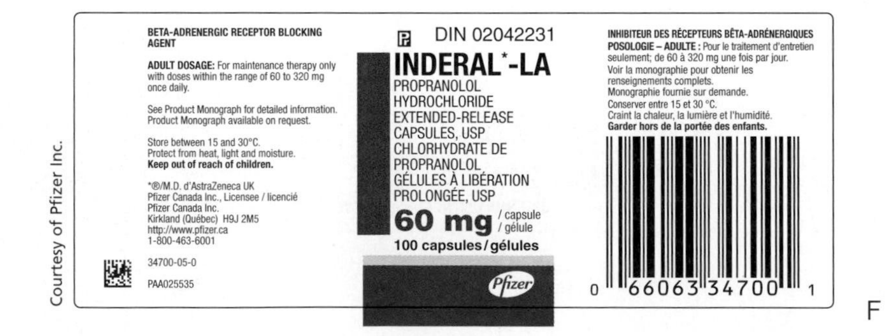
BETA-ADRENERGIC RECEPTOR BLOCKING AGENT
ADULT DOSAGE: For maintenance therapy only with doses within the range of 60 to 320 mg once daily.
See Product Monograph for detailed information. Product Monograph available on request.
Store between 15 and 30°C.
Protect from heat, light and moisture.
Keep out of reach of children.
*®/M.D. d'AstraZeneca UK
Pfizer Canada Inc., Licensee / licencié
Pfizer Canada Inc.
Kirkland (Québec) H9J 2M5
http://www.pfizer.ca
1-800-463-6001
34700-05-0
PAA025535
DIN 02042231
INDERAL*-LA
PROPRANOLOL HYDROCHLORIDE EXTENDED-RELEASE CAPSULES, USP
CHLORHYDRATE DE PROPRANOLOL GÉLULES À LIBÉRATION PROLONGÉE, USP
60 mg / capsule / gélule
100 capsules / gélules
Pfizer
INHIBITEUR DES RÉCEPTEURS BÊTA-ADRÉNERGIQUES
POSOLOGIE – ADULTE : Pour le traitement d'entretien seulement; de 60 à 320 mg une fois par jour.
Voir la monographie pour obtenir les renseignements complets.
Monographie fournie sur demande.
Conserver entre 15 et 30 °C.
Craint la chaleur, la lumière et l'humidité.
Garder hors de la portée des enfants.
0 66063 34700 1
Courtesy of Pfizer Inc.

F

Label G:

19. The dosage strength of the Epi-PenJr is ____________________.
20. The dosage strength of the Epi-Pen is ____________________.

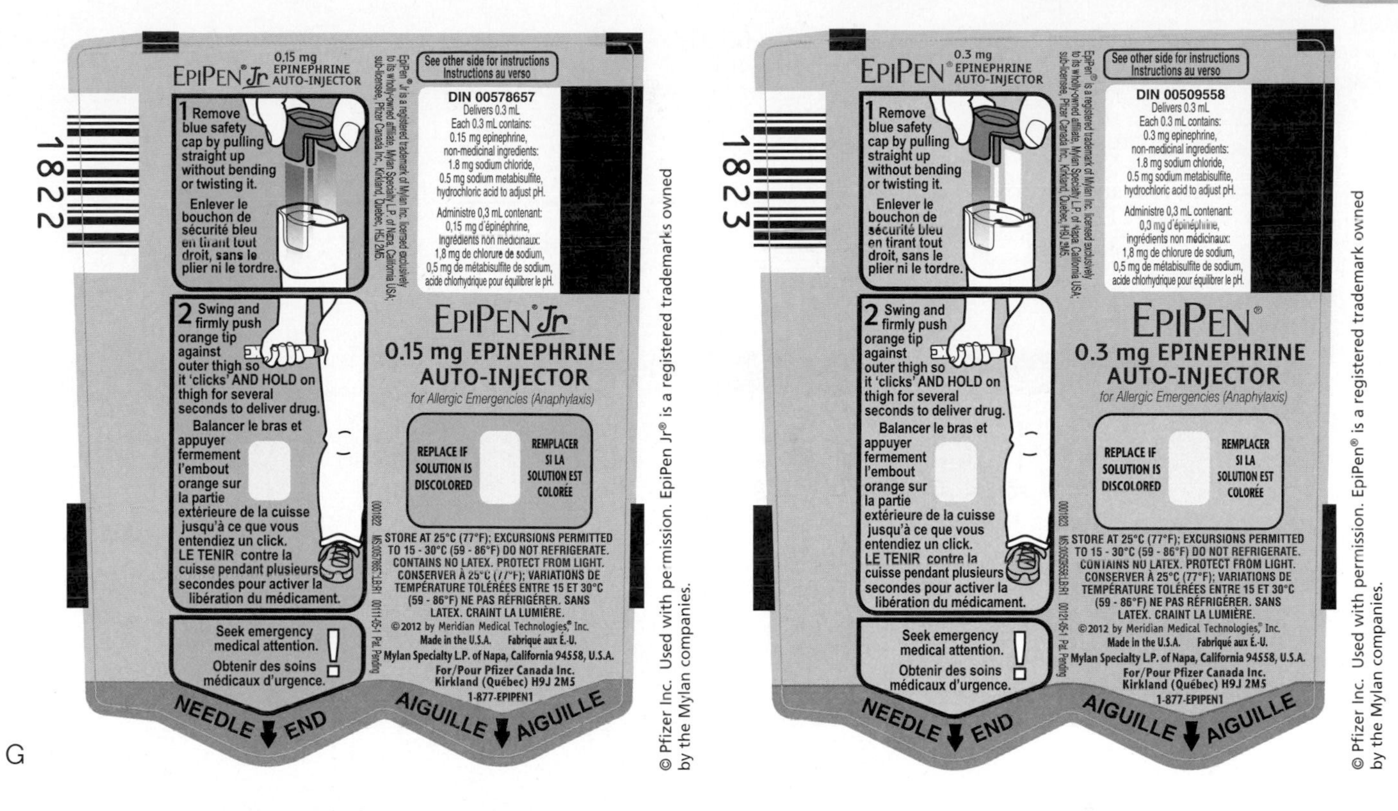

G

Match drug label H or I with each statement 21 through 23.

21. This drug contains 25 mg of spironolactone per tablet. ________
22. This is a label for a combination drug. ________
23. This is a label for a drug that is usually ordered by the number of tablets to be administered rather than the dosage strength. ________
24. The administration route for the drug labelled I is ________.
25. The drug strength for each of the drugs in label H is ________.

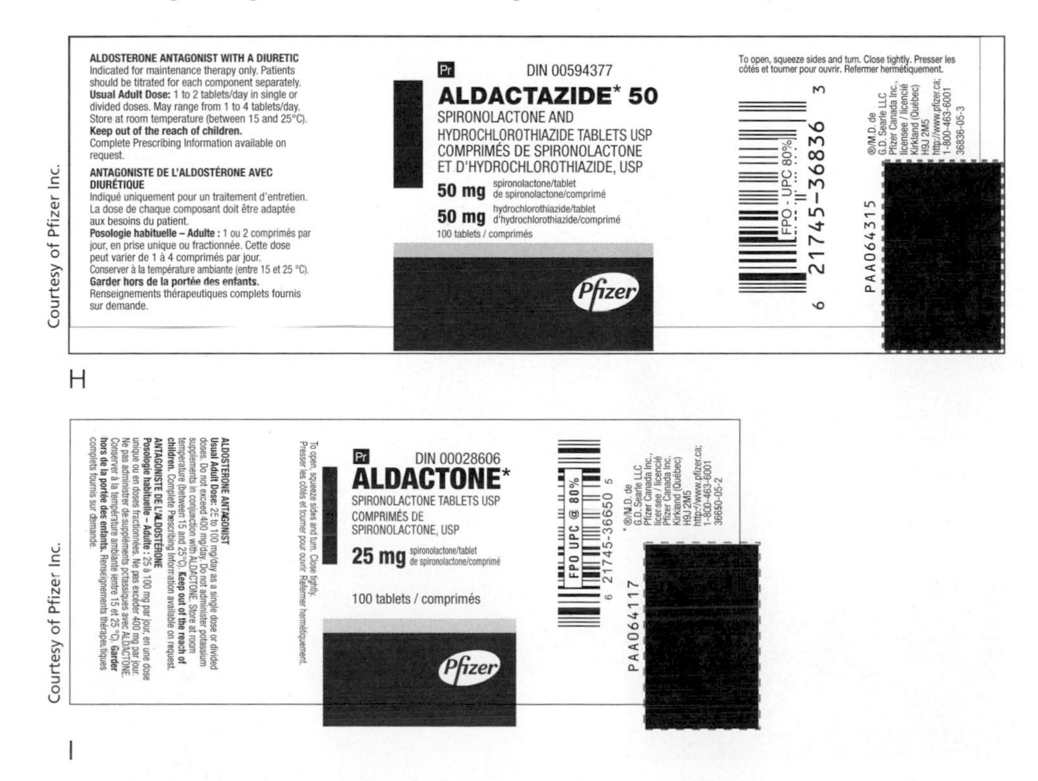

Use drug label J to answer questions 26 and 27.

Label J:

26. Expressed as a percentage, the supply dosage of the drug is ________.
27. The supply dosage is equivalent to ________ g per ________ mL or ________ mg/mL.

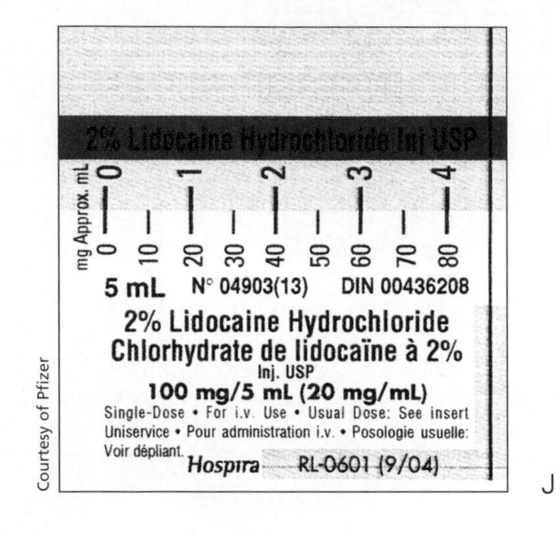

J

Use label K to answer questions 28 and 29.

28. Benadryl is a ________________ formulation and is to be used specifically for this patient population, ________________.
29. The strength of the formulation is ________________.

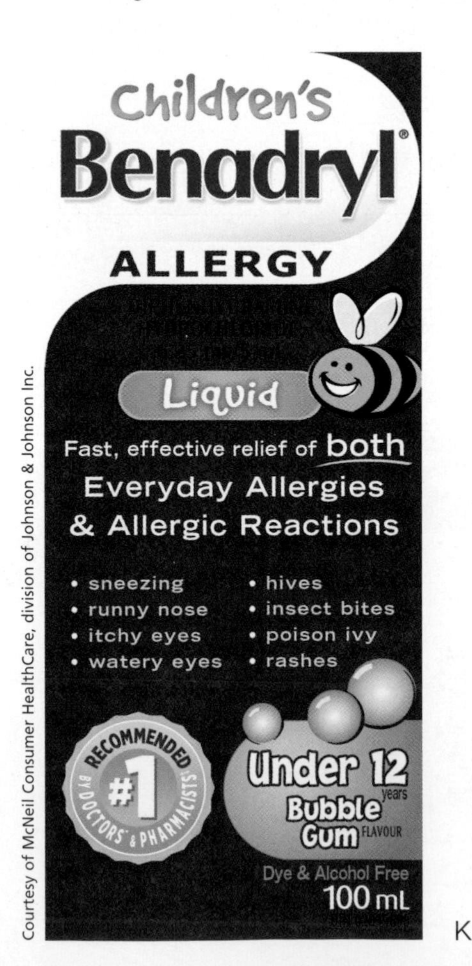

K

APPLICATION OF CLINICAL REASONING

7-1 Describe the clinical reasoning you would implement to prevent this patient safety incident.

Possible Scenario

Suppose the prescriber wrote the order *Celebrex 100 mg PO q12h* (an anti-inflammatory to treat rheumatoid arthritis pain), but the order was difficult to read. The unit nurse, processing the order, and the pharmacist interpreted the order as *Celexa* (an antidepressant), a medication with a similar spelling. Celexa was written on the MAR.

Potential Outcome

The nurse administered the Celexa for several days, and the patient began to experience severe knee and hip pain from rheumatoid arthritis. Also, the patient experienced adverse effects of Celexa, including drowsiness and tremors. A patient safety incident occurred because two healthcare providers misinterpreted the order.

Prevention

What should have alerted the nurse that something was wrong? What should have been considered to prevent this patient safety incident?

____

____

Check your work! Answers to all Application for Clinical Reasoning problems are provided at the end of the book, in the Answers section.

ANSWERS TO REVIEW SETS

Review Set 7-1

1) E **2)** D **3)** C **4)** A **5)** B **6)** F **7)** G **8)** 2.5 mL **9)** IM or IV **10)** A, C, D, E, F **11)** 4 mg/2 mL **12)** 2 tablets **13)** penicillin G sodium **14)** 5 000 000 units per vial; reconstituted to 250 000 units/mL, 500 000 units/mL, or 1 000 000 units/mL **15)** IM or IV **16)** 02220288 **17)** Pharmaceutical Partners of Canada **18)** 2% **19)** 2 g per 100 mL **20)** 20 mg/mL

Directions:

1. Round decimals to two places.
2. Reduce fractions to their lowest terms.

Chapter 5: Equipment Used in Dosage Measurement

Draw an arrow to indicate the correct measurement of the doses given.

1. 1.5 mL

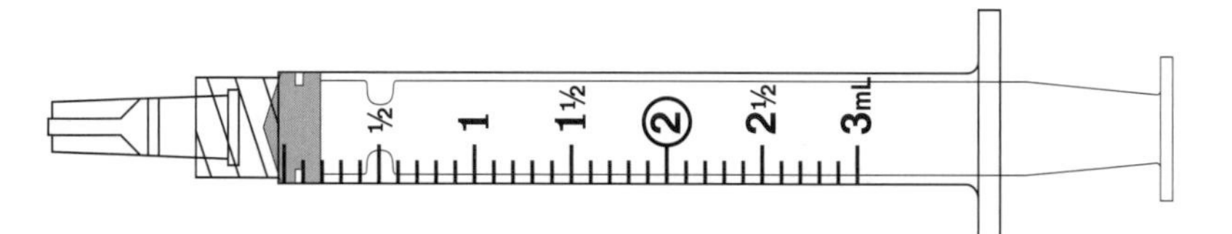

2. 0.33 mL

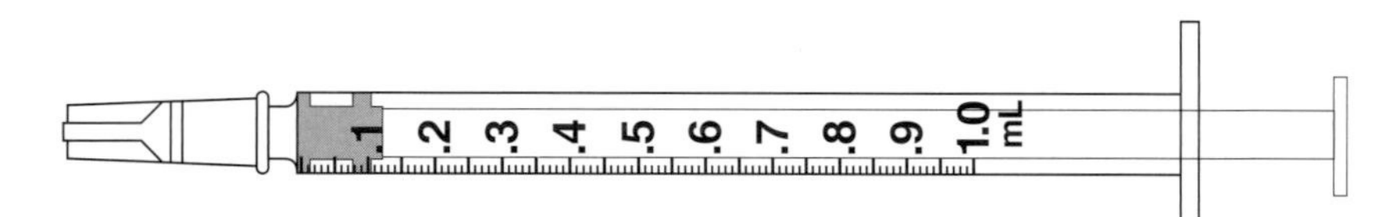

3. 44 units of insulin

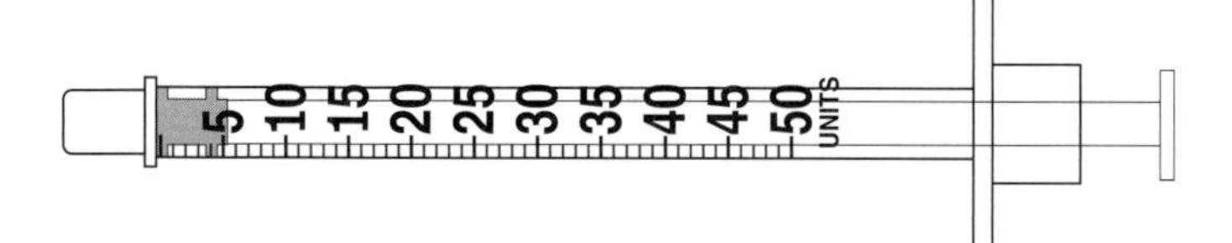

4. 37 units of insulin

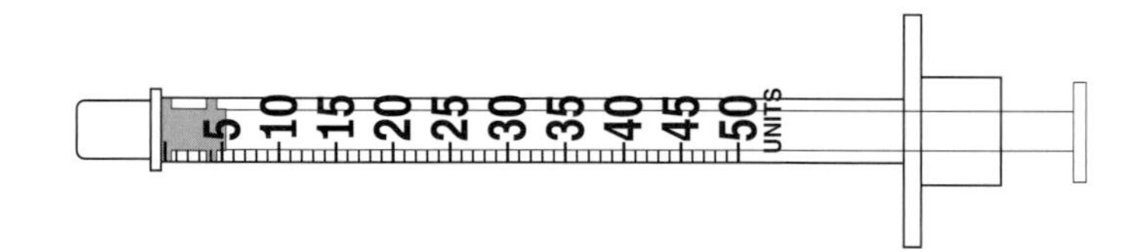

5. 7.5 mL

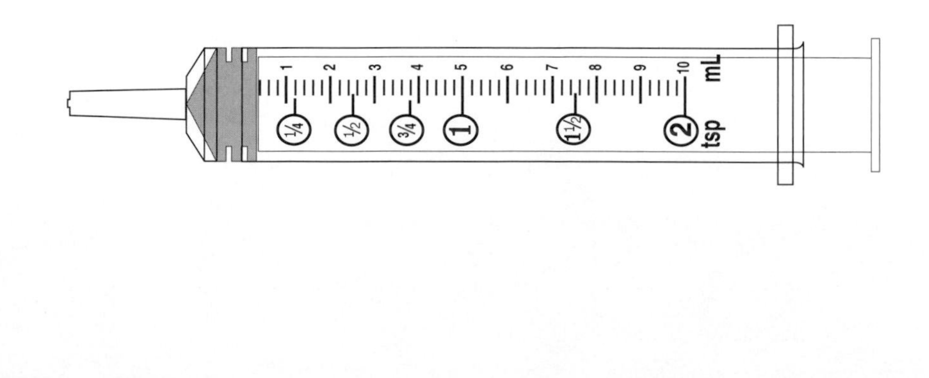

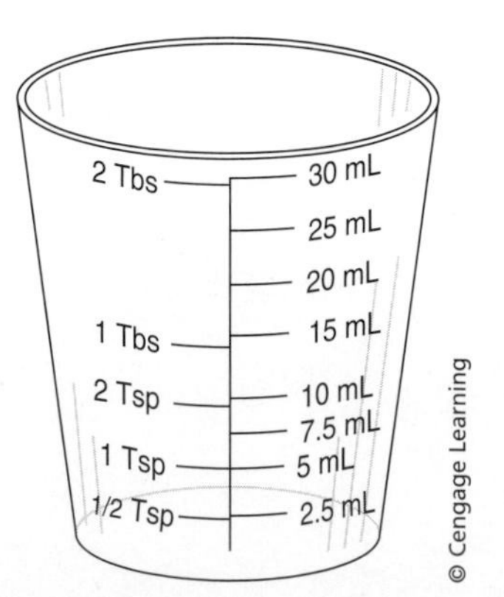

Chapters 6 and 7: Interpreting Drug Orders and Drug Labels

Use drug label A to provide the information requested for questions 6 through 9.

6. The generic name is ____.
7. This drug is an otic and ophthalmic solution and is intended for ________________.
8. The total volume of this container is ____________________________________.
9. Interpret: *Sofracort solution 2 gtt both ears q15 min × 3* ____________________

DIN 02224623
Sofracort®
Sterile ear/eye drops
Gouttes oto-ophtalmiques stériles
8 mL SANOFI
FOR INFORMATION ONLY
POUR INFORMATION SEULEMENT
LOT:

A

Use drug label B to provide the information requested for questions 10 through 12.

10. The supply dosage is __________.
11. The Drug Identification Number is __________.
12. Interpret: *naproxen 750 mg/day PO divided TID* __________.

    ____

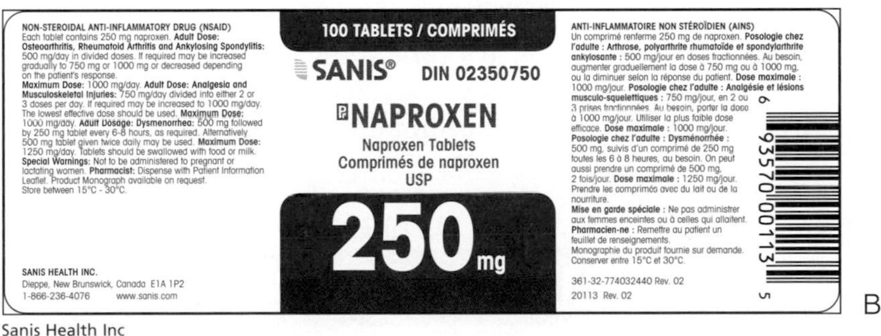

100 TABLETS / COMPRIMÉS
SANIS® DIN 02350750
NAPROXEN
Naproxen Tablets
Comprimés de naproxen
USP
250 mg
SANIS HEALTH INC.
Dieppe, New Brunswick, Canada E1A 1P2
1-866-236-4076 www.sanis.com

B

Sanis Health Inc

Use drug label C to provide the information requested for questions 13 through 15.

ANTIBACTERIAL
Each mL contains 40 mg sulfamethoxazole and 8 mg trimethoprim.
SHAKE WELL BEFORE USING.
Usual Dose for Adults and Children Over 12 Years of Age: 4 teaspoonfuls (20 mL) suspension twice daily.
Children between 6 and 12 years of age: 1 - 2 teaspoonfuls (5 - 10 mL) suspension twice daily.
Children 2 to 5 years of age: 1/2 - 1 teaspoonful (2.5 - 5 mL) suspension twice daily.
Children under 2 years of age: 1/2 teaspoon (2.5 mL) suspension twice daily.
Product monograph available to physicians and pharmacists on request.
Store between 15 - 30C and dispense in a light-resistant container.

DIN 00726540 400 mL
NOVO-TRIMEL
Sulfamethoxazole and Trimethoprim
Sulfaméthoxazole et Triméthoprime
Oral Suspension orale USP
200/40 mg/5 mL
novopharm®
TORONTO, CANADA

ANTIBACTÉRIEN
Chaque mL contient 40 mg de sulfaméthoxazole et 8 mg de triméthoprime.
BIEN AGITER AVANT L'EMPLOI
POSOLOGIE : Adultes et enfants de plus de 12 ans : 4 cuillerées à thé (20 mL) de suspension 2 fois/jour.
Enfants de 6 à 12 ans : 1 à 2 cuillerées à thé (5 à 10 mL) de suspension 2 fois/jour.
Enfants de 2 à 5 ans: 1/2 à 1 cuillerée à thé (2,5 à 5 mL) de suspension 2 fois/jour.
Enfants de moins de 2 ans: 1/2 cuillerée à thé (2,5 mL) de suspension 2 fois/jour.
La monographie du produit est fournie sur demande aux médecins et aux pharmaciens.
Conserver entre 15 C - 30 C et remettre au patient dans un flacon opaque.
6-78503-10-0
85502LA-0066 Rev. 01

C

Novopharm Limited

13. The trade name is ____.
14. The supply dosage is ____________.

15. What amount would be given for one dose if the drug order is for a child under 2 years of age?

    a. __________ mL

    b. Draw an arrow to indicate the dose volume.

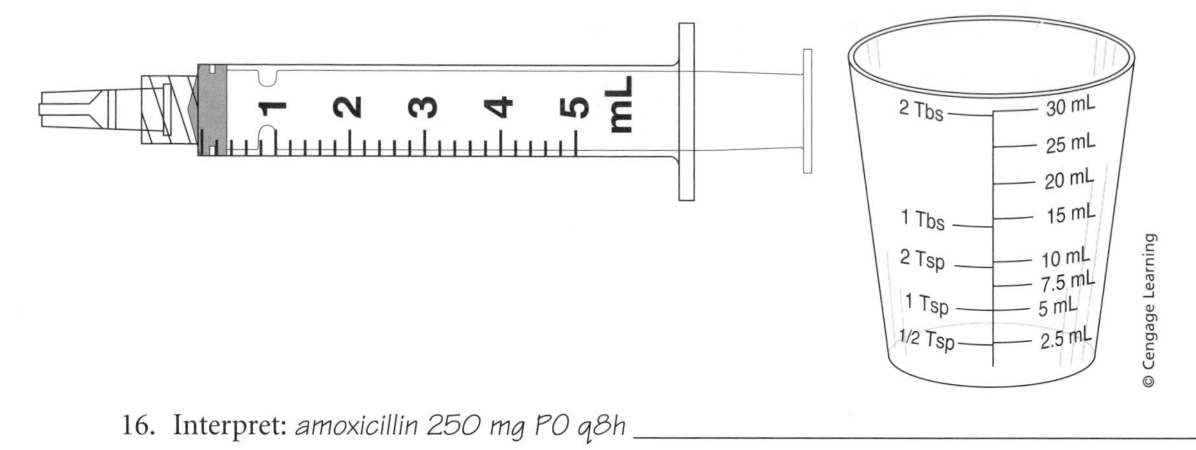

16. Interpret: *amoxicillin 250 mg PO q8h* ________________________________.

Using the information regarding medication abbreviations, symbols, and dosage designations that should NOT be used, identify the mistake in the following orders and correct each order.

17. Prednisone 50 mg p.o. OD ____________________________

18. HCTZ 50.0 mg p.o. bid ____________________________

19. Novolin regular insulin 30U SC daily ____________________________

20. A patient with dysphagia is ordered a variety of oral medications. The patient needs oral drugs to be administered via a nasogastric (NG) tube. Which medications are safe to administer and which are not safe to administer via the NG tube? Explain.

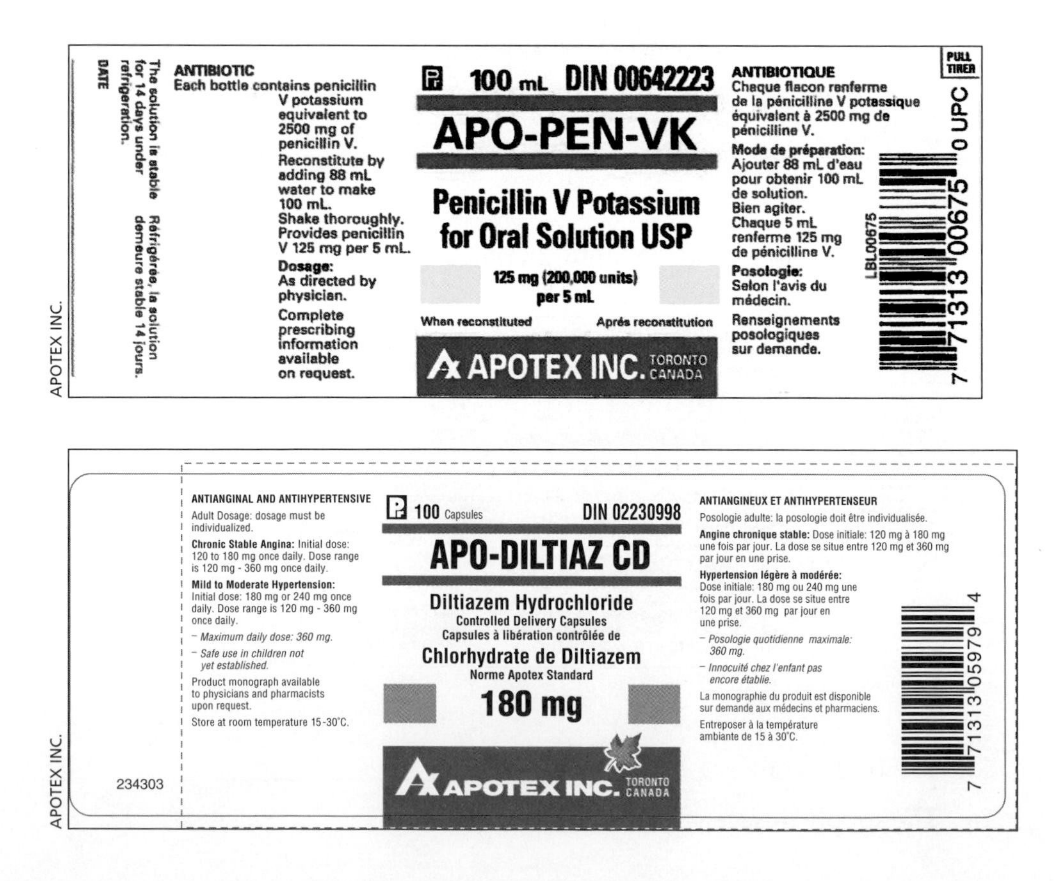

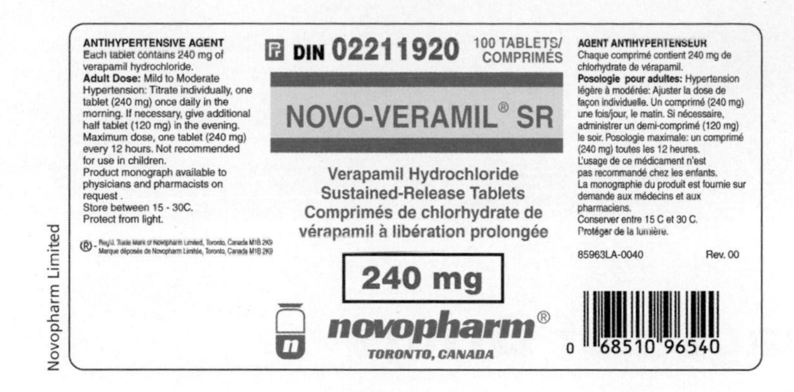
ANTIHYPERTENSIVE AGENT
Each tablet contains 240 mg of verapamil hydrochloride.
Adult Dose: Mild to Moderate Hypertension: Titrate individually, one tablet (240 mg) once daily in the morning. If necessary, give additional half tablet (120 mg) in the evening. Maximum dose, one tablet (240 mg) every 12 hours. Not recommended for use in children.
Product monograph available to physicians and pharmacists on request .
Store between 15 - 30C.
Protect from light.
® - Reg'd. Trade Mark of Novopharm Limited, Toronto, Canada M1B 2K9
Marque déposée de Novopharm Limitée, Toronto, Canada M1B 2K9
DIN 02211920
100 TABLETS/ COMPRIMÉS
NOVO-VERAMIL® SR
Verapamil Hydrochloride Sustained-Release Tablets
Comprimés de chlorhydrate de vérapamil à libération prolongée
240 mg
novopharm®
TORONTO, CANADA
AGENT ANTIHYPERTENSEUR
Chaque comprimé contient 240 mg de chlorhydrate de vérapamil.
Posologie pour adultes: Hypertension légère à modérée: Ajuster la dose de façon individuelle. Un comprimé (240 mg) une fois/jour, le matin. Si nécessaire, administrer un demi-comprimé (120 mg) le soir. Posologie maximale: un comprimé (240 mg) toutes les 12 heures.
L'usage de ce médicament n'est pas recommandé chez les enfants.
La monographie du produit est fournie sur demande aux médecins et aux pharmaciens.
Conserver entre 15 C et 30 C.
Protéger de la lumière.
85963LA-0040
Rev. 00
0 68510 96540
Novopharm Limited

After completing these problems, see the answer section at the back of the book to check your answers. Give yourself 2 points for each correct answer.

Perfect score = 40 My score = ______________________________

Mastery score = 36 or higher (18 or more correct)

Oral Dosages of Drugs

OBJECTIVES

1. Calculate oral dosages of drugs.
2. Use the formula $\frac{D}{H} \times Q = X$ to calculate drug dosages.
3. Calculate the number of tablets or capsules to be administered for a prescribed dosage.
4. Calculate the volume of liquid per dose to be administered for a prescribed dosage in solution form.

Medications for oral administration are supplied in a variety of forms, such as tablets, capsules, and liquids. They are usually ordered to be administered by mouth, or *PO*, the abbreviation for the Latin phrase "*per os.*" To reduce inaccurate dosage calculations, Accreditation Canada criteria for safe medication practice recommend that all medications in acute-care facilities be provided in unit-dose packaging, preferably in the original package from the manufacturer. A unit-dose system includes the preparation and provision of patient-specific oral and injectable drugs in a quantity and formulation that is ready to administer to the patient, as indicated in the prescription requirements. Providing unit-dose packaging may not always be possible, as hospital pharmacies are frequently supplied with large bulk containers of tablets, capsules, and drugs for injection. Whenever possible, hospital pharmacists should repackage medication into unit doses for distribution to inpatient units. Usually a 24-hour supply of drug is provided to the patient care area; however, this time frame can vary among patient care areas and can range from 12 to 72 hours. As part of the hospital pharmacy's unit-dose drug distribution system, a centralized intravenous admixture program makes sterile preparations for injections.

When a liquid form of a drug is unavailable, children and older patients may need to have a tablet crushed or a capsule opened and mixed with a small amount of food or fluid to enable them to swallow the medication. Many of these crushed medications and oral liquids may also be ordered to be given enterally, or into the gastrointestinal tract using a specially placed tube. Such tubes and their associated enteral routes are the *nasogastric* (NG) tube from nares to stomach, the *nasojejunal* (NJ) tube from nares to jejunum, the *gastrostomy tube* (GT) placed directly through the abdomen into the stomach, and the *percutaneous endoscopic gastrostomy* (PEG) tube.

Some solid-form medications, such as Aspirin, are enteric-coated (and also considered a delayed-release formulation). This protective barrier allows the drug to dissolve in the duodenum, avoiding the adverse effect of irritation to the stomach lining. Time-release technology (or sustained-release, extended-release, controlled-release, and so on) allows tablets and capsules to be released over time, which results in a slow, steady release of the drug into the bloodstream and allows for dosing at less frequent intervals. Consequently, enteric-coated and time-release drugs should not be crushed or divided. Consult a drug reference or the pharmacist if you are in doubt about the safety of crushing tablets or opening capsules. The Institute for Safe Medication Practices has a "Do Not Crush" list.

RATIONALE FOR PRACTICE

Do not crush, break, or chew enteric-coated (EC) products. They are formulated to dissolve in the intestine to reduce gastric irritation and to prevent irritation of the mouth, staining of the teeth and oral mucosa, or destruction of the drug by stomach acid. Sustained-release products—controlled-release (CR), extended-release (ER or XL), long-acting (LA), sustained-release (SR), and other products—are formulated to deliver the drug over a 24-hour period. Crushing these formulations may lead to an initial overdose followed by insufficient drug levels to maintain the intended therapeutic effect.

CAUTION

When a drug name lacks a suffix that identifies it as a sustained-release product, do not assume that the product works by immediate release. Some tablets contain pellets within the capsule that are formulated for extended release. For example, Aggrenox is unique because it contains extended-release pellets incorporating dipyridamole and a round white tablet incorporating immediate-release Aspirin in a hard gelatin capsule. It should not be chewed or crushed or opened to release the contents. Always check with the published list of drugs that should not be crushed. The Institute for Safe Medication Practices in the United States posts a list of oral drugs that should not be crushed. To access this list, visit the website at www.ISMP.org, and search for "Do Not Crush" list.

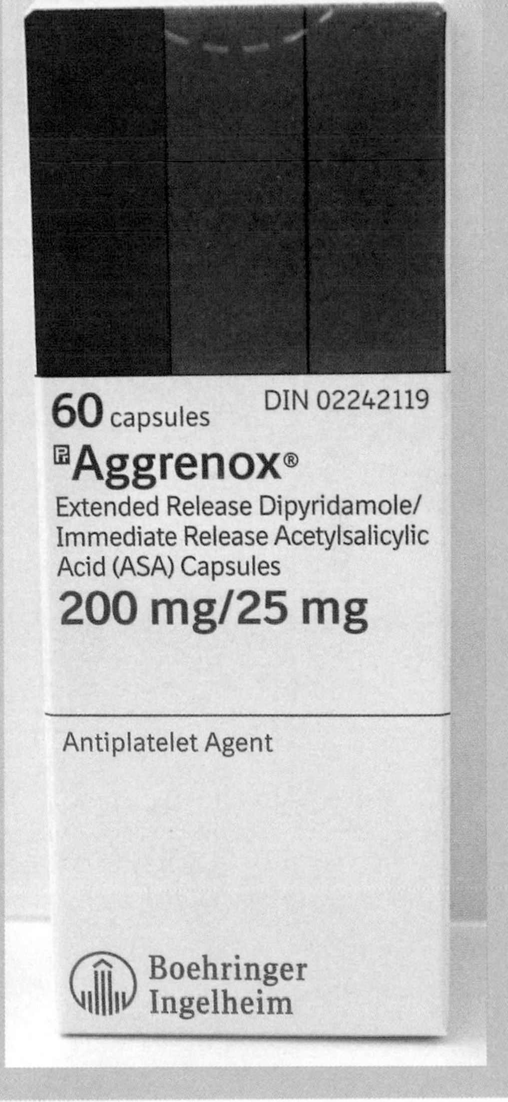

60 capsules
DIN 02242119
Aggrenox®
Extended Release Dipyridamole/
Immediate Release Acetylsalicylic
Acid (ASA) Capsules
200 mg/25 mg
Antiplatelet Agent
Boehringer
Ingelheim

Courtesy of Boehringer Ingelheim

TABLETS AND CAPSULES

Medications prepared in tablet and capsule form are supplied in the strengths or dosages in which they are commonly prescribed (Figure 8-1). It is desirable to obtain the drug in the same strength as the dosage ordered or in multiples of that dosage. When necessary, scored tablets (those marked for division) can be divided into halves or quarters. **Only scored tablets are intended to be divided.**

CAUTION

It is safest and most accurate to give the fewest number of whole, undivided tablets possible.

Area for Lot and Exp.

DIN 02248804 100 TABLETS COMPRIMÉS

TEVA-CLARITHROMYCIN

Clarithromycin Tablets
Comprimés de clarithromycine
Teva Standard Norme Teva

250 mg

TEVA

ANTIBIOTIC Each tablet contains 250 mg clarithromycin. RESPIRATORY TRACT OR SKIN INFECTIONS: Usual dose range for adults and children over 12 years: 250 to 500 mg every 12 hours for 7 to 14 days. MYCOBACTERIAL INFECTIONS (PREVENTION AND TREATMENT): Recommended Adult Dose: 500 mg every 12 hours. HELICOBACTER PYLORI INFECTION: Recommended Adult Dose: Triple Therapy - 500 mg twice daily for 10 days. Pharmacist: Dispense with Patient Information Leaflet. Product Monograph available on request. Store 15 - 30°C in a tightly closed container. Protect from light.

ANTIBIOTIQUE Un comprimé renferme 250 mg de clarithromycine. INFECTIONS RESPIRATOIRES ET CUTANÉES : Schéma posologique habituel chez les adultes et les enfants de plus de 12 ans : 250 mg à 500 mg toutes les 12 heures pendant 7 à 14 jours. INFECTIONS MYCOBACTÉRIENNES (PRÉVENTION ET TRAITEMENT) : Posologie recommandée chez l'adulte : 500 mg toutes les 12 heures. INFECTION À HELICOBACTER PYLORI : Posologie recommandée chez l'adulte : Trithérapie - 500 mg, 2 fois/jour pendant 10 jours. Pharmacien-ne : Remettre au patient un feuillet de renseignements. Monographie de produit fournie sur demande. Conserver entre 15 °C et 30 °C dans un contenant hermétiquement fermé. Garder à l'abri de la lumière.

TEVA is a reg'd trademark of / est une marque déposée de TEVA Pharmaceutical Industries Ltd. used under license by / utilisée sous licence par TEVA Canada Limited / Limitée, Toronto, Canada M1B 2K9

361-32-706230040 Rev 01 323K305390615

0 68510 17140 5

50

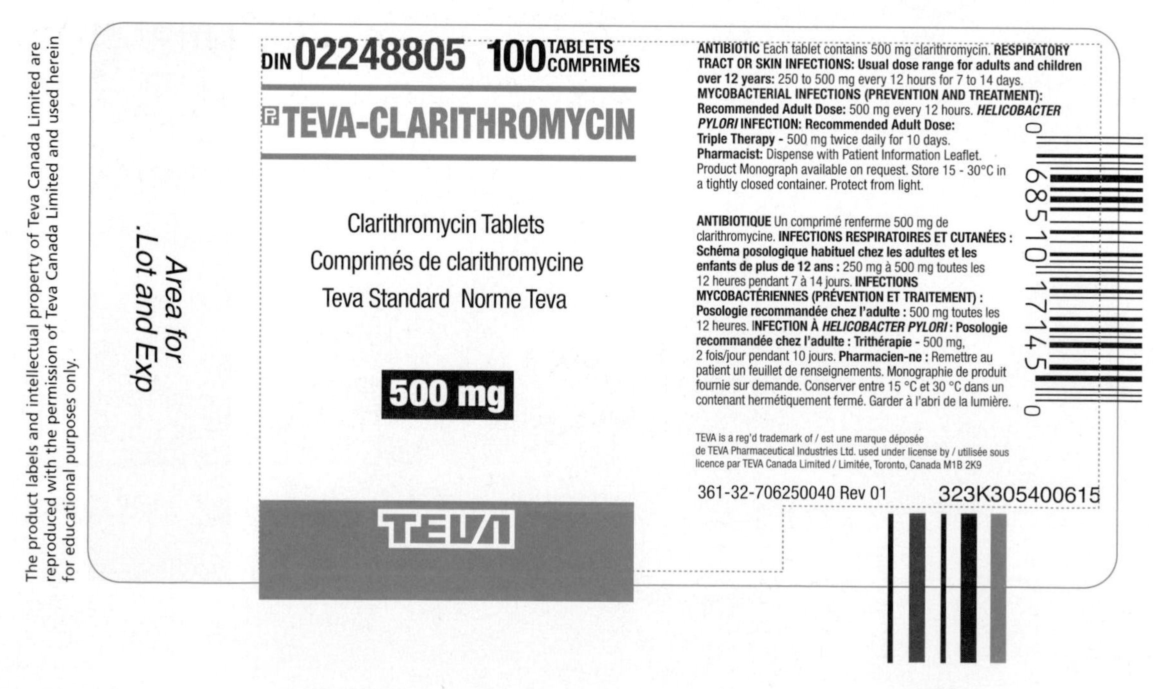

FIGURE 8-1 Clarithromycin 250-mg and 500-mg Tablets

Example 1:

Patient care order: *clarithromycin 500 mg PO q12h*

Clarithromycin is available in tablet strengths of 250 milligrams per tablet and 500 milligrams per tablet. When both strengths are available, the nurse should select the 500-milligram strength, and give 1 whole tablet for each dose.

Example 2:

Patient care order: *lorazepam 1.5 mg PO TID*

Lorazepam is available in strengths of 0.5-mg, 1-mg, and 2-mg tablets (Figure 8-2). When the three strengths are available, the nurse should select one 1-mg tablet and one 0.5-mg tablet (1 mg + 0.5 mg = 1.5 mg). This provides the ordered dosage of 1.5 mg and is the fewest number of tablets (2 tablets total) for the patient to swallow.

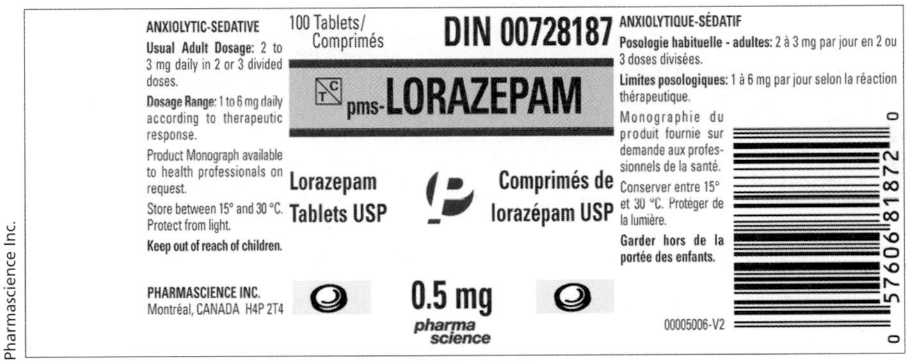

(a)

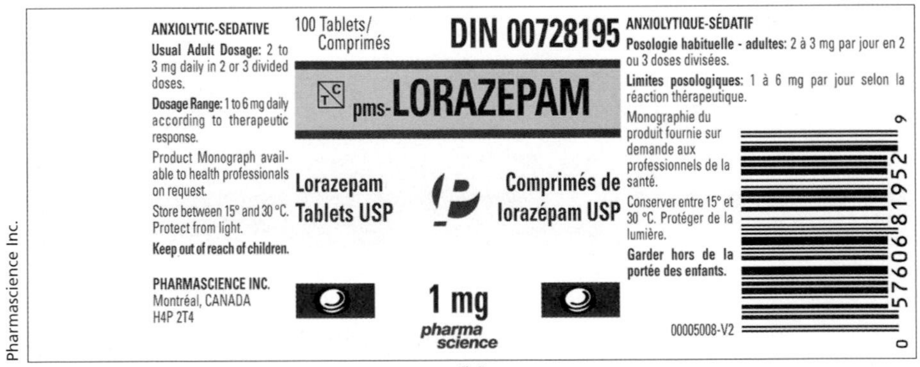

(b)

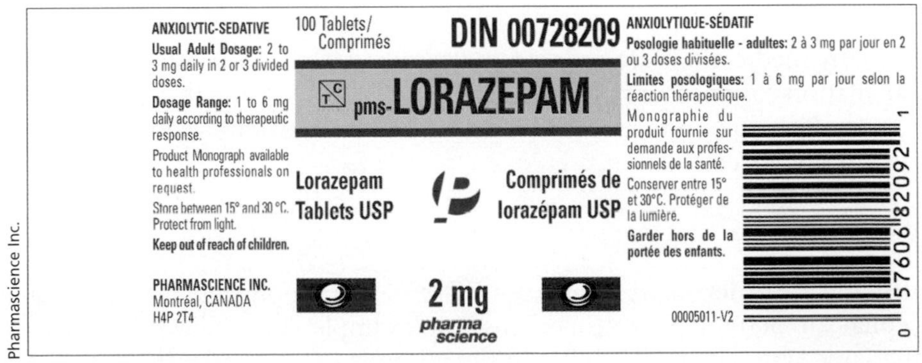

(c)

FIGURE 8-2 Lorazepam: (a) 0.5-mg; (b) 1-mg; (c) 2-mg Tablets

It is also possible to halve the 2-mg tablet to obtain two 1-mg parts and pair one-half with a 0.5-mg tablet. This would also equal 1.5 mg and supply $1\frac{1}{2}$ tablets. However, cutting any tablet in half may produce slightly unequal halves. The patient may not receive the ordered dose as a result. Therefore, it is preferable to give whole, undivided tablets, when they are available.

If the medication from the pharmacy is in the form of a prepackaged unit-dose blister pack, and each tablet is 0.5 mg, then the nurse would administer 3 of the 0.5-mg tablets per dose.

THREE-STEP APPROACH TO DOSAGE CALCULATIONS

The following simple Three-Step Approach has been proven to reduce anxiety about calculations and to ensure accurate results. Note that you will be asked to think and estimate before you apply a formula. Learn this simple Three-Step Approach, and use it for every dosage calculation every time.

REMEMBER

Three-Step Approach to Dosage Calculations

Step 1	**Convert**	Ensure that all measurements are the same unit of measurement. If not, convert before proceeding.
Step 2	**Think**	Estimate a *reasonable amount* of the drug to administer.
Step 3	**Calculate**	Apply the formula $\frac{D}{H} \times Q = X$
		$\frac{\text{D (desired)}}{\text{H (have)}} \times \text{Q (quantity)} = \text{X (amount)}$

Consider each step as an essential and consecutive rule of accurate dosage calculation.

RULE

Step 1	**Convert**	Be sure that all measurements are in the same units, and convert when necessary.

Many medications are ordered and supplied in the same unit of measurement. This makes dosage calculation easy because no conversion is necessary. When this is not the case, it is important to convert to the same units. Examine the following two examples in which conversion is a necessary first step in dosage calculation.

Example 1:

Patient care order: *cephalexin 0.5 g PO q6h*. The supply dosage (what is available) is labelled cephalexin 500 mg per capsule. This is an example of a medication order written and supplied in the same system (metric), but in different units (grams and milligrams). A drug order written in grams but supplied in milligrams will have to be converted so that the units match.

RATIONALE FOR PRACTICE

In most cases, it is more practical to change to the smaller unit (such as grams to milligrams). This requires multiplication and usually eliminates the decimal or fraction, keeping the calculation in whole numbers.

To continue with Example 1, convert 0.5 grams to milligrams. Milligrams is the smaller unit, and converting eliminates the decimal fraction.

Equivalent: 1 g = 1000 mg

Remember, you are converting from a larger unit to a smaller unit. Therefore, you will multiply by the conversion factor of 1000, or move the decimal point three places to the right.

$$0.5 \text{ g} = 0.5 \cancel{\text{g}} \times \frac{1000 \text{ mg}}{1 \cancel{\text{g}}} = 500 \text{ mg}$$

or 0.5 g = 0.500. = 500 mg

Order: *cephalexin 500 mg PO q6h*

Supply: cephalexin 500 mg per capsule

Give the patient 1 cephalexin 500-mg capsule by mouth every 6 hours.

Example 2:

Patient care order: *levothyroxine sodium 75 mcg PO daily*. The supply dosage (what is available) is labelled levothyroxine sodium 0.15 mg, scored tablets. This is another example of a medication ordered and supplied in different units. The order is in micrograms, the smaller unit, but the medication is supplied in milligrams, the larger unit.

Equivalent: 1 mg = 1000 mcg

Remember, convert from the larger unit to the smaller unit. Therefore, multiply by a conversion factor of 1000.

$$0.15 \text{ mg} = 0.15 \cancel{\text{mg}} \times \frac{1000 \text{ mcg}}{1 \cancel{\text{mg}}} = 150 \text{ mcg}$$

Now the example looks like this:

Order: *levothyroxine sodium 75 mcg PO daily*

Supply: levothyroxine sodium 150 mcg, scored tablets

Now solve this problem in your head. That is what Step 2 is about.

RULE

Step 2	Think	Carefully consider a reasonable amount of the drug that should be administered.

Once all the units are the same, Step 2 logically concludes what amount should be given. Before going on to Step 3, picture a reasonable amount of medication to be administered, as was demonstrated in the previous example. A close approximation, such as more or less than 1 tablet (or capsule or millilitre), can usually be estimated. Essentially, Step 2 requires a "*stop and think approach*" before going any further.

In the levothyroxine example, the patient should receive less than 1 tablet. In fact, $\frac{1}{2}$ of the 150-mcg tablet would be administered to fill the order for 75 mcg.

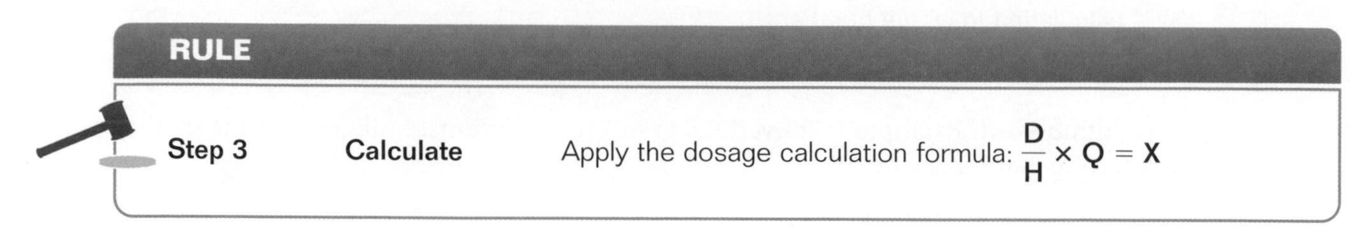

RULE
Step 3
Calculate
Apply the dosage calculation formula: $\frac{D}{H} \times Q = X$

Always double-check the estimated amount from Step 2 with the simple formula $\frac{D}{H} \times Q = X$. In this formula, *D* represents the *desired* dosage or the dosage ordered in the patient care order. *H* represents the dosage *available* on hand per a *quantity*, Q. Both *H* and *Q* constitute the *supply dosage* found on the label of the drug available.

RATIONALE FOR PRACTICE

When solving dosage problems for drugs supplied in tablets or capsules, Q (quantity) is always 1 because the supply dosage is per one tablet or capsule. Therefore, Q = 1 tablet or capsule.

Use the $\frac{D}{H} \times Q = X$ formula to double-check the process, and calculate the dosage needed for levothyroxine sodium.

Order: *levothyroxine sodium 75 mcg PO daily*

Supply: levothyroxine sodium 0.15 mg, converted to levothyroxine 150 mcg, scored tablets

D = desired = 75 mcg

H = have = 150 mcg

Q = quantity = 1 tablet

$$\frac{D}{H} \times Q = \frac{75 \text{ mcg}}{150 \text{ mcg}} \times 1 \text{ tablet}$$

$$\frac{\overset{1}{\cancel{75 \text{ mcg}}}}{\underset{2}{\cancel{150 \text{ mcg}}}} \times 1 \text{ tablet} = \frac{1}{2} \times 1 \text{ tablet} = \frac{1}{2} \text{ or } 0.5 \text{ tablet (Note that mcg cancels out.)}$$

Give $\frac{1}{2}$ (0.5) of the levothyroxine sodium 0.15-mg tablets orally once a day. The calculations verify the estimate from Step 2.

It is wise to get into the habit of always inserting the *quantity* value in the formula, even when Q is 1. Then you will be prepared to accurately calculate dosages for oral liquid or parenteral injection drugs that may be supplied in a solution strength quantity of more or less than 1 (mL).

Notice that the formula is set up with D (*desired dosage*) as the numerator and H (dosage *strength* you *have* on hand) as the denominator of a fraction. You are calculating for some portion of Q (*quantity* on hand). Setting up a dosage calculation like this makes sense. Now examine two more examples to reinforce this concept.

Example 3:

Order: *furosemide 10 mg PO BID*

Supply: furosemide 20 mg per tablet

$$\frac{D}{H} \times Q = \frac{10\text{ mg}}{20\text{ mg}} \times 1\text{ tablet}$$

$$\frac{\overset{1}{\cancel{10\text{ mg}}}}{\underset{2}{\cancel{20\text{ mg}}}} \times 1\text{ tablet} = \frac{1}{2} \times 1\text{ tablet} = \frac{1}{2}\text{ tablet}$$

Notice that you want to give $\frac{1}{2}$ of the Q (quantity of the supply dosage on hand, which in this case is 1 tablet). Therefore, give $\frac{1}{2}$ tablet of a furosemide 20-mg tablet orally twice daily.

Example 4:

Order: *acetaminophen 650 mg PO q4h prn for headache*

Supply: acetaminophen 325 mg per tablet

$$\frac{D}{H} \times Q = \frac{650\text{ mg}}{325\text{ mg}} \times 1\text{ tablet}$$

$$\frac{\overset{2}{\cancel{650\text{ mg}}}}{\underset{1}{\cancel{325\text{ mg}}}} \times 1\text{ tablet} = 2 \times 1\text{ tablet} = 2\text{ tablets}$$

Notice that 2 times the amount of Q will be administered; that is, give 2 of the acetaminophen 325-mg tablets orally every 4 hours as needed for headache.

Now apply all three steps of this logical approach to dosage calculations. The same three steps will be used to solve both oral and parenteral dosage calculation problems. It is most important to develop the ability to reason the answer or estimate before applying the $\frac{D}{H} \times Q = X$ formula.

Note to Learner

Healthcare providers can unknowingly make medication miscalculations if they rely solely on a formula rather than first asking themselves what the answer should be. The expectation is that healthcare providers are able to reason sensibly, problem solve, and justify their judgments rationally. While you are sharpening your math skills, your ability to think and estimate is your best resource for avoiding miscalculations. Use the formula as a calculation tool to validate the dose amount you anticipate should be given, rather than the reverse. If your reasoning is sound, you will find the dosages you calculate make sense and are accurate. For example, question any calculation that directs you to administer 15 tablets of any medication.

CAUTION

Recheck your calculation if a single dose seems unreasonable. Although not impossible, amounts less than $\frac{1}{2}$ tablet or greater than 3 tablets or capsules are uncommon and should be reassessed.

The next four examples of oral dosages supplied in capsules and tablets will help reinforce the three basic steps.

Example 1:

Patient care order: *allopurinol 200 mg PO BID*. The drug container is labelled allopurinol 100 mg per tablet. Calculate one dose.

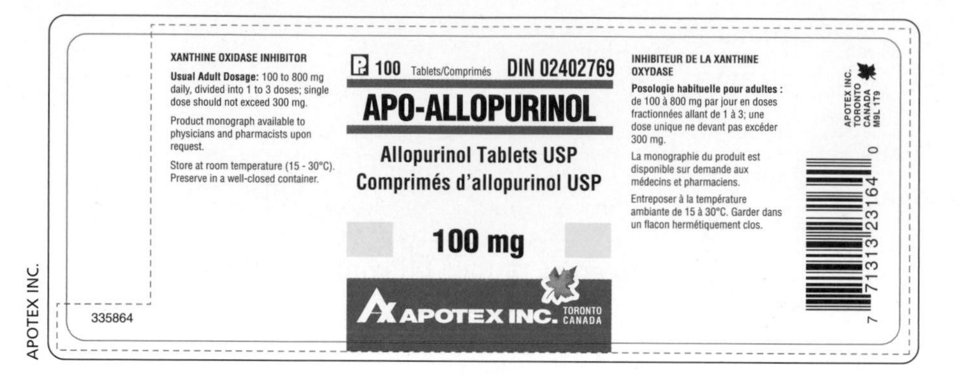
XANTHINE OXIDASE INHIBITOR
Usual Adult Dosage: 100 to 800 mg daily, divided into 1 to 3 doses; single dose should not exceed 300 mg.
Product monograph available to physicians and pharmacists upon request.
Store at room temperature (15 - 30°C). Preserve in a well-closed container.
100 Tablets/Comprimés DIN 02402769
APO-ALLOPURINOL
Allopurinol Tablets USP
Comprimés d'allopurinol USP
100 mg
APOTEX INC. TORONTO CANADA
INHIBITEUR DE LA XANTHINE OXYDASE
Posologie habituelle pour adultes : de 100 à 800 mg par jour en doses fractionnées allant de 1 à 3; une dose unique ne devant pas excéder 300 mg.
La monographie du produit est disponible sur demande aux médecins et pharmaciens.
Entreposer à la température ambiante de 15 à 30°C. Garder dans un flacon hermétiquement clos.
APOTEX INC. TORONTO CANADA M9L 1T9
7 71313 23164 0
335864
APOTEX INC.

Step 1 Convert No conversion is necessary. The units are the same (milligrams).

Step 2 Think You want to administer 200 milligrams, and you have 100 milligrams in each tablet. You want to give twice the equivalent of each tablet, or you want to administer 2 tablets per dose.

Step 3 Calculate $\frac{D}{H} \times Q = \frac{200 \text{ mg}}{100 \text{ mg}} \times 1 \text{ tablet}$

$$\frac{\overset{2}{\cancel{200}\ \cancel{\text{mg}}}}{\underset{1}{\cancel{100}\ \cancel{\text{mg}}}} \times 1 \text{ tablet} = 2 \times 1 \text{ tablet} = 2 \text{ tablets; given orally twice daily}$$

Double-check to be sure the calculated dosage matches the *reasonable* dosage from Step 2. If, for example, you had calculated to give more or less than 2 tablets of allopurinol, a calculation error would be suspected.

Example 2:

Patient care order: *amoxicillin 0.5 g PO QID*. The dosage available is amoxicillin 250 mg per capsule. How many capsules per dose should the nurse give to the patient?

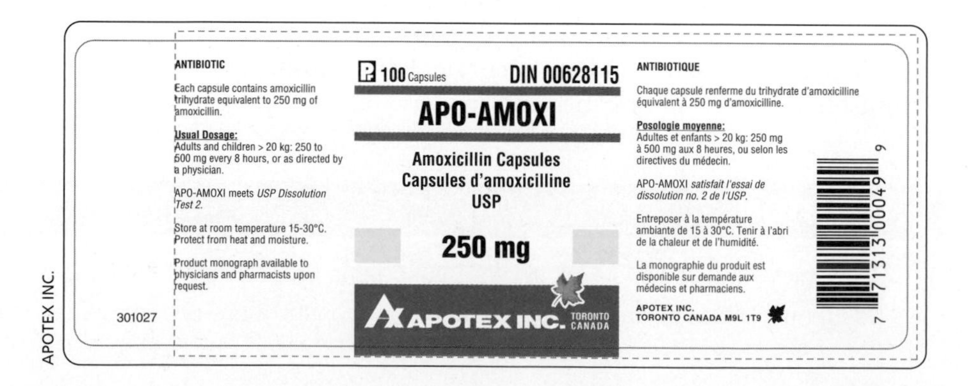
ANTIBIOTIC
Each capsule contains amoxicillin trihydrate equivalent to 250 mg of amoxicillin.
Usual Dosage:
Adults and children > 20 kg: 250 to 500 mg every 8 hours, or as directed by a physician.
APO-AMOXI meets USP Dissolution Test 2.
Store at room temperature 15-30°C. Protect from heat and moisture.
Product monograph available to physicians and pharmacists upon request.
100 Capsules DIN 00628115
APO-AMOXI
Amoxicillin Capsules
Capsules d'amoxicilline
USP
250 mg
APOTEX INC. TORONTO CANADA
ANTIBIOTIQUE
Chaque capsule renferme du trihydrate d'amoxicilline équivalent à 250 mg d'amoxicilline.
Posologie moyenne:
Adultes et enfants > 20 kg: 250 mg à 500 mg aux 8 heures, ou selon les directives du médecin.
APO-AMOXI satisfait l'essai de dissolution no. 2 de l'USP.
Entreposer à la température ambiante de 15 à 30°C. Tenir à l'abri de la chaleur et de l'humidité.
La monographie du produit est disponible sur demande aux médecins et pharmaciens.
APOTEX INC. TORONTO CANADA M9L 1T9
7 71313 00049 6
301027
APOTEX INC.

Step 1 Convert To the same units. Convert 0.5 grams to milligrams. Remember the math tip: Convert the larger unit (g) to the smaller unit (mg).

Equivalent: 1 g = 1000 mg. Conversion factor is 1000.

Larger → Smaller: (×)

$$0.5 \text{ g} = 0.5 \cancel{\text{g}} \times \frac{1000 \text{ mg}}{1 \cancel{\text{g}}} = 500 \text{ mg}$$

or 0.500. g = 500 mg

Now you have the order and supply measured in the same units.

Order: *amoxicillin 0.5 g = 500 mg*

Supply: amoxicillin 250-mg capsule

By now, you can probably do conversions like this from memory.

Step 2 Think 500 mg is twice as much as 250 mg. You want to give 2 capsules.

Step 3 Calculate $\frac{D}{H} \times Q = \frac{500 \text{ mg}}{250 \text{ mg}} \times 1 \text{ capsule}$

$$\frac{\overset{2}{\cancel{500}} \cancel{\text{mg}}}{\underset{1}{\cancel{250}} \cancel{\text{mg}}} \times 1 \text{ capsule} = 2 \times 1 \text{ capsule} = 2 \text{ capsules; given orally 4 times daily}$$

Example 3:

Patient care order: *levothyroxine sodium 0.05 mg PO daily*. Levothyroxine sodium 50-mcg tablets are available. How many tablets will you give?

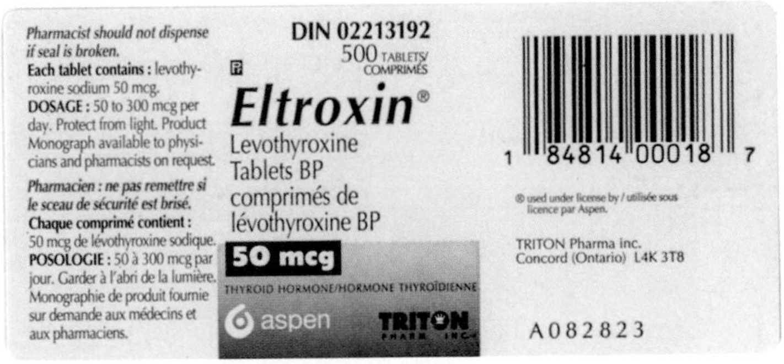

TRITON PHARMA INC.

Step 1 Convert To the same units. Remember, convert the larger unit (mg) to the smaller unit (mcg).

Equivalent: 1 mg = 1000 mcg. Conversion factor is 1000.

Larger → Smaller: (×)

$$0.5 \text{ mg} = 0.05 \cancel{\text{mg}} \times \frac{1000 \text{ mcg}}{1 \cancel{\text{mg}}} = 50 \text{ mcg}$$

Order: *levothyroxine sodium 0.05 mg = 50 mcg*

Supply: levothyroxine sodium 50-mcg tablets

Step 2 Think As soon as the ordered dosage of levothyroxine sodium 0.05 mg is converted to levothyroxine sodium 50 mcg, you realize that you want to give 1 tablet for each dose.

Avoid being confused by the way the original problem is presented. Be sure to recognize which is the dosage ordered (D—desired) and which is the supply dosage (H—have on hand) per the quantity on hand (Q). A common error is to misread the information and mix up the calculations in Step 3. This emphasizes the importance of thinking (Step 2) before calculating.

Step 3 Calculate $\frac{D}{H} \times Q = \frac{50 \text{ mcg}}{50 \text{ mcg}} \times 1 \text{ tablet}$

$$\frac{\overset{1}{\cancel{50 \text{ mcg}}}}{\underset{1}{\cancel{50 \text{ mcg}}}} \times 1 \text{ tablet} = 1 \text{ tablet; given orally once a day}$$

Example 4:

Patient care order: *hydrochlorothiazide 37.5 mg PO each morning*. The label on the available Apo-Hydro (hydrochlorothiazide) container tells you that each tablet provides 25 mg. How much will be given to the patient?

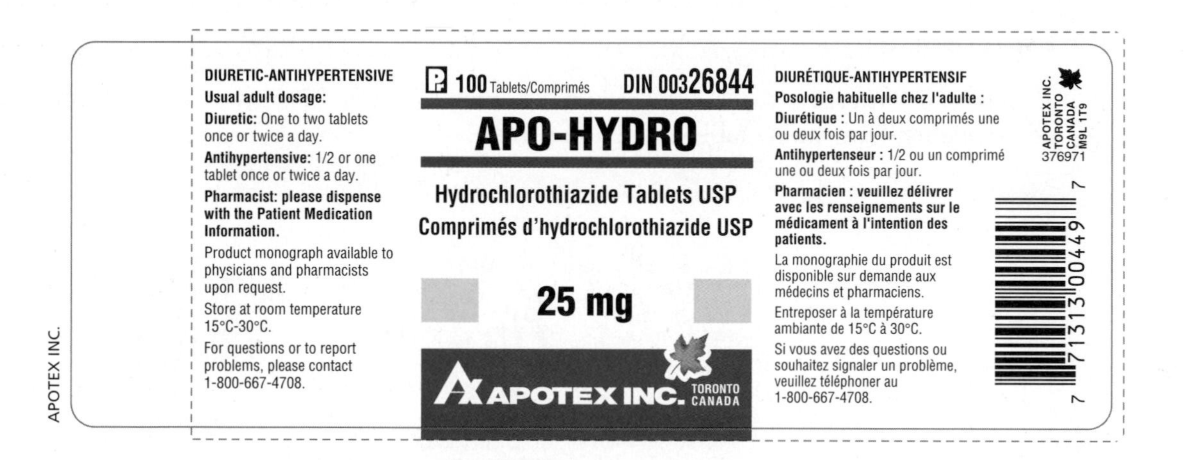

Step 1 Convert The desired dose and the supply dose are in same units. No conversion required.

Step 2 Think Look at the supply dosage and compare the ordered dosage of 37.5 mg with the supply dosage of 25 mg per tablet. You can reason that you want to give more than 1 tablet. Further, you can see that if you move the decimal point to make numbers whole, you want to give $1\frac{1}{2}$ tablet. Check your reasoning in Step 3.

Step 3 Calculate Move the decimal point to make D a whole number. Move the decimal point similarly in H by adding "0" (as per Chapter 1).

$$\frac{D}{H} \times Q = \frac{37.5 \text{ mg}}{25 \text{ mg}} \times 1 \text{ tablet}$$

$$\frac{\overset{3}{\cancel{375 \text{ mg}}}}{\underset{2}{\cancel{250 \text{ mg}}}} \times 1 \text{ tablet} = 1\frac{1}{2} \text{ tablets; given orally each morning}$$

QUICK REVIEW

Simple Three-Step Approach to Dosage Calculations

Step 1	**Convert**	To the same units.
Step 2	**Think**	Estimate a reasonable amount to give.
Step 3	**Calculate**	$\frac{D}{H} \times Q = X$

$$\frac{\text{D (desired)}}{\text{H (have)}} \times \text{Q (quantity)} = \text{X (amount)}$$

For most dosage calculation problems,

- Convert to the smaller unit. Example: g → mg
- Consider the reasonableness of the calculated amount to give. Example: You would question giving less than $\frac{1}{2}$ tablet or more than 3 tablets or capsules per dose for oral administration.

REVIEW SET 8-1

Calculate the correct number of tablets or capsules to be administered per dose. Tablets are scored.

1. The prescriber orders *nitrofurantoin 0.1 g PO QID*. The drug container label reads nitrofurantoin 100-mg tablets.

   Give: ________ tablet(s)

2. cephalexin 500-mg tablets available. The order is for *cephalexin 0.5 g PO BID.*

   Give: ________ tablet(s)

3. bethanechol chloride 10-mg tablets available. Order: *bethanechol chloride 15 mg PO TID*

   Give: ________ tablet(s)

4. Order: *hydrochlorothiazide 12.5 mg PO TID.* Available: hydrochlorothiazide 25-mg tablets

   Give: ________ tablet(s)

5. Order: *digoxin 0.125 mg PO daily*

   Supply: digoxin 0.25-mg tablets

   Give: ________ tablet(s)

6. Order: *ibuprofen 600 mg PO BID*

   Supply: ibuprofen 300-mg tablets

   Give: ________ tablet(s)

7. Order: *potassium chloride 16 mEq PO stat*

   Supply: potassium chloride 8-mEq tablets

   Give: ________ tablet(s)

8. cyclophosphamide 25-mg tablets available. Order: *cyclophosphamide 50 mg PO daily*

   Give: ________ tablet(s)

9. metolazone 2.5-mg tablets available. Order: *metolazone 7.5 mg PO BID*

   Give: ________ tablet(s)

10. *warfarin sodium 5 mg PO daily* ordered. Warfarin sodium 2.5-mg tablets available

    Give: ________ tablet(s)

11. levofloxacin is available in 500-mg tablets. Ordered dose is *levofloxacin 0.5 g PO daily.*

    Give ________ tablet(s)

12. Order: *labetalol hydrochloride 150 mg PO BID*

    Supply: labetalol hydrochloride 300-mg tablets

    Give: ________ tablet(s)

13. Order: *cephalexin 1 g PO BID*

    Supply: cephalexin 500-mg capsules

    Give: ________ capsule(s)

14. levothyroxine sodium 50-mcg tablets available. Order: *levothyroxine sodium 0.1 mg PO daily*

    Give: ________ tablet(s)

15. *riociquat 2.5 mg PO TID* is ordered, and you have 0.5-mg riociguat tablets available.

    Give: ________ tablet(s)

16. Order: *atenolol 100 mg BID*

    Supply: atenolol 50-mg tablets

    Give: ________

17. The doctor orders *minoxidil 7.5 mg PO stat,* and you have available minoxidil 10-mg and 2.5-mg scored tablets. Select ________ mg tablets and give ________ tablet(s).

18. Order: *metoclopramide 15 mg PO 1 h ac and at bedtime.* You have available metoclopramide 10-mg and metoclopramide 5-mg scored tablets. Select ________ mg tablets and give ________ tablet(s). How many doses of metoclopramide will the patient receive in 24 hours? ________ dose(s).

19. Order: *phenobarbital sodium 45 mg PO daily*

    Supply: phenobarbital *sodium* 30-mg and 60-mg scored tablets

    Select ________ mg tablets and give ________ tablet(s).

20. Order: *acetaminophen 300 mg/codeine 60 mg PO q4h prn for pain*

    Supply: acetaminophen 300 mg with codeine 7.5-mg, 15-mg, 30-mg, and 60-mg tablets

    Select ________ mg tablets and give ________ tablet(s).

Calculate one dose for each of the medication orders 21 through 30. The drug labels lettered A through K are the drugs you have available. Indicate the letter corresponding to the label you select.

21. Order: *verapamil hydrochloride sustained release 240 mg PO daily*

    Select: ________

    Give: ________

22. Order: *carbamazepine 0.2 g PO TID*

    Select: ________

    Give: ________

23. Order: *metoprolol 50 mg PO BID*

    Select: ________

    Give: ________

24. Order: *potassium chloride 40 mEq PO BID*

    Select: ________

    Give: ________

25. Order: *gemfibrozil 600 mg PO q6h*

    Select: ________

    Give: ________

26. Order: *cephalexin 0.5 g PO QID*

    Select: ________

    Give: ________

27. Order: *levothyroxine sodium 0.2 mg PO daily*

    Select: ________

    Give: ________

28. Order: *allopurinol 0.1 g PO TID*

    Select: ________

    Give: ________

29. Order: *diltiazem 180 mg PO daily*

    Select: ________

    Give: ________

    Provide rationale for your answer: ___________

30. Order: *lisinopril 10 mg PO daily*

    Select: ___________

    Give: ___________

Check your work! Answers to all Review Sets are provided at the end of each chapter. Worked solutions for selected Review Sets are also available there.

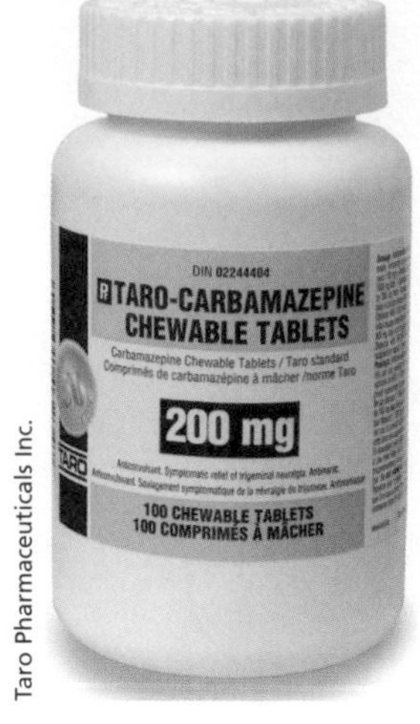

DIN 02244404
TARO-CARBAMAZEPINE
CHEWABLE TABLETS
200 mg
100 CHEWABLE TABLETS
100 COMPRIMÉS À MÂCHER

Taro Pharmaceuticals Inc.

A

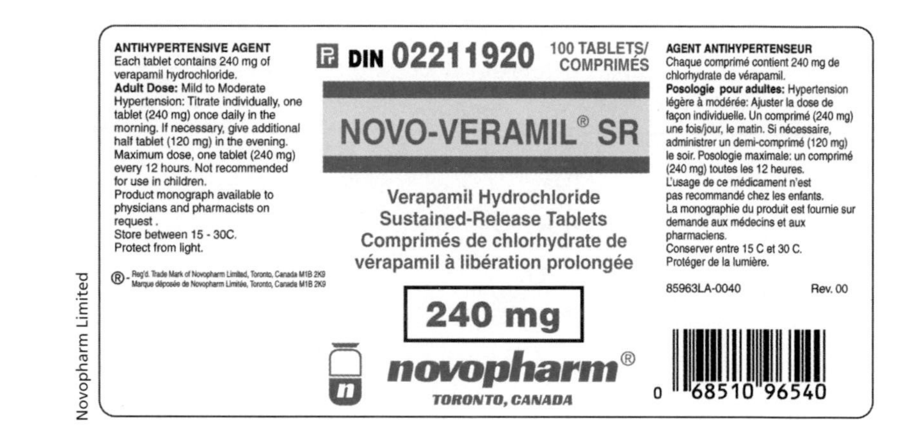

ANTIHYPERTENSIVE AGENT
Each tablet contains 240 mg of verapamil hydrochloride.
Adult Dose: Mild to Moderate Hypertension: Titrate individually, one tablet (240 mg) once daily in the morning. If necessary, give additional half tablet (120 mg) in the evening. Maximum dose, one tablet (240 mg) every 12 hours. Not recommended for use in children.
Product monograph available to physicians and pharmacists on request .
Store between 15 - 30C.
Protect from light.
DIN 02211920
100 TABLETS/ COMPRIMÉS
NOVO-VERAMIL® SR
Verapamil Hydrochloride Sustained-Release Tablets
Comprimés de chlorhydrate de vérapamil à libération prolongée
240 mg
novopharm®
TORONTO, CANADA
AGENT ANTIHYPERTENSEUR
Chaque comprimé contient 240 mg de chlorhydrate de vérapamil.
Posologie pour adultes: Hypertension légère à modérée: Ajuster la dose de façon individuelle. Un comprimé (240 mg) une fois/jour, le matin. Si nécessaire, administrer un demi-comprimé (120 mg) le soir. Posologie maximale: un comprimé (240 mg) toutes les 12 heures.
L'usage de ce médicament n'est pas recommandé chez les enfants.
La monographie du produit est fournie sur demande aux médecins et aux pharmaciens.
Conserver entre 15 C et 30 C.
Protéger de la lumière.
85963LA-0040 Rev. 00
0 68510 96540

Novopharm Limited

B

CLEAR AREA FOR IMPRINTING LOT NO. & EXP DATE

*TM/M.C. de Warner-Lambert Company Pfizer Canada Inc., licensee/licencié Kirkland (Québec) H9J 2M5

FOR POSITION ONLY 0 60093 34995 0

Pr DIN 00659606

Lopid*

GEMFIBROZIL TABLETS U.S.P. / COMPRIMÉS DE GEMFIBROZIL, USP

600 mg

100 tablets / comprimés

Pfizer

349H846 34995-05-0

ANTIHYPERLIPIDEMIC/HYPOLIPIDÉMIANT

Adult Dose: The recommended dose for adults is 1200 mg/day administered in two divided doses (one 600 mg tablet twice a day) 30 minutes before the morning and evening meal. The maximum daily dose should not exceed 1500 mg.
Prescribing Information available on request.
Store at controlled room temperature (15-30°C).

Dose pour adultes : La dose recommandée pour les adultes est de 1 200 mg/jour, administrés en deux prises égales (1 comprimé de 600 mg, deux fois par jour), 30 minutes avant les repas du matin et du soir. La dose quotidienne ne doit pas dépasser 1 500 mg.
Renseignements thérapeutiques fournis sur demande.
Conserver à une température ambiante contrôlée (15 - 30 °C).

Courtesy of Pfizer Inc.

C

Pharmacist should not dispense if seal is broken.

Each tablet contains : levothyroxine sodium 100 mcg.
DOSAGE : 50 to 300 mcg per day. Protect from light. Product Monograph available to physicians and pharmacists on request.

Pharmacien : ne pas remettre si le sceau de sécurité est brisé.

Chaque comprimé contient : 100 mcg de lévothyroxine sodique.
POSOLOGIE : 50 à 300 mcg par jour. Garder à l'abri de la lumière. Monographie de produit fournie sur demande aux médecins et aux pharmaciens.

DIN 02213206

500 TABLETS/ COMPRIMÉS

Eltroxin®

levothyroxine sodium tablets USP

comprimés de lévothyroxine sodique USP

100 mcg

THYROID HORMONE/HORMONE THYROÏDIENNE

aspen TRITON PHARMA INC.

® used under license by / utilisée sous licence par Aspen.

TRITON Pharma inc.
Concord (Ontario) L4K 3T8

A065532

TRITON PHARMA INC.

D

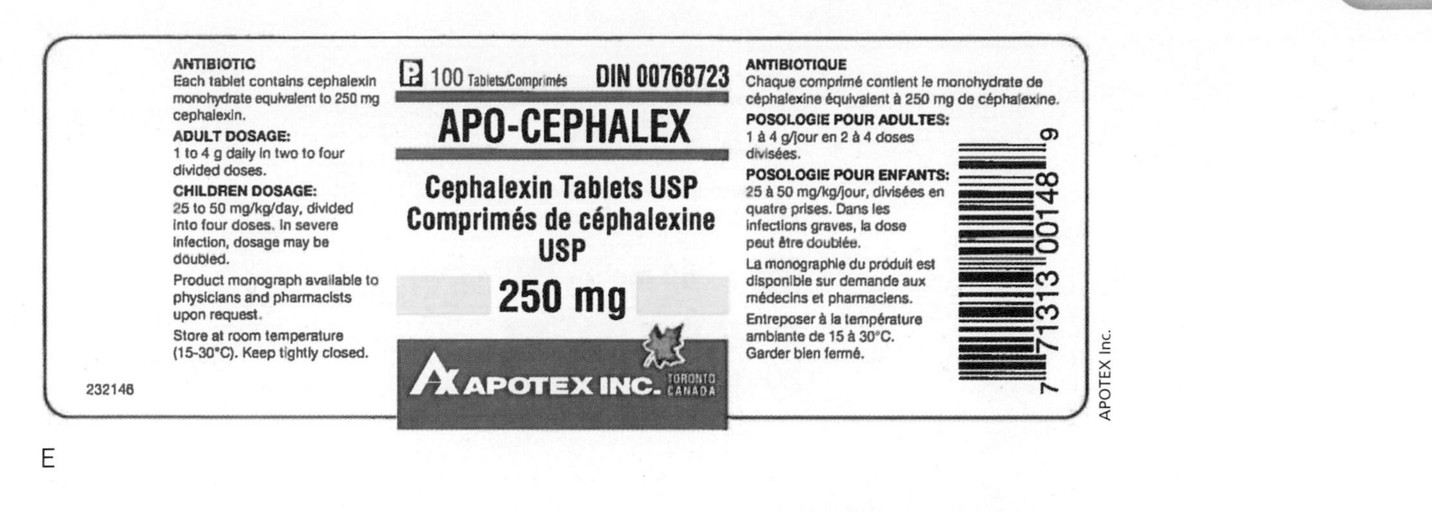

ANTIBIOTIC
Each tablet contains cephalexin monohydrate equivalent to 250 mg cephalexin.
ADULT DOSAGE:
1 to 4 g daily in two to four divided doses.
CHILDREN DOSAGE:
25 to 50 mg/kg/day, divided into four doses. In severe infection, dosage may be doubled.
Product monograph available to physicians and pharmacists upon request.
Store at room temperature (15-30°C). Keep tightly closed.
232146
100 Tablets/Comprimés DIN 00768723
APO-CEPHALEX
Cephalexin Tablets USP
Comprimés de céphalexine USP
250 mg
APOTEX INC. TORONTO CANADA
ANTIBIOTIQUE
Chaque comprimé contient le monohydrate de céphalexine équivalent à 250 mg de céphalexine.
POSOLOGIE POUR ADULTES:
1 à 4 g/jour en 2 à 4 doses divisées.
POSOLOGIE POUR ENFANTS:
25 à 50 mg/kg/jour, divisées en quatre prises. Dans les infections graves, la dose peut être doublée.
La monographie du produit est disponible sur demande aux médecins et pharmaciens.
Entreposer à la température ambiante de 15 à 30°C.
Garder bien fermé.
7 71313 00148 9
APOTEX Inc.

E

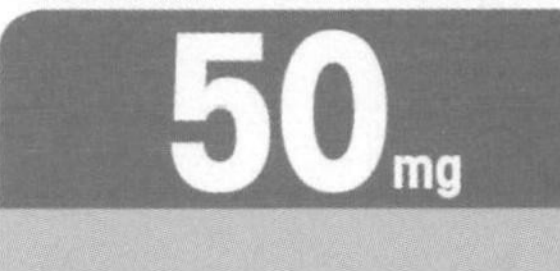

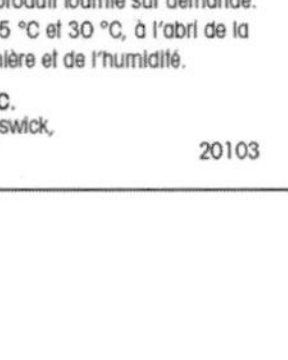

β-ADRENORECEPTOR BLOCKING AGENT
Each coated tablet contains 50 mg metoprolol tartrate.
Adult Dosage: Hypertension and Angina: Individual titration required, starting with 50 mg twice daily. Maintenance Dose: Hypertension: 100 – 200 mg/day. Angina: 200 mg/day, given in divided doses. Maximum Dose: 400 mg/day.
Myocardial Infarction: Early Treatment: Initiate with 25 – 50 mg, 4 times daily, orally 15 minutes after last intravenous dose or as soon as clinical condition allows. Continue for 48 hours. Late Treatment and Maintenance Dosing: 100 mg twice daily.
No experience for use in children.
Keep this and all medicine out of the reach of children.
Product Monograph available on request.
Store 15°C - 30°C. Protect from heat, light and humidity.
361-32-765852440 Rev. 01

METOPROLOL
Metoprolol Tartrate Tablets
Comprimés de tartrate de métoprolol USP
COATED TABLETS / COMPRIMÉS ENROBÉS
50 mg

INHIBITEUR DES RÉCEPTEURS β-ADRÉNERGIQUES
Un comprimé enrobé contient 50 mg de tartrate de métoprolol.
Posologie chez l'adulte : Hypertension et angine de poitrine : Ajuster la posologie en fonction des besoins du patient en commençant par une dose de 50 mg, 2 fois/jour. Posologie d'entretien : Hypertension : 100 mg à 200 mg/jour ; Angine de poitrine : 200 mg/jour en prises fractionnées.
Dose maximale : 400 mg/jour.
Infarctus du myocarde : Traitement précoce : Instaurer le traitement en administrant une dose orale de 25 à 50 mg, 4 fois/jour, 15 minutes après la dernière dose i.v. ou dès que l'état du patient le permet. Continuer ainsi pendant 48 heures. Traitement tardif et d'entretien : 100 mg, 2 fois/jour. Aucune expérience clinique chez les enfants. Comme tout médicament, ranger ce produit hors de la portée des enfants.
Monographie du produit fournie sur demande.
Conserver entre 15 °C et 30 °C, à l'abri de la chaleur, de la lumière et de l'humidité.
SANIS HEALTH INC.
Dieppe, New Brunswick,
Canada E1A 1P2
20103
9 93570 00103 6
Sanis Health Inc.

F

Each tablet contains: **Medicinal Ingredient:** Potassium Chloride 1500 mg (20 mEq) in an extended-release formulation.
Non-Medicinal Ingredients: colloidal silicon dioxide, ethylcellulose, hydrogenated vegetable oil, hypromellose, methacrylic acid polymer, silica, sodium bicarbonate, sodium lauryl sulfate, talc, titanium dioxide, triacetin, triethyl citrate.
Contains no preservatives, artificial flavor, lactose, yeast, sugar, starch or gluten.
Indications: Treatment or prevention of hypokalemia (potassium depletion) which does not result from dietary deficiency • Potassium replacement therapy • Electrolyte replenisher • For the treatment of metabolic alkalosis. To be taken only on the advice of a physician.
Adult Dosage: For the prevention of hypokalemia, 1 tablet 1-2 times per day (20 to 40 mEq/day). For the treatment of hypokalemia, potassium replacement therapy, electrolyte replenisher, and for the treatment of metabolic alkalosis, 1 tablet 2-5 times per day (40 to 100 mEq/day). Swallow tablets whole with a glass of water. Do not break, crush or chew tablets. Adjust dosage on an individual basis. Prescribing information is available to physicians and pharmacists on request. Take this medicine immediately after meals or with food to lessen possible stomach upset or laxative action. ● **WARNING:** A probable association exists between the use of coated tablets containing potassium salts, with or without thiazide diuretics, and the incidence of serious small bowel ulceration. Such preparations should be used only when adequate dietary supplementation is not practical, and should be discontinued if abdominal pain, distention, nausea, vomiting or gastrointestinal bleeding occur. For therapeutic use only. Keep out of reach of children. Keep container tightly closed. Store at room temperature (15-30 °C). Bottle is sealed for your protection. Do not use if seal is broken.

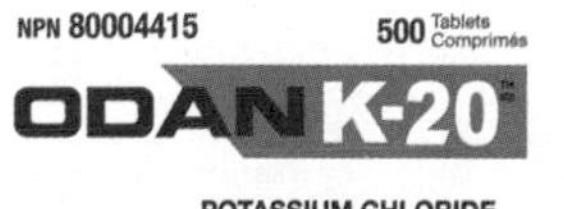

NPN 80004415 500 Tablets Comprimés

POTASSIUM CHLORIDE SUSTAINED RELEASE TABLETS
COMPRIMÉS DE CHLORURE DE POTASSIUM À LIBÉRATION PROLONGÉE
SMALLER SIZE TABLETS / COMPRIMÉS PLUS PETITS

1500 mg

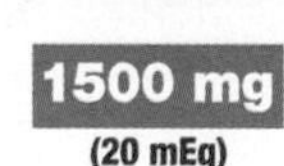

(20 mEq)
POTASSIUM SUPPLEMENT
ODAN
www.odanlab.com

Chaque comprimé contient : **Ingrédient Médicinal :** Chlorure de potassium 1500 mg (20 mEq) – formule longue action. **Ingrédients non médicinaux :** bicarbonate de sodium, citrate de triéthyle, dioxyde de silicium colloïdal, dioxyde de titane, éthylcellulose, huile végétale hydrogénée, hypromellose, lauryl sulfate de sodium, polymère d'acide méthacrylique, silice, talc, triacétine.
Ne contient aucun préservatif, saveur artificielle, lactose, levure, sucre, amidon ou gluten.
Indications : Traitement ou prévention de l'hypokaliémie (déficit en potassium) non attribuable à une carence alimentaire • Traitement de remplacement potassique • Recharge électrolytique • Traitement de l'alcalose métabolique. À consommer que sur l'avis d'un médecin.
Posologie Adulte : Pour la prévention de l'hypokaliémie, 1 comprimé 1 à 2 fois par jour (20 à 40 mEq/jour). Pour le traitement de l'hypokaliémie, le traitement de remplacement potassique, la recharge électrolytique et pour le traitement de l'alcalose métabolique, 1 comprimé 2 à 5 fois par jour (40 à 100 mEq/jour). Avaler les comprimés en entier avec un verre d'eau. Ne pas rompre, écraser ou mâcher les comprimés. Ajuster la dose sur une base individuelle. Renseignements thérapeutiques disponibles pour les médecins et les pharmaciens sur demande. À consommer immédiatement après le repas ou avec un aliment afin de réduire les possibilités d'inconfort gastrique ou d'effet laxatif.
● **MISE EN GARDE :** Il existe un lien probable entre l'emploi de comprimés enrobés contenant des sels de potassium avec ou sans diurétiques de thiazide et l'incidence de l'ulcération grave de l'intestin grêle. Ces préparations ne sont à utiliser que s'il n'est pas possible de suppléer convenablement au régime alimentaire; il faut en cesser l'emploi dès qu'apparaissent des douleurs abdominales, une distension abdominale, des nausées, des vomissements ou des hémorragies gastro-intestinales.
Pour usage thérapeutique seulement. Garder hors de la portée des enfants. Garder le contenant bien fermé. Conserver à température ambiante (15-30 °C). Ce contenant est scellé pour votre sécurité. Ne pas utiliser si le sceau est brisé.

INFO? 1-888-666-ODAN
LABORATOIRES ODAN LABORATORIES LTÉE LTD, MONTREAL, QC, CANADA, H9R 2V6

7 76097 42077 8
ODAN LABORATORIES LTD

G

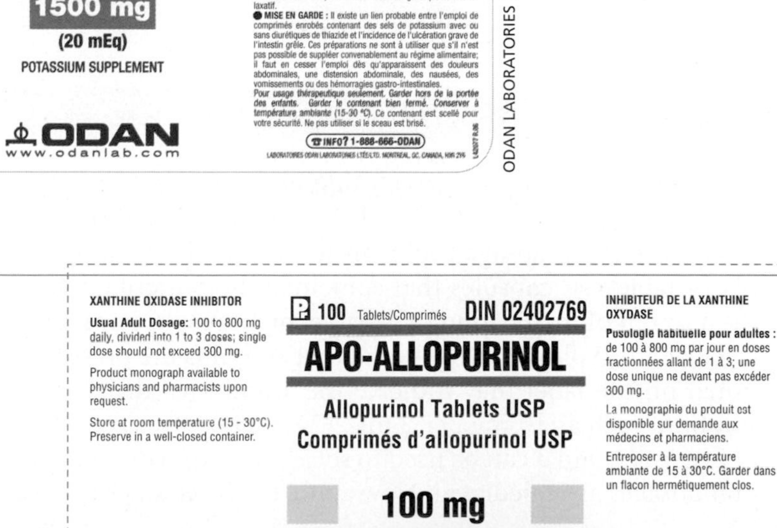

XANTHINE OXIDASE INHIBITOR
Usual Adult Dosage: 100 to 800 mg daily, divided into 1 to 3 doses; single dose should not exceed 300 mg.
Product monograph available to physicians and pharmacists upon request.
Store at room temperature (15 - 30°C). Preserve in a well-closed container.
335864
100 Tablets/Comprimés DIN 02402769
APO-ALLOPURINOL
Allopurinol Tablets USP
Comprimés d'allopurinol USP
100 mg
APOTEX INC. TORONTO CANADA
INHIBITEUR DE LA XANTHINE OXYDASE
Posologie habituelle pour adultes : de 100 à 800 mg par jour en doses fractionnées allant de 1 à 3; une dose unique ne devant pas excéder 300 mg.
La monographie du produit est disponible sur demande aux médecins et pharmaciens.
Entreposer à la température ambiante de 15 à 30°C. Garder dans un flacon hermétiquement clos.
APOTEX INC. TORONTO CANADA M9L 1T9
7 71313 23164 0
APOTEX INC.

H

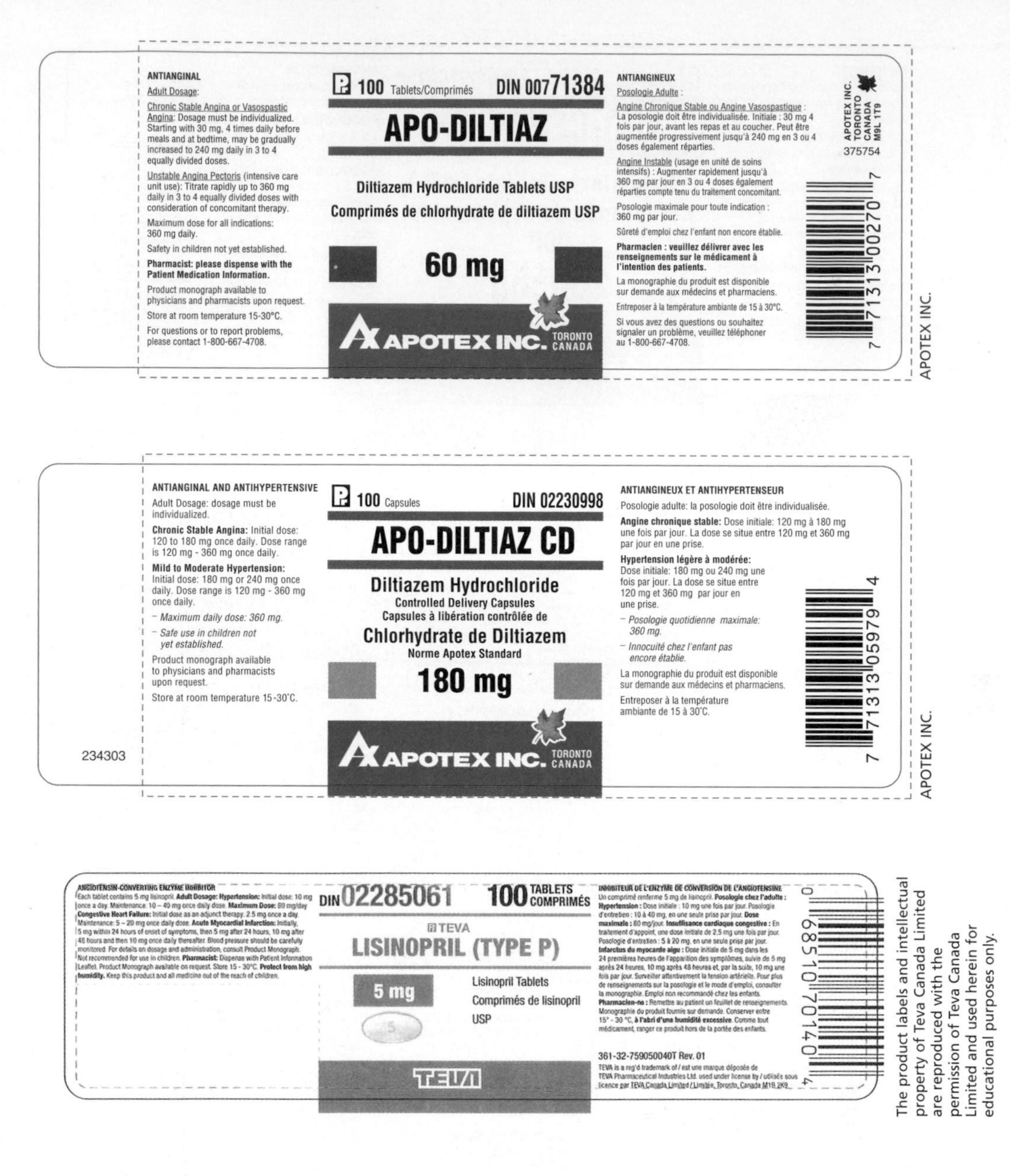

ORAL LIQUIDS

Oral liquids are supplied in solution form and contain a specific amount of drug in a given amount of solution as stated on the label (Figures 8-3(a) and (b)).

When solving dosage problems for a drug that is supplied in solid form, you calculated the number of tablets or capsules that contained the prescribed dosage. The supply container label indicates the amount of medication per 1 tablet or 1 capsule. For medications supplied in liquid form, you must calculate the volume of the liquid that contains the prescribed dosage of the drug. The supply dosage noted on the label may indicate the amount of drug per 1 millilitre or per multiple millilitres of solution, such as 10 mg per 2 mL, 125 mg per 5 mL, or 1.2 g per 30 mL.

Steps 1, 2, and 3 can be used to solve liquid oral dosage calculations in the same way that solid-form oral dosages are calculated. Now apply the three steps to dosage calculations in a few examples.

Example 1:

Patient care order: *cephalexin 100 mg PO QID*. Look at the cephalexin labels available in Figure 8-3. You choose cephalexin 125 mg per 5 mL. Follow the three steps to calculate the dosage.

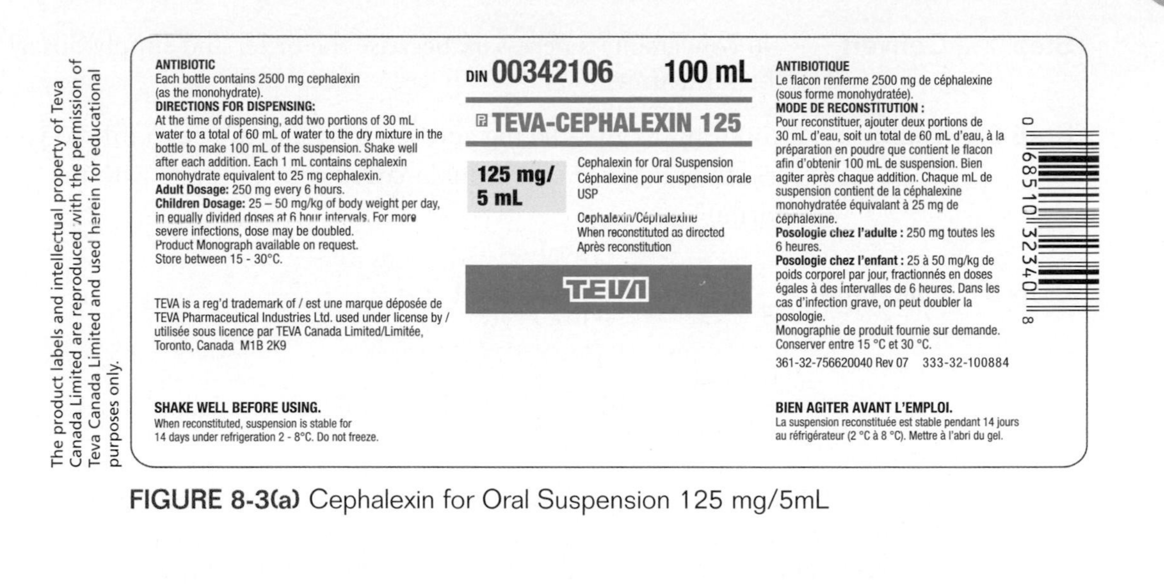

FIGURE 8-3(a) Cephalexin for Oral Suspension 125 mg/5mL

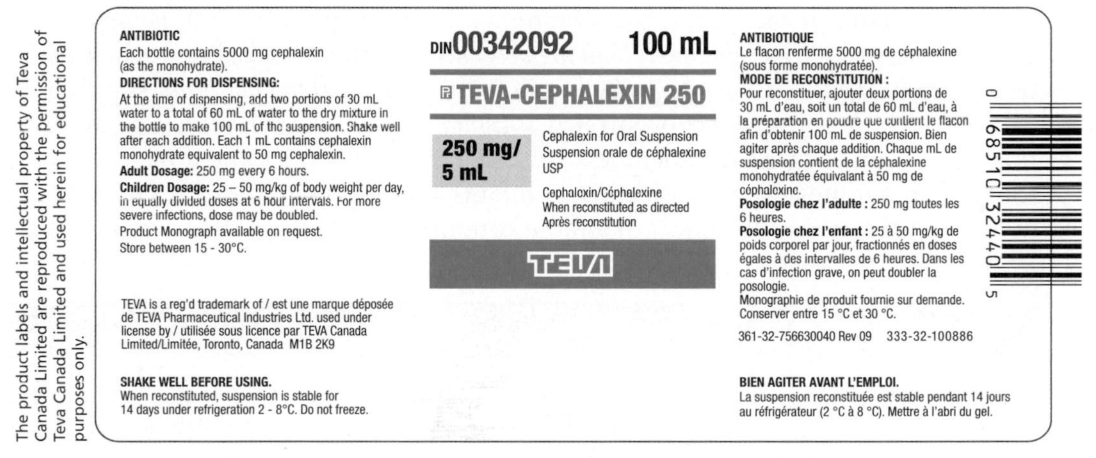

FIGURE 8-3(b) Cephalexin for Oral Suspension, 250 mg/5 mL

Step 1 **Convert** No conversion is necessary because the order and supply dosage are both in the same units.

Step 2 **Think** You want to give less than 125 mg, so you want to give less than 5 mL. Double-check your thinking with the $\frac{D}{H} \times Q = X$ formula.

Step 3 **Calculate** $\frac{D}{H} \times Q = \frac{100 \text{ mg}}{125 \text{ mg}} \times 5 \text{ mL}$

$$\frac{\overset{4}{\cancel{100}} \cancel{\text{mg}}}{\underset{5}{\cancel{125}} \cancel{\text{mg}}} \times 5 \text{ mL} = \frac{4}{\cancel{5}} \times \overset{1}{\cancel{5}} \text{ mL} = 4 \text{ mL; given orally 4 times a day}$$

You will give 4 mL of the cephalexin with the dosage strength of 125 mg per 5 mL. Double-check to be sure your calculated dosage is consistent with your *reasonable* dosage estimate from Step 2. If, for instance, you calculate to give *more* than 5 mL, then you should suspect a calculation error.

Example 2:

Suppose, using the same patient care order in Example 1, *cephalexin 100 mg PO QID*, you choose a stronger (more concentrated) solution, cephalexin 250 mg per 5 mL. Follow the three steps to calculate the dosage.

Step 1 Convert No conversion is necessary because the order and supply dosage are both in the same units.

Step 2 Think You want to give 100 mg and you have 250 mg per 5 mL, so you will give less than half of 5 mL. Double-check your thinking with the $\frac{D}{H} \times Q = X$ formula.

Step 3 Calculate $\frac{D}{H} \times Q = \frac{100 \text{ mg}}{250 \text{ mg}} \times 5 \text{ mL}$

$$\frac{\overset{2}{\cancel{100}\ \cancel{\text{mg}}}}{\underset{5}{\cancel{250}\ \cancel{\text{mg}}}} \times 5 \text{ mL} = \frac{2}{\cancel{5}} \times \overset{1}{\cancel{5}} \text{ mL} = 2 \text{ mL; given orally 4 times a day}$$

Notice that in both Example 1 and Example 2, the supply quantity is the same (5 mL), but the dosage strength (weight) of medication is different (125 mg per 5 mL vs. 250 mg per 5 mL). This results in the calculated dose volume (amount to give) being different (4 mL compared to 2 mL). This difference is the result of each liquid's *concentration. Cephalexin penicillin V potassium 125 mg per 5 mL* is half as concentrated as *cephalexin 250 mg per 5 mL*. In other words, there is half as much drug in 5 mL of the *125 mg per 5 mL* supply as there is in 5 mL of the *250 mg per 5 mL* supply. Likewise, *cephalexin 250 mg per 5 mL* is twice as concentrated as *cephalexin 125 mg per 5 mL*. The more concentrated solution allows you to give the patient less volume per dose for the same dosage. This difference is significant when administering medication to infants and small children who will likely require a smaller quantity. Think about the effect of a more concentrated solution carefully until it is clear.

CAUTION

Think before you calculate. It is important to estimate before you apply any formula. In this way, if you make a careless math error or if you set up the problem incorrectly, your thinking will alert you to *try again*.

Example 3:

Patient care order: *azithromycin monohydrate 150 mg PO daily.* The label on the package is azithromycin monohydrate 250 mg/5 mL. How many mL should you administer?

Step 1 Convert No conversion is necessary.

Step 2 Think You want to give less than 5 mL. Continue to Step 3 to double-check your thinking. You know that 150 mg is less than the amount available, which is 250 mL. Therefore, you need to divide 150 mg by 250 mg, then multiply by the amount available, which is 5 mL.

Step 3 Calculate $\frac{D}{H} \times Q = \frac{\overset{3}{\cancel{150}\ \cancel{\text{mg}}}}{\underset{5}{\cancel{250}\ \cancel{\text{mg}}}} \times 5 \text{ mL} = 3 \text{ mL; given orally once a day}$

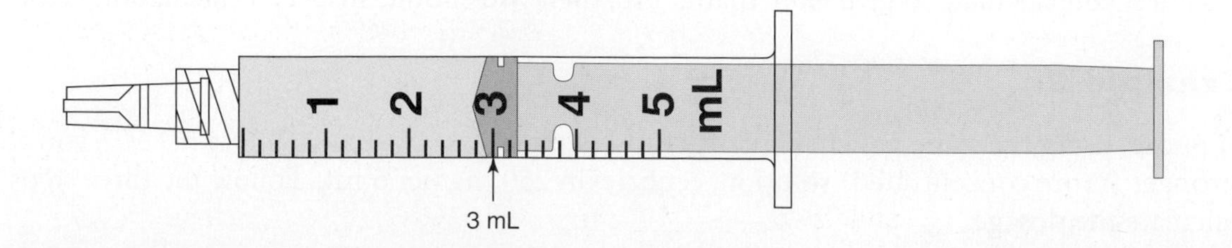

Measuring Liquid Medications

It is important to measure liquid medicine accurately to get the right dose. In the three examples above, an oral syringe would be used for accuracy. However, for doses of 2.5, 5 mL, and 10 mL or greater, a calibrated medication cup (described in Chapter 5) would be used. To ensure an accurate dose, make sure that the medication cup is at eye level when pouring the liquid. The liquid should be poured to the lower level of the meniscus, a U-shaped or concave curve that forms against the side of the glass container (Figure 8-4). To read the amount, hold the container at eye level and note the level at the bottom of the curve. Note that the meniscus is an optical illusion seen only when using a glass medication cup. When using a plastic medication cup, a meniscus will not form, so the reading will be at the level of the measurement.

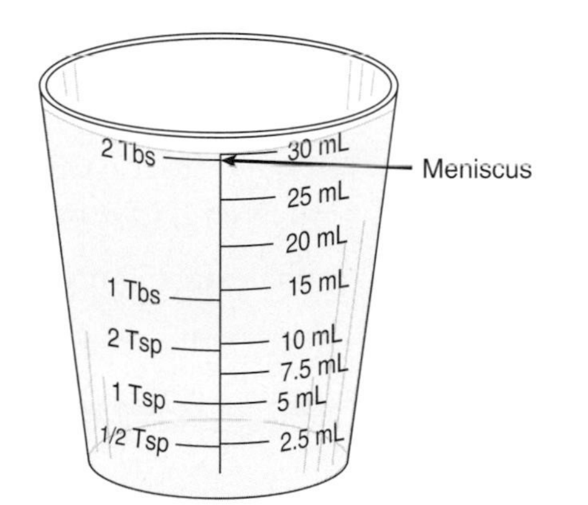

FIGURE 8-4 Calibrated Glass Medication Cup Showing Meniscus

QUICK REVIEW

Look again at Steps 1 through 3, and think of the steps as a valuable dosage calculation checklist.

Step 1	**Convert**	Be sure that all measurement are the same units.
Step 2	**Think**	Carefully estimate a reasonable amount of the drug that you should administer.
Step 3	**Calculate**	$\frac{D}{H} \times Q = X$; $\frac{\text{D (desired)}}{\text{H (have)}} \times \text{Q (quantity)} = \text{X (amount)}$

REVIEW SET 8-2

Calculate one dose of the drugs ordered.

1. Order: *amoxicillin trihydrate 200 mg PO q8h*

   Supply: amoxicillin dihydrate 250 mg/5 mL

   Give: ________ mL

2. Order: *lorazepam 1.5 mg SL stat*

   Supply: lorazepam sublingual tablets 0.5 mg, 1 mg, 2 mg

   Give: ________ tablets of ________ mg

3. Order: *penicillin V potassium 1 g PO*

   Supply: penicillin V potassium suspension 300 mg (500 000 units)/5 mL

   Give: ________ mL

4. Order: *amoxicillin trihydrate 100 mg PO q8h*

   Supply: 80-mL bottle of amoxicillin trihydrate oral suspension 125 mg/5 mL

   Give: ________ mL

5. Order: *acetaminophen 0.16 g PO q4h prn for pain*

   Supply: acetaminophen 160 mg/5 mL

   Give: ________ mL

6. Order: *amoxicillin trihydrate/clavulanate potassium 25 mg PO q8h*

   Supply: Apo-Amoxi Clav 125 mg/5 mL

   Give: ________ mL

7. Order: *perphenazine 4 mg PO q8h*

   Supply: perphenazine concentrate 3.2 mg/mL

   Give: ________ mL

8. Order: *erythromycin ethylsuccinate suspension 600 mg PO q6h*

   Supply: erythromycin ethylsuccinate 400 mg/5 mL

   Give: ________ mL

9. Order: *cefaclor suspension 225 mg PO BID*

   Supply: cefaclor suspension 375 mg/5 mL

   Give: ________ mL

10. Order: *sulfamethoxazole/trimethoprim suspension 100 mg PO BID*

    Supply: sulfamethoxazole/trimethoprim suspension 40 mg/mL

    Give: ________ mL

11. Order: *theophylline elixir 0.1 g PO stat*

    Supply: theophylline elixir 80 mg/15 mL

    Give: ________ mL

12. Order: *ampicillin suspension 750 mg PO TID*

    Supply: ampicillin suspension 250 mg/5 mL

    Give: ________ mL

13. Order: *fluoxetine hydrochloride solution 45 mg PO daily 0800*

    Supply: fluoxetine hydrochloride 20 mg/5 mL solution

    Give: ________ mL

14. Order: *nystatin suspension 400 000 units PO QID*

    Supply: nystatin suspension 100 000 units/mL

    Give: ________ mL

15. Order: *digoxin elixir 0.25 mg PO daily*

    Supply: digoxin elixir 50 mcg/mL

    Give: ________ mL

16. Order: *phenobarbital elixir 15 mg PO TID*

    Supply: phenobarbital 5 mg/mL

    Give: ________ mL

17. Order: *cephalexin 375 mg PO TID*

    Supply: cephalexin 250 mg/5 mL

    Give: ________ mL

18. Order: *lactulose 20 g via gastric tube BID today*

    Supply: lactulose 10 g/15 mL

    Give: ________ mL

19. Order: *erythromycin ethylsuccinate 1.2 g PO q8h*

    Supply: erythromycin ethylsuccinate 400 mg/5 mL

    Give: ________ mL

20. Order: *cloxacillin sodium 0.25 g PO q8h*

    Supply: cloxacillin sodium 125 mg/5 mL

    Give: ________ mL

21. Order: *amoxicillin suspension 100 mg PO q6h*

    Supply: amoxicillin suspension 250 mg/5 mL

    Give: ________ mL

Use the drug labels A, B, and C below to calculate one dose of the orders in questions 22 through 24. Indicate the letter corresponding to the label you select.

22. Order: *erythromycin estolate 125 mg PO TID*

    Select: ________

    Give: ________

23. Order: *cephalexin 50 mg PO q6h*

    Select: ________

    Give: ________

24. Order: *hydroxyzine 10 mg PO QID*

    Select: ________

    Give: ________

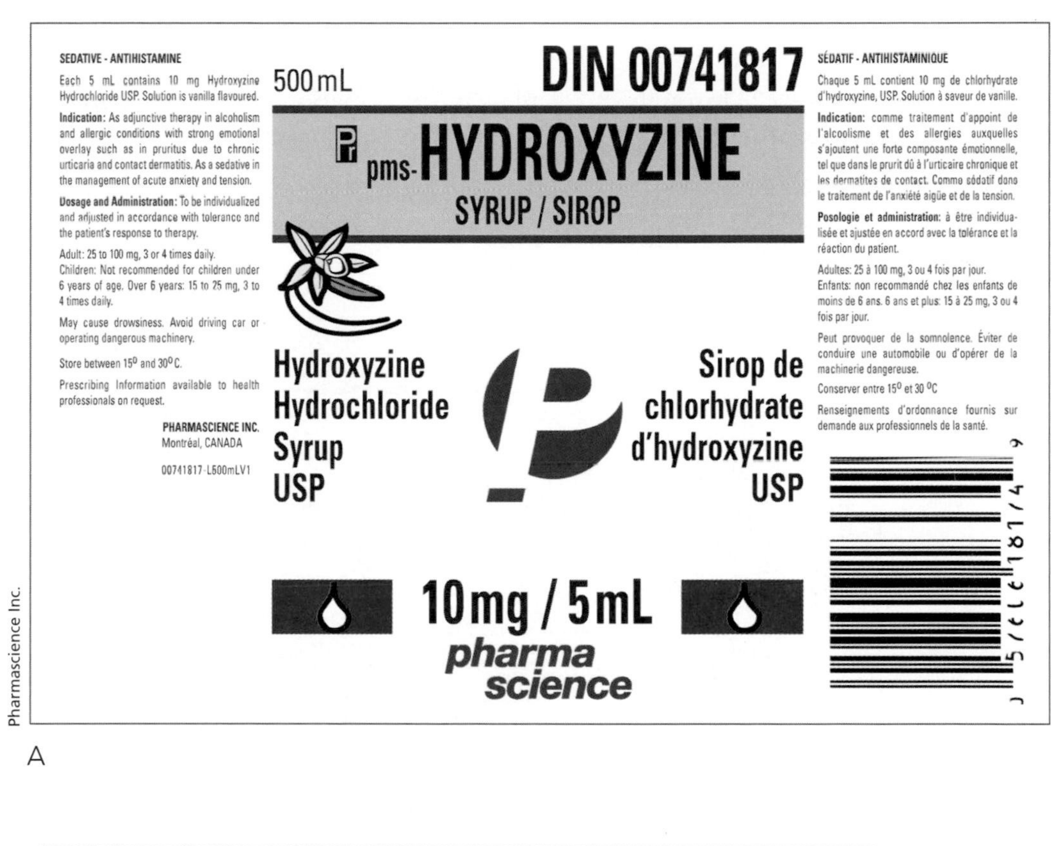

SEDATIVE - ANTIHISTAMINE
Each 5 mL contains 10 mg Hydroxyzine Hydrochloride USP. Solution is vanilla flavoured.
Indication: As adjunctive therapy in alcoholism and allergic conditions with strong emotional overlay such as in pruritus due to chronic urticaria and contact dermatitis. As a sedative in the management of acute anxiety and tension.
Dosage and Administration: To be individualized and adjusted in accordance with tolerance and the patient's response to therapy.
Adult: 25 to 100 mg, 3 or 4 times daily.
Children: Not recommended for children under 6 years of age. Over 6 years: 15 to 25 mg, 3 to 4 times daily.
May cause drowsiness. Avoid driving car or operating dangerous machinery.
Store between 15° and 30° C.
Prescribing Information available to health professionals on request.
PHARMASCIENCE INC.
Montréal, CANADA
00741817-L500mLV1
500 mL
DIN 00741817
pms-HYDROXYZINE
SYRUP / SIROP
Hydroxyzine Hydrochloride Syrup USP
Sirop de chlorhydrate d'hydroxyzine USP
10 mg / 5 mL
pharma science
SÉDATIF - ANTIHISTAMINIQUE
Chaque 5 mL contient 10 mg de chlorhydrate d'hydroxyzine, USP. Solution à saveur de vanille.
Indication: comme traitement d'appoint de l'alcoolisme et des allergies auxquelles s'ajoutent une forte composante émotionnelle, tel que dans le prurit dû à l'urticaire chronique et les dermatites de contact. Comme sédatif dans le traitement de l'anxiété aigüe et de la tension.
Posologie et administration: à être individualisée et ajustée en accord avec la tolérance et la réaction du patient.
Adultes: 25 à 100 mg, 3 ou 4 fois par jour.
Enfants: non recommandé chez les enfants de moins de 6 ans. 6 ans et plus: 15 à 25 mg, 3 ou 4 fois par jour.
Peut provoquer de la somnolence. Éviter de conduire une automobile ou d'opérer de la machinerie dangereuse.
Conserver entre 15° et 30 °C
Renseignements d'ordonnance fournis sur demande aux professionnels de la santé.

Pharmascience Inc.

A

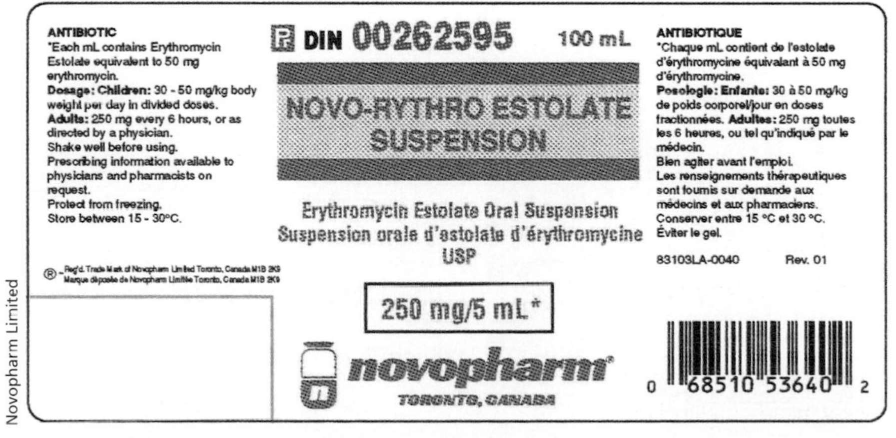

ANTIBIOTIC
*Each mL contains Erythromycin Estolate equivalent to 50 mg erythromycin.
Dosage: Children: 30 - 50 mg/kg body weight per day in divided doses.
Adults: 250 mg every 6 hours, or as directed by a physician.
Shake well before using.
Prescribing information available to physicians and pharmacists on request.
Protect from freezing.
Store between 15 - 30°C.
DIN 00262595
100 mL
NOVO-RYTHRO ESTOLATE SUSPENSION
Erythromycin Estolate Oral Suspension
Suspension orale d'estolate d'érythromycine
USP
250 mg/5 mL*
novopharm
TORONTO, CANADA
ANTIBIOTIQUE
*Chaque mL contient de l'estolate d'érythromycine équivalant à 50 mg d'érythromycine.
Posologie: Enfants: 30 à 50 mg/kg de poids corporel/jour en doses fractionnées. Adultes: 250 mg toutes les 6 heures, ou tel qu'indiqué par le médecin.
Bien agiter avant l'emploi.
Les renseignements thérapeutiques sont fournis sur demande aux médecins et aux pharmaciens.
Conserver entre 15 °C et 30 °C.
Éviter le gel.
83103LA-0040
Rev. 01
0 68510 53640 2

Novopharm Limited

B

ANTIBIOTIC
Each bottle contains 2500 mg cephalexin (as the monohydrate).
DIRECTIONS FOR DISPENSING:
At the time of dispensing, add two portions of 30 mL water to a total of 60 mL of water to the dry mixture in the bottle to make 100 mL of the suspension. Shake well after each addition. Each 1 mL contains cephalexin monohydrate equivalent to 25 mg cephalexin.
Adult Dosage: 250 mg every 6 hours.
Children Dosage: 25 – 50 mg/kg of body weight per day, in equally divided doses at 6 hour intervals. For more severe infections, dose may be doubled.
Product Monograph available on request.
Store between 15 - 30°C.

TEVA is a reg'd trademark of / est une marque déposée de TEVA Pharmaceutical Industries Ltd. used under license by / utilisée sous licence par TEVA Canada Limited/Limitée, Toronto, Canada M1B 2K9

DIN 00342106 100 mL
TEVA-CEPHALEXIN 125
125 mg/ 5 mL
Cephalexin for Oral Suspension
Céphalexine pour suspension orale USP
Cephalexin/Céphalexine
When reconstituted as directed
Après reconstitution
TEVA

ANTIBIOTIQUE
Le flacon renferme 2500 mg de céphalexine (sous forme monohydratée).
MODE DE RECONSTITUTION :
Pour reconstituer, ajouter deux portions de 30 mL d'eau, soit un total de 60 mL d'eau, à la préparation en poudre que contient le flacon afin d'obtenir 100 mL de suspension. Bien agiter après chaque addition. Chaque mL de suspension contient de la céphalexine monohydratée équivalant à 25 mg de céphalexine.
Posologie chez l'adulte : 250 mg toutes les 6 heures.
Posologie chez l'enfant : 25 à 50 mg/kg de poids corporel par jour, fractionnés en doses égales à des intervalles de 6 heures. Dans les cas d'infection grave, on peut doubler la posologie.
Monographie de produit fournie sur demande.
Conserver entre 15 °C et 30 °C.
361-32-756620040 Rev 07 333-32-100884

0 68510 32340 8

SHAKE WELL BEFORE USING.
When reconstituted, suspension is stable for 14 days under refrigeration 2 - 8°C. Do not freeze.

BIEN AGITER AVANT L'EMPLOI.
La suspension reconstituée est stable pendant 14 jours au réfrigérateur (2 °C à 8 °C). Mettre à l'abri du gel.

C

For questions 25 through 28, calculate the information requested based on the drugs ordered. The drug labels provided are the drugs available.

25. Order: *furosemide oral solution 40 mg PO TID*

    Give: ________ mL

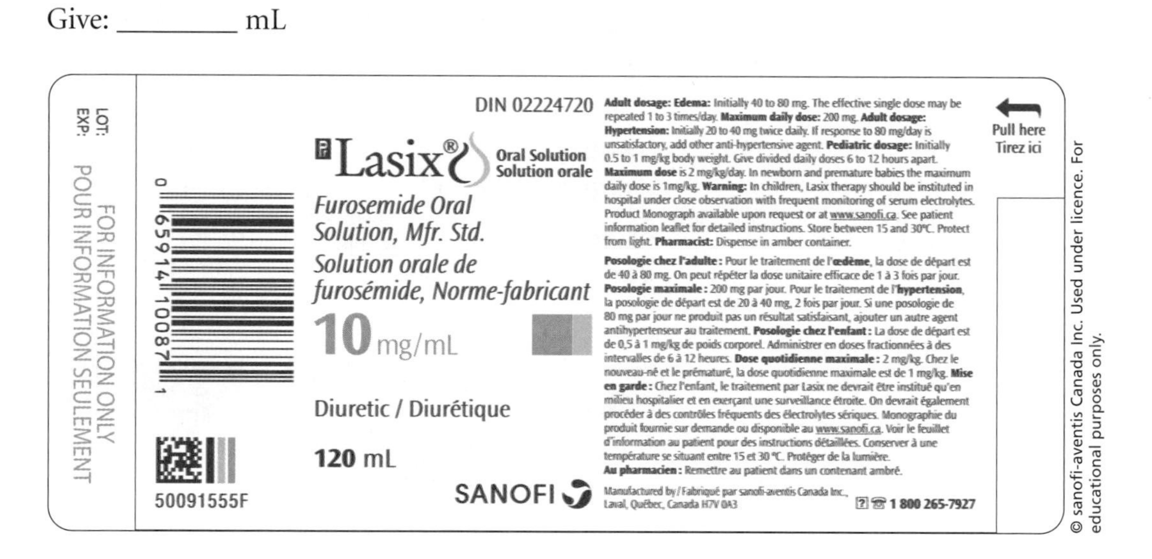

LOT:
EXP:
FOR INFORMATION ONLY
POUR INFORMATION SEULEMENT
DIN 02224720
Lasix® Oral Solution Solution orale
Furosemide Oral Solution, Mfr. Std.
Solution orale de furosémide, Norme-fabricant
10 mg/mL
Diuretic / Diurétique
120 mL
50091555F
SANOFI
Pull here
Tirez ici
1 800 265-7927

26. Order: *dilantin 175 mg PO TID*

    Give: ________ mL

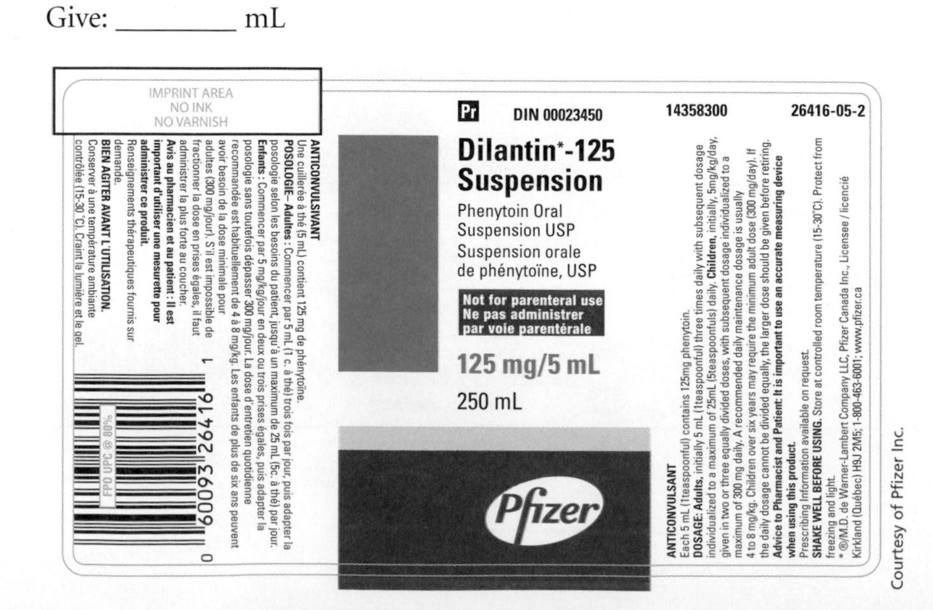

27. Order: *valproic acid 0.5 g PO TID*

Give: ________ mL

How many full doses are available in this bottle? ________ full doses

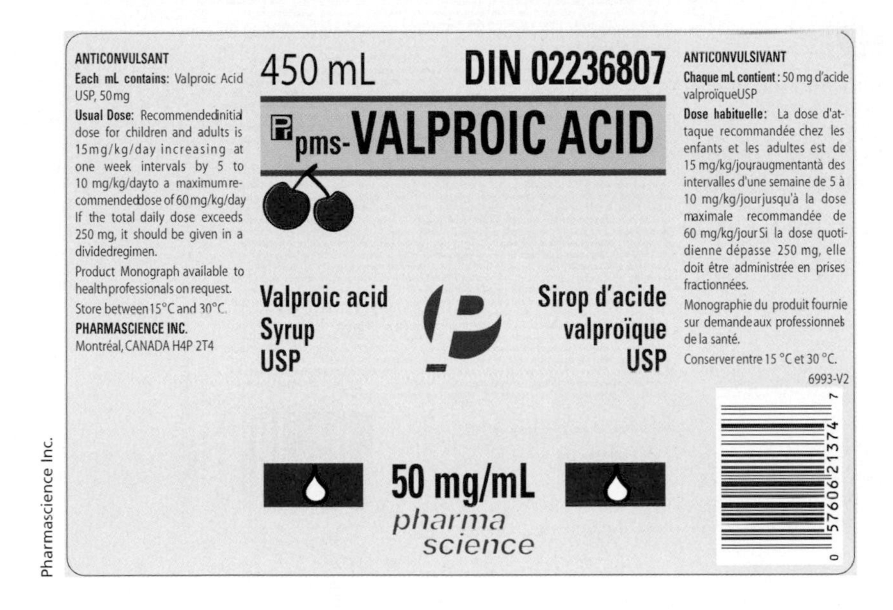

Pharmascience Inc.

28. Order: *clarithromycin 75 mg PO q12h*

Available: clarithromycin 125 mg/5 mL

Give: ________ mL

29. Order: *phenytoin oral suspension 225 mg/day divided BID*

Give: ___________mL

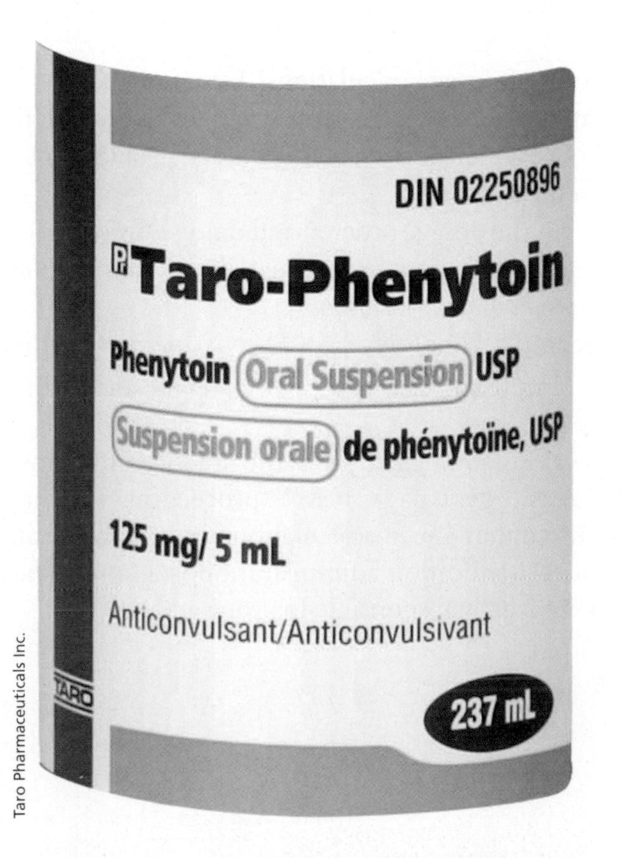

Taro Pharmaceuticals Inc.

30. Order: *potassium chloride oral solution 20 mEq BID, dissolved in 100 mL of cold water*

Give: __________ mL

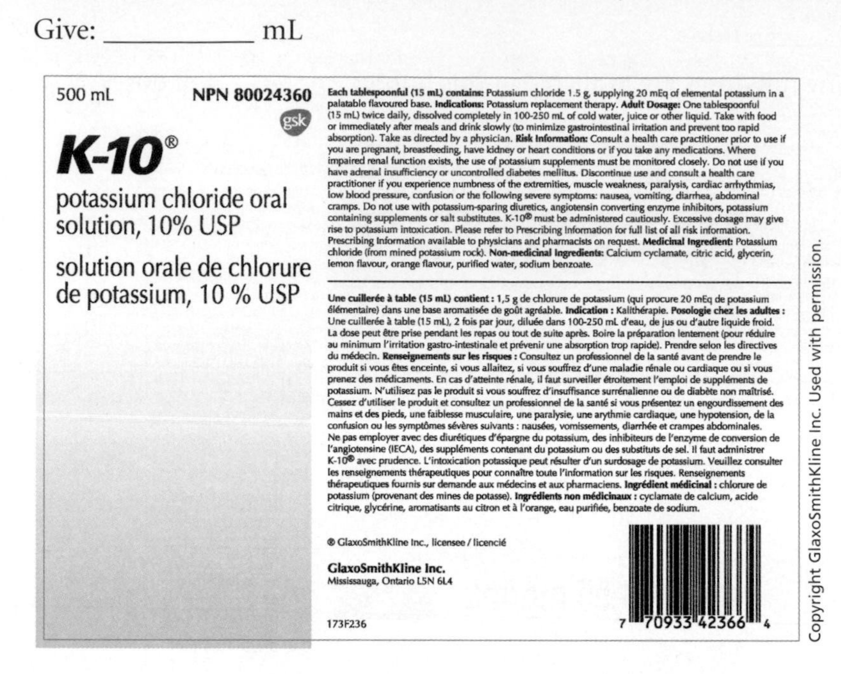

Check your work! Answers to all Review Sets are provided at the end of the chapter. Worked solutions for selected Review Sets are also available there.

CHECK POINT

Where are you in mastering the skill of dosage calculations? First, you learned to convert equivalent units within the metric systems. You applied this conversion skill to the calculation of oral dosages—both solid and liquid forms. By now, you know that solving dosage problems requires that all units of measurement first be expressed in the same unit.

Next, you learned to think through the dosage ordered and dosage supplied to estimate the amount to be given. *To minimize patient safety incidents, it is essential that you consider the reasonableness of the amount before applying a calculation method or formula.*

Finally, you learned the formula method $\frac{D}{H} \times Q = X$ (*desired* over *have* times *quantity* = *amount to give*). This method is so simple and easy to recall that it will stick with you throughout your career.

Review the Application of Clinical Reasoning and work the practice problems for Chapter 8. If you are having difficulty, get help on the next page, before proceeding to Chapter 9. Continue to concentrate on accuracy. Keep in mind that one miscalculation can be a serious mistake when you are calculating the dosages of medicines. Medication administration is a *legal responsibility*. Remember, when you give a medication, you are legally responsible for your action.

APPLICATION OF CLINICAL REASONING

Patient safety incidents are often attributed to inaccuracy in dosage calculation. By first asking the question, "What is the reasonable amount to give?" many patient safety incidents can be avoided.

Potential Patient Safety Incident

Incorrect calculation and not assessing the reasonableness of the calculation before administering the medication.

Possible Scenario

The prescriber ordered *phenobarbital 60 mg PO BID* for a patient with a seizure disorder. The pharmacy supplied *phenobarbital 30 mg per tablet*. The nurse did not use Step 2 to think about the reasonable dosage and calculated the dosage this way:

$$\frac{\text{D (desired)}}{\text{H (have)}} \times \text{Q (quantity)} = \text{A (amount)}$$

$$\frac{60 \text{ mg}}{30 \text{ mg}} \times 1 \text{ tab} = 20 \text{ tab (incorrect)}$$

Suppose the nurse then gave the patient 20 tablets of the 30-mg tablet of phenobarbital. The patient would then have received 600 mg of phenobarbital, or 10 times the correct dosage. This scenario would have led to an extremely serious patient safety incident.

Potential Outcome

The patient would likely develop signs of phenobarbital toxicity, such as nystagmus (rapid eye movement), ataxia (lack of coordination), central nervous system depression, respiratory depression, hypothermia, and hypotension. When the error was caught and the prescriber notified, the patient would likely be given activated charcoal to hasten elimination of the drug. Depending on the severity of the symptoms, the patient might have been moved to the intensive care unit for monitoring of respiratory and neurological status.

Prevention

This patient safety incident could have been prevented if the nurse had used the Three-Step Approach and estimated a reasonable dosage of the drug to give. The order was for 60 mg of phenobarbital and the available drug was 30 mg per tablet, so the nurse should have given 2 tablets. The incorrect calculation that indicated such a large number of tablets to give per dose should have alerted the nurse to a possible patient safety incident. The formula $\frac{D}{H} \times Q = X$ should have been used to verify the *reasonable* dosage. Further, the nurse should have double-checked the math and found the error.

$$\frac{D}{H} \times Q = \frac{60 \text{ mg}}{30 \text{ mg}} \times 1 \text{ tablet}$$

$$\frac{\overset{2}{\cancel{60}} \cancel{\text{mg}}}{\underset{1}{\cancel{30}} \cancel{\text{mg}}} \times 1 \text{ tablet} = 2 \text{ tablets, not 20 tablets}$$

Application of Critical Reasoning Additional application problems are provided at the end of the chapter. Answers are provided at the end of the book.

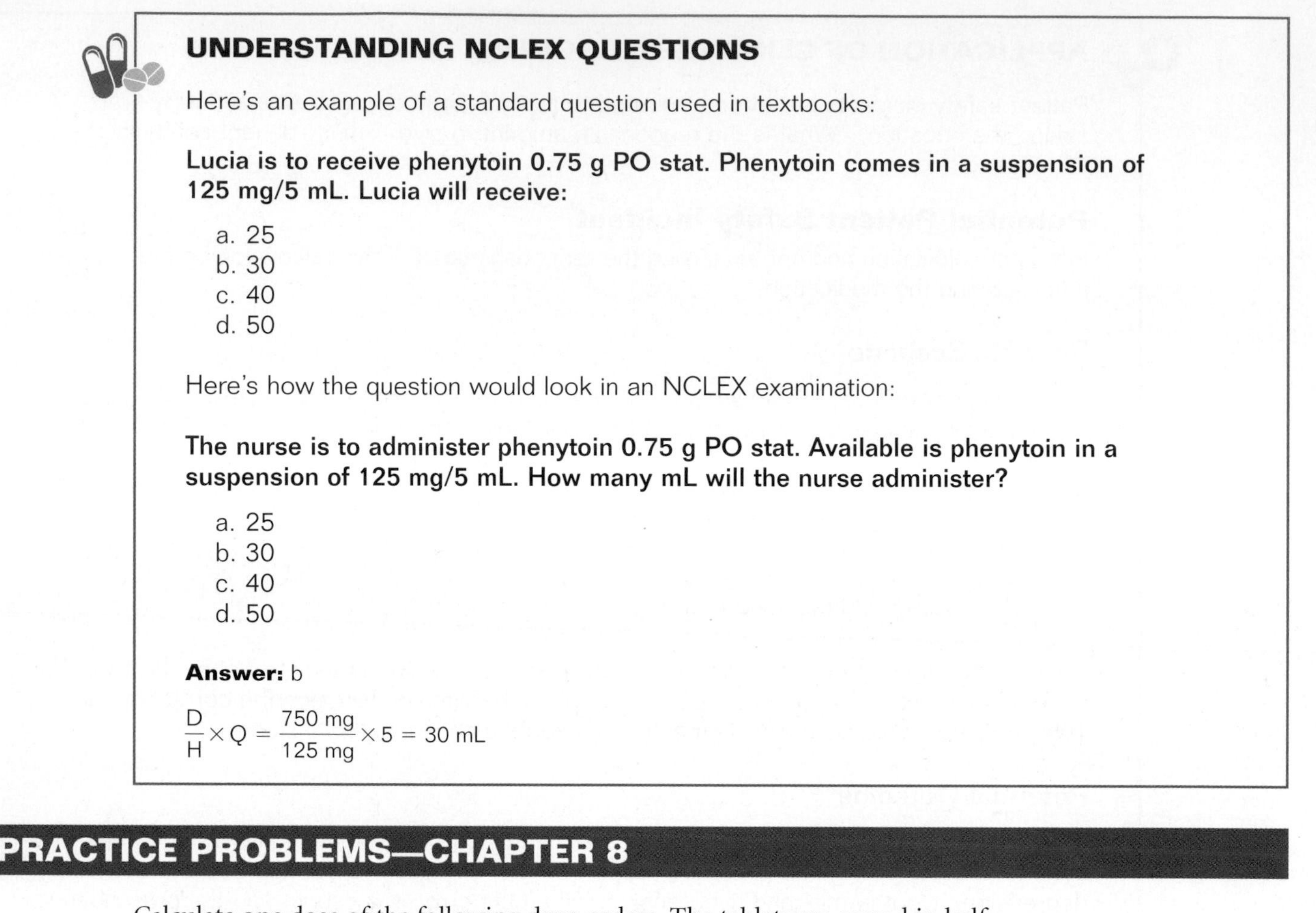

UNDERSTANDING NCLEX QUESTIONS

Here's an example of a standard question used in textbooks:

Lucia is to receive phenytoin 0.75 g PO stat. Phenytoin comes in a suspension of 125 mg/5 mL. Lucia will receive:

a. 25
b. 30
c. 40
d. 50

Here's how the question would look in an NCLEX examination:

The nurse is to administer phenytoin 0.75 g PO stat. Available is phenytoin in a suspension of 125 mg/5 mL. How many mL will the nurse administer?

a. 25
b. 30
c. 40
d. 50

Answer: b

$$\frac{D}{H} \times Q = \frac{750 \text{ mg}}{125 \text{ mg}} \times 5 = 30 \text{ mL}$$

PRACTICE PROBLEMS—CHAPTER 8

Calculate one dose of the following drug orders. The tablets are scored in half.

1. Order: *metformin 250 mg PO BID*

   Supply: metformin 0.5-g tablets

   Give: ________ tablet(s)

2. Order: *codeine phosphate 45 mg PO q4h prn for pain*

   Supply: codeine phosphate 15-mg tablets

   Give: ________ tablet(s)

3. Order: *levothyroxine sodium 0.075 mg PO daily*

   Supply: levothyroxine sodium 150-mcg tablets

   Give: ________ tablet(s)

4. Order: *diphenhydramine hydrochloride elixir 25 mg PO q4h*

   Supply: diphenhydramine hydrochloride 12.5 mg/5 mL

   Give: ________ mL

5. Order: *cephalexin 500 mg PO QID*

   Supply: cephalexin 250 mg/5 mL

   Give: ________ mL

6. Order: *propranolol hydrochloride 20 mg PO QID*

   Supply: propranolol hydrochloride 10-mg tablets

   Give: ________ tablet(s)

7. Order: *amoxicillin 400 mg PO q6h*

   Supply: amoxicillin 250 mg/5 mL

   Give: ________ mL

8. Order: *gliclazide 120 mg PO BID*

   Supply: gliclazide 80-mg tablets

   Give: ________ tablet(s)

9. Order: *acetylsalicylic acid (Aspirin) 650 mg PO daily*

   Supply: acetylsalicylic acid 325-mg tablets

   Give: ________ tablet(s)

10. Order: *codeine phosphate 15 mg PO daily*

    Supply: codeine phosphate 30-mg tablets

    Give: ________ tablet(s)

11. Order: *propranolol hydrochloride 30 mg PO QID*

    Supply: propranolol hydrochloride 20-mg tablets

    Give: ________ tablet(s)

12. Order: *levothyroxine sodium 300 mcg PO daily*

    Supply: levothyroxine sodium 0.3-mg tablets

    Give: ________ tablet(s)

13. Order: *furosemide 60 mg PO daily*

    Supply: furosemide 40-mg tablets

    Give: ________ tablet(s)

14. Order: *penicillin V potassium 400 000 units PO QID*

    Supply: penicillin V potassium 250-mg (400 000 units) tablets

    Give: ________ tablet(s)

15. Order: *enalapril maleate 7.5 mg PO daily*

    Supply: enalapril maleate 5-mg and 10-mg tablets

    Select: ________ mg tablets

    Give ________ tablet(s)

16. Order: *penicillin V potassium 300 000 units PO QID*

    Supply: penicillin V potassium 200 000 units/5 mL

    Give: ________ mL

17. Order: *pyrazinamide 0.75 g PO BID*

    Supply: pyrazinamide 500-mg tablets

    Give: ________ tablet(s)

18. Order: *triazolam 0.25 mg PO at bedtime*

    Supply: triazolam 0.125-mg tablets

    Give: ________ tablet(s)

19. Order: *morphine hydrochloride 5 mg PO q3h for pain*

    Supply: morphine hydrochloride 10 mg/mL

    Give: ________ mL

20. Order: *dexamethasone 750 mcg PO BID*

    Supply: dexamethasone 0.5-mg and 0.75-mg tablets

    Select: ________ mg tablets

    Give: ________ tablet(s)

21. Order: *ethacrynic acid 12.5 mg PO BID*

    Supply: ethacrynic acid 25-mg tablets

    Give: ________ tablet(s)

22. Order: *bethanechol chloride 50 mg PO TID*

    Supply: bethanechol chloride 25-mg tablets

    Give: ________ tablet(s)

23. Order: *erythromycin 0.5 g PO q12h*

    Supply: erythromycin 250 mg tablets

    Give: ________ tablet(s)

24. Order: *glyburide 2.5 mg PO daily*

    Supply: glyburide 1.25-mg tablets

    Give: ________ tablet(s)

25. Order: *clorazepate dipotassium 7.5 mg PO qAM*

    Supply: clorazepate dipotassium 3.75-mg capsules

    Give: ________ capsules

26. Order: *oxazepam 45 mg PO at bedtime*

    Supply: oxazepam 10-mg, 15-mg, and 30-mg scored tablets

    Which strength of tablet(s) would you select, and how much would you give?

    Select: ________ mg tablets

    Give: ________ tablet(s)

27. Order: *acetaminophen 240 mg PO q4h prn for pain or T greater than 38.5°C*

    Supply: acetaminophen elixir 160 mg/5 mL

    Give: ________ mL

28. Order: *acetaminophen 160 mg PO q4h prn for pain or T greater than 38.5°C*

    Supply: acetaminophen drops 80 mg/mL

    Give: ________ mL

29. Order: *warfarin sodium 7.5 mg PO daily*

    Supply: warfarin sodium 2.5-mg tablets

    Give: ________ tablet(s)

See the three medication administration records and accompanying drug labels on the following pages for questions 30 through 42.

Calculate one dose of each of the drugs prescribed. Drug labels A through N provided on pages 187–194 are the drugs available. Indicate the letter corresponding to the label you select.

PAGE ____ of ____

MEDICATION ADMINISTRATION RECORD

	ORIGINAL ORDER DATE	DATE STARTED / RENEWED	MEDICATION - DOSAGE	ROUTE	SCHEDULE 23-07	SCHEDULE 07-15	SCHEDULE 15-23	DATE 1/5/xx 23-07	07-15	15-23	DATE 23-07	07-15	15-23	DATE 23-07	07-15	15-23	DATE 23-07	07-15	15-23
30.	1/5/xx	1/5	sucralfate 1000 mg	PO		09			ZW 09										
31.	1/5/xx	1/5	glyburide 5 mg daily	PO		09			ZW 09										
32.	1/5/xx	1/5	erythromycin ethylsuccinate 0.6 g q12h	PO		08	18		ZW 08	MS 18									
33.	1/5/xx	1/5	spironolactone 0.1 g daily	PO		09			ZW 09										
			PRN																

PRINTED BY STANDARD REGISTER U.S.A. ZIPSET ®

INJECTION SITES: B - RIGHT ARM; C - RIGHT ABDOMEN; D - RIGHT ANTERIOR THIGH; G - LEFT ARM; H - LEFT ABDOMEN; J - LEFT ANTERIOR THIGH; L - LEFT BUTTOCKS; M - RIGHT BUTTOCKS

DATE GIVEN	TIME	INT.	ONE - TIME MEDICATION - DOSAGE	RT.

SIGNATURE OF NURSE ADMINISTERING MEDICATIONS	DATE 1/5/xx	DATE	DATE	DATE
23-07				
07-15	ZW Zada Winthrop, RN			
15-23	MS M. Smith, RN			

DATE GIVEN	TIME	INT.	MEDICATION-DOSAGE-CONT.	RT.
			RECOPIED BY:	
			CHECKED BY:	

LITHO IN U.S.A. K6508 (7-92) D09553B

Patient, John Q.

ALLERGIES:

602-31 (7-XX) (MPC# 1355)

1 ORIGINAL COPY

30. Select: ________

    Give: ________

31. Select: ________

    Give: ________

32. Select: ________

    Give: ________

33. Select: ________

    Give: ________

PAGE ______ of ______

MEDICATION ADMINISTRATION RECORD

	ORIGINAL ORDER DATE	DATE STARTED / RENEWED	MEDICATION - DOSAGE	ROUTE	SCHEDULE 23-07	SCHEDULE 07-15	SCHEDULE 15-23	DATE 1/5/xx 23-07	07-15	15-23	DATE 23-07	07-15	15-23	DATE 23-07	07-15	15-23	DATE 23-07	07-15	15-23
34.	1/5/xx	1/5	lorazepam 1 mg BID	PO		09			ZW 09										
35.	1/5/xx	1/5	glyburide 5 mg daily	PO		09			ZW 09										
36.	1/5/xx	1/5	clarithromycin 500 mg BID	PO		08	18		ZW 08	MS 18									
37.	1/5/xx	1/5	spironolactone 0.1 g daily	PO		09			ZW 09										
			PRN																

PRINTED BY STANDARD REGISTER U.S.A. ZIPSET ®

INJECTION SITES

B - RIGHT ARM
C - RIGHT ABDOMEN
D - RIGHT ANTERIOR THIGH
G - LEFT ARM
H - LEFT ABDOMEN
J - LEFT ANTERIOR THIGH
L - LEFT BUTTOCKS
M - RIGHT BUTTOCKS

DATE GIVEN	TIME	INT.	ONE - TIME MEDICATION - DOSAGE	RT.

SIGNATURE OF NURSE ADMINISTERING MEDICATIONS	DATE 1/5/xx	DATE	DATE	DATE
23-07				
07-15	ZW Zada Winthrop			
15-23	MS M. Smith, RN			

DATE GIVEN	TIME	INT.	MEDICATION-DOSAGE-CONT.	RT.
			RECOPIED BY:	
			CHECKED BY:	

LITHO IN U.S.A. K6508 (7-92) D095538

Patient, John Q.

ALLERGIES:

602-31 (7-XX) (MPC# 1355)

1 ORIGINAL COPY

34. Select: ________

    Give: ________

35. Select: ________

    Give: ________

36. Select: ________

    Give: ________

37. Select: ________

    Give: ________

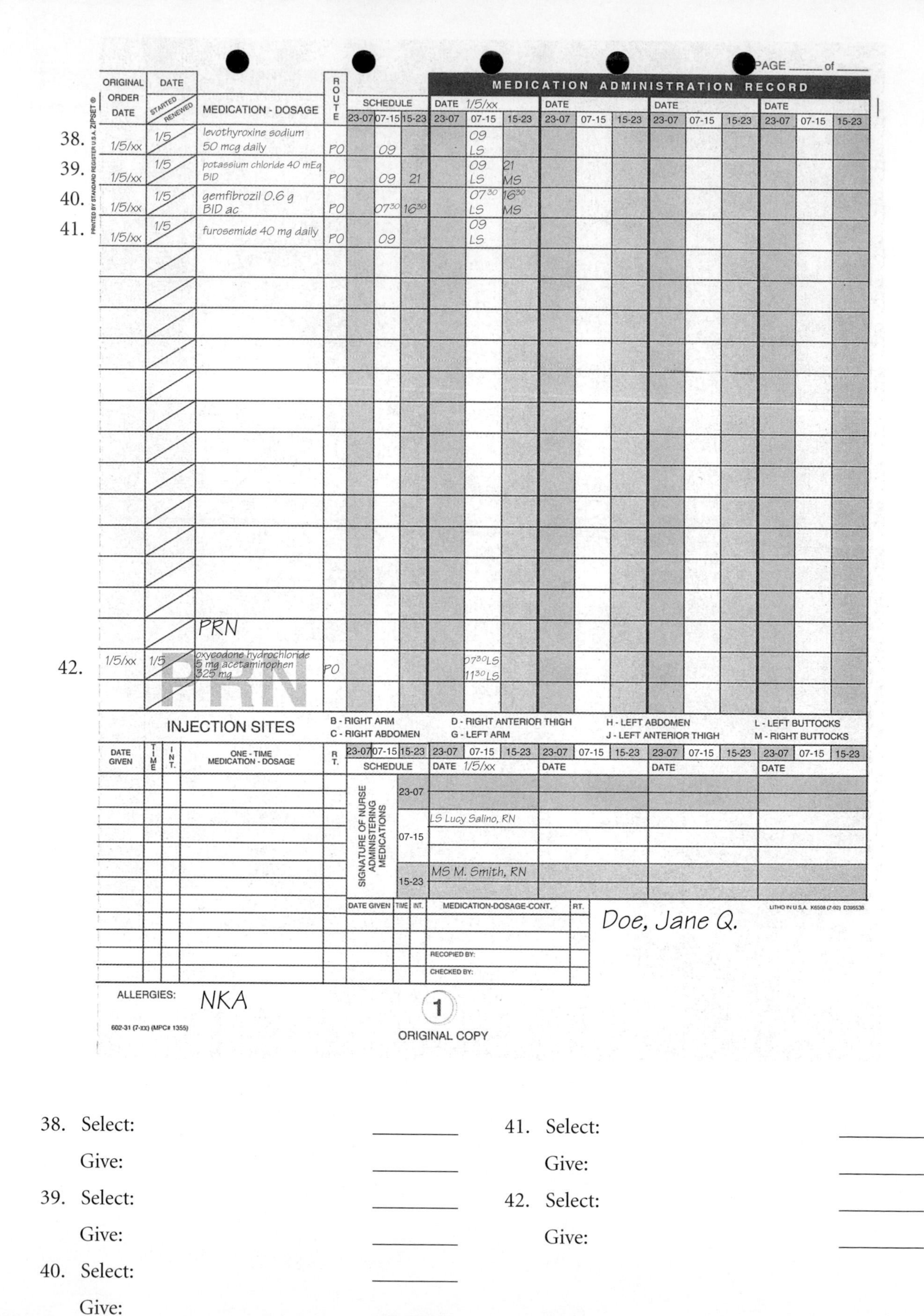

PAGE ___ of ___

MEDICATION ADMINISTRATION RECORD

	ORIGINAL ORDER DATE	DATE STARTED / RENEWED	MEDICATION - DOSAGE	ROUTE	SCHEDULE 23-07	SCHEDULE 07-15	SCHEDULE 15-23	DATE 1/5/xx 23-07	07-15	15-23
38.	1/5/xx	1/5	levothyroxine sodium 50 mcg daily	PO		09			09 LS	
39.	1/5/xx	1/5	potassium chloride 40 mEq BID	PO		09	21		09 LS	21 MS
40.	1/5/xx	1/5	gemfibrozil 0.6 g BID ac	PO		07^{30}	16^{30}		07^{30} LS	16^{30} MS
41.	1/5/xx	1/5	furosemide 40 mg daily	PO		09			09 LS	
			PRN							
42.	1/5/xx	1/5	oxycodone hydrochloride 5 mg acetaminophen 325 mg	PO					07^{30} LS 11^{30} LS	

INJECTION SITES

B - RIGHT ARM
C - RIGHT ABDOMEN
D - RIGHT ANTERIOR THIGH
G - LEFT ARM
H - LEFT ABDOMEN
J - LEFT ANTERIOR THIGH
L - LEFT BUTTOCKS
M - RIGHT BUTTOCKS

DATE GIVEN | TIME | INT. | ONE - TIME MEDICATION - DOSAGE | RT.

SIGNATURE OF NURSE ADMINISTERING MEDICATIONS

SCHEDULE	DATE 1/5/xx
23-07	
07-15	LS Lucy Salino, RN
15-23	MS M. Smith, RN

DATE GIVEN | TIME | INT. | MEDICATION-DOSAGE-CONT. | RT.

RECOPIED BY:

CHECKED BY:

Doe, Jane Q.

ALLERGIES: NKA

602-31 (7-xx) (MPC# 1355)

1 ORIGINAL COPY

38. Select: ________

    Give: ________

39. Select: ________

    Give: ________

40. Select: ________

    Give: ________

41. Select: ________

    Give: ________

42. Select: ________

    Give: ________

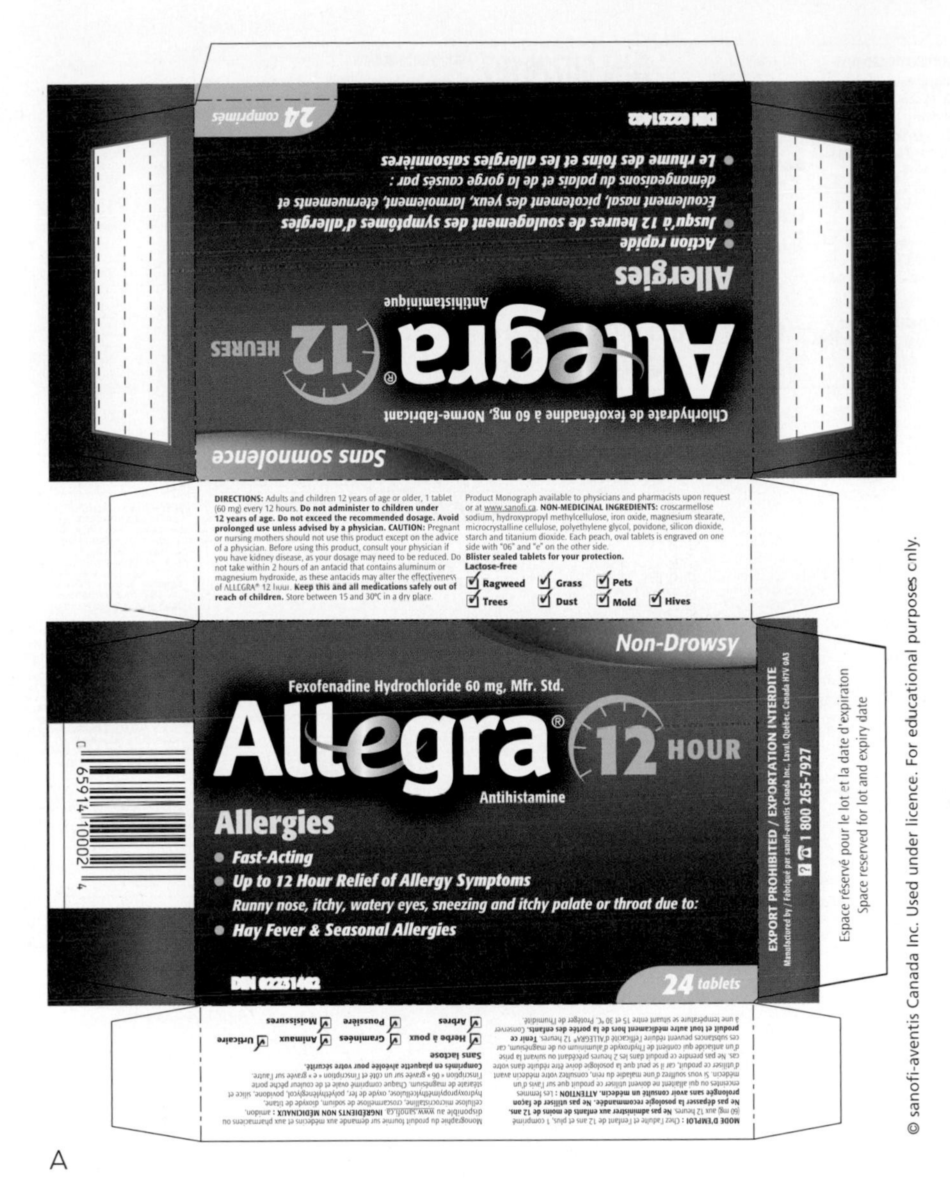
24 comprimés
DIN 02251462
Le rhume des foins et les allergies saisonnières
Jusqu'à 12 heures de soulagement des symptômes d'allergies
Écoulement nasal, picotement des yeux, larmoiement, éternuements et démangeaisons du palais et de la gorge causés par :
Action rapide
Allergies
Allegra 12 HEURES
Antihistaminique
Chlorhydrate de fexofénadine à 60 mg, Norme-fabricant
Sans somnolence
DIRECTIONS: Adults and children 12 years of age or older, 1 tablet (60 mg) every 12 hours. Do not administer to children under 12 years of age. Do not exceed the recommended dosage. Avoid prolonged use unless advised by a physician. CAUTION: Pregnant or nursing mothers should not use this product except on the advice of a physician. Before using this product, consult your physician if you have kidney disease, as your dosage may need to be reduced. Do not take within 2 hours of an antacid that contains aluminum or magnesium hydroxide, as these antacids may alter the effectiveness of ALLEGRA® 12 hour. Keep this and all medications safely out of reach of children. Store between 15 and 30°C in a dry place.
Product Monograph available to physicians and pharmacists upon request or at www.sanofi.ca. NON-MEDICINAL INGREDIENTS: croscarmellose sodium, hydroxypropyl methylcellulose, iron oxide, magnesium stearate, microcrystalline cellulose, polyethylene glycol, povidone, silicon dioxide, starch and titanium dioxide. Each peach, oval tablets is engraved on one side with "06" and "e" on the other side.
Blister sealed tablets for your protection.
Lactose-free
Ragweed
Grass
Pets
Trees
Dust
Mold
Hives
Non-Drowsy
Fexofenadine Hydrochloride 60 mg, Mfr. Std.
Allegra® 12 HOUR
Antihistamine
Allergies
Fast-Acting
Up to 12 Hour Relief of Allergy Symptoms
Runny nose, itchy, watery eyes, sneezing and itchy palate or throat due to:
Hay Fever & Seasonal Allergies
DIN 02251462
24 tablets
EXPORT PROHIBITED / EXPORTATION INTERDITE
1 800 265-7927
Espace réservé pour le lot et la date d'expiration
Space reserved for lot and expiry date
C 65914 10002 4

A

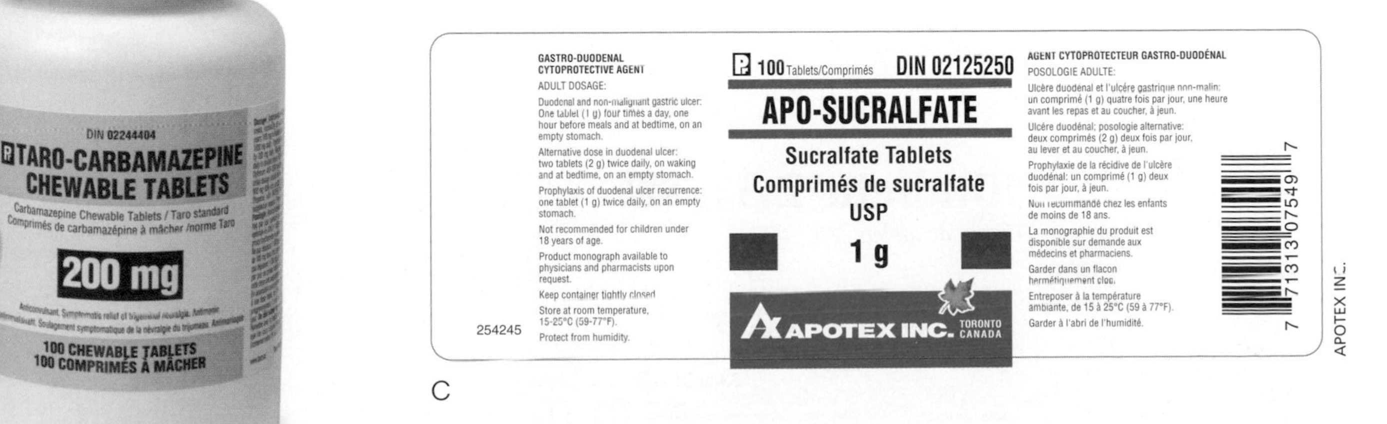
DIN 02244404
TARO-CARBAMAZEPINE CHEWABLE TABLETS
Carbamazepine Chewable Tablets / Taro standard
Comprimés de carbamazépine à mâcher /norme Taro
200 mg
100 CHEWABLE TABLETS
100 COMPRIMÉS À MÂCHER
GASTRO-DUODENAL CYTOPROTECTIVE AGENT
ADULT DOSAGE:
Duodenal and non-malignant gastric ulcer: One tablet (1 g) four times a day, one hour before meals and at bedtime, on an empty stomach.
Alternative dose in duodenal ulcer: two tablets (2 g) twice daily, on waking and at bedtime, on an empty stomach.
Prophylaxis of duodenal ulcer recurrence: one tablet (1 g) twice daily, on an empty stomach.
Not recommended for children under 18 years of age.
Product monograph available to physicians and pharmacists upon request.
Keep container tightly closed
Store at room temperature, 15-25°C (59-77°F).
Protect from humidity.
254245
100 Tablets/Comprimés
DIN 02125250
APO-SUCRALFATE
Sucralfate Tablets
Comprimés de sucralfate
USP
1 g
APOTEX INC. TORONTO CANADA
AGENT CYTOPROTECTEUR GASTRO-DUODÉNAL
POSOLOGIE ADULTE:
Ulcère duodénal et l'ulcère gastrique non-malin: un comprimé (1 g) quatre fois par jour, une heure avant les repas et au coucher, à jeun.
Ulcère duodénal; posologie alternative: deux comprimés (2 g) deux fois par jour, au lever et au coucher, à jeun.
Prophylaxie de la récidive de l'ulcère duodénal: un comprimé (1 g) deux fois par jour, à jeun.
Non recommandé chez les enfants de moins de 18 ans.
La monographie du produit est disponible sur demande aux médecins et pharmaciens.
Garder dans un flacon hermétiquement clos.
Entreposer à la température ambiante, de 15 à 25°C (59 à 77°F).
Garder à l'abri de l'humidité.
7 71313 07549 7

B

C

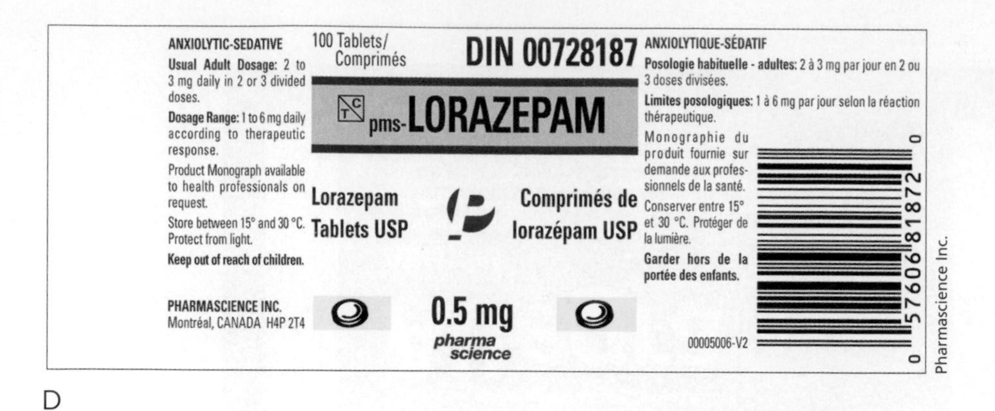

ANXIOLYTIC-SEDATIVE
Usual Adult Dosage: 2 to 3 mg daily in 2 or 3 divided doses.
Dosage Range: 1 to 6 mg daily according to therapeutic response.
Product Monograph available to health professionals on request.
Store between 15° and 30 °C. Protect from light.
Keep out of reach of children.
PHARMASCIENCE INC.
Montréal, CANADA H4P 2T4
100 Tablets/ Comprimés
DIN 00728187
pms-LORAZEPAM
Lorazepam Tablets USP
Comprimés de lorazépam USP
0.5 mg
pharma science
ANXIOLYTIQUE-SÉDATIF
Posologie habituelle - adultes: 2 à 3 mg par jour en 2 ou 3 doses divisées.
Limites posologiques: 1 à 6 mg par jour selon la réaction thérapeutique.
Monographie du produit fournie sur demande aux professionnels de la santé.
Conserver entre 15° et 30 °C. Protéger de la lumière.
Garder hors de la portée des enfants.
00005006-V2
0 57606 81872 0
Pharmascience Inc.

D

The product labels and intellectual property of Teva Canada Limited are reproduced with the permission of Teva Canada Limited and used herein for educational purposes only.

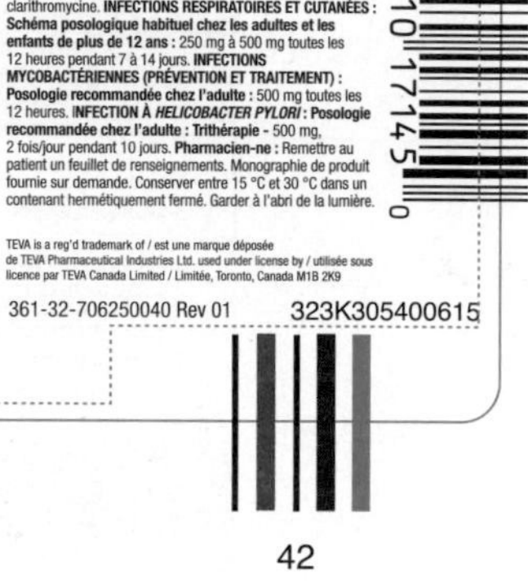

Area for Lot and Exp
DIN 02248805 100 TABLETS COMPRIMÉS
TEVA-CLARITHROMYCIN
Clarithromycin Tablets
Comprimés de clarithromycine
Teva Standard Norme Teva
500 mg
TEVA
ANTIBIOTIC Each tablet contains 500 mg clarithromycin. RESPIRATORY TRACT OR SKIN INFECTIONS: Usual dose range for adults and children over 12 years: 250 to 500 mg every 12 hours for 7 to 14 days. MYCOBACTERIAL INFECTIONS (PREVENTION AND TREATMENT): Recommended Adult Dose: 500 mg every 12 hours. HELICOBACTER PYLORI INFECTION: Recommended Adult Dose: Triple Therapy - 500 mg twice daily for 10 days. Pharmacist: Dispense with Patient Information Leaflet. Product Monograph available on request. Store 15 - 30°C in a tightly closed container. Protect from light.
ANTIBIOTIQUE Un comprimé renferme 500 mg de clarithromycine. INFECTIONS RESPIRATOIRES ET CUTANÉES : Schéma posologique habituel chez les adultes et les enfants de plus de 12 ans : 250 mg à 500 mg toutes les 12 heures pendant 7 à 14 jours. INFECTIONS MYCOBACTÉRIENNES (PRÉVENTION ET TRAITEMENT) : Posologie recommandée chez l'adulte : 500 mg toutes les 12 heures. INFECTION À HELICOBACTER PYLORI : Posologie recommandée chez l'adulte : Trithérapie - 500 mg, 2 fois/jour pendant 10 jours. Pharmacien-ne : Remettre au patient un feuillet de renseignements. Monographie de produit fournie sur demande. Conserver entre 15 °C et 30 °C dans un contenant hermétiquement fermé. Garder à l'abri de la lumière.
361-32-706250040 Rev 01
323K305400615
0 68510 17145 0
42

E

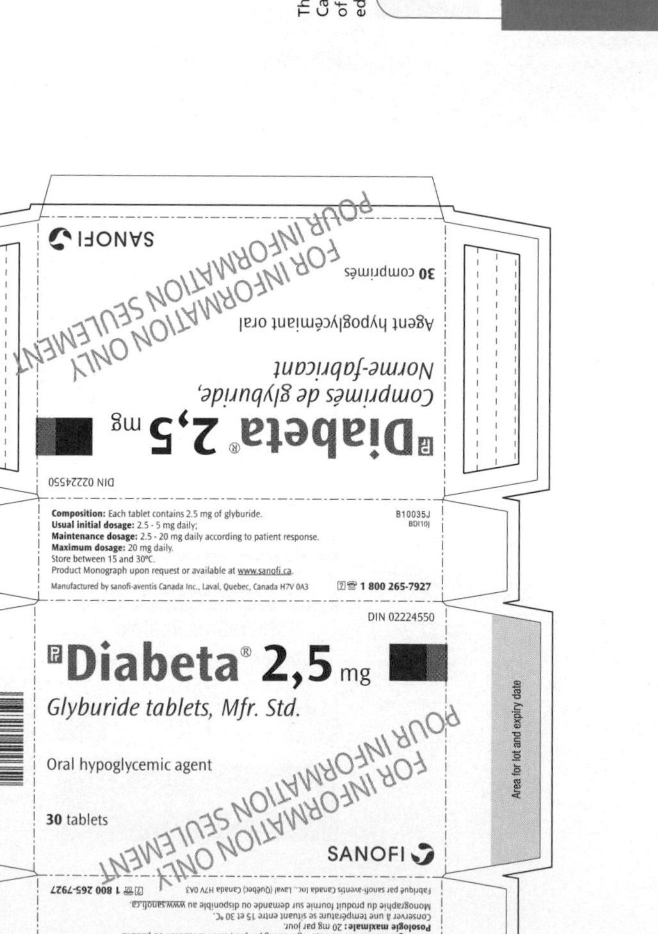

DIN 02224550
Diabeta® 2,5 mg
Glyburide tablets, Mfr. Std.
Oral hypoglycemic agent
30 tablets
SANOFI
Area for lot and expiry date
FOR INFORMATION ONLY
POUR INFORMATION SEULEMENT
Composition: Each tablet contains 2.5 mg of glyburide.
Usual initial dosage: 2.5 - 5 mg daily;
Maintenance dosage: 2.5 - 20 mg daily according to patient response.
Maximum dosage: 20 mg daily.
Store between 15 and 30°C.
Product Monograph upon request or available at www.sanofi.ca.
Manufactured by sanofi-aventis Canada Inc., Laval, Quebec, Canada H7V 0A3
1 800 265-7927
B10035J
Diabeta® 2,5 mg
Comprimés de glyburide, Norme-fabricant
Agent hypoglycémiant oral
30 comprimés

F

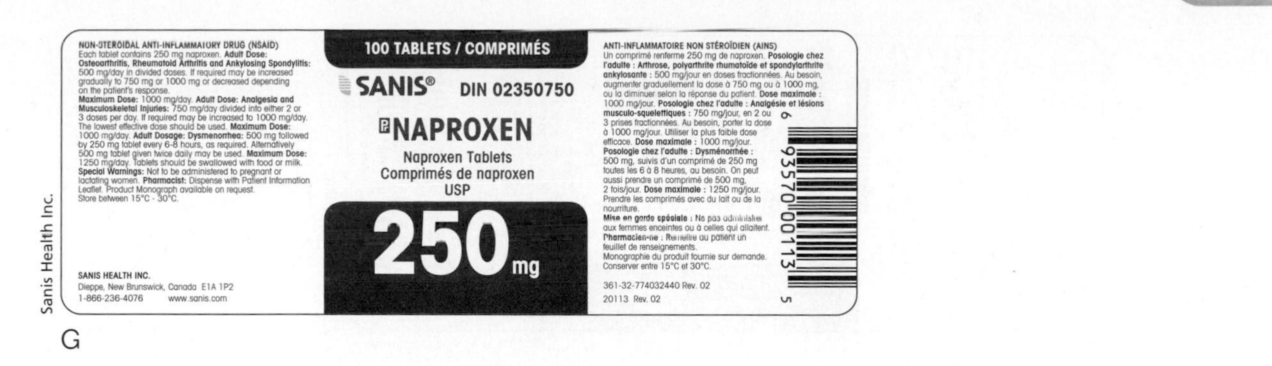
NON-STEROIDAL ANTI-INFLAMMATORY DRUG (NSAID)
Each tablet contains 250 mg naproxen. Adult Dose: Osteoarthritis, Rheumatoid Arthritis and Ankylosing Spondylitis: 500 mg/day in divided doses. If required may be increased gradually to 750 mg or 1000 mg or decreased depending on the patient's response.
Maximum Dose: 1000 mg/day. Adult Dose: Analgesia and Musculoskeletal Injuries: 750 mg/day divided into either 2 or 3 doses per day. If required may be increased to 1000 mg/day. The lowest effective dose should be used. Maximum Dose: 1000 mg/day. Adult Dosage: Dysmenorrhea: 500 mg followed by 250 mg tablet every 6-8 hours, as required. Alternatively 500 mg tablet given twice daily may be used. Maximum Dose: 1250 mg/day. Tablets should be swallowed with food or milk.
Special Warnings: Not to be administered to pregnant or lactating women. Pharmacist: Dispense with Patient Information Leaflet. Product Monograph available on request.
Store between 15°C - 30°C.
SANIS HEALTH INC.
Dieppe, New Brunswick, Canada E1A 1P2
1-866-236-4076 www.sanis.com
100 TABLETS / COMPRIMÉS
SANIS® DIN 02350750
NAPROXEN
Naproxen Tablets
Comprimés de naproxen
USP
250 mg
ANTI-INFLAMMATOIRE NON STÉROÏDIEN (AINS)
Un comprimé renferme 250 mg de naproxen. Posologie chez l'adulte : Arthrose, polyarthrite rhumatoïde et spondylarthrite ankylosante : 500 mg/jour en doses fractionnées. Au besoin, augmenter graduellement la dose à 750 mg ou à 1000 mg, ou la diminuer selon la réponse du patient. Dose maximale : 1000 mg/jour. Posologie chez l'adulte : Analgésie et lésions musculo-squelettiques : 750 mg/jour, en 2 ou 3 prises fractionnées. Au besoin, porter la dose à 1000 mg/jour. Utiliser la plus faible dose efficace. Dose maximale : 1000 mg/jour.
Posologie chez l'adulte : Dysménorrhée : 500 mg, suivis d'un comprimé de 250 mg toutes les 6 à 8 heures, au besoin. On peut aussi prendre un comprimé de 500 mg, 2 fois/jour. Dose maximale : 1250 mg/jour. Prendre les comprimés avec du lait ou de la nourriture.
Mise en garde spéciale :
aux femmes enceintes ou à celles qui allaitent.
feuillet de renseignements.
Monographie du produit fournie sur demande.
Conserver entre 15°C et 30°C.
361-32-774032440 Rev. 02
20113 Rev. 02
6 93570 00113 5

G

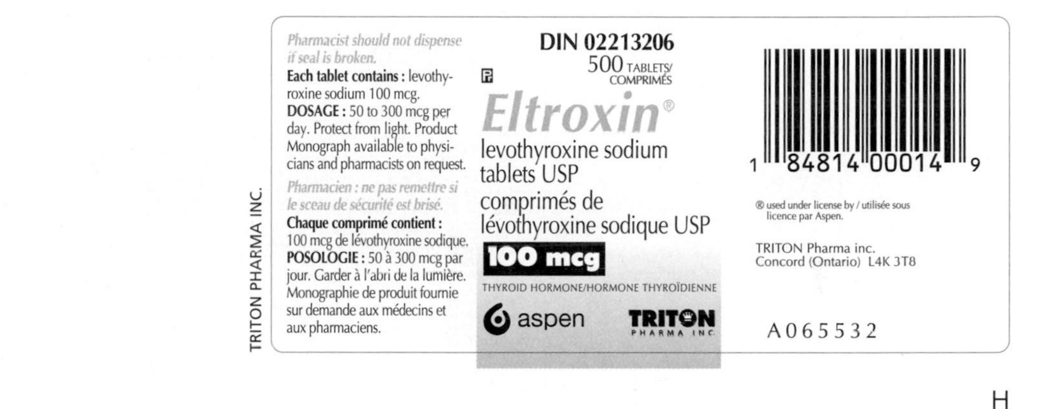
Pharmacist should not dispense if seal is broken.
Each tablet contains : levothyroxine sodium 100 mcg.
DOSAGE : 50 to 300 mcg per day. Protect from light. Product Monograph available to physicians and pharmacists on request.
Pharmacien : ne pas remettre si le sceau de sécurité est brisé.
Chaque comprimé contient : 100 mcg de lévothyroxine sodique.
POSOLOGIE : 50 à 300 mcg par jour. Garder à l'abri de la lumière. Monographie de produit fournie sur demande aux médecins et aux pharmaciens.
DIN 02213206
500 TABLETS/COMPRIMÉS
Eltroxin®
levothyroxine sodium tablets USP
comprimés de lévothyroxine sodique USP
100 mcg
THYROID HORMONE/HORMONE THYROÏDIENNE
aspen
TRITON PHARMA INC
1 84814 00014 9
® used under license by / utilisée sous licence par Aspen.
TRITON Pharma inc.
Concord (Ontario) L4K 3T8
A065532

H

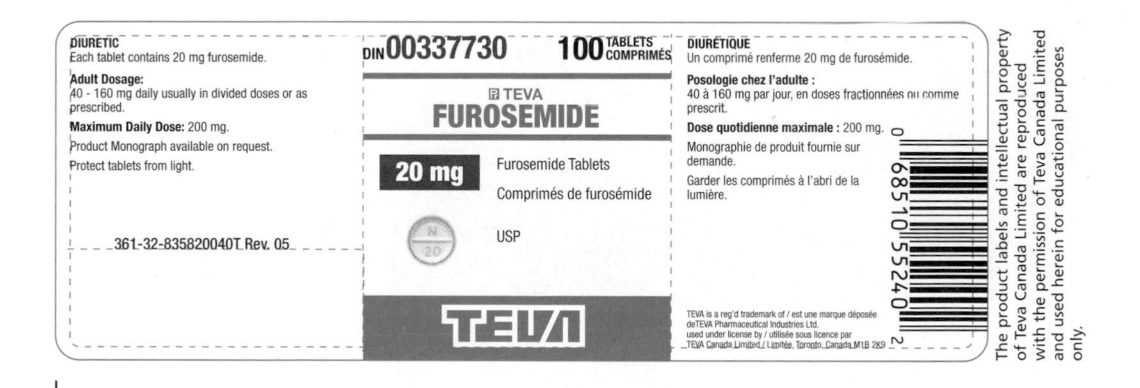
DIURETIC
Each tablet contains 20 mg furosemide.
Adult Dosage:
40 - 160 mg daily usually in divided doses or as prescribed.
Maximum Daily Dose: 200 mg.
Product Monograph available on request.
Protect tablets from light.
361-32-835820040T Rev. 05
DIN 00337730 100 TABLETS COMPRIMÉS
TEVA
FUROSEMIDE
20 mg
Furosemide Tablets
Comprimés de furosémide
USP
N 20
TEVA
DIURÉTIQUE
Un comprimé renferme 20 mg de furosémide.
Posologie chez l'adulte :
40 à 160 mg par jour, en doses fractionnées ou comme prescrit.
Dose quotidienne maximale : 200 mg.
Monographie de produit fournie sur demande.
Garder les comprimés à l'abri de la lumière.
TEVA is a reg'd trademark of / est une marque déposée de TEVA Pharmaceutical Industries Ltd.
used under license by / utilisée sous licence par TEVA Canada Limited / Limitée, Toronto, Canada M1B 2K9
0 68510 55240 2

I

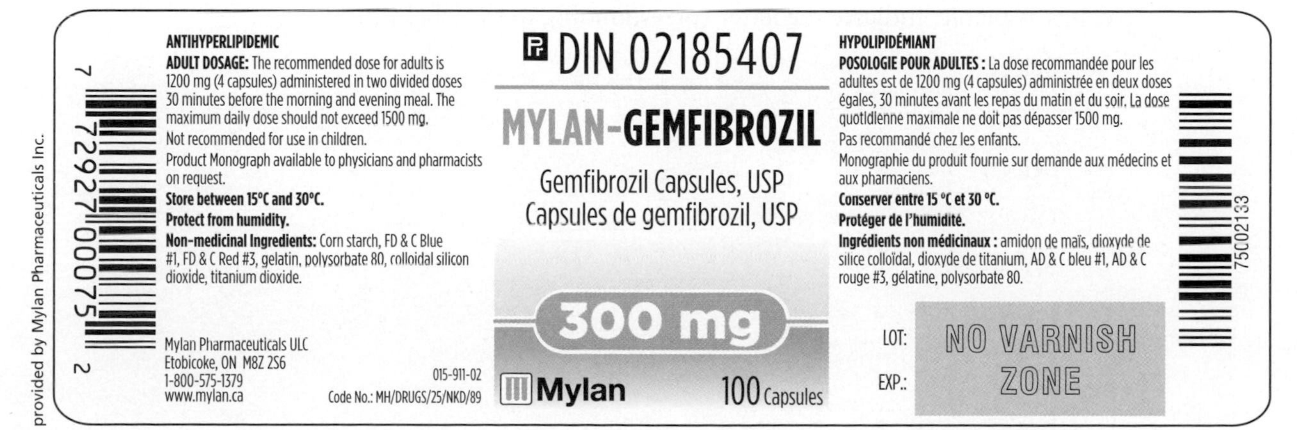
7 72927 00075 2
ANTIHYPERLIPIDEMIC
ADULT DOSAGE: The recommended dose for adults is 1200 mg (4 capsules) administered in two divided doses 30 minutes before the morning and evening meal. The maximum daily dose should not exceed 1500 mg.
Not recommended for use in children.
Product Monograph available to physicians and pharmacists on request.
Store between 15°C and 30°C.
Protect from humidity.
Non-medicinal Ingredients: Corn starch, FD & C Blue #1, FD & C Red #3, gelatin, polysorbate 80, colloidal silicon dioxide, titanium dioxide.
Mylan Pharmaceuticals ULC
Etobicoke, ON M8Z 2S6
1-800-575-1379
www.mylan.ca
015-911-02
Code No.: MH/DRUGS/25/NKD/89
DIN 02185407
MYLAN-GEMFIBROZIL
Gemfibrozil Capsules, USP
Capsules de gemfibrozil, USP
300 mg
Mylan
100 Capsules
HYPOLIPIDÉMIANT
POSOLOGIE POUR ADULTES : La dose recommandée pour les adultes est de 1200 mg (4 capsules) administrée en deux doses égales, 30 minutes avant les repas du matin et du soir. La dose quotidienne maximale ne doit pas dépasser 1500 mg.
Pas recommandé chez les enfants.
Monographie du produit fournie sur demande aux médecins et aux pharmaciens.
Conserver entre 15 °C et 30 °C.
Protéger de l'humidité.
Ingrédients non médicinaux : amidon de maïs, dioxyde de silice colloïdal, dioxyde de titanium, AD & C bleu #1, AD & C rouge #3, gélatine, polysorbate 80.
LOT:
EXP.:
NO VARNISH ZONE
75C02133

J

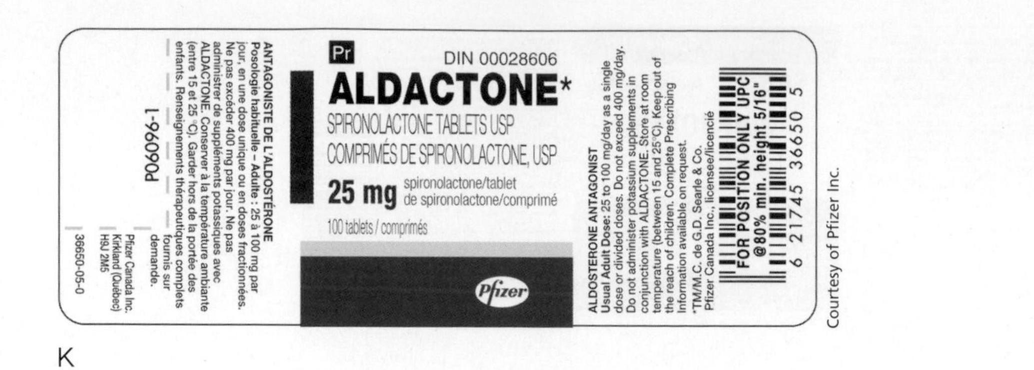

Pr
DIN 00028606
ALDACTONE*
SPIRONOLACTONE TABLETS USP
COMPRIMÉS DE SPIRONOLACTONE, USP
25 mg spironolactone/tablet de spironolactone/comprimé
100 tablets / comprimés
Pfizer
ALDOSTERONE ANTAGONIST
Usual Adult Dose: 25 to 100 mg/day as a single dose or divided doses. Do not exceed 400 mg/day. Do not administer potassium supplements in conjunction with ALDACTONE. Store at room temperature (between 15 and 25°C). Keep out of the reach of children. Complete Prescribing Information available on request.
TM/M.C. de G.D. Searle & Co. Pfizer Canada Inc., licensee/licencié
FOR POSITION ONLY UPC @80% min. height 5/16"
6 21745 36650 5
ANTAGONISTE DE L'ALDOSTÉRONE
P06096-1
Pfizer Canada Inc. Kirkland (Québec) H9J 2M5
36650-05-0

Courtesy of Pfizer Inc.

K

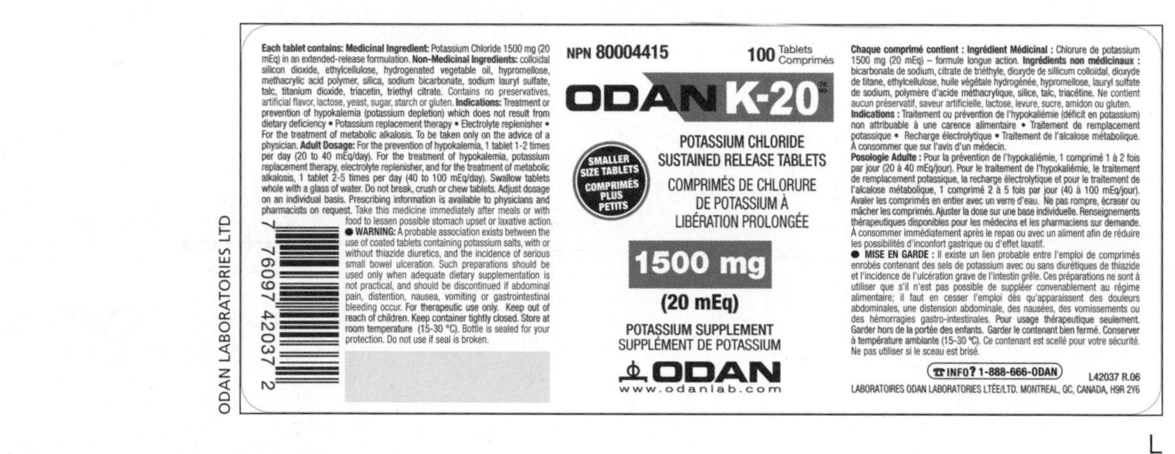

ODAN LABORATORIES LTD

L

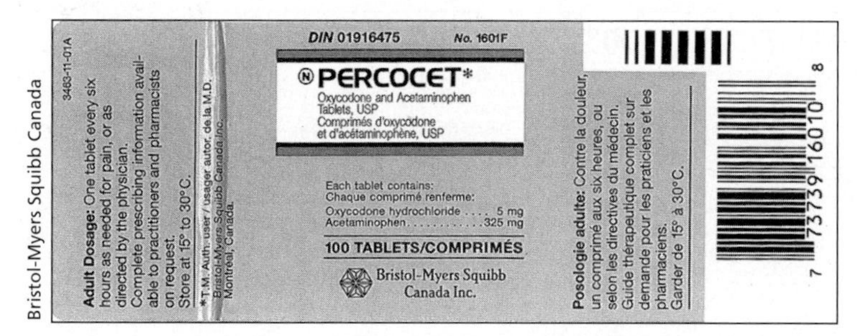

DIN 01916475
No. 1601F
PERCOCET*
Oxycodone and Acetaminophen Tablets, USP
Comprimés d'oxycodone et d'acétaminophène, USP
Each tablet contains:
Chaque comprimé renferme:
Oxycodone hydrochloride . . . . 5 mg
Acetaminophen . . . . 325 mg
100 TABLETS/COMPRIMÉS
Bristol-Myers Squibb Canada Inc.
Adult Dosage: One tablet every six hours as needed for pain, or as directed by the physician. Complete prescribing information available to practitioners and pharmacists on request. Store at 15° to 30°C.
Posologie adulte: Contre la douleur, un comprimé aux six heures, ou selon les directives du médecin. Guide thérapeutique complet sur demande pour les praticiens et les pharmaciens. Garder de 15° à 30°C.
7 73739 16010 8

Bristol-Myers Squibb Canada

M

For questions 43 through 46, calculate one dose of the medications indicated on the medication administration record that follows. Drug labels O through Q provided on the following pages are the drugs available. Indicate the letter corresponding to the label you select.

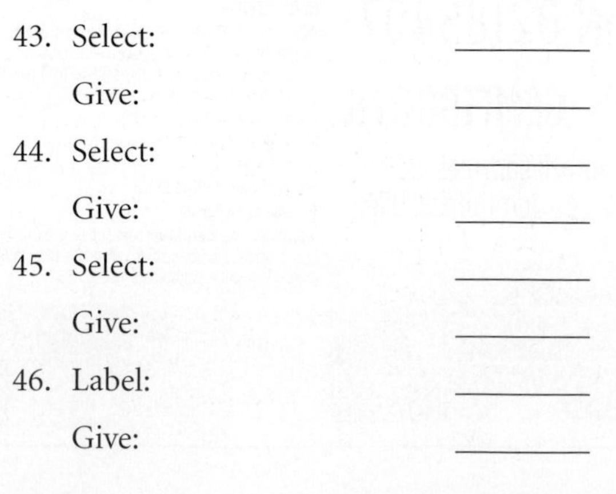

43. Select: ________

    Give: ________

44. Select: ________

    Give: ________

45. Select: ________

    Give: ________

46. Label: ________

    Give: ________

PAGE ____ of ____

MEDICATION ADMINISTRATION RECORD

	ORIGINAL ORDER DATE	DATE STARTED / RENEWED	MEDICATION - DOSAGE	ROUTE	SCHEDULE 23-07	SCHEDULE 07-15	SCHEDULE 15-23	DATE 3/8/xx 23-07	07-15	15-23	DATE 23-07	07-15	15-23	DATE 23-07	07-15	15-23	DATE 23-07	07-15	15-23
43.	3/8/xx	3-8	ranitidine hydrochloride 300 mg bedtime	PO			22			22 MS									
44.	3/8/xx	3-8	propranolol hydrochloride LA 120 mg OD	PO		09			09 MK										
45.	3/8/xx	3-8	furosemide 20 mg BID	PO		09	21		09 MK	21 MS									
46.	3/8/xx	3-8	potassium chloride oral solution 20 mEq BID	PO		09	21		09 MK	21 MS									
			PRN																

PRINTED BY STANDARD REGISTER U.S.A. ZIPSET ®

INJECTION SITES

B - RIGHT ARM
C - RIGHT ABDOMEN
D - RIGHT ANTERIOR THIGH
G - LEFT ARM
H - LEFT ABDOMEN
J - LEFT ANTERIOR THIGH
L - LEFT BUTTOCKS
M - RIGHT BUTTOCKS

DATE GIVEN	TIME	INT.	ONE - TIME MEDICATION - DOSAGE	RT.

SIGNATURE OF NURSE ADMINISTERING MEDICATIONS	DATE	DATE	DATE	DATE
23-07	MK M. King, RN			
07-15	MS M. Smith, RN			
15-23				

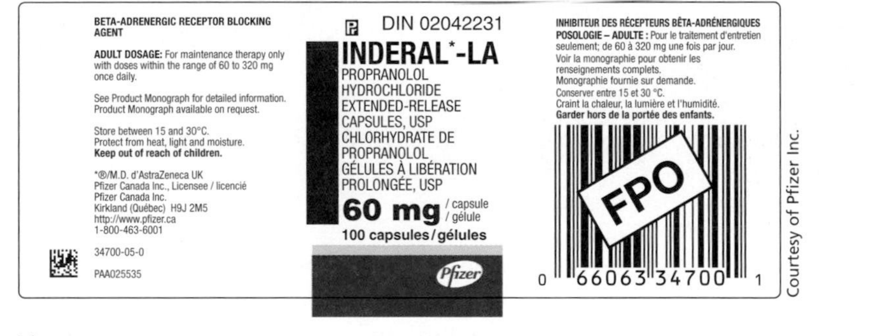

BETA-ADRENERGIC RECEPTOR BLOCKING AGENT
ADULT DOSAGE: For maintenance therapy only with doses within the range of 60 to 320 mg once daily.
See Product Monograph for detailed information. Product Monograph available on request.
Store between 15 and 30°C. Protect from heat, light and moisture. Keep out of reach of children.
*®/M.D. d'AstraZeneca UK
Pfizer Canada Inc., Licensee / licencié
Pfizer Canada Inc.
Kirkland (Québec) H9J 2M5
http://www.pfizer.ca
1-800-463-6001
34700-05-0
PAA025535
DIN 02042231
INDERAL*-LA
PROPRANOLOL HYDROCHLORIDE EXTENDED-RELEASE CAPSULES, USP
CHLORHYDRATE DE PROPRANOLOL GÉLULES À LIBÉRATION PROLONGÉE, USP
60 mg / capsule / gélule
100 capsules / gélules
Pfizer
INHIBITEUR DES RÉCEPTEURS BÊTA-ADRÉNERGIQUES
POSOLOGIE – ADULTE : Pour le traitement d'entretien seulement; de 60 à 320 mg une fois par jour.
Voir la monographie pour obtenir les renseignements complets.
Monographie fournie sur demande.
Conserver entre 15 et 30 °C.
Craint la chaleur, la lumière et l'humidité.
Garder hors de la portée des enfants.
FPO
0 66063 34700 1

N

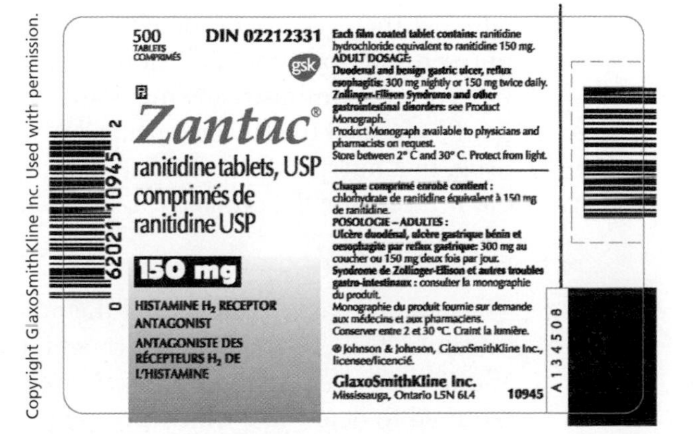

500 TABLETS COMPRIMÉS
DIN 02212331
gsk
Zantac®
ranitidine tablets, USP
comprimés de ranitidine USP
150 mg
HISTAMINE H2 RECEPTOR ANTAGONIST
ANTAGONISTE DES RÉCEPTEURS H2 DE L'HISTAMINE
Each film coated tablet contains: ranitidine hydrochloride equivalent to ranitidine 150 mg.
ADULT DOSAGE:
Duodenal and benign gastric ulcer, reflux esophagitis: 300 mg nightly or 150 mg twice daily.
Zollinger-Ellison Syndrome and other gastrointestinal disorders: see Product Monograph.
Product Monograph available to physicians and pharmacists on request.
Store between 2° C and 30° C. Protect from light.
Chaque comprimé enrobé contient : chlorhydrate de ranitidine équivalent à 150 mg de ranitidine.
POSOLOGIE – ADULTES :
Ulcère duodénal, ulcère gastrique bénin et oesophagite par reflux gastrique: 300 mg au coucher ou 150 mg deux fois par jour.
Syndrome de Zollinger-Ellison et autres troubles gastro-intestinaux : consulter la monographie du produit.
Monographie du produit fournie sur demande aux médecins et aux pharmaciens.
Conserver entre 2 et 30 °C. Craint la lumière.
® Johnson & Johnson, GlaxoSmithKline Inc., licensee/licencié.
GlaxoSmithKline Inc.
Mississauga, Ontario L5N 6L4
10945
0 62021 10945 2
A134508

O

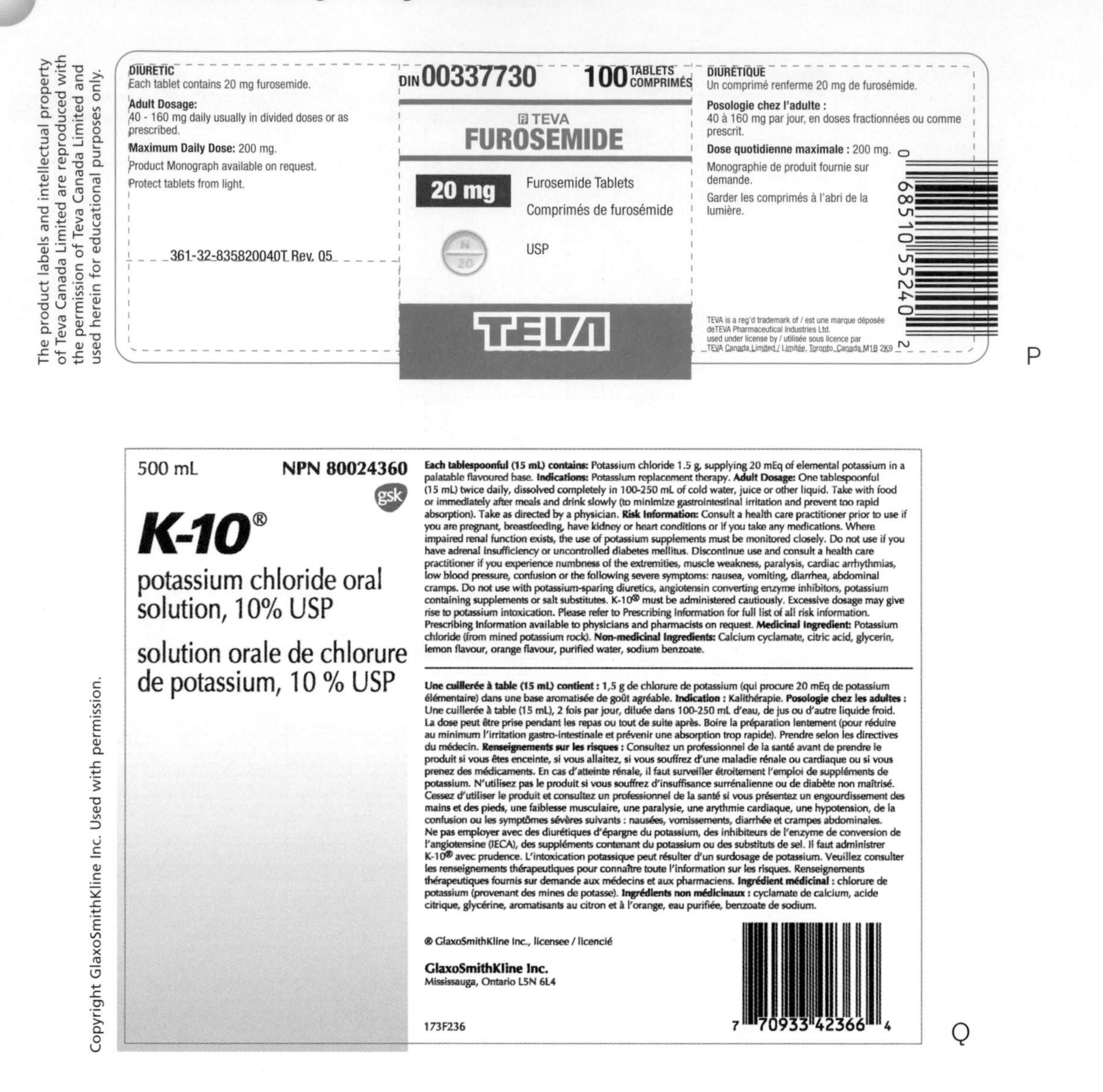

Check your work! Answers to all problems are provided at the end of the book, in the Answers section. Worked solutions for some Practice Problems are also provided there.

APPLICATION OF CLINICAL REASONING

8-1. Describe the strategy to prevent this patient safety incident.

Possible Scenario

Suppose the prescriber ordered *penicillin V potassium 5 mL (250 mg) PO QID* for a patient with an upper respiratory tract infection. The pharmacy supplied penicillin V potassium 125 mg per 5 mL. In a rush to administer the medication on time, the nurse read the order as "penicillin V potassium 5 mL," checked the label for penicillin V potassium, poured that amount, and administered the drug. In a hurry, the nurse failed to recognize that 5 mL of the supply dosage of 125 mg per 5 mL did not provide the ordered dosage of 250 mg and underdosed the patient.

Potential Outcome

The patient received one-half of the ordered dosage of antibiotic needed to treat the respiratory infection. If this error were not caught, the patient's infection would not be halted, which would add to the patient's illness time and might lead to a more severe infection. Additional tests might be required to determine why the patient was not responding to the medication.

Prevention

____

____

Check your work! Answers to all Application of Clinical Reasoning problems are provided at the end of the book, in the Answers section.

ANSWERS TO REVIEW SETS

Review Set 8-1

1) 1 **2)** 1 **3)** $1\frac{1}{2}$ **4)** $\frac{1}{2}$ **5)** $\frac{1}{2}$ **6)** 2 **7)** 2 **8)** 2 **9)** 3 **10)** 2 **11)** 1 **12)** $\frac{1}{2}$ **13)** 2 **14)** 2 **15)** 5 **16)** 2 **17)** 2.5, 3 **18)** 10 and 5; 1 of each (or 3 of 5 mg or $1\frac{1}{2}$ of 10 mg); 4 **19)** 30, 1.5 **20)** 60, 1 **21)** B, 1 tablet **22)** A, 1 tablet **23)** F, 1 tablet **24)** G, 2 tablets **25)** C, 1 tablet **26)** E, 2 capsules **27)** D, 2 tablets **28)** H, 1 tablet **29)** I, 3 tablets 60 mg, the order is for diltiazem 180 mg not for controlled delivery; therefore, 3 tablets of 60 mg should be administered, not 1 controlled-delivery 180-mg capsule **30)** K, 2 tablets

Review Set 8-2

1) 4 **2)** Give one 0.5 mg and one 1 mg (or 3 of the 0.5 mg) **3)** 16.7 **4)** 4 **5)** 5 **6)** 1 **7)** 1.25 **8)** 7.5 **9)** 3 **10)** 2.5 **11)** 18.75 mL or 18.8 mL **12)** 15 **13)** 11.25 mL or 11.3 mL **14)** 4 **15)** 5 **16)** 3 **17)** 7.5 **18)** 30 **19)** 15 **20)** 10 **21)** 2 **22)** B; 2.5 mL **23)** C; 2 mL **24)** A; 5 mL **25)** 4 mL **26)** 7 mL **27)** 10; 45 **28)** 3 mL **29)** 9 mL **30)** 15 mL

SELECTED SOLUTIONS TO REVIEW SETS

Review Set 8-1

1) Order: 0.1 g = 0.1 × 1000 = 100 mg

Supply: 100 mg/tab

$$\frac{D}{H} \times Q = \frac{\overset{1}{\cancel{100\text{ mg}}}}{\underset{1}{\cancel{100\text{ mg}}}} \times 1\text{ tab} = 1\text{ tab}$$

5) Order: 0.125 mg

Supply: 0.25 mg/tab = 0.250 mg/tab

$$\frac{D}{H} \times Q = \frac{\overset{1}{\cancel{0.125\text{ mg}}}}{\underset{2}{\cancel{0.250\text{ mg}}}} \times 1\text{ tab} = \frac{1}{2}\text{ tab}$$

10) Order: 5 mg = 5.0 mg

Supply: 2.5 mg/tab

$$\frac{D}{H} \times Q = \frac{\overset{2}{\cancel{5.0\text{ mg}}}}{\underset{1}{\cancel{2.5\text{ mg}}}} \times 1\text{ tab} = 2\text{ tabs}$$

14) Order: 0.1 mg = 0.1 × 1000 = 100 mcg

Supply: 50 mcg/tab

$$\frac{D}{H} \times Q = \frac{\overset{2}{\cancel{100\text{ mg}}}}{\underset{1}{\cancel{50\text{ mg}}}} \times 1\text{ tab} = 2\text{ tabs}$$

Review Set 8-2

4) Order: 100 mg

Supply: $\frac{125\text{ mg}}{5\text{ mL}}$

$$\frac{D}{H} \times Q = \frac{\overset{4}{\cancel{100\text{ mg}}}}{\underset{5}{\cancel{125\text{ mg}}}} \times \text{mL} = \frac{\overset{4}{\cancel{20}}}{\underset{1}{\cancel{5}}}\text{ mL} = 4\text{ mL}$$

6) Order: 25 mg

Supply: $\frac{125\text{ mg}}{5\text{ mL}}$

$$\frac{D}{H} \times Q = \frac{25\cancel{\text{ mg}}}{125\cancel{\text{ mg}}} \times 5\text{ mL} = 1\text{ mL}$$

7) Order: 4 mg

Supply: $\frac{3.2\text{ mg}}{\text{mL}}$

$$\frac{D}{H} \times Q = \frac{\overset{1}{\cancel{4\text{ mg}}}}{\underset{0.8}{\cancel{3.2\text{ mg}}}} \times 1\text{ mL} = 1.25\text{ mL}$$

11) Order: 0.1 g = 100 mg

Supply: $\frac{80\text{ mg}}{15\text{ mL}}$

$$\frac{D}{H} \times Q = \frac{\overset{20}{\cancel{100\text{ mg}}}}{\underset{16}{\cancel{80\text{ mg}}}} \times 15\text{ mL} = \frac{300}{16} = 18.75\text{ mL}$$

15) Order: 0.25 mg = 0.25 × 1000 = 250 mcg

Supply: $\frac{50\text{ mcg}}{1\text{ mL}}$

$$\frac{D}{H} \times Q = \frac{\overset{5}{\cancel{250\text{ mcg}}}}{\underset{1}{\cancel{50\text{ mcg}}}} \times 1\text{ mL} = 5\text{ mL}$$

17) Order: 375 mg

Supply: $\frac{250\text{ mg}}{5\text{ mL}}$

$$\frac{D}{H} \times Q = \frac{375\ \cancel{\text{mg}}}{\underset{50}{\cancel{250\text{ mg}}}} \times \overset{1}{\cancel{5}}\text{ mL} = \frac{375}{50}\text{ mL} = 7.5\text{ mL}$$

19) Order: 1.2 g = 1.2 × 1000 = 1200 mg

Supply: $\frac{400\text{ mg}}{5\text{ mL}}$

$$\frac{D}{H} \times Q = \frac{\overset{3}{\cancel{1200\text{ mg}}}}{\underset{1}{\cancel{400\text{ mg}}}} \times 5\text{ mL} = 15\text{ mL}$$

20) Order: 0.25 g = 250 mg

Supply: $\frac{125\text{ mg}}{5\text{ mL}}$

Supply: $\frac{\overset{2}{\cancel{125\text{ mg}}}}{\underset{1}{\cancel{125\text{ mg}}}} \times 5\text{ mL} = 10\text{ mL}$

$$\frac{\cancel{250\text{ mg}}}{\cancel{125\text{ mg}}} \times 5\text{ mL} = 10\text{ mL}$$

21) Order: 100 mg

Supply: $\frac{250\text{ mg}}{5\text{ mL}}$

$$\frac{D}{H} \times Q = \frac{100\ \cancel{\text{mg}}}{\underset{50}{\cancel{250\text{ mg}}}} \times \overset{1}{\cancel{5}}\text{ mL} = \frac{\overset{2}{\cancel{100}}}{\underset{1}{\cancel{50}}}\text{ mL} = 2\text{ mL}$$

CHAPTER 9

Parenteral Dosages of Drugs

OBJECTIVES

1. Apply the Three-Step Approach for parenteral dosage calculations: convert, think, and calculate using $\frac{D}{H} \times Q = X$.
2. Identify high-alert medications.
3. Calculate and assess safe hourly heparin sodium dosage.
4. Measure insulin in the appropriate insulin syringe.

The term *parenteral* is used to designate routes of administration such as the injection routes of intramuscular (IM), subcutaneous, intradermal (ID), and intravenous (IV). In this chapter, IM, subcutaneous, and IV injections will be emphasized. Intravenous flow-rate calculations are discussed in Chapters 12 through 14.

An *intramuscular* injection is given into a muscle, for example, meperidine hydrochloride given IM for pain. *Subcutaneous* refers to an injection given into the subcutaneous tissue, such as an insulin injection for the management of diabetes. *Intravenous* refers to an injection given directly into a vein, either by direct injection (IV push) or an injection diluted in a larger volume of IV fluid and administered as part of an IV infusion. When a patient has an IV site or IV infusing, the IV injection route is preferred over the IM route when administering parenteral drugs. *Intradermal* means an injection given under the skin, such as an allergy test or tuberculin skin test.

INJECTABLE SOLUTIONS

Most parenteral medications are supplied in liquid or solution form, and packaged in dosage vials, ampules, or prefilled syringes (Figure 9-1). Injectable drugs are measured in syringes.

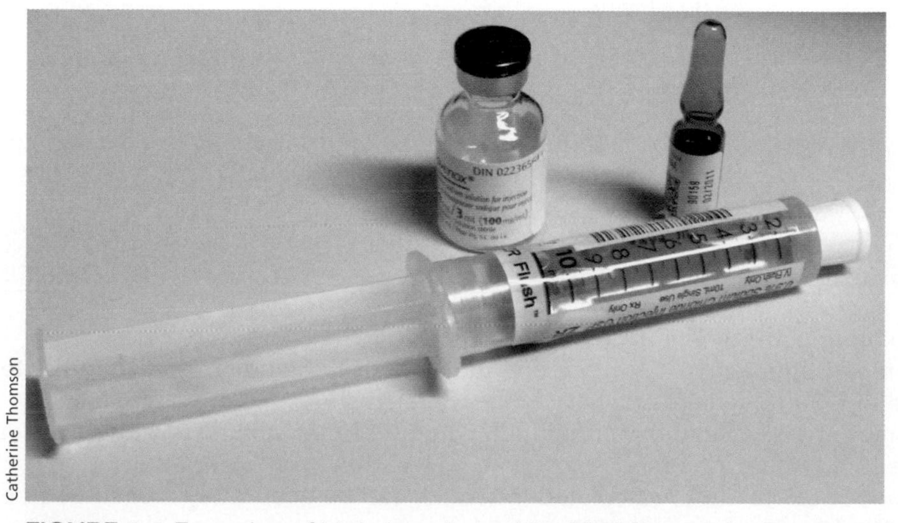

Catherine Thomson

FIGURE 9-1 Examples of Vial, Ampule, and Prefilled Syringe for Parenteral Medications

An IM injection is the choice when two things are required: a reasonably rapid systemic uptake of the drug (usually within 15 to 20 minutes) and a relatively prolonged action. There are various recommendations in the literature regarding the maximum volume that can be administered in one injection site. However, in general, the amount of solution that can be given depends on the amount of the muscle (i.e., the ventrogluteal site is free of nerves and blood vessels and can usually accommodate a larger volume) and subcutaneous mass, and ranges from 1 mL to 5 mL for adults. Smaller volumes are acceptable in children (see the Rules box).

RULES

The maximum dose volumes to be administered in an IM injection site are as follows:

1. **An average adult weighing 75 kg receives a maximum dose volume of 5 mL (with lower maximums proposed for adult patients with less-developed or small muscle mass). The maximum for the deltoid is 1 mL.**
2. **Children ages 6 through 12 years receive a maximum dose volume of 2 mL.**
3. **Children between birth and 6 years receive a maximum dose volume of 1 mL.**

Note: These are recommended ages and doses. Always check the institution policy prior to administering any injection.

Drugs administered intravenously may be injected directly into the infusion port located on the side of the IV tubing. For safety, other drugs may need to be diluted further so that all the concentrated solution enters the vein. The nurse is responsible for ensuring that the medication is infused at the recommended rate. Some medications are given rapidly (as quickly as 1 minute), others as a slow push over a few minutes, while others are injected into a small piggyback bag to infuse over a slower rate. In this chapter, the first skill of calculating and measuring the ordered dose will be covered. In later chapters, additional skills for diluting and managing the flow rate of IV medications and solutions will be covered.

To solve parenteral dosage problems, apply the same Three-Step Approach used for the calculation of oral doses.

REMEMBER

Step 1	**Convert**	All units of measurement to the same units.
Step 2	**Think**	Estimate the logical dosage.
Step 3	**Calculate**	$\frac{\text{D (desired)}}{\text{H (have)}} \times \text{Q (quantity)} = \text{X (amount)}$

Use the following recommendations to help decide the appropriate size of syringe to administer parenteral dosages.

RULES

When calculating parenteral dosages,

1. **For an amount greater than 1 mL, round the amount to be administered to the tenths. Measure in a 3-mL syringe.**
2. **For an amount less than 0.5 mL, round the amount to be administered to the hundredths. Measure in a 1-mL syringe.**
3. **An amount of 0.5 to 1 mL, calculated in tenths, can be accurately measured in either a 1-mL or 3-mL syringe.**

The administration of IM and IV injections requires the important skill of calculating and measuring the ordered dosage. Now examine some examples of appropriate syringe selections for the dosages to be measured, and review how to read the calibrations. Chapter 5, *Equipment Used in Dosage Measurement,* covers how to measure medication in a syringe. However, to review: the top black ring should align with the desired calibration, not the raised midsection and not the bottom ring. Look carefully at the illustrations given below.

Example 1:

Measure 0.33 mL in a 1-mL syringe. The exact amount is measured with this syringe. No rounding is necessary.

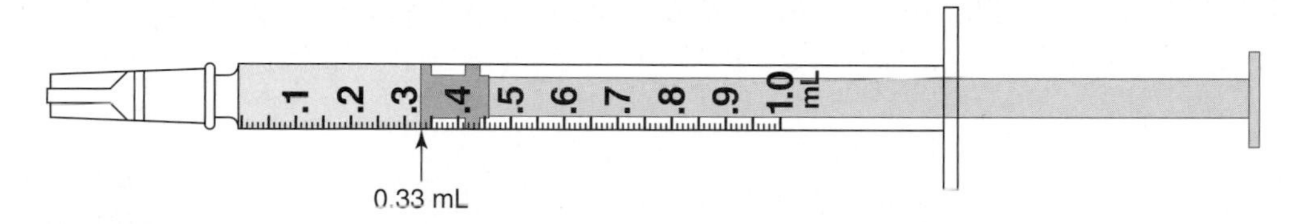

Example 2:

Round 1.33 mL to 1.3 mL, and measure in a 3-mL syringe. The syringe is calibrated in tenths, so rounding is necessary to measure the desired amount.

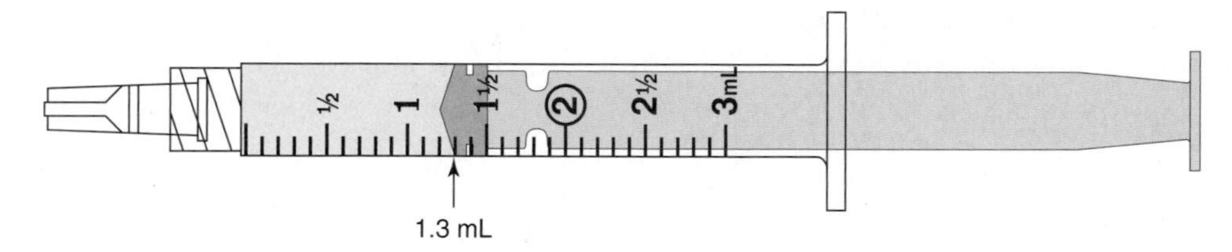

Example 3:

Measure 0.6 mL in either a 1-mL or 3-mL syringe. (Notice that the amount is measured in tenths and is greater than 0.5 mL, so the 3-mL syringe is preferable.)

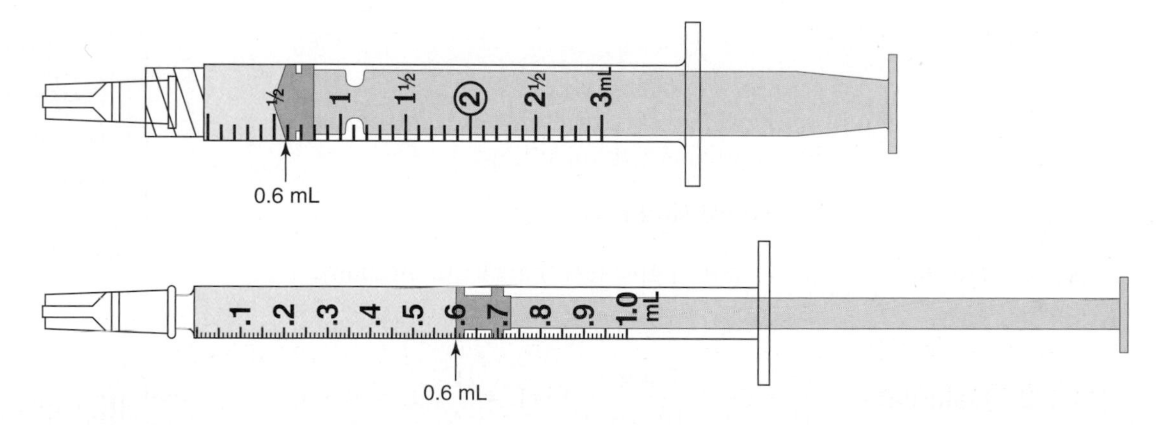

Example 4:

Measure 0.65 mL in a 1-mL syringe. (Notice that the amount is measured in hundredths and is less than 1 mL.) The volume would need to be rounded if a 3-mL syringe is used. However, the 1-mL syringe would provide a more accurate dose.

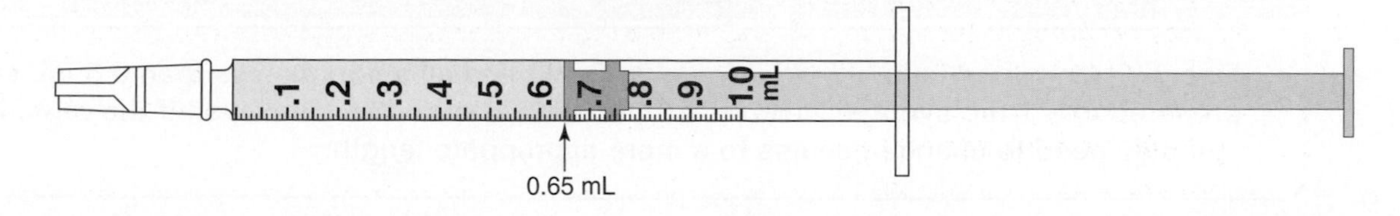

An amber colour has been added to selected syringe drawings throughout the text *to simulate a specific amount of medication*, as specified in the example or problem. Because the colour used may not correspond to the actual colour of the medications named, **it must not be used as a reference for identifying medications.**

Examine some examples of parenteral dosage calculations applying the Three-Step Approach to dosage calculation.

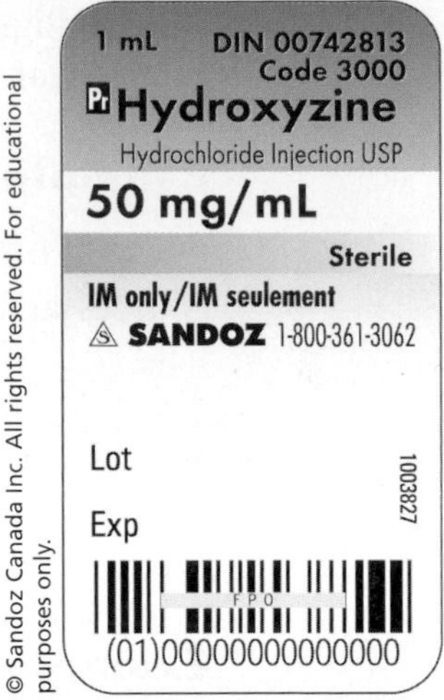

Example 1:

The patient care order is for *hydroxyzine hydrochloride 100 mg IM stat.* Available is hydroxyzine hydrochloride for injection 50 mg/mL in a 1-mL vial. How many millilitres should be administered to the patient?

Step 1 Convert No conversion is necessary.

Step 2 Think You want to give more than 1 mL. In fact, you want to give twice as much because 100 mg is twice as much as 50 mg.

Step 3 Calculate $\frac{D}{H} \times Q = \frac{\overset{2}{\cancel{100\text{ mg}}}}{\underset{1}{\cancel{50\text{ mg}}}} \times 1\text{ mL} = 2\text{ mL}$; to be given intramuscularly immediately

Select a *3-mL syringe and measure 2 mL* of hydroxyzine hydrochloride 50 mg/mL. Look carefully at the illustration to clearly identify the part of the black rubber stopper that measures the exact dosage.

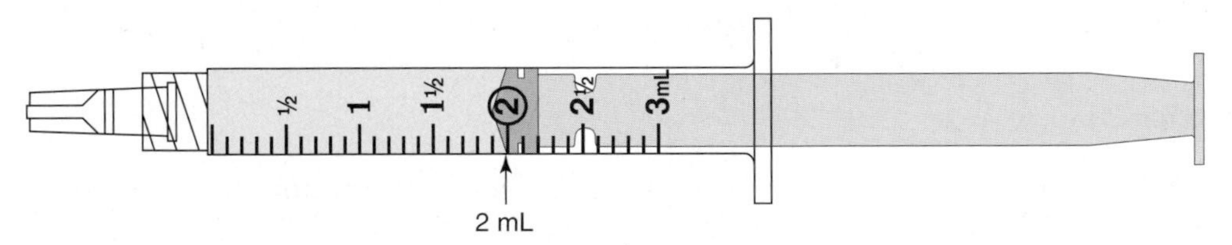

Example 2:

The patient care order is for *nalbuphine hydrochloride 5 mg subcutaneously q3h prn for pain.* The 1-mL unit dose vial is labelled nalbuphine hydrochloride 10 mg per mL injection.

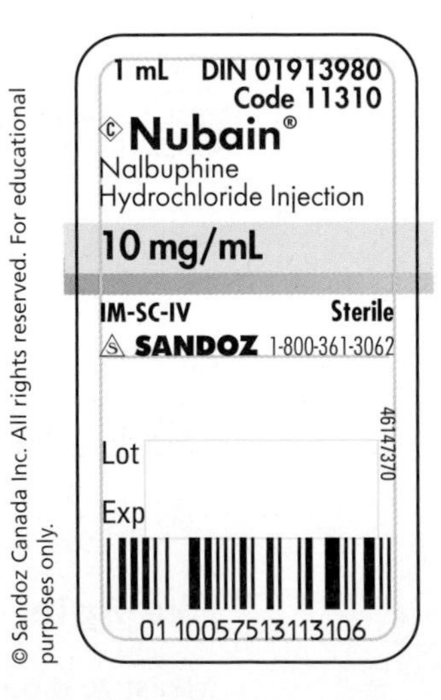

Step 1 Convert No conversion necessary.

Step 2 Think You want to give less than 1 mL. Actually, you want to give $\frac{1}{2}$ or 0.5 of a mL.

Step 3 Calculate $\frac{D}{H} \times Q = \frac{\overset{1}{\cancel{5\text{ mg}}}}{\underset{2}{\cancel{10\text{ mg}}}} \times 1\text{ mL} = \frac{1}{2}\text{ mL} = 0.5\text{ mL}$;

to be given subcutaneously as needed for pain every 3 hours

KEY POINT

Dosages measured in hundredths (e.g., 0.25 mL) and all amounts less than 0.5 mL should be prepared in a 1-mL syringe, which is calibrated in hundredths. However, if the route is IM, you may need to change needles to a more appropriate length.

Select a *1-mL syringe and measure 0.5 mL* of nalbuphine hydrochloride 10 mg/mL. Look carefully at the illustration to clearly identify the part of the black rubber stopper that measures the exact dosage.

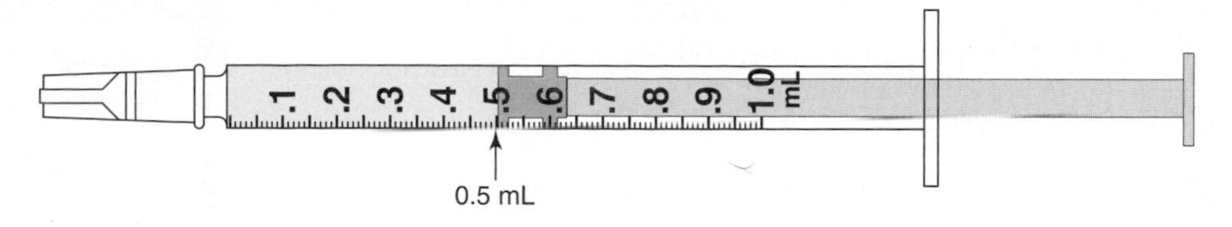

Example 3:

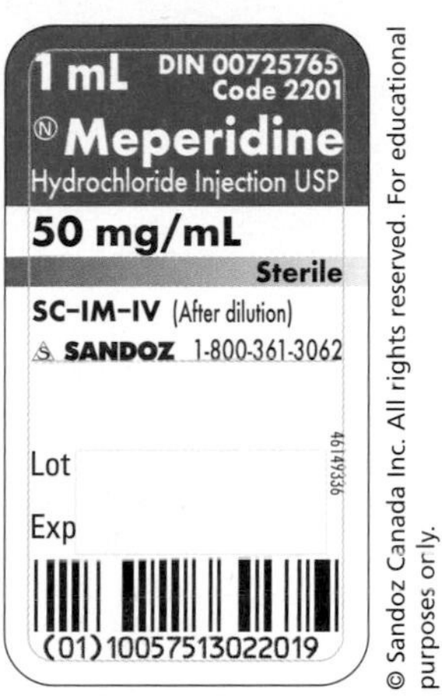

Order: *meperidine hydrochloride 40 mg IM q4h prn for pain*

Supply: meperidine hydrochloride injection 50 mg/mL

Step 1 Convert No conversion is necessary.

Step 2 Think You want to give less than 1 mL but more than 0.5 mL.

Step 3 Calculate $\frac{D}{H} \times Q = \frac{\overset{4}{\cancel{40}}\ \cancel{mg}}{\underset{5}{\cancel{50}}\ \cancel{mg}} \times 1\text{ mL} = \frac{4}{5}\text{ mL} = 0.8\text{ mL}$; to be given intramuscularly every 4 hours as needed for pain

Select *a 1-mL or a 3-mL syringe,* and draw up all of the contents of the 1-mL vial. Then *discard 0.2 mL to administer 0.8 mL* of meperidine hydrochloride 75 mg/mL. Meperidine hydrochloride is a controlled substance. Therefore, you must discard the 0.2 mL in the presence of another nurse; the 0.2 mL cannot be left in the single-dose vial.

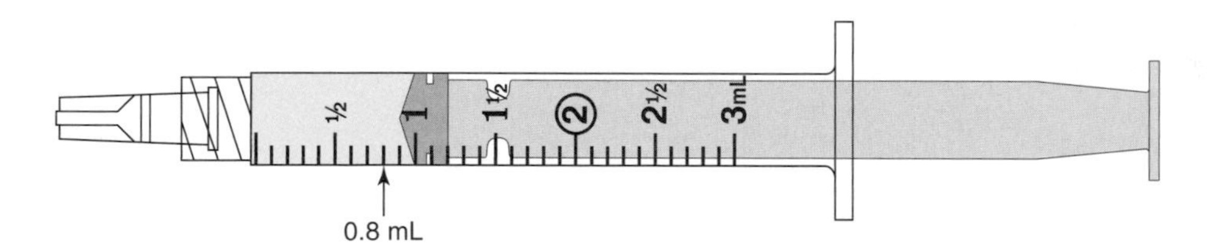

Example 4:

5 mL DIN: 00579718
Heparin LEO*
Heparin Sodium Injection B.P.
Héparine sodique injectable B.P.
L E O
10,000 i.u./mL
*Regd User
LEO Pharma Inc.,
Thornhill, Ontario
I.V./S.C.
006176-05
LEO
LOT:
EXP:

Order: *heparin sodium 8000 units subcutaneously BID*

Supply: a vial of heparin sodium injection 10 000 units/mL

Step 1 Convert No conversion is necessary.

Step 2 Think You want to give less than 1 mL but more than 0.5 mL.

Step 3 Calculate $\frac{D}{H} \times Q = \frac{8\,\cancel{000}\ \cancel{unit}}{10\,\cancel{000}\ \cancel{unit}} \times 1\text{ mL} = \frac{8}{10}\text{ mL} = 0.8\text{ mL}$; given subcutaneously twice daily

Select a *1-mL or a 3-mL syringe and measure 0.8 mL* of heparin sodium 10 000 units/mL. Heparin sodium is a potent anticoagulant drug. It is safest to measure it in a 1-mL syringe.

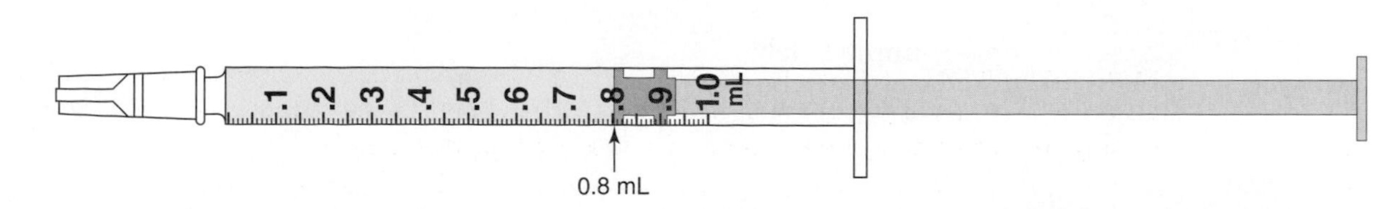

Example 5:

Order: *clindamycin phosphate 150 mg IM q12h*

Supply: clindamycin phosphate injection 300 mg/2 mL

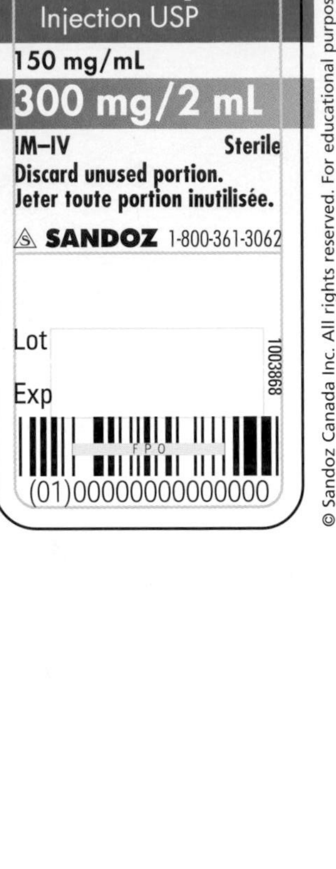

Step 1 Convert No conversion is necessary.

Step 2 Think You want to give less than 2 mL. Actually, you want to give 150 mg, which is $\frac{1}{2}$ of 300 mg and $\frac{1}{2}$ of 2 mL, or 1 mL. Calculate to double-check your estimate.

Step 3 Calculate $\frac{D}{H} \times Q = \frac{\overset{1}{\cancel{150}\ \cancel{mg}}}{\underset{2}{\cancel{300}\ \cancel{mg}}} \times 2\ mL = \frac{2}{2}\ mL = 1\ mL$; given intramuscularly every 12 hours

Select a *3-mL syringe and measure 1 mL* of clindamycin injection 300 mg/2 mL.

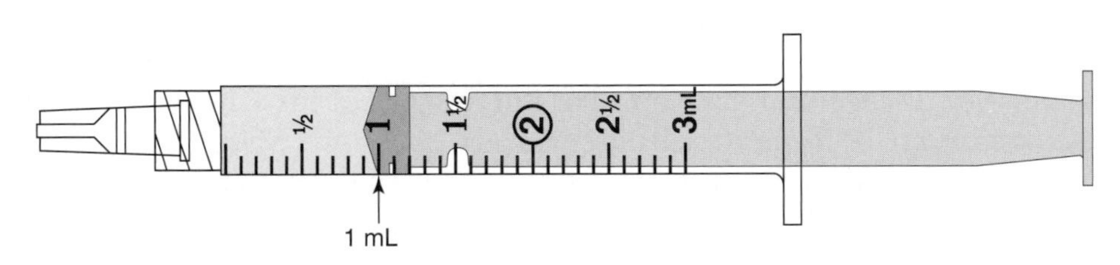

Example 6:

Order: *glycopyrrolate 150 mcg IM stat*

Supply: glycopyrrolate 0.4 mg/2 mL

Step 1 Convert Order: *glycopyrrolate 150 mcg*

Equivalent: 1 mg = 1000 mcg

Supply: glycopyrrolate 0.4 mg $= 0.4\ \cancel{mg} \times \frac{1000\ mcg}{1\ \cancel{mg}}$

$= 400$ mcg

Step 2 Think You want to give less than 1 mL but more than 0.5 mL. Be careful with the units and decimals. Do not be fooled into thinking 0.4 mg is less than 150 mcg. After conversion, you can clearly see that 0.2 mg is more than 150 mcg because 0.4 mg = 400 mcg, which is more than 150 mcg.

Step 3 Calculate $\frac{D}{H} \times Q = \frac{\overset{3}{\cancel{150}\ \cancel{mg}}}{\underset{8}{\cancel{400}\ \cancel{mg}}} \times 2\ mL = \frac{6}{8}\ mL = 0.75\ mL$; to be given intramuscularly immediately

Select a *1-mL syringe, and measure 0.75 mL* of glycopyrrolate 0.4 mg/2 mL. You may have to change needles because this is an IM injection, and the needle gauge on a 1-mL syringe is insufficient for an IM injection.

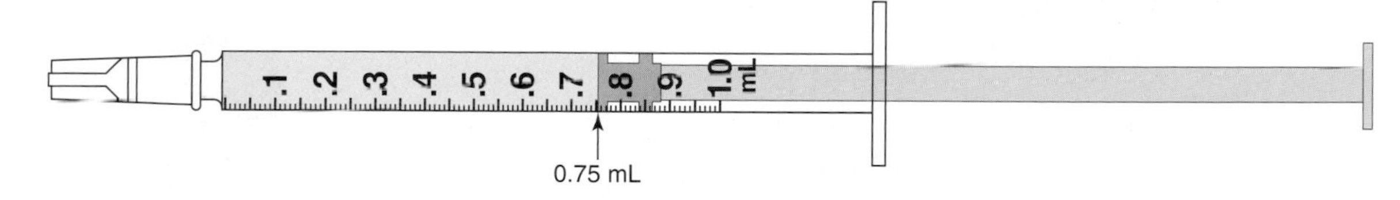

Example 7:

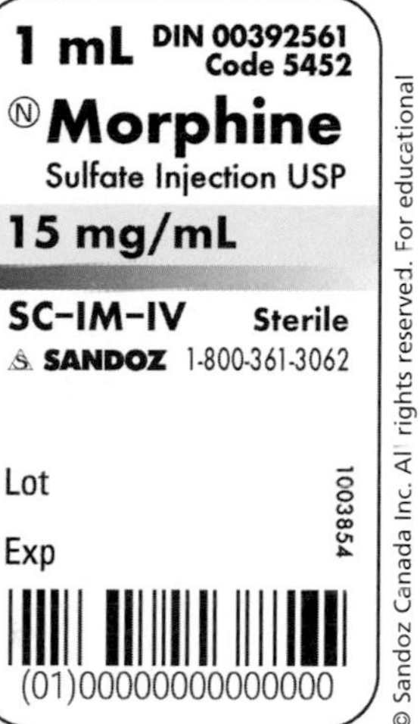

The patient care order is for *morphine sulfate 10 mg IM q4h prn for pain,* and the label on the vial indicates *morphine sulfate 15 mg/mL.*

Step 1 Convert No conversion is necessary.

Supply: morphine sulfate 15 mg/mL

Step 2 Think You want to give less than 1 mL. Actually, you want to give 0.67 mL.

Step 3 Calculate $\frac{D}{H} \times Q = \frac{\overset{2}{\cancel{10}\ \cancel{\text{mg}}}}{\underset{3}{\cancel{15}\ \cancel{\text{mg}}}} \times 1\text{ mL} = 0.666 = 0.67\text{ mL};$

given intramuscularly every 4 hours as needed for pain

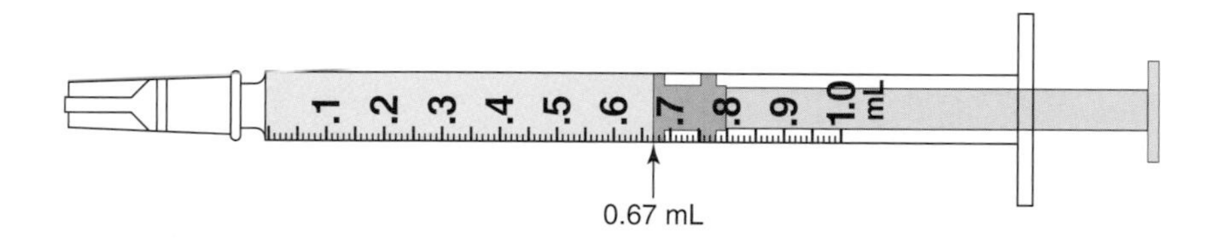

QUICK REVIEW

- To solve parenteral dosage problems, apply the Three-Step Approach to dosage calculations:
  Step 1 **Convert**
  Step 2 **Think**
  Step 3 **Calculate** $\frac{\text{D (desired)}}{\text{H (have)}} \times \text{Q (quantity)} = \text{X (amount)}$
- Prepare a maximum of 5 mL per IM injection site for an average-size adult, 2 mL per site for children age 6 through 12, and 1 mL for children between birth and 6 years.
- Calculate dose volumes and prepare injectable fractional doses in a syringe using these guidelines:
  - Standard doses more than 1 mL: Round to *tenths* and measure in a 3-mL syringe. The 3-mL syringe is calibrated in 0.1-mL increments. Example: 1.53 mL is rounded to 1.5 mL and drawn up in a 3-mL syringe.
  - Small (less than 0.5 mL) doses: Round to *hundredths* and measure in a 1-mL syringe. Critical care and children's doses less than 1 mL calculated in hundredths should also be measured in a 1-mL syringe. The 1-mL syringe is calibrated in 0.01-mL increments. Example: 0.257 mL is rounded to 0.26 mL and drawn up in a 1-mL syringe.
  - Amounts of 0.5 mL to 1 mL, calculated in tenths, can be accurately measured in either a 1-mL or a 3-mL syringe.

REVIEW SET 9-1

Calculate the amount you will prepare for each dose. The labels provided represent the drugs available. Draw an arrow to the syringe calibration that corresponds to the amount you will administer. Indicate doses that have to be divided.

1. Order: *medroxyprogesterone acetate 100 mg IM every 2 weeks*

   Give: ________ mL

DIN 00585092 1 mL
DEPO-PROVERA™
MEDROXYPROGESTERONE ACETATE
INJECTABLE SUSPENSION USP
150 mg/mL medroxyprogesterone acetate
Sterile Aqueous Suspension
Pfizer Canada Inc. Kirkland, Quebec H9J 2M5

Courtesy of Pfizer Canada Inc.

.1 .2 .3 .4 .5 .6 .7 .8 .9 1.0 mL

2. Order: *oxytocin 10 units IM after delivery of placenta*

   Give: ________ mL

1 mL Sterile DIN 00497398
Oxytocin Inj. USP
10 USP Units/mL
I.M., I.V.
K184105Q Hospira
(L) Exp.:

Courtesy of Pfizer Inc.

½ 1 1½ 2 2½ 3mL

3. Order: *haloperidol 2 mg IV stat*

   Give: ________ mL

1 mL DIN 00808652
Code 2900
Haloperidol
Injection USP
5 mg/mL
Sterile
IM only–Not for IV use.
SANDOZ 1-800-361-3062
Lot
Exp
(01)100575131029001

.1 .2 .3 .4 .5 .6 .7 .8 .9 1.0 mL

4. Order: *dexamethasone sodium phosphate 1.5 mg IM q12h*

   Give: ________ mL

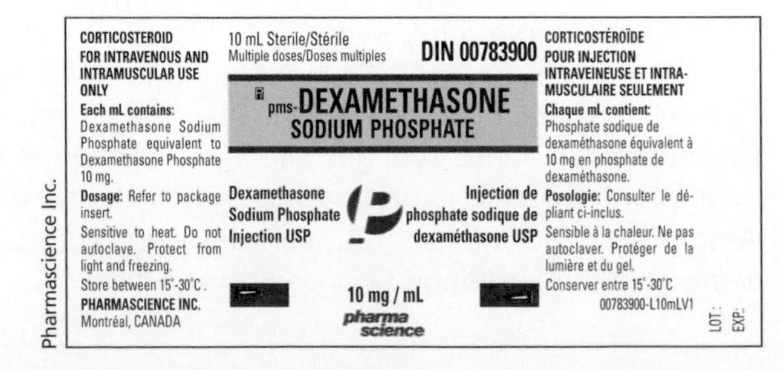

CORTICOSTEROID
FOR INTRAVENOUS AND INTRAMUSCULAR USE ONLY
Each mL contains:
Dexamethasone Sodium Phosphate equivalent to Dexamethasone Phosphate 10 mg.
Dosage: Refer to package insert.
Sensitive to heat. Do not autoclave. Protect from light and freezing.
Store between 15°-30°C.
PHARMASCIENCE INC.
Montréal, CANADA
10 mL Sterile/Stérile
Multiple doses/Doses multiples
DIN 00783900
pms-DEXAMETHASONE
SODIUM PHOSPHATE
Dexamethasone Sodium Phosphate Injection USP
Injection de phosphate sodique de dexaméthasone USP
10 mg / mL
pharma science
CORTICOSTÉROÏDE
POUR INJECTION INTRAVEINEUSE ET INTRAMUSCULAIRE SEULEMENT
Chaque mL contient:
Phosphate sodique de dexaméthasone équivalent à 10 mg en phosphate de dexaméthasone.
Posologie: Consulter le dépliant ci-inclus.
Sensible à la chaleur. Ne pas autoclaver. Protéger de la lumière et du gel.
Conserver entre 15°-30°C
00783900-L10mLV1
LOT:
EXP:

Pharmascience Inc.

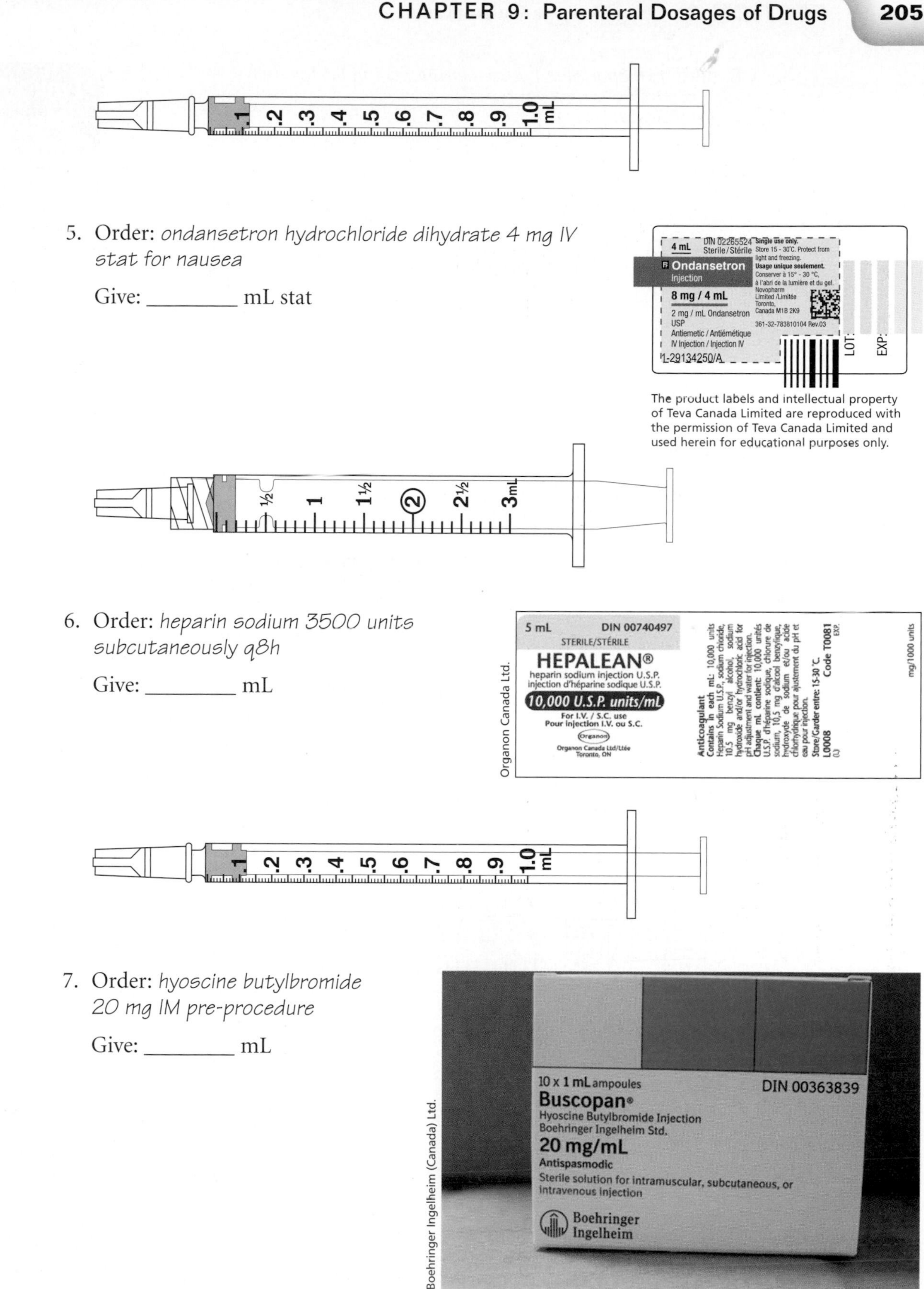

5. Order: *ondansetron hydrochloride dihydrate 4 mg IV stat for nausea*

   Give: ________ mL stat

The product labels and intellectual property of Teva Canada Limited are reproduced with the permission of Teva Canada Limited and used herein for educational purposes only.

6. Order: *heparin sodium 3500 units subcutaneously q8h*

   Give: ________ mL

7. Order: *hyoscine butylbromide 20 mg IM pre-procedure*

   Give: ________ mL

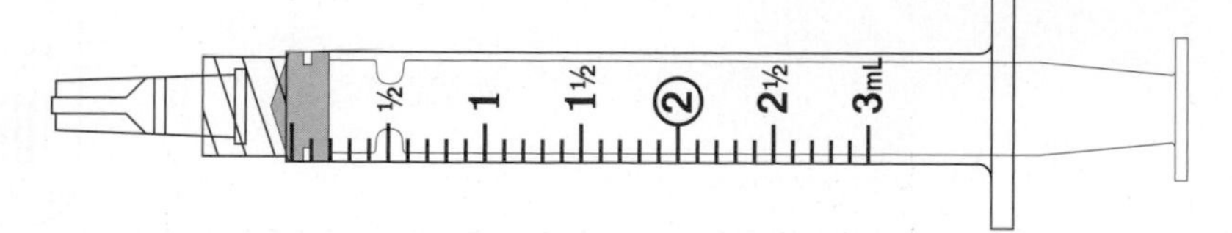

8. Order: *meperidine hydrochloride 35 mg IM for pain*

   Give: ________ mL

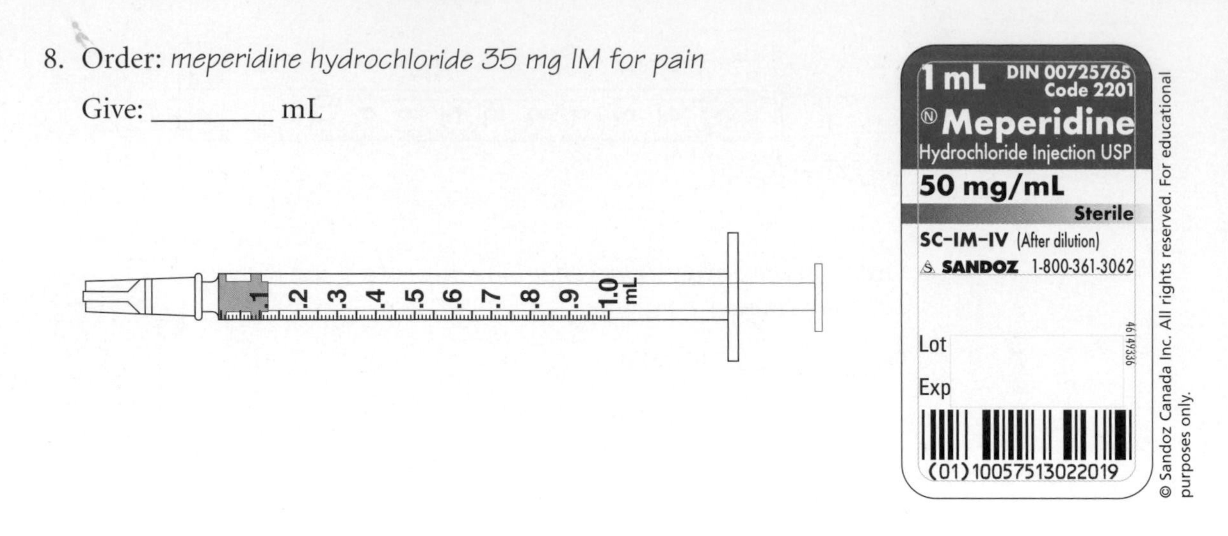

9. Order: *furosemide 40 mg IV bolus stat*

   Give: ________ mL

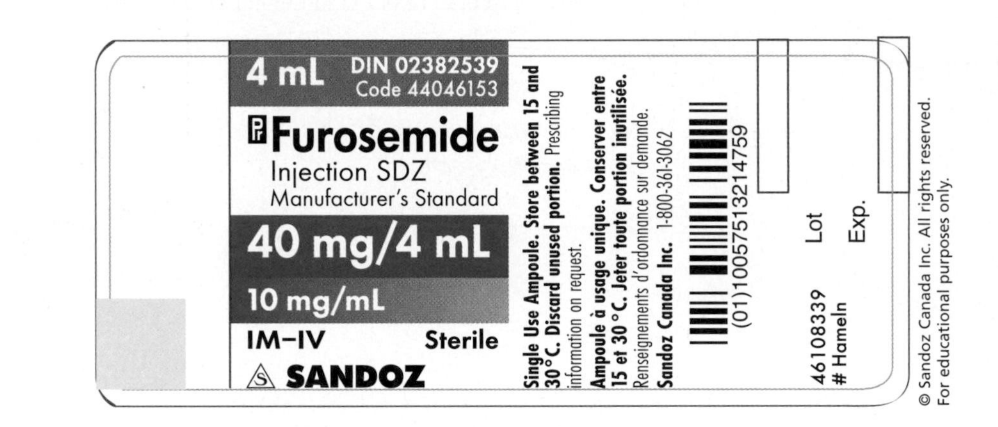

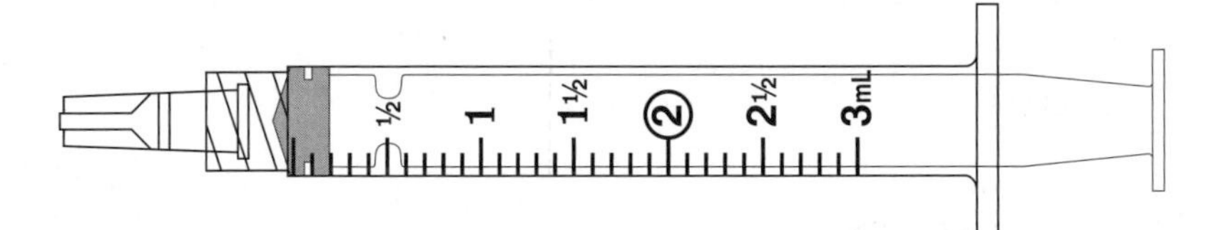

10. Order: *morphine sulfate 15 mg IM q3h prn for pain*

    Give: ________ mL

1 mL DIN 00392561 Code 5452

Morphine

Sulfate Injection USP

15 mg/mL

SC-IM-IV Sterile

SANDOZ 1-800-361-3062

Lot

Exp

(01)00000000000000

11. Order: *hyoscine hydrobromide 15 mg IM daily*

    Give: ________ mL

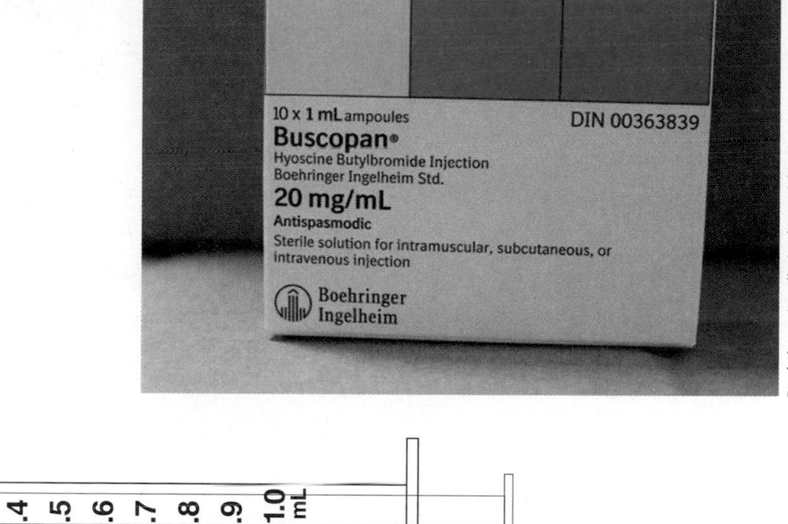

Boehringer Ingelheim (Canada) Ltd.

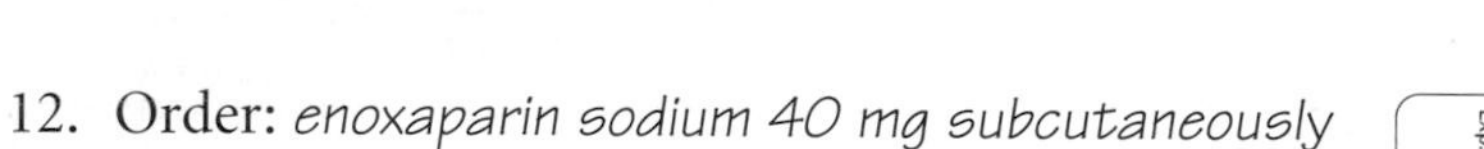

12. Order: *enoxaparin sodium 40 mg subcutaneously daily*

    Give: ________ mL

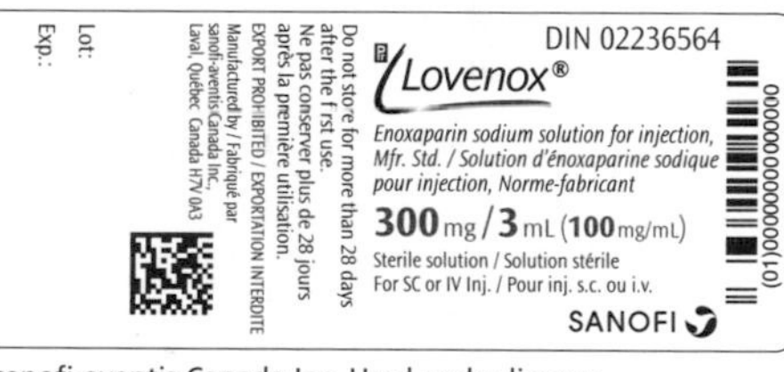

© sanofi-aventis Canada Inc. Used under licence.
For educational purposes only.

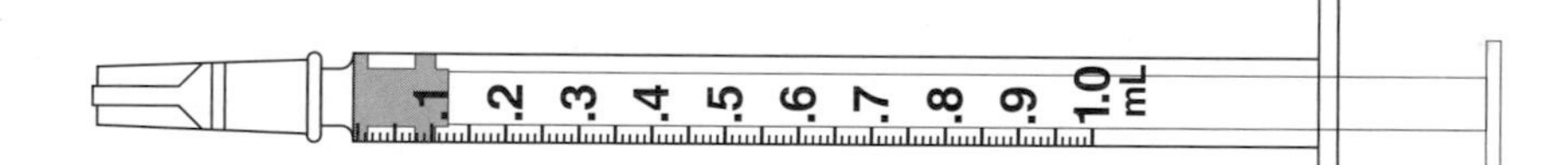

13. Order: *midazolam 2.5 mg IM 30 min preoperatively*

    Give: ________ mL

DIN 02423758
Midazolam Injection
midazolam (as hydrochloride) solution for injection
midazolam (sous forme de chlorhydrate) solution pour injection

5 mg/5 mL
1 mg/mL

For slow IV or IM use / Pour injection i.v. lente ou i.m.
Sterile / Stérile

10 x 5 mL Steriluer™ Single Use Ampoules
10 ampoules Steriluer^MC de 5 mL à usage unique

Pfizer Injectables

Courtesy of Pfizer Inc.

½ 1 1½ 2 2½ 3mL

14. Order: *hydroxyzine hydrochloride 25 mg IM q4h prn for nausea*

    Give: ________ mL

1 mL DIN 00742813
Code 3000
Pr Hydroxyzine
Hydrochloride Injection USP
50 mg/mL
Sterile
IM only/IM seulement
SANDOZ 1-800-361-3062
Lot
Exp
1003827
(01)00000000000000

.1 .2 .3 .4 .5 .6 .7 .8 .9 1.0 mL

15. Order: *tinzaparin sodium 50 units/kg subcut 2 h before hip surgery. Patient weighs 100 kg.*

    Give: ________ mL

LEO
LEO Pharma Inc.,
Thornhill,
L3T 7W8
LEO®
010112-09
2 mL DIN 02167840
Pr innohep®
Sterile Tinzaparin sodium injection
Tinzaparine sodique injectable stérile
20,000 anti-Xa IU/2 mL
(10,000 anti-Xa IU/mL)
Subcutaneous/sous-cutaneé
(01)00623041000237
Imprinting area
LOT:
EXP:

16. Order: *calcitriol 1.5 mcg IV 3 times/week once daily M-W-F*

    Give: ________ mL

½ 1 1½ 2 2½ 3mL

1 mL DIN 02245686
C730101
Pr CALCITRIOL
Injection/Injectable
1 μg/mL
Sterile/Stérile
For IV Use/Pour usage IV
PPC
646692
LOT
EXP

17. Order: *cyanocobalamin 0.5 mg IM once/week*

    Give: ________ mL

10 mL DIN 00521515
Code 9051
Vitamin B_{12}
Cyanocobalamin Injection USP
1 000 mcg/mL
10 000 mcg/10 mL
IM-Deep SC
For therapeutic use only.
IM – SC profonde
Pour usage thérapeutique seulement.
Sterile/Stérile
Fiole Multidose Vial
SANDOZ
Contains benzyl alcohol 1.5%.
Store between 15 and 30°C.
Contient 1,5 % d'alcool benzylique.
Conserver entre 15 et 30 °C.
Sandoz Canada Inc. 1-800-361-3062
46081859
(01)10057513090513
Lot
Exp

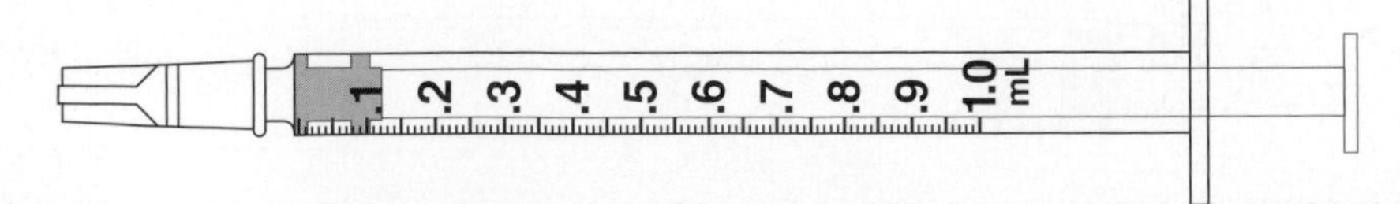

18. Order: *ranitidine hydrochloride 25 mg IV BID*

    Give: ________ mL

2 mL DIN 02256711 Code 7250
Ranitidine
Injection USP
25 mg/mL
50 mg/2 mL
IM–IV Sterile
Single Dose Vial
Fiole unidose
SANDOZ 1-800-361-3062
Lot
Exp

19. Order: *hydromorphone hydrochloride 2 mg IM stat*

    Give: ________ mL

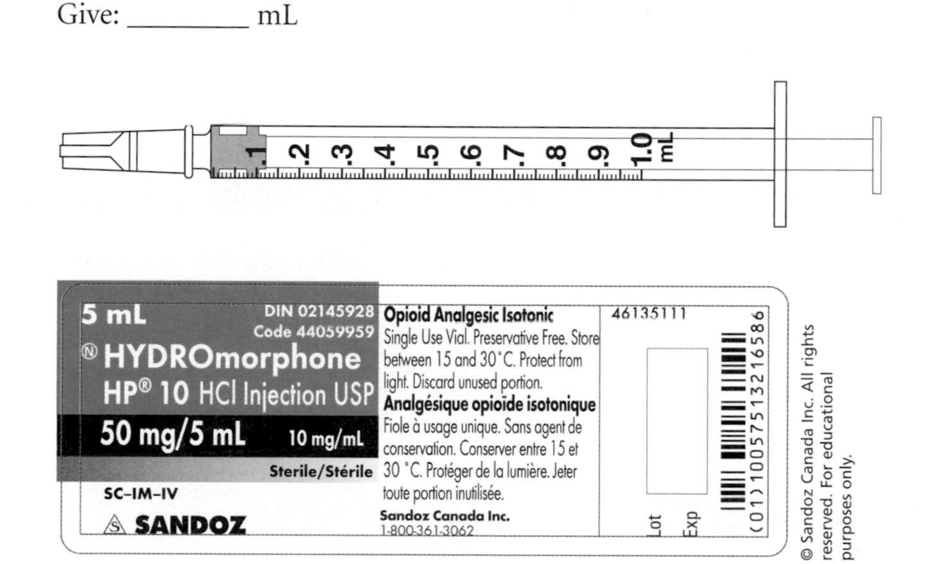

20. Order: *famotidine 20 mg IV q6h IV daily*

    Give: ________ mL

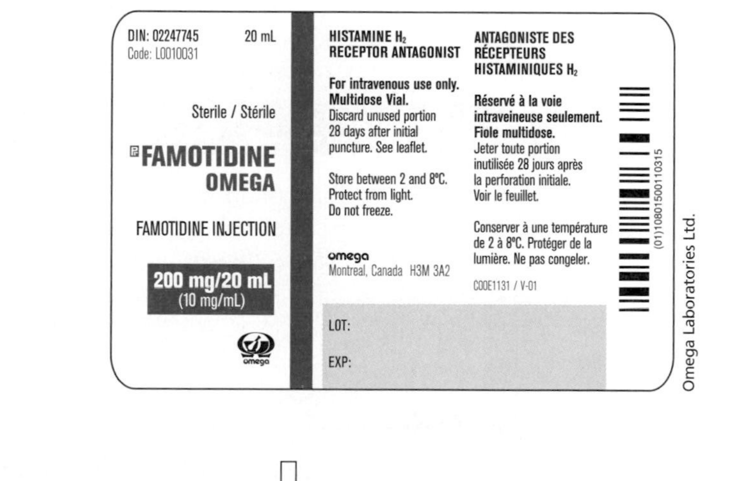

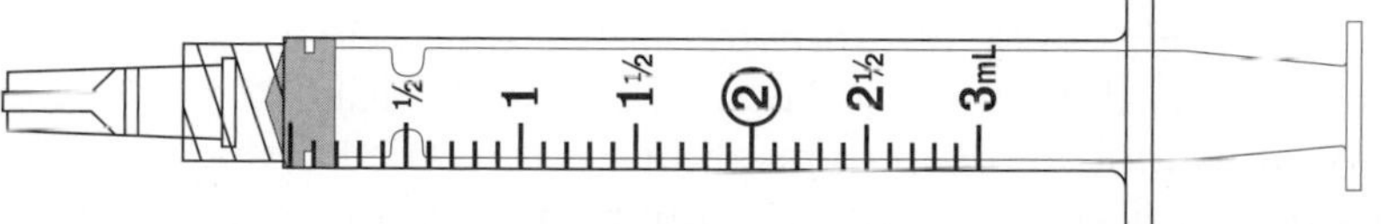

Check your work! Answers to all Review Sets are provided at the end of each chapter. Worked solutions for select Review Sets are also provided there.

HIGH-ALERT PARENTERAL MEDICATIONS

The Institute for Safe Medication Practices Canada (ISMP, 2016) defines high-alert medications as "drugs that bear a heightened risk of causing significant patient harm when they are used in error." The ISMP has published a list of classes/categories of high-alert medications and specific medications that require safeguards to reduce the risk of patient safety incidents leading to devastating consequences. These high-alert or high-risk medications have a narrow margin of safety. High-alert medications usually cause severe patient harm when implicated in a medication incident. Heparin sodium and insulin have been identified as two such medications with the greatest safety risk. In addition to dosage miscalculations, confusing various concentrations of the drug and reading drug labels incorrectly have been associated with fatal dosing errors. Heparin sodium and insulin are both measured in units, administered subcutaneously or intravenously, and supplied in multidose vials that may look similar. Many hospitals require independent double verification before administration of high-alert drugs. When double-checking, the nurse should check the patient care order, the product selected, the calculated dose, and the dose drawn up.

INSULIN

Insulin, a hormone produced by the pancreas, is necessary for the metabolism of glucose, proteins, and fats. Patients who are deficient in insulin are required to take insulin daily by injection. Insulin is a ready-to-use solution that is measured in units. The most common supply dosage is 100 units per mL, which is often seen on the label as U-100. It is important to note that "U" is recognized as an error-prone abbreviation; therefore, it should always be written as "unit."

MATH TIP

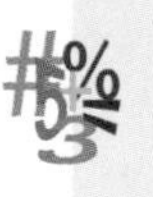

The supply dosage of insulin is **100 units per mL** (which is abbreviated on some labels as **U-100**). Think: U-100 = 100 units per mL.

CAUTION

Accuracy when preparing and administering insulin is critical. Inaccuracy is potentially life-threatening. It is essential for nurses to *understand the information on the insulin label*, to correctly *interpret the insulin order*, and to *select the correct syringe* to measure insulin for administration.

Insulin Labels

The insulin label includes important information. For example, as shown in Figure 9-2, the *trade* and *generic names*, the *supply dosage* or *concentration*, and the *storage* instructions are details commonly found on most parenteral drug labels. These and other typical drug label components are described in Chapter 7. We now look at different insulin types classified by the insulin *action times* and insulin *species*, which are critical identifiers of this important hormone supplement.

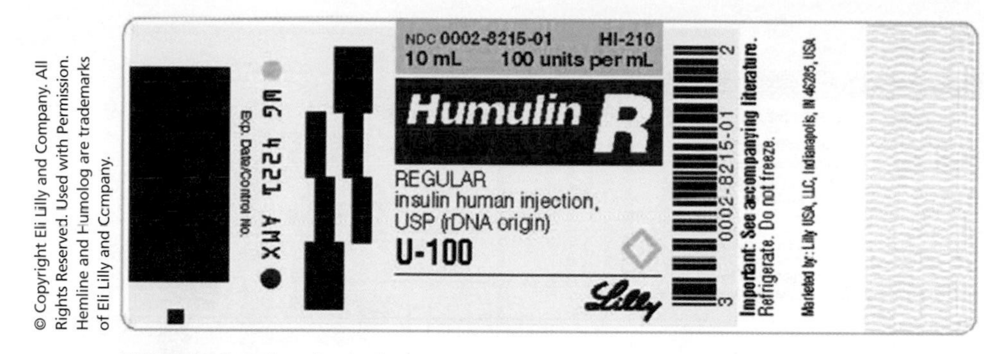

FIGURE 9-2 Insulin Label

Insulin Action Times

Insulins vary in onset, peak, and duration of action. A sampling of insulin labels arranged by the four action times—rapid-acting, short-acting, intermediate-acting, and long-acting—is shown in Figure 9-3, on page 212. In Figure 9-2, notice the upper case, bold letter R for regular insulin, and in Figure 9-3, the upper case bold letter N on the Humulin label for NPH insulin.

A short-acting insulin or a rapid-acting insulin analogue is usually administered at each meal and for continuous subcutaneous insulin infusions. An intermediate-acting insulin or a long-acting insulin analogue is administered once or twice daily to manage normal daily blood glucose fluctuations. Intermediate insulins (e.g., Humulin N and Novolin® ge NPH) are crystalline zinc suspensions of human regular insulin combined with the polypeptide protamine (protein taken from salmon) in a phosphate buffer. They have a milky white or cloudy appearance. The protamine delays the onset of NPH insulin.

An *analogue* is defined as a chemical compound that is structurally similar to another compound, but differs slightly in composition. Insulin analogues are produced by recombinant DNA technology by altering the amino acid sequencing on the A and B chains of the human insulin. Such structural changes can influence the drug's pharmacokinetics (absorption, distribution, metabolism, and excretion). For example, insulin lispro (Humalog), insulin aspart (NovoRapid), and insulin glulisine (Apidra) are rapid-acting insulin analogues that have a faster onset of action and a shorter duration time. Insulin glargine (Lantus) and detemer (Levemir and Toujeo; 100-unit and 300-unit insulins) are long-acting insulin analogues that are released steadily and continuously over 24 hours with no peak of action after once-daily subcutaneous administration. They should be administered at the same time each day. Touleo has a duration of up to 30 hours. They are alternatives to the use of NPH insulin. Long-acting insulins are not mixed with any other insulin. The long-acting insulins are clear and colourless and *should not be confused* with rapid- or short-acting insulins, which are also clear.

CAUTION

Do not confuse trade names for aspart (NovoRapid) and lispro (Humalog) with the trade names for regular insulins (Humulin R and Novolin® ge). Also avoid confusing the trade names for the long-acting insulin detemir (Levemir) with the anticoagulant enoxaparin (Lovenox).

Species of Insulin

Human biosynthetic insulin is the most commonly used insulin. It is also called *recombinant* or *DNA-derived.* It is made from bacteria such as *Escherichia coli* or from yeast cells that have been genetically altered to create human insulin. Pork regular insulin (Hypurin Regular Insulin Pork) and pork isophane insulin (Hypurin NPH Insulin Isophane) are available but are rarely used.

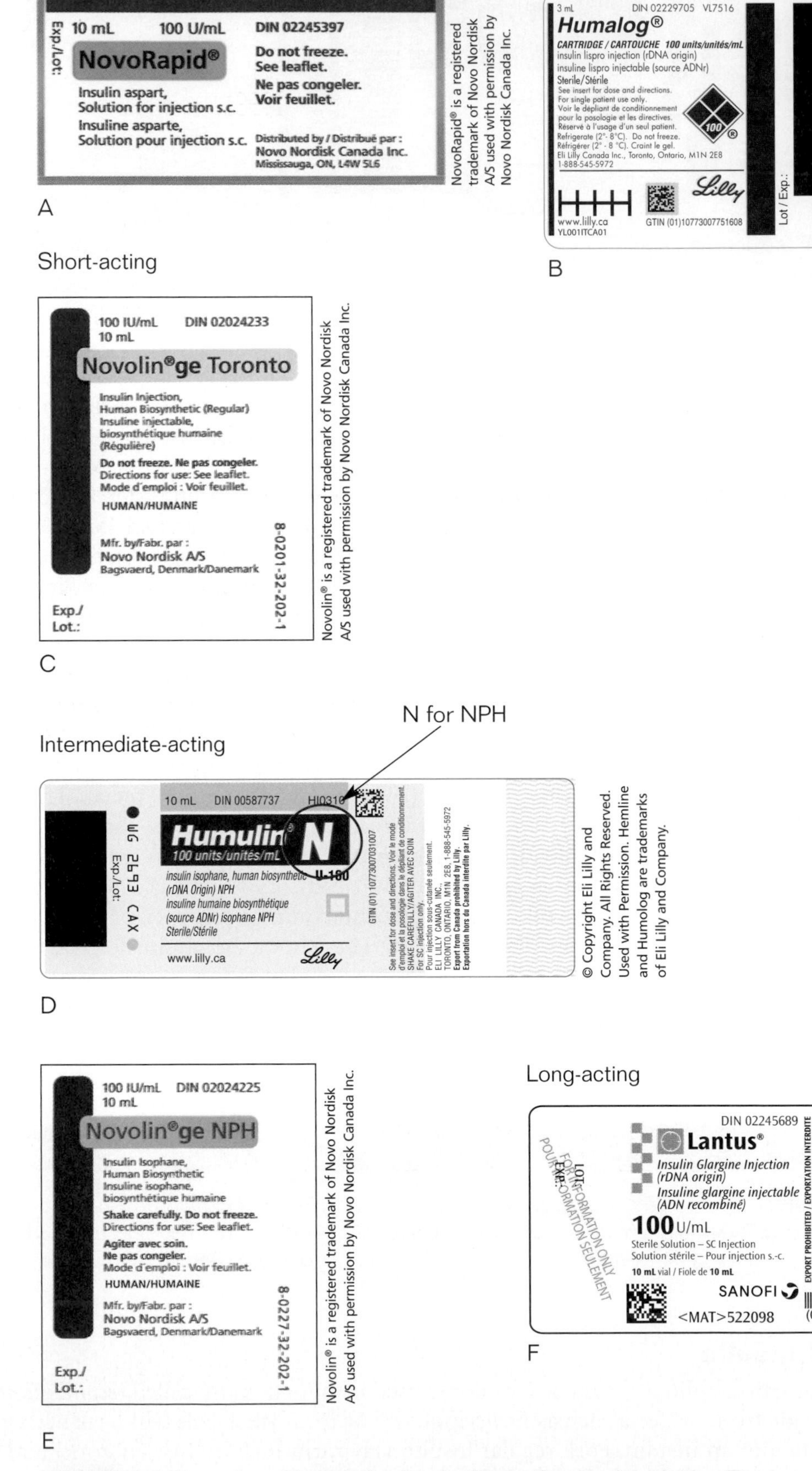

FIGURE 9-3 Examples of Labels for Insulin Types Grouped by Action Times

CAUTION

Avoid a potentially life-threatening patient safety incident. Carefully read the medication label, and compare it to the drug order to ensure that you select the correct action time and species of insulin.

Premixed Combination Insulins

Commercially available premixed insulin combinations contain a combination of a rapid- or short-acting insulin and an intermediate-acting insulin in fixed proportions in an insulin vial or pen (Figure 9-4). These product combinations are convenient for patients who are in a treatment plan that uses a standard ratio of these insulins because the number of injections required is reduced. However, premixed insulin preparations are not suitable for patients with type 1 diabetes who require intensive therapy and frequent adjustments of insulin.

Several different premixed combinations containing 10% to 50% short-acting insulin and 70% to 50% intermediate-acting insulin are available. It is important to carefully read the labels to understand which types of insulin are included in each combination. For example, the 30/70-insulin concentration contains 30% short-acting insulin and 70% intermediate-acting insulin in each unit. Therefore, if the order is 10 units of 30/70 insulin, the patient would receive 3 units of short-acting insulin (30% or 0.3×10 units = 3 units) and 7 units of intermediate-acting insulin (70% or 0.7×10 units = 7 units). If the order is 20 units of 30/70 insulin, the patient would receive 6 units of short-acting insulin ($0.3 \times 20 = 6$) and 14 units ($0.7 \times 20 = 14$) of intermediate-acting insulin.

The 50/50 insulin concentration contains 50% NPH insulin and 50% regular insulin in each unit. Therefore, if the prescriber orders 12 units of 50/50 insulin, the patient would receive 6 units of NPH insulin (50% or 0.5×12 units = 6 units) and 6 units of regular insulin (50% or 0.5×12 units = 6 units).

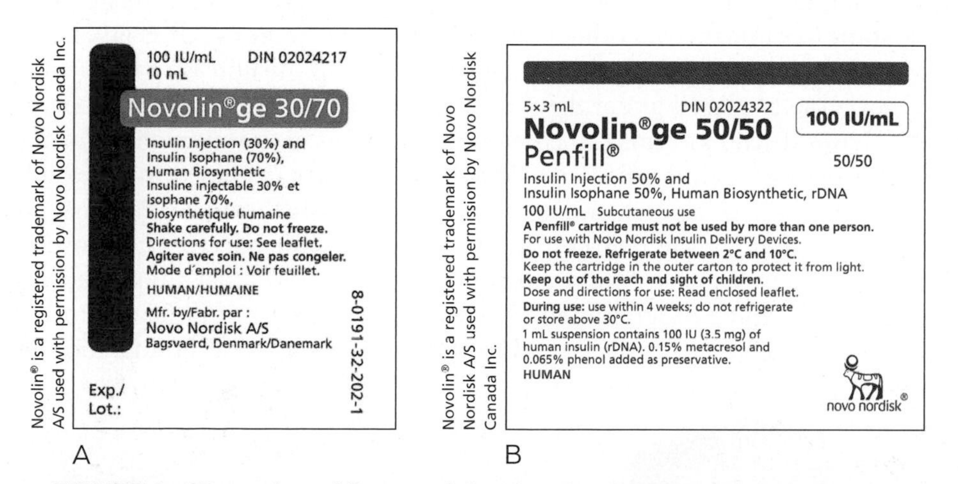

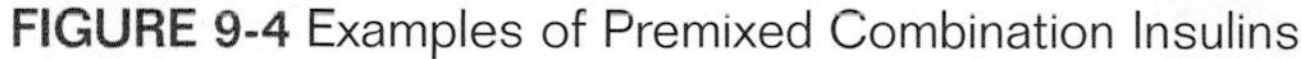

FIGURE 9-4 Examples of Premixed Combination Insulins

CAUTION

Long-acting types of insulin should not be combined or diluted with any other insulin preparations. Combining long-acting insulin with other insulin solutions may interfere with blood glucose control, which can be life-threatening.

Interpreting the Insulin Order

Insulin orders must be written clearly and contain specific information to ensure correct administration and prevent patient safety incidents. An insulin order should contain the following:

1. The *trade* and generic *names, and the action time.* Patients are instructed to stay with the same manufacturer's trade-name insulin. Slight variations between trade names can affect an individual's response. Before administration, verify with the patient both the usual trade name used and the actual insulin supplied. Look for one of the four action times: rapid-acting (e.g., lispro, aspart, and glulisine), short-acting (e.g., Novolin® ge Toronto and Humulin R), intermediate-acting (e.g., Humulin N and Novolin® ge NPH), or long-acting (e.g., insulin glargine and insulin detemir).
2. The *supply dosage (concentration) and the number of units* to be given, for example, 100-unit insulin regular 40 units.
3. The *route of administration and time or frequency.* All insulin may be administered by the subcutaneous route, and regular 100-unit insulin may additionally be administered intravenously (IV).

Examples:

Humulin R insulin regular 14 units subcutaneously stat

Humulin N NPH insulin 24 units subcutaneously 30 min before breakfast

Insulin Delivery Systems

Insulin is administered by syringe, pen, or pump (continuous subcutaneous insulin infusion [CSII]). Insulin regular can also be administered intravenously to manage hyperglycemic episodes. Insulin administration regimens (schedule and frequency) are individualized based on the needs of the patient. Insulin pen devices facilitate management requiring multiple injections of insulin. CSII is considered a safe and effective method to deliver flexible insulin therapy for patients with type 1 diabetes. CSII therapy may provide some advantages over other methods of flexible therapy such as NPH-based regimens. Insulin delivery systems deliver rapid- or short-acting insulins (e.g., insulin aspart or insulin lispro) over 24 hours through a catheter placed under the skin. The pump is usually worn on a belt and resembles a standard pager. Newer deliver systems can combine continuous blood sugar monitoring with insulin pump delivery. The newest device, called an OMNIPOD, delivers insulin through a tubeless insulin reservoir attached to the skin by a patch and is controlled wirelessly through a Personal Diabetes Manager. Pumps can be programmed to deliver a basal rate and/or bolus doses. Basal insulin is delivered continuously over 24 hours to keep blood glucose levels within a target range between meals and overnight. The basal rate can be programmed to deliver different rates at different times of the day or night. Bolus doses can be delivered at mealtimes to provide control for additional food intake.

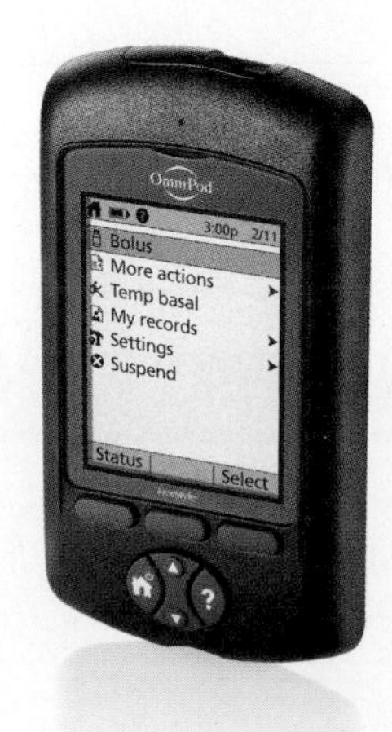

Courtesy Insulet Corporation

Measuring Insulin in an Insulin Syringe

The insulin syringe and measurement of insulin were introduced in Chapter 5. This critical skill warrants attention again. Once you understand how insulin is packaged and how to use the insulin syringe, you will find insulin dosage simple.

RATIONALE FOR PRACTICE

- **Measure insulin in an insulin syringe only. Do not use a 3-mL or 1-mL syringe to measure insulin.**
- **Do not measure other drugs supplied in units in an insulin syringe.**

Measuring insulin with an insulin syringe is simple. The insulin syringe makes it possible to obtain the correct dosage without mathematical calculation. There are three different insulin syringes: the *standard* 100-unit capacity, the *lo-dose* 50-unit capacity, and the *lo-dose* 30-unit capacity.

The Standard Insulin Syringe

The standard insulin syringe in Figure 9-5 is a dual-scale syringe with 100-unit capacity. It is calibrated on one side in *even*-numbered, 2-unit increments (2, 4, 6, . . .) with every 10 units labelled (10, 20, 30, . . .). It is calibrated on the reverse side in *odd*-numbered, 2-unit increments (1, 3, 5, . . .) with every 10 units labelled (5, 15, 25, . . .). It is not necessary to use the dosage calculations formula to measure the volume to prepare insulin. The insulin syringe is specially designed to measure a dose of insulin in units. The important skill is to correctly read the syringe calibrations. The measurement of 73 units of insulin is illustrated in Figure 9-5.

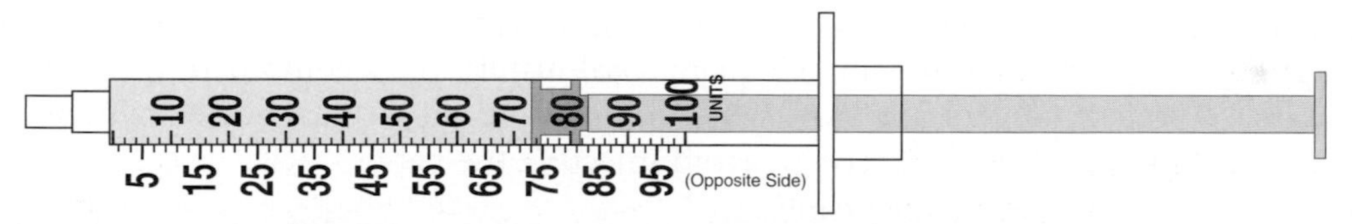

FIGURE 9-5 Standard Insulin Syringe Measuring 73 Units

CAUTION

Look carefully at the increments on the dual scale. The volume from one mark to the next (on either side) is 2 units. You are probably comfortable counting by 2s for even numbers. Pay close attention when counting by 2s with odd numbers.

Lo-Dose Insulin Syringes

The lo-dose insulin syringe in Figure 9-6 is a single-scale syringe with 50-unit capacity. It is calibrated in 1-unit increments with every 5 units (5, 10, 15, . . .) labelled up to 50 units. The enlarged 50-unit calibration of this syringe makes it easy to read and use to measure low dosages of insulin. To measure 32 units, for example, withdraw insulin to the 32-unit mark (Figure 9-6).

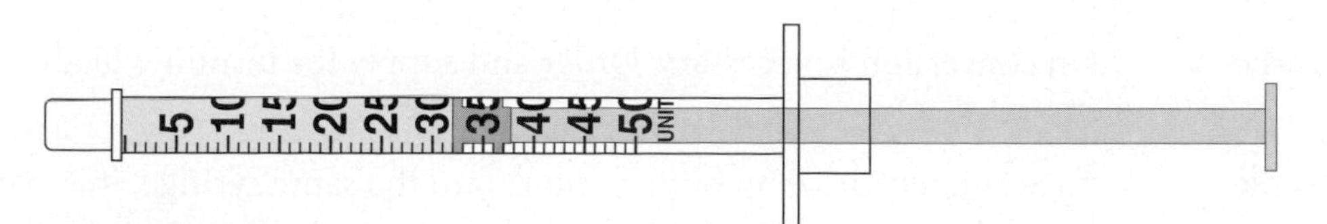

FIGURE 9-6 Fifty-Unit Lo-Dose Insulin Syringe Measuring 32 Units

The lo-dose insulin syringe in Figure 9-7 is a single-scale syringe with 30-unit/0.3 mL capacity. It is calibrated in 1-unit increments with every 5 units (5, 10, 15, . . .) labelled up to 30 units. The enlarged 30-unit calibration accurately measures very small amounts of insulin, such as for children. To measure 12 units, for example, withdraw insulin to the 12-unit mark (Figure 9-7).

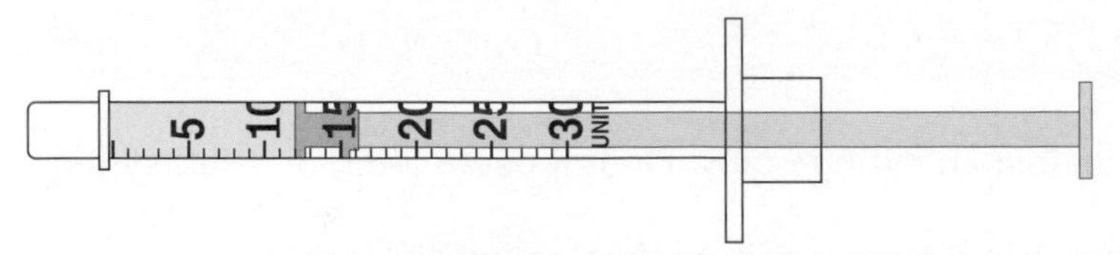

FIGURE 9-7 Thirty-Unit Lo-Dose Insulin Syringe Measuring 12 Units

CAUTION

Always choose the *smallest*-capacity insulin syringe available for accurate insulin measurement. Use standard and lo-dose syringes to measure insulin. Although the lo-dose insulin syringes measure a maximum of only 30 or 50 units, they are still intended for the measurement of 100-unit insulin.

Be cautious when measuring. The lo-dose syringe is calibrated in 1-unit increments; the standard insulin syringe is calibrated in 2-unit increments on the even and odd scales.

Combination Insulin Dosage

The patient may have two types of insulin prescribed to be administered at the same time: a rapid- or short-acting insulin combined with an intermediate-acting insulin. The Canadian Diabetes Association Clinical Practice Guidelines (McGibbon et al., 2013) recommend insulin aspart, insulin glulisine, or insulin lispro in combination with adequate basal insulin. This combination results in improved postprandial glycemic control and A1C while minimizing the occurrence of hypoglycemia (when using insulin lispro or insulin aspart). To avoid injecting the patient twice, it is common practice to draw up both insulins in the same syringe.

RATIONALE FOR PRACTICE

1. **Draw up *rapid- or short-acting insulin first*, then draw up *intermediate-acting insulin*.**
2. **Rapid- and short-acting (regular, lispro, and aspart) insulins are clear. Intermediate-acting (NPH) insulin is cloudy.**
3. **Think: *First* rapid- or *short-acting* insulin, *then intermediate-acting insulin*.**

Example 1:

Order: *Novolin® ge Toronto insulin 12 units with Novolin® ge NPH insulin 40 units subcutaneously before breakfast*

The patient in this scenario requires an injection of both Novolin® ge Toronto, a short-acting insulin, and the intermediate-acting isophane suspension Novolin® ge NPH.

Step 1 Convert No conversion is necessary. Order and supply for insulin will always be in units.

Step 2 Think To accurately draw up both insulins into the same syringe, it is critical to know the total units of both insulins: 12 units + 40 units = 52 units.

Withdraw 12 units of the Novolin® ge Toronto insulin and then withdraw 40 units of the Novolin® ge NPH insulin up to the 52-unit mark (Figure 9-8). In this case, the smallest-capacity syringe that can be used is the standard insulin syringe.

Step 3 Calculate 10 units + 2 units = 12 units. Draw up 12 units. One calibration line equals 2 units. Starting at 10 units, count 1 calibration line toward 12 units on the even-numbered side of the syringe. 50 units + 2 units = 52 units on the even-numbered side. Starting at 50 units, count 1 calibration line toward 52 units on the even-numbered side. The filled syringe in Figure 9-8 shows the measurement. Notice that the NPH insulin is drawn up last and is closest to the needle in the figure. In reality, the drugs mix right away. Give the order, vials, and syringe to another nurse for independent verification after drawing up each insulin.

CAUTION

When withdrawing two insulins into the same syringe,

1. Take care to accurately withdraw both amounts, especially with the second draw; and
2. Inject air into both insulin vials equal to the amount of insulin required to increase pressure in the vials to make it easier to withdraw accurate doses.

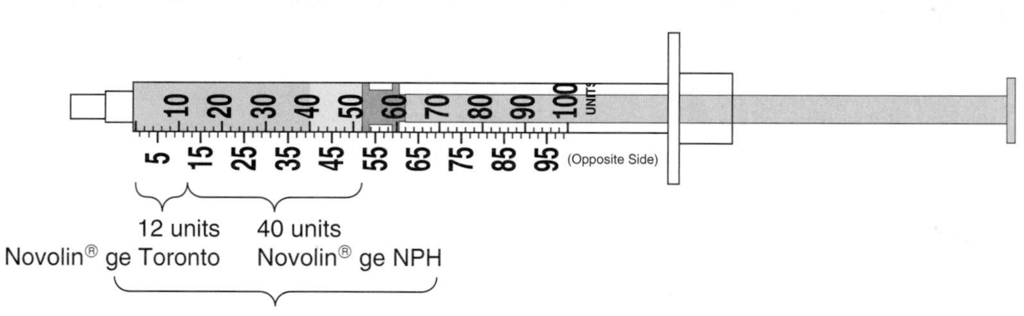

FIGURE 9-8 Combination Insulin Dosage

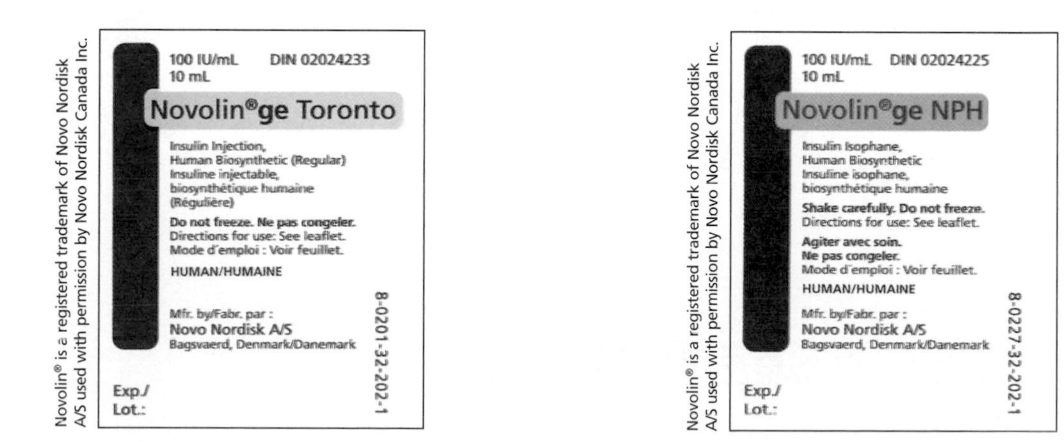

Example 2:

The prescriber orders *Novolin® ge Toronto insulin 10 units with Novolin® ge NPH insulin 30 units subcutaneously 30 min before dinner.*

This example gives step-by-step directions for this procedure. Look closely at Figures 9-9 and 9-10 (on the next page), which illustrate the procedure. Notice that to withdraw Novolin® ge Toronto

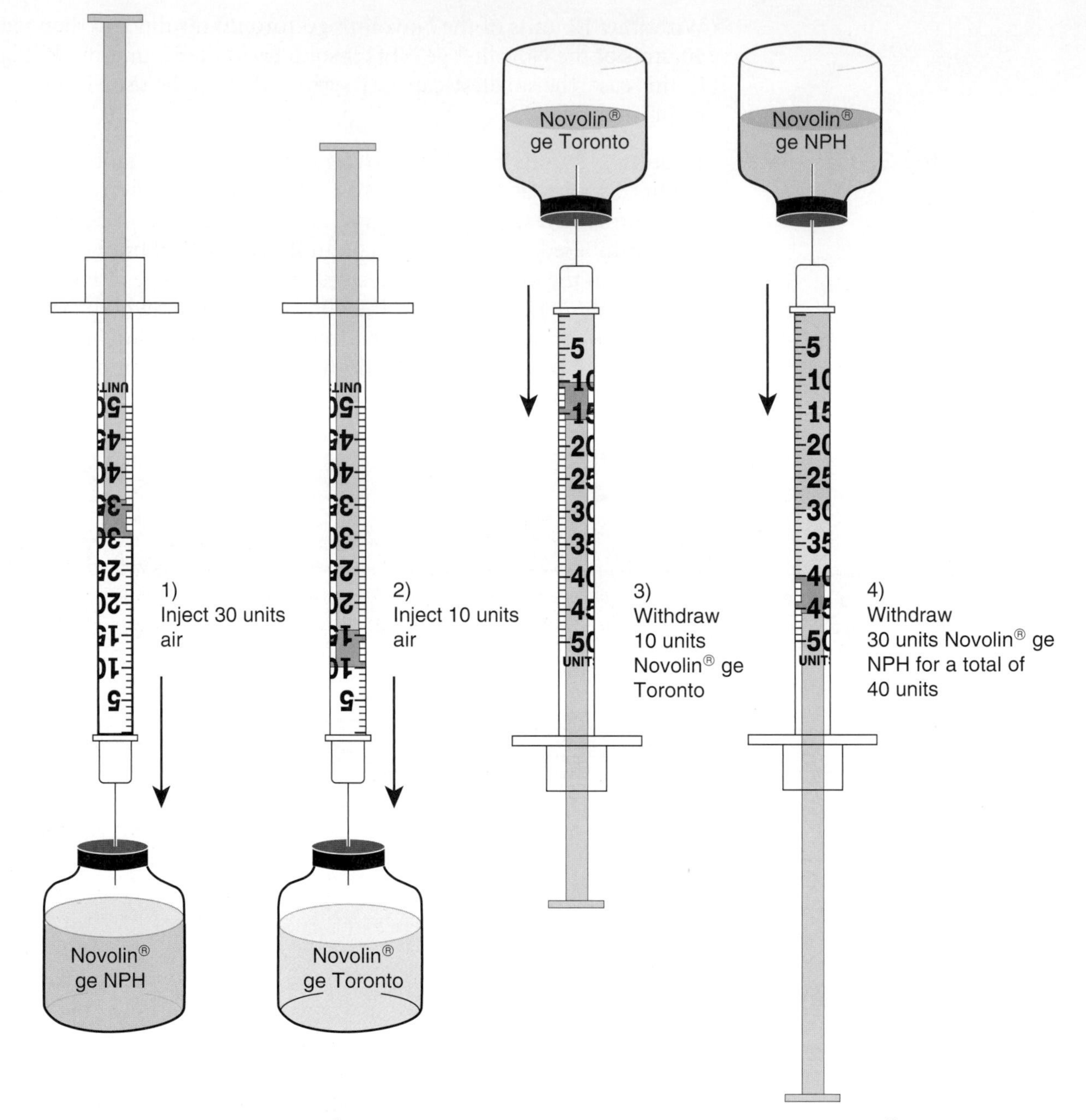

FIGURE 9-9 Procedure for Drawing Up Combination Insulin Dosage: 10 Units Novolin® ge Toronto (short-acting) Insulin with 30 Units Novolin® ge NPH (intermediate-acting) Insulin

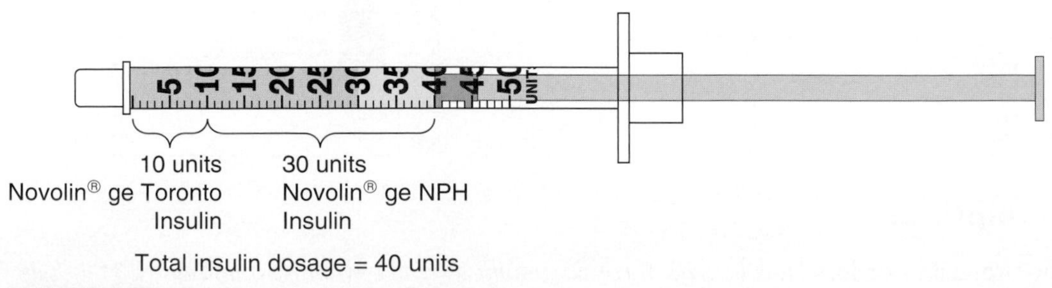

FIGURE 9-10 Combination Insulin Dosage

insulin first and then Novolin® ge NPH insulin, you must inject the dose amount of air into the Novolin® ge NPH insulin *before* you inject the dose amount of air into the regular insulin.

1. Draw back and inject 30 units of air into the Novolin® ge NPH insulin vial. Remove the needle.
2. Roll the vial of the NPH insulin in your hands to mix; do not shake it. Draw back and inject 10 units of air into the Novolin® ge Toronto insulin vial and leave the needle in the vial.
3. Turn the vial of Novolin® ge Toronto insulin upside down, and draw out the insulin to the 10-unit mark on the syringe. Make sure all air bubbles are removed.
4. Insert the needle into the Novolin® ge NPH insulin vial, turn the vial upside down, and slowly draw back to the 40-unit mark, being careful not to exceed the 40-unit calibration. If more NPH insulin is withdrawn, discard and begin again with a new syringe. The cloudy solution contaminates the regular insulin and an accurate amount cannot be determined. Ten units of Novolin® ge Toronto + 30 units of Novolin® ge NPH = 40 units of insulin total (Figure 9-10).

CAUTION

If you withdraw too much of the Novolin® ge NPH, you must discard the entire medication and start over. With a combined insulin medication, another nurse must be present to view steps 1 to 4 of the procedure.

Insulin Coverage—the "Sliding Scale"

Sometimes, hyperglycemia in a hospitalized patient is not yet regulated, and a special insulin order is needed to "cover" the sugar level. Sliding scale is a reactive approach to rising blood glucose levels rather than a proactive approach and allows for hyperglycemia to occur before responding. A sliding scale consists of the administration of a predetermined amount of short-acting insulin in response to hyperglycemia in the hospital setting. Capillary blood glucose is checked 4 times a day for patients on insulin, 30 minutes prior to meals and at bedtime (around 2130 to 2200). For patients who are on nothing by mouth (NPO), blood glucose is checked every 4 hours (0400, 0800, 1200, 1600, 2000, 2400). *Only* regular insulin is used because of its rapid action. The prescriber will specify the amount of insulin in units, which "slide" up or down based on the specific blood glucose level range. Sliding scales are individualized for each patient. The goal is to use as little sliding-scale insulin as possible. A sliding scale is not used during ketoacidosis or if a patient is on IV insulin. Figure 9-11 is an example of a sliding-scale order.

Insulin Dose	Glucose Reading (mmol/L)
No coverage	Glucose less than 8
2 units	10.1–12
4 units	12.1–14
6 units	14.1–16
8 units	16.1–18
10 units	18.1–19.9
Hold insulin; call prescriber stat	20 and above

FIGURE 9-11 Sample Insulin Sliding Scale Order

Example:

Humulin R is a trade name for regular insulin, a short-acting agent with an onset within 30 minutes. For this example, the patient is an adult who had major abdominal surgery and is slowly returning to a regular diet. Yesterday, pharmacy delivered a multidose 10-mL vial of Humulin R (Figure 9-12). Until the patient fully recovers, the blood glucose levels will be monitored before each meal (ac) and at bedtime. The dose of insulin the nurse will administer will be based on a sliding scale (Figure 9-11). The glucose measurement before the evening meal was 15 mmol/L.

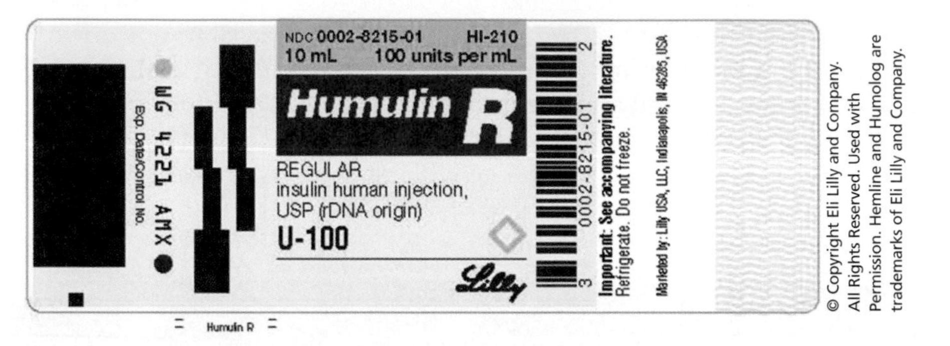

FIGURE 9-12 Humulin R

Order: *Humulin R insulin regular subcutaneously ac and at bedtime per sliding scale*

Apply the Three-Step Approach.

Step 1 Convert No conversion needed. Order and supply for insulin will always be in units.

Step 2 Think There is a glucose range of 14.1 to 16 mmol/L; 15 is greater than 14.1 but less than 16, so the insulin coverage for this range should be used. The amount of coverage, 6 units, is a small amount. The most appropriate choice of syringe to use to draw up 6 units would be a lo-dose syringe. Choose the 30-unit lo-dose syringe if available; otherwise, a 50-unit lo-dose syringe can be used. The 6-unit increment should fall between 5 and 10 units. Note that the lo-dose syringe is calibrated in 1-unit increments; the standard syringe is calibrated in 2-unit increments on the even and odd scales.

Step 3 Calculate No calculation is necessary, but accurate measurement is necessary. It may appear obvious how to fill the syringe to the correct calibration. Remember, though, that this is a high-alert medication and simple insulin measurement errors with potentially fatal consequences are quite common. Avoid distractions, and take your time when measuring insulin and other high-alert medications. Once the insulin has been drawn up into the syringe, give the order, the glucose measurement, vial, and syringe to another nurse for independent validation and documentation.

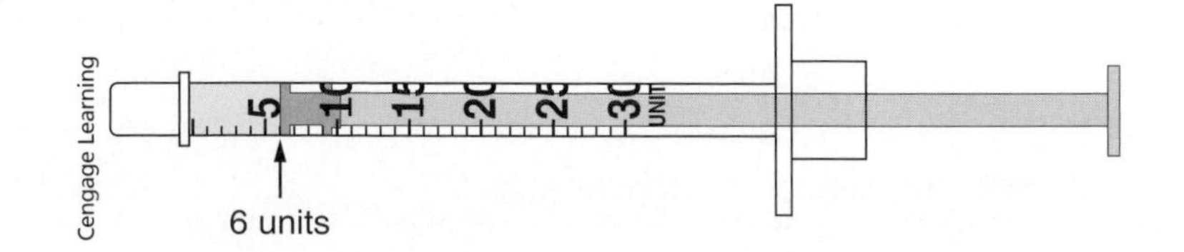

Prefilled 100-Unit Insulin Pen Devices

A variety of insulin pen devices are currently available for patient use (Figures 9-13 and 9-14). Insulin pen devices facilitate the use of multiple injections of insulin. An insulin pen combines an insulin container and a syringe in a single unit, which allows for the precise and convenient delivery of insulin. Although there are many brands and models, insulin pens come in two basic types: (a) disposable prefilled devices and (b) reusable devices that are loaded with new insulin cartridges when the old ones are used up. Each cartridge is filled with 3 mL of a single insulin (e.g., glulisine, Humulin N isophane insulin, or Humulin N insulin regular) or a premixed combination of insulin (e.g., Humalog Mix 25, Humalog Mix 50, Humulin 30/70, or NovoMix 30). Needles come in a variety of sizes and lengths. Newer pen devices have a memory function and other added features.

Pen devices are a safe, convenient, easy, and accurate method for self-administration of insulin. They also improve patient comfort and provide optimal glycemic control. Some newer pens allow for easy correction of doses without wasting insulin. Some also have larger, easy-to-read numbers or click as the dose is dialed or the plunger is depressed. However, only premixed combinations of insulin or a single insulin can be used, as different insulins cannot be mixed in an insulin pen device.

All devices require patient involvement to attach a disposable needle, prime the pen, dial up the dose, and depress a plunger to deliver the dose. It is recommended to leave the needle in the skin for at least 5 seconds to ensure complete delivery of insulin into the subcutaneous depot.

The insulin pen cartridge is marked to estimate the amount used or remaining for additional doses but is not intended to measure individual doses. To administer the correct dose, after adding a new cartridge and before each additional dose, the pen must be primed by releasing 2 units of insulin.

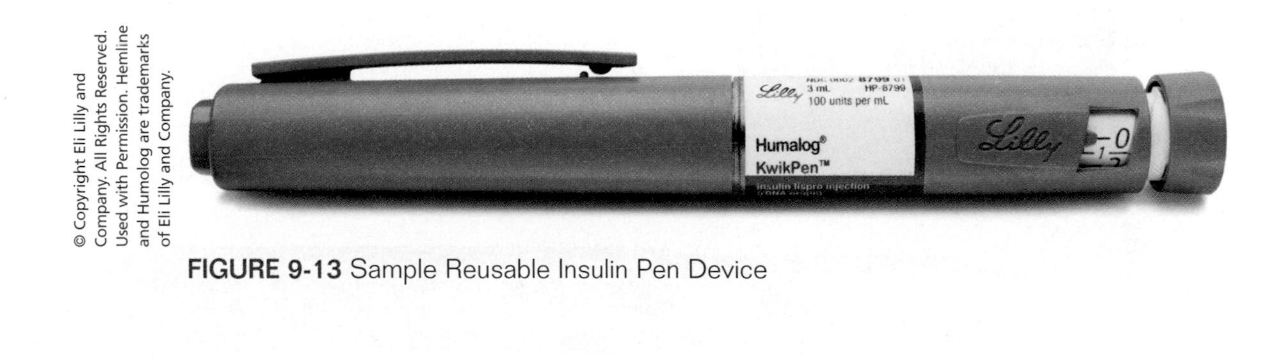

FIGURE 9-13 Sample Reusable Insulin Pen Device

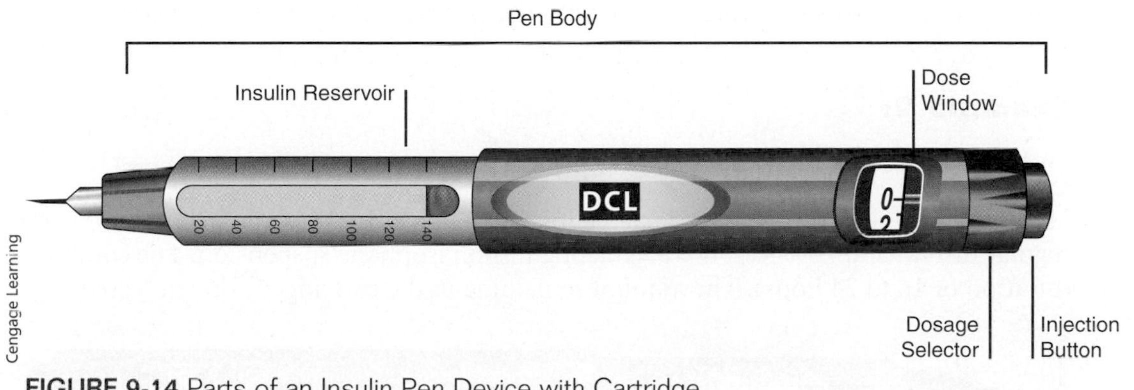

FIGURE 9-14 Parts of an Insulin Pen Device with Cartridge

Example 1:

Order: *Humalog insulin 12 units subcutaneously ac breakfast*

Humalog is the trade name for the rapid-acting insulin lispro, with an onset of action within 15 minutes. The amount remaining in the cartridge is shown below.

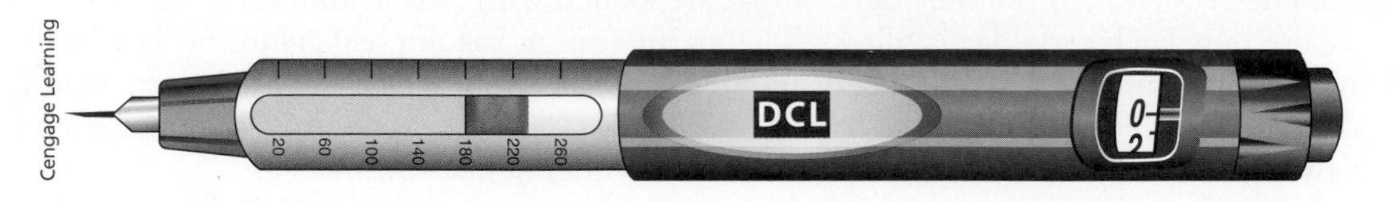

Apply the Three-Step Approach.

Step 1 Convert No conversion needed. Order and supply for insulin will always be in units.

Step 2 Think There are 180 units of insulin remaining in the cartridge. After administering the 12 units ordered dose, the remaining amount should be between the 180-unit and 140-unit marks.

Step 3 Calculate 180 units − 12 units = 168 units (estimated amount remaining)

Dial the ordered amount until the dosage window reaches the correct number of units. After dialing the insulin amount, give the order and insulin pen to another nurse for independent verification and documentation.

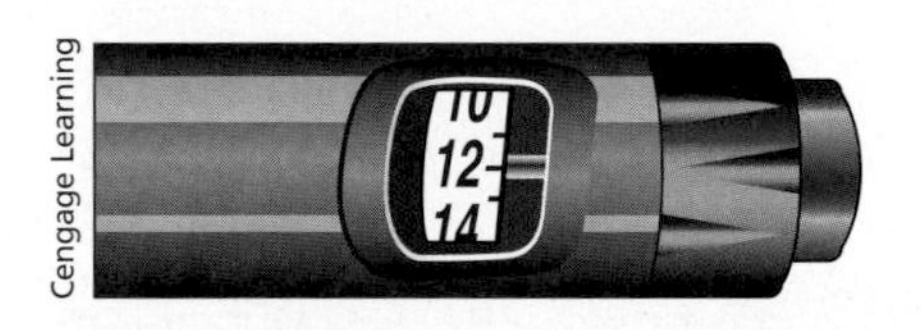

The amount remaining in the cartridge after administration of the insulin dose is shown below.

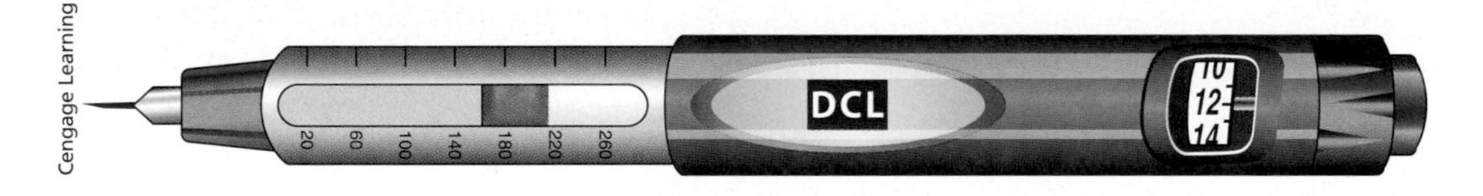

The remaining volume approximates the calculated amount; the amount injected is correct, and the pen functioned properly. Store the pen with the cartridge attached for later use. Discard the needle.

Example 2:

Order: *Humulin 30/70 insulin 36 units subcutaneously at 1700*

Humulin 30/70 insulin is the trade name for the premixed combination containing 30% short-acting regular insulin and 70% intermediate-acting insulin isophane suspension. The combined action has a duration of 16 to 24 hours. The amount remaining in the cartridge is shown below.

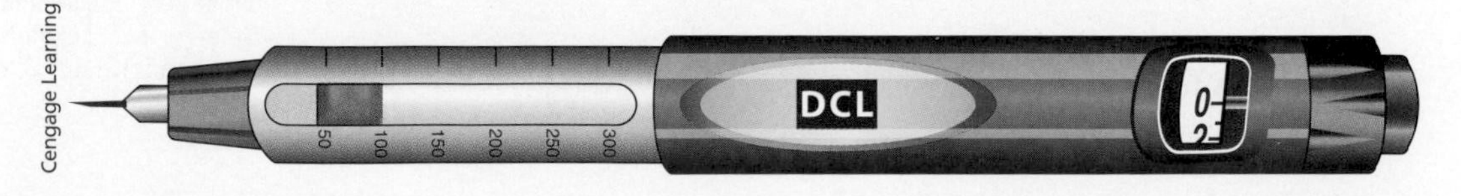

Apply the Three-Step Approach.

Step 1 Convert No conversion needed. Order and supply for insulin will also be in units.

Step 2 Think Slightly less than 50 units of insulin remain in the cartridge. There should be sufficient quantity to administer the 36-unit dose. The pen should not allow the dial to be turned farther than the amount left in the cartridge. After administration of the 36-unit insulin dose, the remaining amount should be slightly above the zero mark, with a volume of less than dose.

Step 3 Calculate 45 units − 36 units = 9 units (verifies estimated amount remaining)

Dial the ordered amount until the dosage window reaches the correct number of units. After dialing the insulin amount, give the order and insulin pen to another nurse for independent verification and documentation.

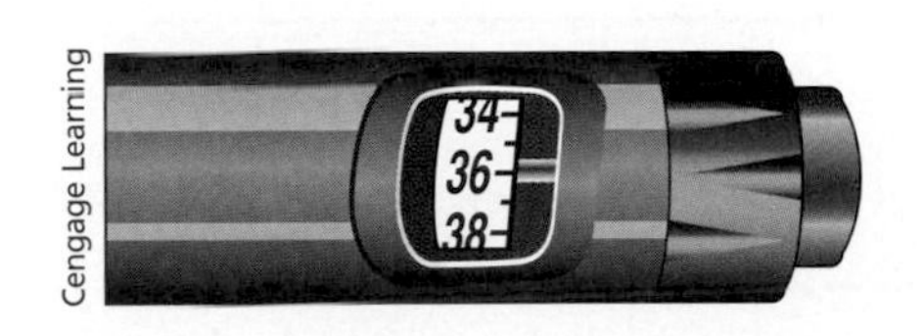

The amount remaining in the cartridge after administration of the insulin dose is shown below.

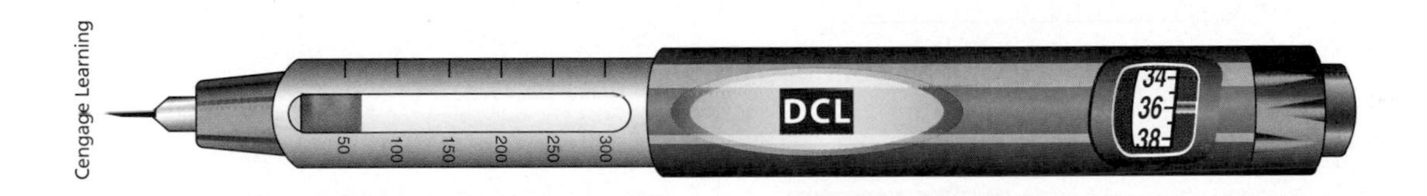

The remaining volume approximates the calculated amount; the amount injected is correct, and the pen functioned properly. There is an insufficient amount for another dose. Discard the cartridge and needle safely. Store the pen for later use.

Avoiding Insulin Dosage Patient Safety Incidents

Insulin dosage patient safety incidents are serious and, unfortunately, too common. They can be avoided by following three important rules.

RATIONALE FOR PRACTICE

1. **Best practice recommendations are that two nurses check insulin dosages to prevent patient safety incidents.**
2. **When combination dosages are prepared, best practice is that two nurses verify each step of the process.**
3. **In the community setting, when a second nurse is not available, an alert patient or family member may do the second independent check.**

QUICK REVIEW

- Carefully read the patient care order, and match the supply dosage for type, trade, and species of insulin.
- Always measure insulin in an insulin syringe.
- An insulin syringe is used to measure only 100-unit insulin. Insulin syringes must not be used to measure other medications measured in units.
- Use the smallest-capacity insulin syringe possible to most accurately measure insulin doses.
- When drawing up combination insulin doses, think *short- or rapid-acting first, then intermediate-acting.*
- Avoid insulin dosage patient safety incidents. Obtain independent verification by a second nurse.
- Do not mix long-acting insulin with any other insulin or solution.
- There are 100 units per mL for 100-unit insulin.

REVIEW SET 9-2

For questions 1 through 3, for each of the heparin sodium labels, match the letter(s) of the concentrations of the supply dosage with the most appropriate use. Select all that apply.

1. IV bolus of 7500 units to treat thrombosis: ______________________
2. Prepare IVPB bag for continuous infusion 40 000 units in 1 L D_5W to treat thrombosis: ______________________
3. Subcutaneous injection of 5000 units to prevent thrombosis: ______________________

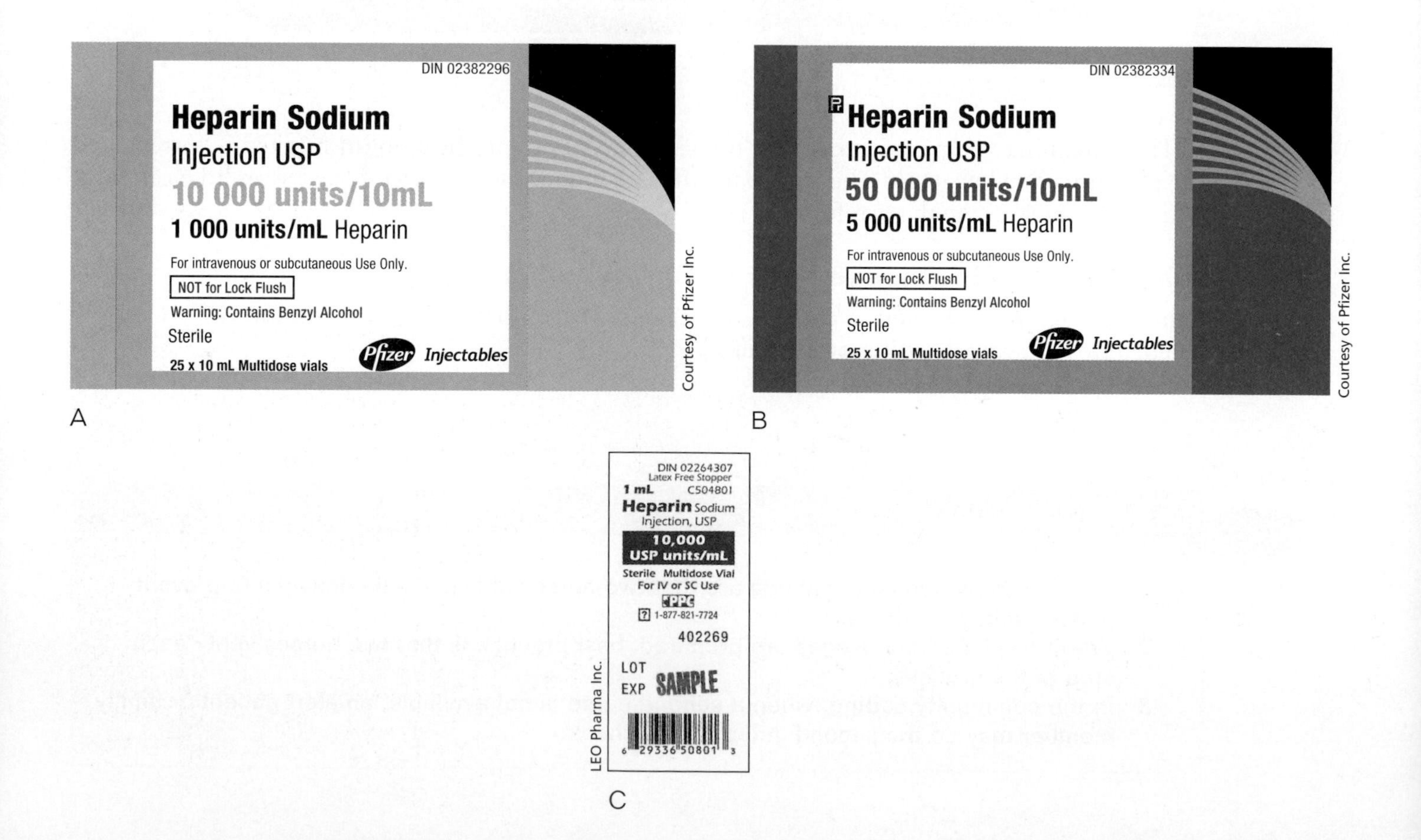

For questions 4 through 8, for each of the following labels, identify the brand name and the action time.

4. Insulin brand name: ________

   Action time: ________

5. Insulin brand name: ________

   Action time: ________

6. Insulin brand name: ________

   Action time: ________

7. Insulin brand name: ________

   Action time: ________

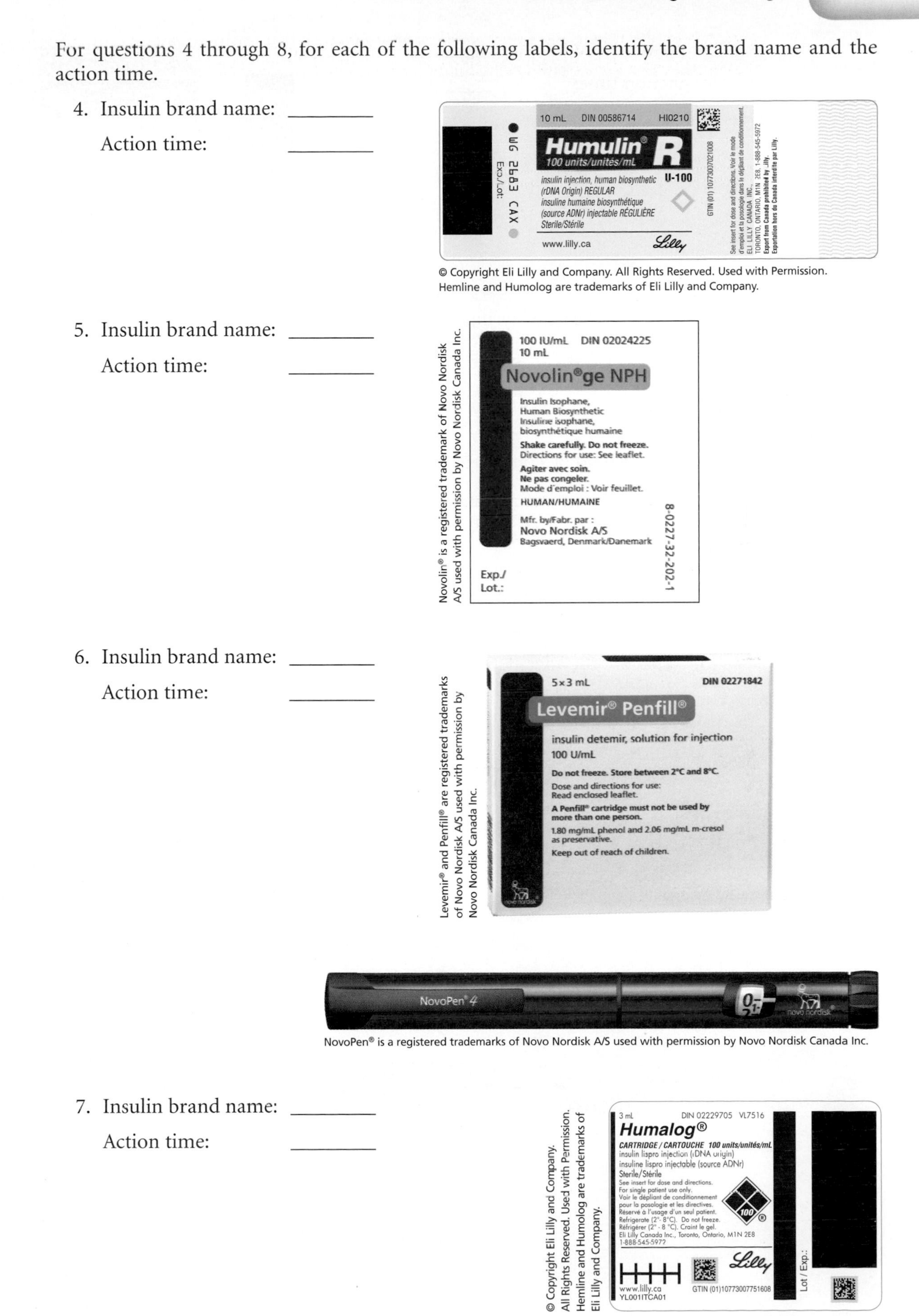

8. Insulin brand name: ________
   Action time: ________

10 mL DIN 00795879 HI-710
Humulin® 30/70
100 U/mL
30% insulin injection,
70% insulin isophane human
biosynthetic (rDNA Origin)
30 % insuline injectable
70 % insuline humaine
biosynthétique (source ADNr) isophane
www.lilly.ca
Lilly
U-100
Exp./Lot:

9. Describe the three syringes available to measure 100-unit insulin. ____________________
____
10. What would be your preferred syringe choice to measure 24 units of insulin?
____
11. What would be your preferred syringe choice to measure 35 units of insulin?
____
12. Sixty-five units of insulin should be measured in a(n) ________ syringe.
13. The 50-unit lo-dose insulin syringe is intended to measure 50-unit insulin only. ________ (True) (False)
14. Explain the purpose of an insulin sliding scale.
15. What are the advantages of an insulin pump?

For questions 16 through 18, refer to the label provided for each question and identify the heparin sodium dosage indicated by the coloured area of the syringe.

16. ____________________ units of heparin sodium.

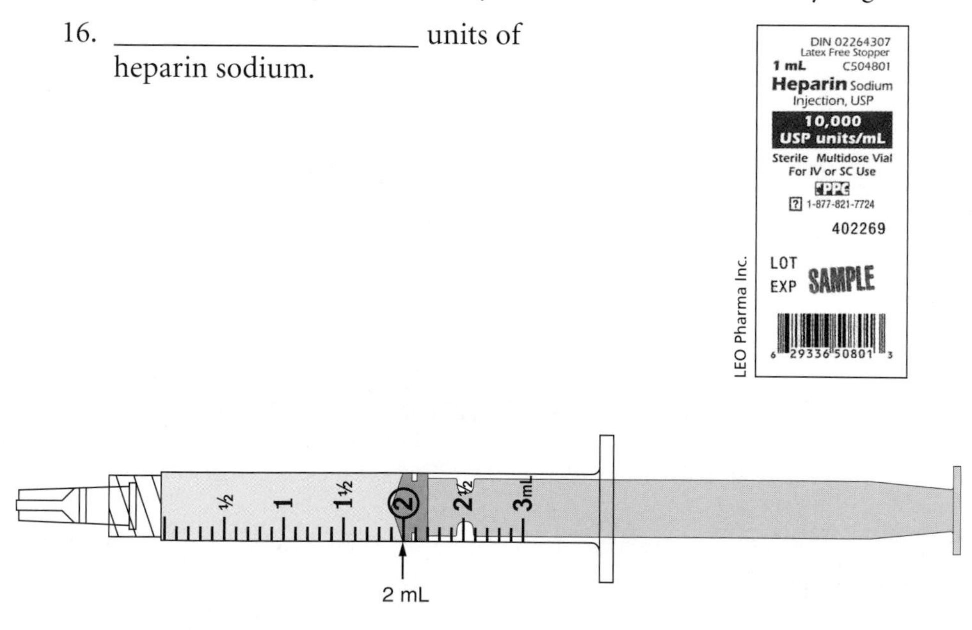

17. ______________________ units of heparin sodium.

18. ______________________ units of heparin sodium.

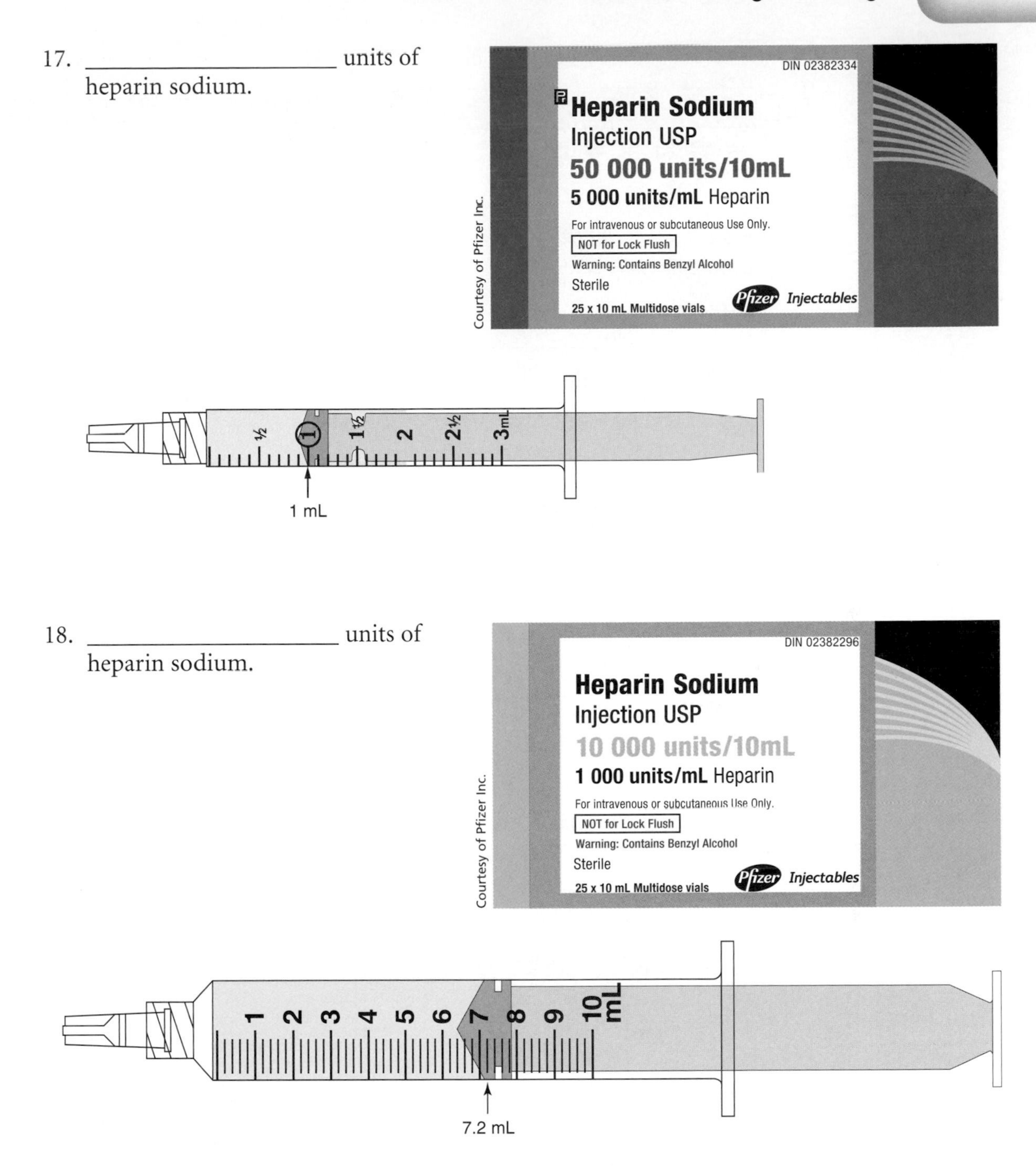

For questions 19 through 22, provide independent verification for high-alert dosages. Your nurse colleague provides you with the drug order, a labelled vial used to prepare the dosage, and the syringe filled with the dose amount. Determine whether or not the drug drawn up is the correct dosage.

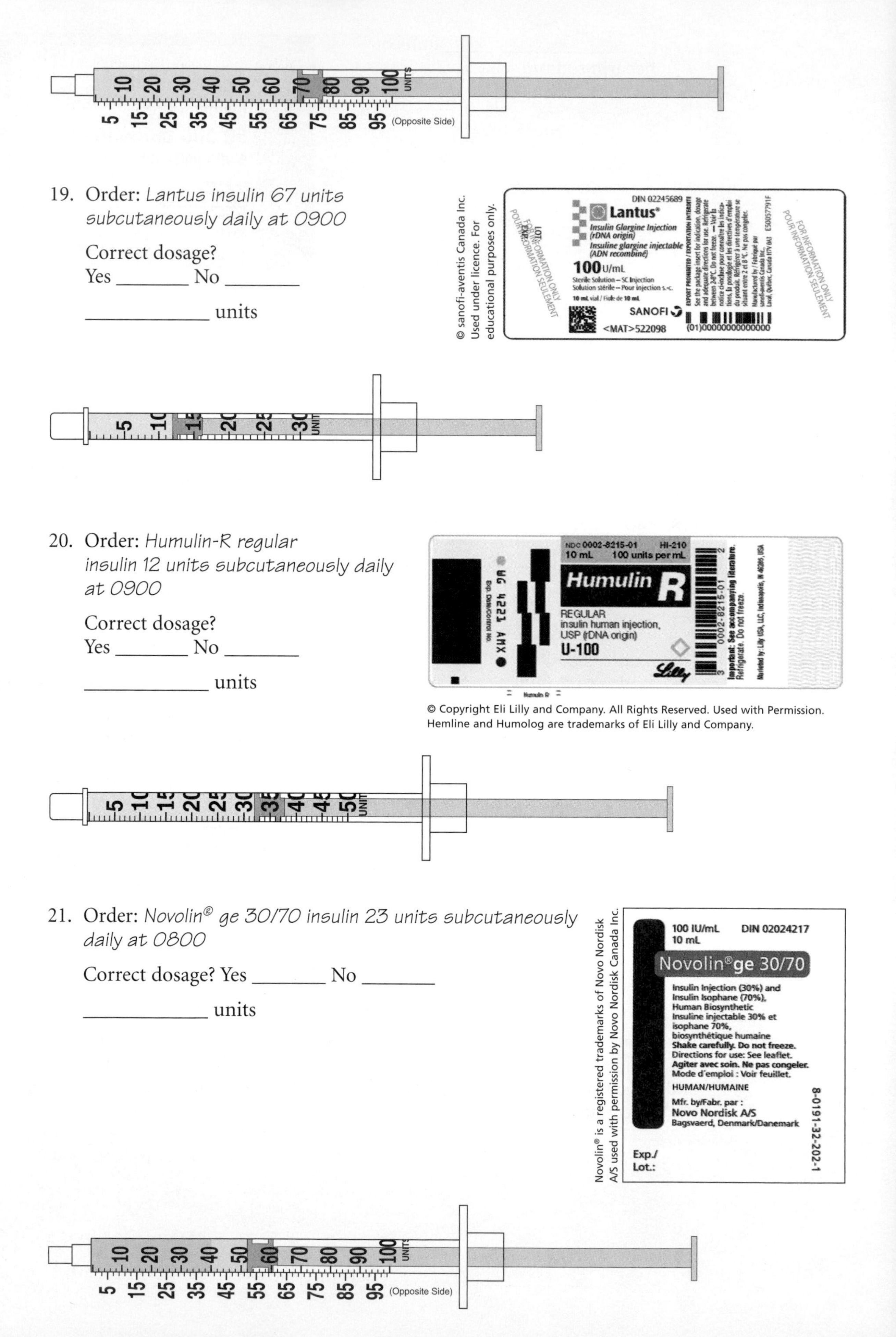

19. Order: *Lantus insulin 67 units subcutaneously daily at 0900*

    Correct dosage?
    Yes _______ No _______

    ___________ units

20. Order: *Humulin-R regular insulin 12 units subcutaneously daily at 0900*

    Correct dosage?
    Yes _______ No _______

    ___________ units

21. Order: *Novolin® ge 30/70 insulin 23 units subcutaneously daily at 0800*

    Correct dosage? Yes _______ No _______

    ___________ units

22. Order: *Humulin R insulin 52 units subcutaneously daily at 0800*

Correct dosage? Yes ________
No ________

____________ units

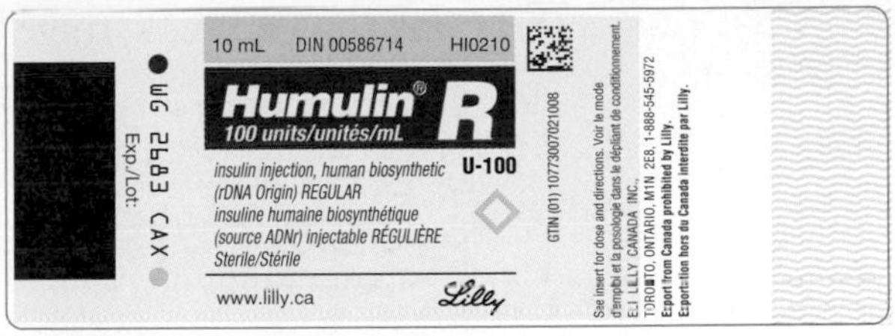

For questions 23 through 29, draw an arrow on the syringe to identify the ordered dosages.

23. Order: *heparin sodium 7200 units IV bolus stat prior to initiation of continuous heparin sodium infusion*

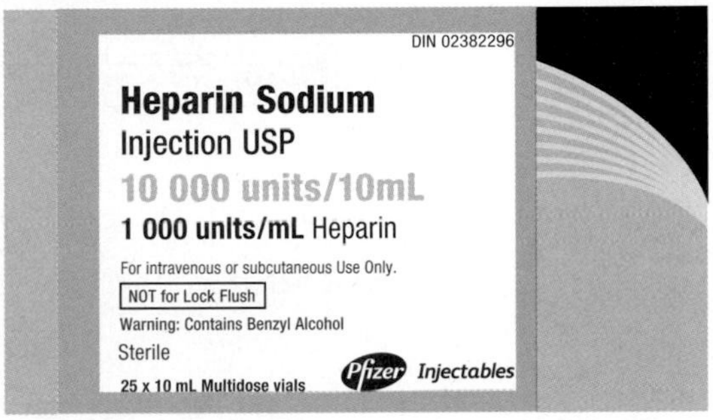

Courtesy of Pfizer Inc.

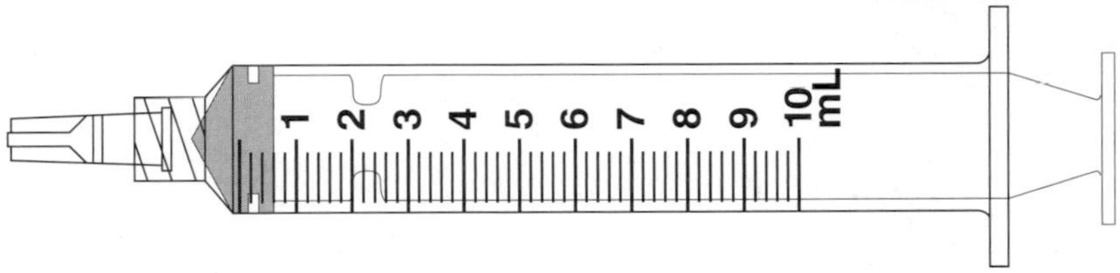

24. Order: *heparin sodium 4000 units subcutaneously 2 h prior to surgery*

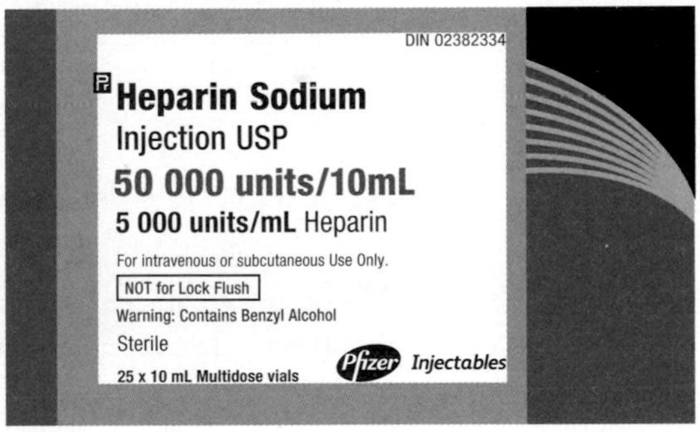

Courtesy of Pfizer Inc.

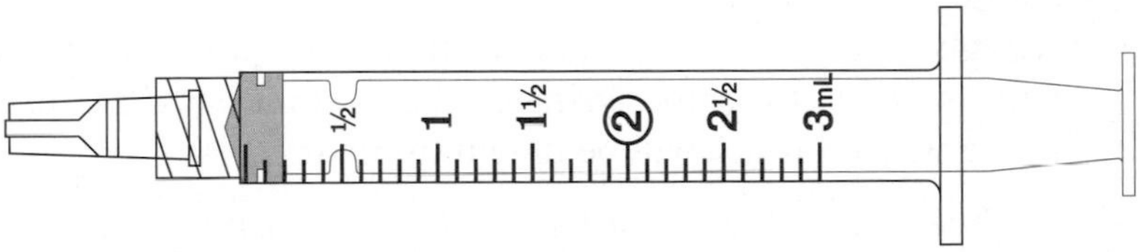

25. Order: *D_5W 500 mL IVPB with heparin sodium 50 000 units*

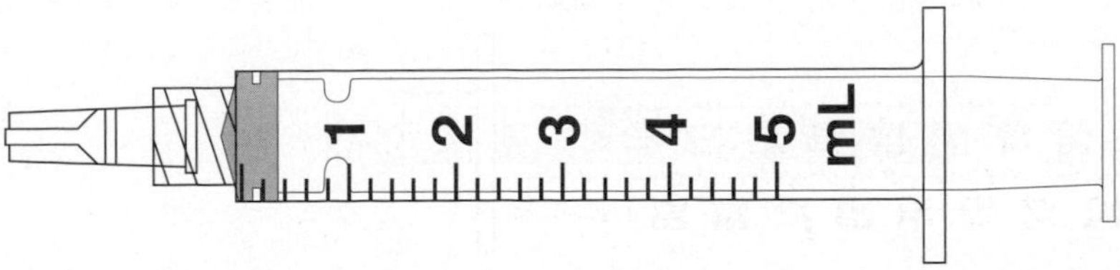

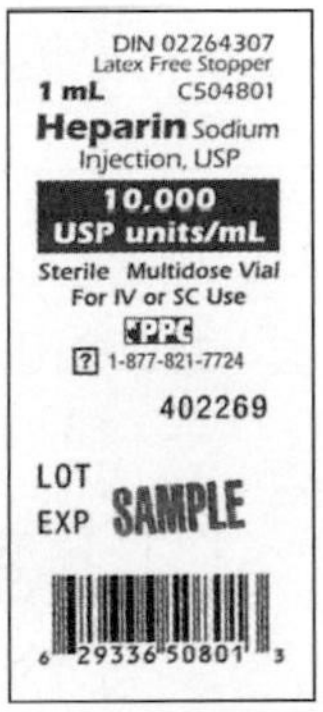

LEO Pharma Inc.

Draw an arrow on the syringe to identify the given dosages.

26. Order: *glargine insulin 35 units subcutaneously*

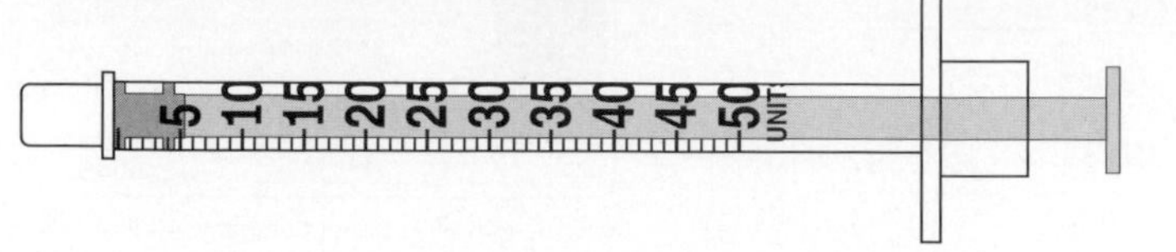

27. Order: *glulisine insulin 15 units subcutaneously*

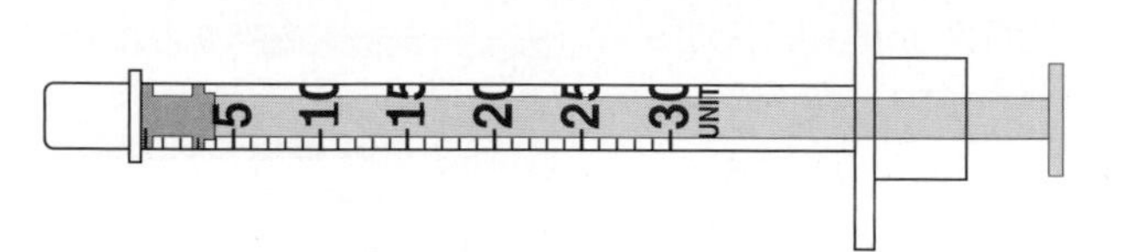

28. Order: *aspart insulin 20 units subcutaneously*

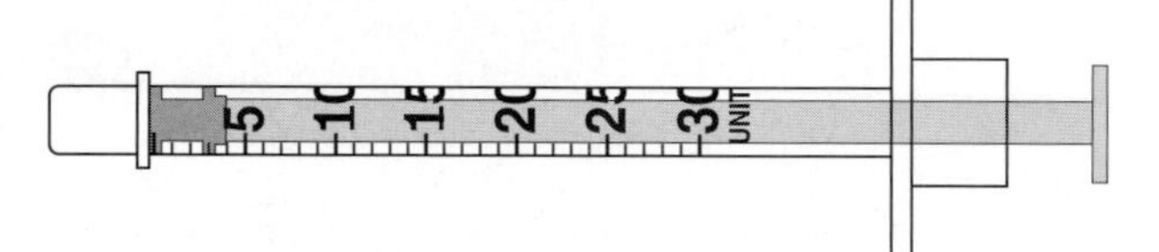

29. Order: *lispro insulin 16 units subcutaneously*

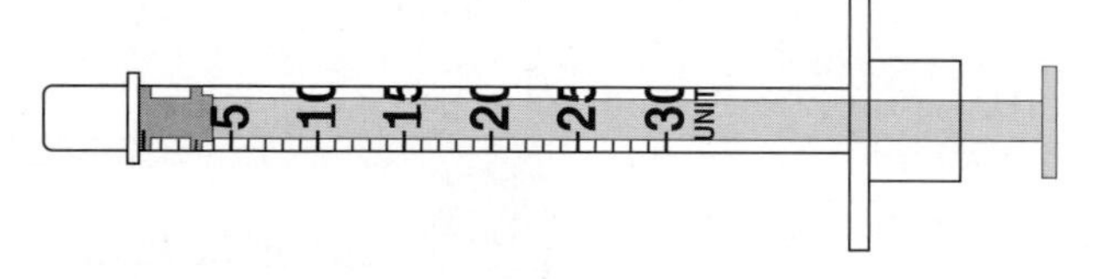

30. Order: *Humulin N insulin 32 units subcutaneously*

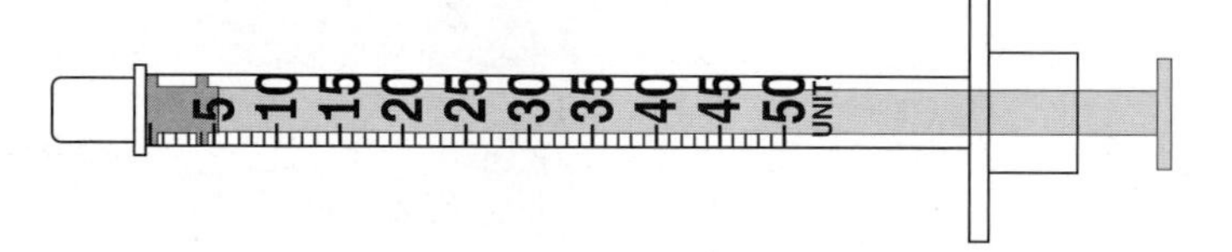

For questions 31 through 34, draw arrows, and label the dosage for each of the combination insulin orders to be measured in the same syringe. Label and measure the insulins in the correct order, indicating which insulin will be drawn up first.

31. Order: *Humulin R insulin 21 units with Humulin N NPH insulin 15 units subcutaneously stat*

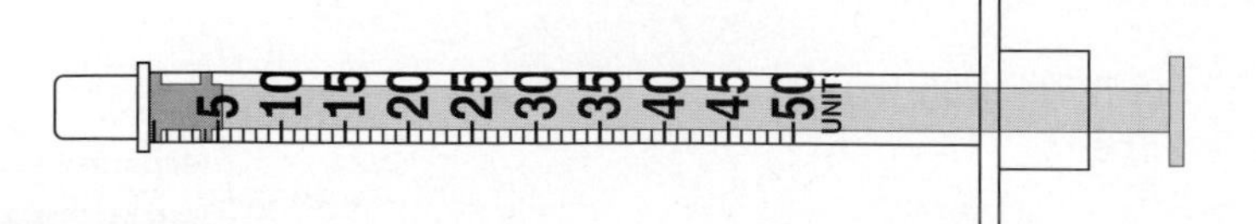

32. Order: *NovoRapid insulin 16 units with Novolin® ge NPH insulin 42 units subcutaneously stat*

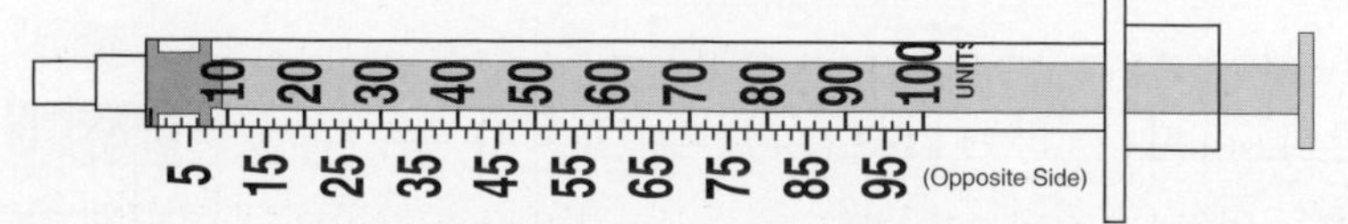

33. Order: *Humulin R insulin 32 units with Humulin N NPH insulin 40 units subcutaneously before dinner*

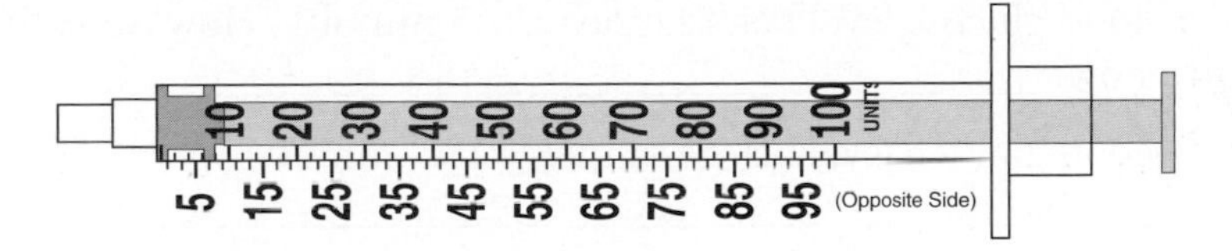

34. Order: *Novolin® ge Toronto insulin 8 units with Novolin® ge NPH insulin 12 units subcutaneously stat*

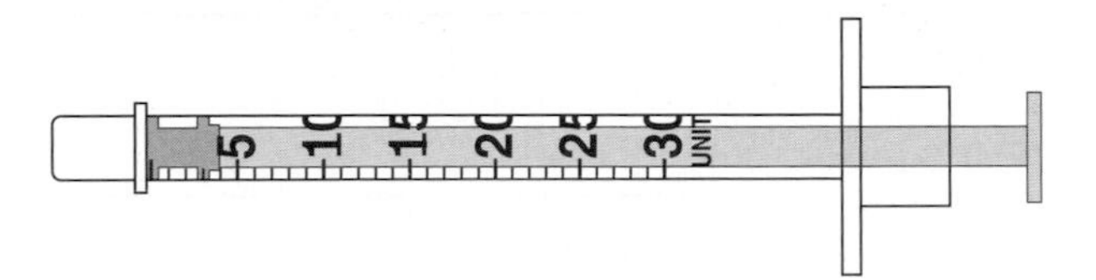

For questions 35 and 36, identify the dose of insulin displayed in the dose window of the insulin pen.

35. ____________ units

36. ____________ units

To answer questions 37 to 41, refer to the following insulin sliding scale and medication order.

Insulin Sliding Scale

Insulin Dose	Glucose Reading (mmol/L)
No coverage	Glucose less than 8
2 units	8.1–12
4 units	12.1–14
6 units	14.1–16
8 units	16.1–18
10 units	18.1–19.9
Hold insulin; call prescriber stat	Glucose greater than 20

Order: *Humulin R insulin subcutaneously before meals per sliding scale*

37. When will the nurse check the patient's blood glucose level to determine the amount of insulin to give? ____________

38. At what range of blood glucose levels will the nurse administer insulin? ____________

39. The patient's blood glucose level before breakfast is 13 mmol/L. What should the nurse do? ______

40. The patient's blood glucose level before lunch is 7.5 mmol/L. How much insulin should the nurse give now? ______

41. The patient's blood glucose level before dinner is 18.2 mmol/L. What should the nurse do now? ______

Check your work! Answers to all Review Sets are provided at the end of each chapter. Worked solutions for selected Review Sets are also available there.

APPLICATION OF CLINICAL REASONING

Many patient safety incidents involving insulin occur when the nurse fails to clarify an incomplete order. Let us look at an example of a patient safety incident involving insulin when the order did not include the type of insulin to be given.

Potential Patient Safety Incident

Failing to clarify an insulin order when the type of insulin is not specified.

Possible Scenario

Suppose the prescriber wrote an insulin order this way:

Humulin insulin 50 units before breakfast

Because the prescriber did not specify the type of insulin, the nurse assumed it was short-acting insulin and noted that on the medication administration record. Suppose the patient was given the short-acting insulin for 3 days. On the morning of the third day, the patient developed signs of hypoglycemia (low blood glucose), including shakiness, tremors, confusion, and sweating.

Potential Outcome

A stat blood glucose test would likely reveal a dangerously low glucose level. The patient would be given a glucose infusion to increase the blood sugar. The nurse may not realize the incident until she and the prescriber check the original order and find that the incomplete order was filled in by the nurse. When the prescriber did not specify the type of insulin, the nurse assumed the prescriber meant regular, which is short-acting, when in fact intermediate-acting NPH insulin was desired.

Prevention

This patient safety incident could have been avoided by remembering all the essential components of an insulin order: species, type of insulin (such as short-acting or NPH), supply dosage, the amount to give in units, and the frequency. When the nurse fills in an incomplete order, the nurse is essentially practising medicine outside the scope of practice. This would be a clear harmful incident, as it resulted in harm to the patient. It does not make sense to put you and your patient in such jeopardy. Communicating with the prescriber verbally or by phone would clarify the situation for everyone involved. Further, the nurse should have double-checked the dosage with another registered healthcare provider. Had the nurse done so, the harmful incident would have been discovered prior to administration.

Application of Critical Reasoning Additional application problems are provided at the end of the chapter. Answers are provided at the end of the book.

CHECK POINT

This chapter has provided many different examples of dosage calculations to solve that you will encounter in your healthcare career. Oral and parenteral drug orders, written in the forms presented thus far, account for a large percentage of prescriptions. Remember that a high percentage of patient safety incidents involve high-alert drugs and that extreme caution is required.

You have learned to think through the process from order, to supply, to amount administered, and to apply the Three-Step Approach and the dosage calculation formula method:

$$\frac{\text{D (desired)}}{\text{H (have)}} \times \text{Q (quantity)} = \text{X (amount)}$$

Work through the practice problems for Chapter 9. Once completed, you should feel comfortable and confident working through dosage calculations. Concentrate on accuracy. Remember, one error in dosage calculation can result in serious risk to your patient.

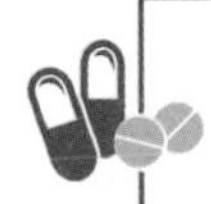

UNDERSTANDING NCLEX QUESTIONS

Here's an example of a standard question used in textbooks:

The physician orders 36 units of NPH and 12 units of regular insulin. The nurse plans to administer these drugs in 1 syringe. Identify the steps in this procedure by listing them in priority order. 1. Inject air equal to NPH dose into NPH vial 2. Invert regular insulin bottle and withdraw regular insulin dose 3. Inject air equal to regular dose into regular dose 4. Invert NPH vial and withdraw NPH dose.

a. 1, 2, 3, 4
b. 1, 4, 3, 2
c. 1, 4, 2, 3
d. 1, 3, 2, 4

Here's how the question would look in an NCLEX examination:

The nurse is to administer 36 units of NPH and 12 units of regular insulin. Identify the steps the nurse would take in order of priority to prepare this dosage of insulin.

1. Inject air equal to NPH dose into NPH vial
2. Invert regular insulin bottle and withdraw regular insulin dose
3. Inject air equal to regular dose into regular dose
4. Invert NPH vial and withdraw NPH dose.

a. 1, 2, 3, 4
b. 1, 4, 3, 2
c. 1, 4, 2, 3
d. 1, 3, 2, 4

Answer: d

Rationale: The intermediate insulin is withdrawn first and the regular insulin is withdrawn second.

PRACTICE PROBLEMS—CHAPTER 9

Calculate the amount you will prepare for one dose. Indicate the syringe you will select to measure the medication.

1. Order: *hydromorphone hydrochloride 4 mg slow IV push (over 10 min) 4h prn for severe pain*

   Supply: hydromorphone hydrochloride 10 mg/mL

   Give: ________ mL Select ________ syringe

2. Order: *morphine sulfate 15 mg slow IV push (over 5 min) stat*

   Supply: morphine sulfate 10 mg/mL

   Give: ________ mL Select ________ syringe

3. Order: *haloperidol 2.5 mg IV stat*

   Supply: haloperidol 5 mg/mL

   Give: ________ mL Select ________ syringe

4. Order: *hydroxyzine hydrochloride 20 mg IM stat*

   Supply: hydroxyzine hydrochloride 50 mg/mL

   Give: ________ mL Select ________ syringe

5. Order: *clindamycin phosphate 300 mg IM QID*

   Supply: clindamycin phosphate 150 mg/mL

   Give: ________ mL Select ________ syringe

6. Order: *naloxolone hydrochloride 0.3 mg IM stat*

   Supply: naloxolone hydrochloride 0.4 mg/mL

   Give: ________ mL Select ________ syringe

7. Order: *ketorolac tromethamine 20 mg IM q4h prn for pain*

   Supply: ketorolac tromethamine 30 mg/mL

   Give: ________ mL Select ________ syringe

8. Order: *midazolam 5 mg IM 60 minutes pre-operatively*

   Supply: midazolam 5 mg/mL

   Give: ________ mL Select ________ syringe

9. Order: *ondansetron hydrochloride dihydrate 8 mg IV over 15 min given 30 min prior to chemotherapy*

   Supply: ondansetron hydrochloride dihydrate 2 mg/mL

   Give: ________ mL Select ________ syringe

10. Order: *chlorpromazine hydrochloride 25 mg IM stat*

    Supply: chlorpromazine hydrochloride 25 mg/mL

    Give: ________ mL Select ________ syringe

11. Order: *atropine sulfate 0.6 mg IM on call to the operating room*

    Supply: atropine sulfate 0.6 mg/mL

    Give: ________ mL Select ________ syringe

12. Order: *glycopyrrolate 200 mcg IM 60 min pre-op*

    Supply: glycopyrrolate 0.2 mg/mL

    Give: ________ mL Select ________ syringe

13. Order: *heparin sodium 6000 units subcut q12h*

    Supply: heparin sodium 10 000 units/mL vial

    Give: ________ mL Select ________ syringe

14. Order: *tobramycin sulfate 75 mg IM q8h*

    Supply: tobramycin sulfate 80 mg/2 mL

    Give: ________ mL Select ________ syringe

15. Order: *digoxin 0.6 mg slow IV push stat*

    Supply: digoxin 0.25 mg/mL

    Give: ________ mL Select ________ syringe

16. Order: *atropine sulfate 0.4 mg IM on call to the operating room*

    Supply: atropine sulfate 0.4 mg/mL

    Give: ________ mL Select ________ syringe

17. Order: *enoxaparin sodium 40 mg subcut BID*

    Supply: enoxaparin sodium 300 mg/mL multidose vial

    Give: ________ mL Select ________ syringe

18. Order: *penicillin G sodium 4 000 000 units IM stat*

    Supply: penicillin G sodium 5 000 000 units/mL

    Give: ________ mL Select ________ syringe

19. Order: *hydromorphone 3 mg slow IV push (over 5 to 10 min) q4h prn for severe pain*

    Supply: hydromorphone 10 mg/mL

    Give: ________ mL Select ________ syringe

20. Order: *dalteparin sodium 5000 units subcut, pre-operatively*

    Supply: dalteparin sodium 25 000 units/mL

    Give: ________ mL Select: ________ syringe

21. Order: *cyanocobalamin 0.75 mg IM daily*

    Supply: cyanocobalamin 1000 mcg/mL

    Give: ________ mL Select ________ syringe

22. Order: *vitamin K 15 mg subcut stat*

    Supply: vitamin K 10 mg per mL

    Give: ________ mL Select ________ syringe

23. Order: *promethazine hydrochloride 35 mg IM q4h prn for nausea and vomiting*

    Supply: promethazine hydrochloride 50 mg/mL

    Give: ________ mL Select ________ syringe

24. Order: *magnesium sulfate 500 mg IV stat*

    Supply: magnesium sulfate 1 g/2 mL

    Give: ________ mL Select ________ syringe

25. Order: *methylprednisolone acetate, 60 mg IM, daily for 1 week*

    Supply: methylprednisolone acetate 80 mg/mL

    Give: ________ mL Select ________ syringe

26. Order: *haloperidol 2.5 mg IV stat*

    Supply: haloperidol 5 mg/mL

    Give: ________ mL Select ________ syringe

27. Order: *furosemide 60 mg IV stat*

    Supply: furosemide 10 mg/mL

    Give: ________ mL Select ________ syringe

28. Order: *heparin sodium 4000 units subcut q6h*

    Supply: heparin sodium 5000 units/mL

    Give: ________ mL Select ________ syringe

29. Order: *hydralazine hydrochloride 30 mg IV q6h*

    Supply: hydralazine hydrochloride 20 mg/mL

    Give: ________ mL Select ________ syringe

30. Order: *lidocaine hydrochloride 2% 50 mg IV stat*

    Supply: lidocaine hydrochloride 2% 20 mg/mL

    Give: ________ mL Select ________ syringe

31. Order: *verapamil hydrochloride 2.5 mg IV push stat*

    Supply: verapamil hydrochloride 5 mg/2 mL

    Give: ________ mL Select ________ syringe

32. Order: *phenytoin sodium 100 mg IV stat*

    Supply: phenytoin sodium 50 mg/mL

    Give: ________ mL Select ________ syringe

33. Order: *neostigmine methylsulfate 0.5 mg IM TID*

    Supply: neostigmine methylsulfate 1 mg/mL

    Give: ________ mL Select ________ syringe

34. Order: *amikacin sulfate 125 mg IV BID*

    Supply: amikacin sulfate 250 mg/mL

    Give: ________ mL Select ________ syringe

35. Order: *Humulin R insulin 16 units subcut*

    Supply: Humulin R insulin, with standard 100-unit and lo-dose 30 units insulin syringes

    Give: ________ units Select ________ syringe

36. Order: *Novolin® ge NPH insulin 25 units subcut before breakfast*

    Supply: Novolin® ge NPH insulin with standard 100-unit and lo-dose 50 units insulin syringes

    Give: ________ units Select ________ syringe

Calculate one dose of each of the drug orders numbered 37 through 48. Draw an arrow on the syringe to indicate the calibration line that corresponds to the dose to be administered. The labels are the medications you have available. Indicate dosages that must be divided.

37. Order: *haloperidol 1.5 mg IM q8h*

    Give: ________ mL

38. Order: *clindamycin phosphate 900 mg IV q8h*

    Give: ________ mL

39. Order: *midazolam 1 mg IV stat*

    Give: ________ mL

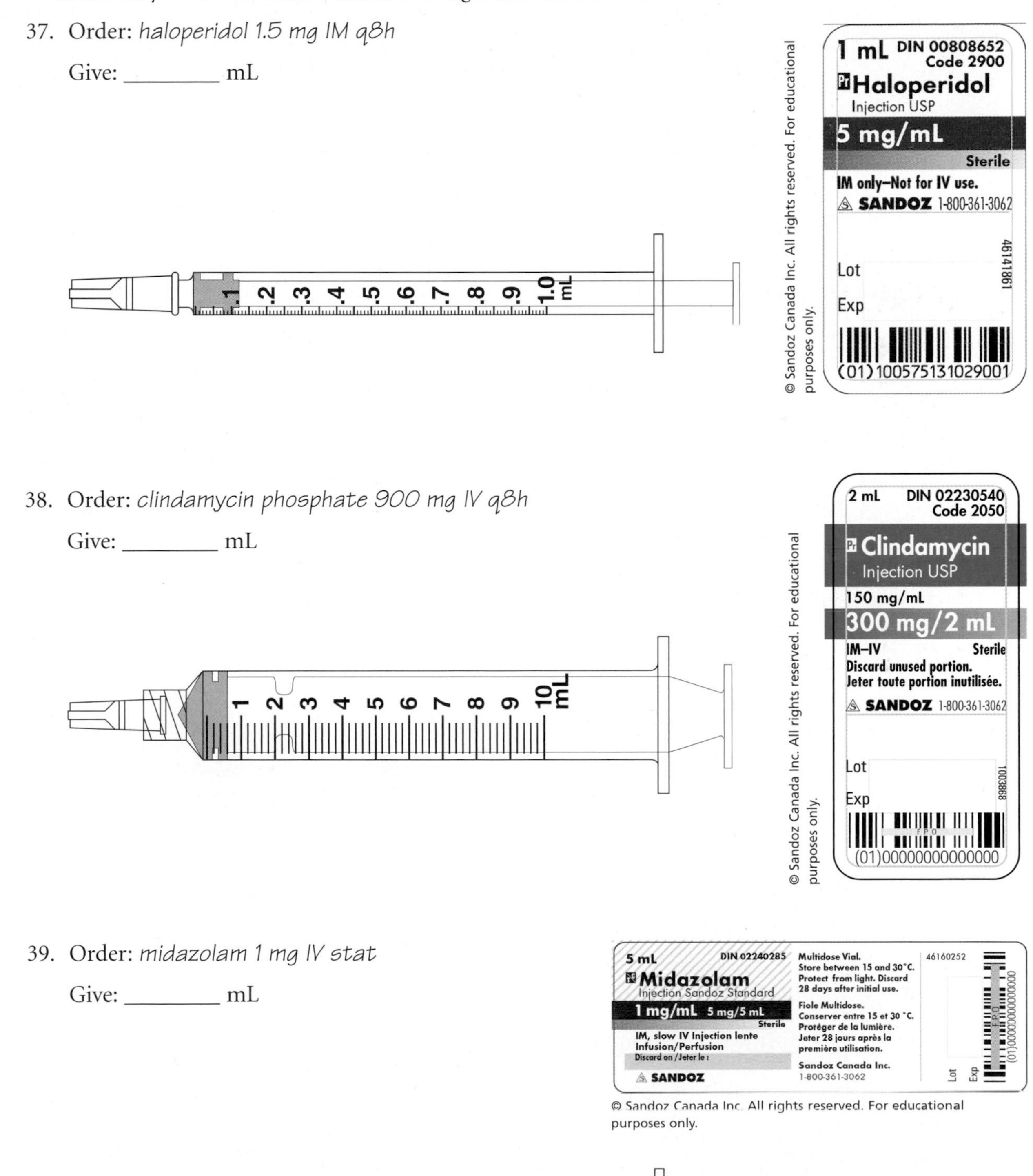

1 mL DIN 00808652
Code 2900
Haloperidol
Injection USP
5 mg/mL
Sterile
IM only—Not for IV use.
SANDOZ 1-800-361-3062
Lot
Exp
(01)10057513102900
2 mL DIN 02230540
Code 2050
Clindamycin
Injection USP
150 mg/mL
300 mg/2 mL
IM–IV
Sterile
Discard unused portion.
Jeter toute portion inutilisée.
SANDOZ 1-800-361-3062
Lot
Exp
5 mL
DIN 02240285
Midazolam
Injection Sandoz Standard
1 mg/mL 5 mg/5 mL
Sterile
IM, slow IV Injection lente
Infusion/Perfusion
SANDOZ
Multidose Vial.
Store between 15 and 30°C.
Protect from light. Discard 28 days after initial use.
Fiole Multidose.
Conserver entre 15 et 30 °C.
Protéger de la lumière.
Jeter 28 jours après la première utilisation.
Sandoz Canada Inc.
1-800-361-3062

40. Order: *tobramycin 80 mg IV q8h*

Give: ________ mL

2 mL DIN 02241210
Code 8650
SA PF
Tobramycin
Injection USP
40 mg/mL
80 mg/2 mL
IM–IV Sterile
Single use vial
Fiole à usage unique
SANDOZ 1-800-361-3062
Lot
Exp
(01)00000000000000

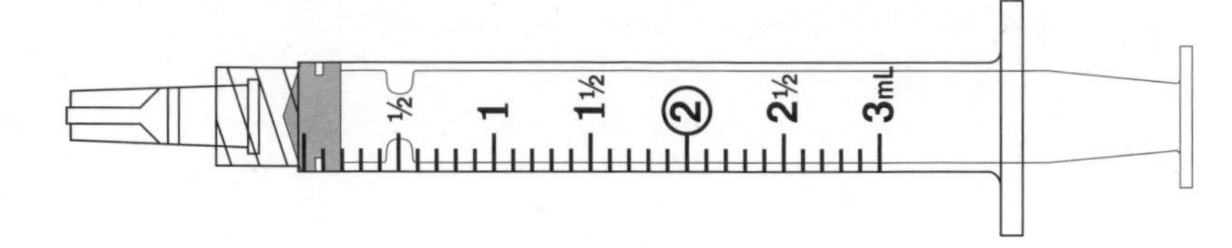

41. Order: *epoetin alfa 12 000 units subcutaneously daily × 10 days*

Give: ________ mL

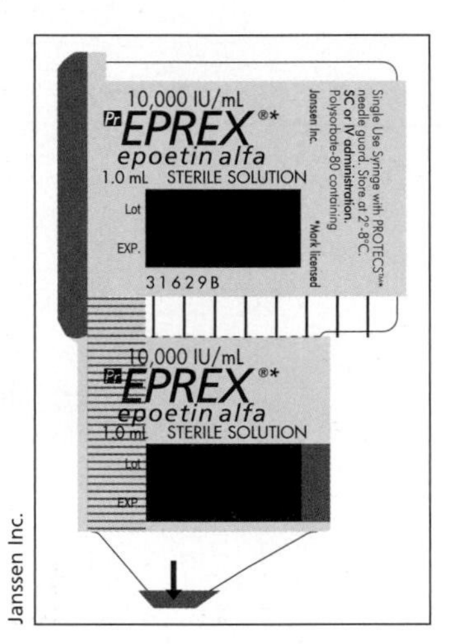

42. Order: *Humulin R insulin 22 units subcutaneously stat*

Give: ________ units

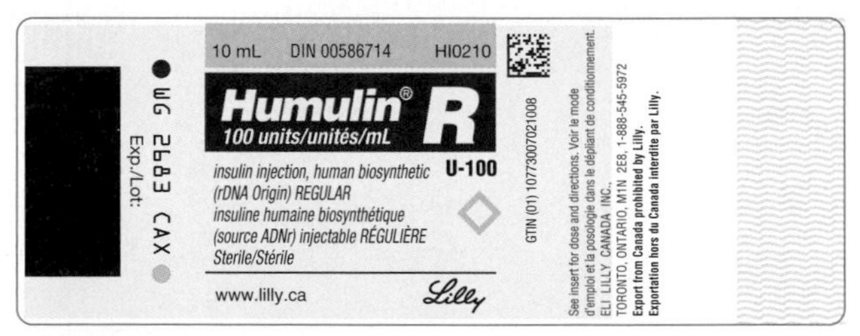

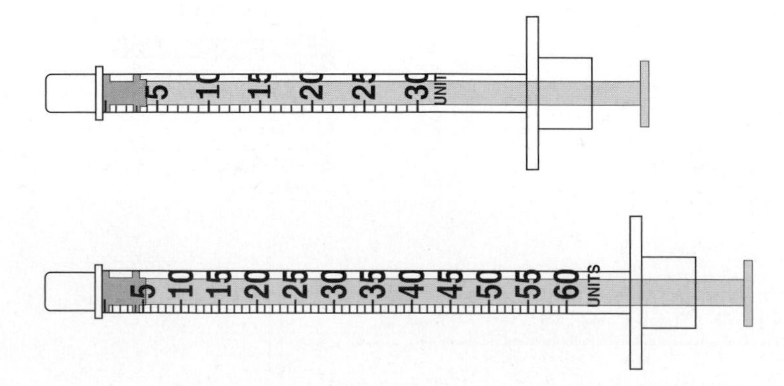

43. Order: *meperidine hydrochloride 45 mg IM q4h prn for pain*

    Give: ________ mL

44. Order: *triamcinolone acetonide 20 mg IM q4h daily*

    Give: ________ mL

45. Order: *metoclopramide hydrochloride 7 mg IM stat*

    Give: ________ mL

46. Order: *filgrastim 225 mcg subcut daily × 2 weeks*

    Give: ________ mL

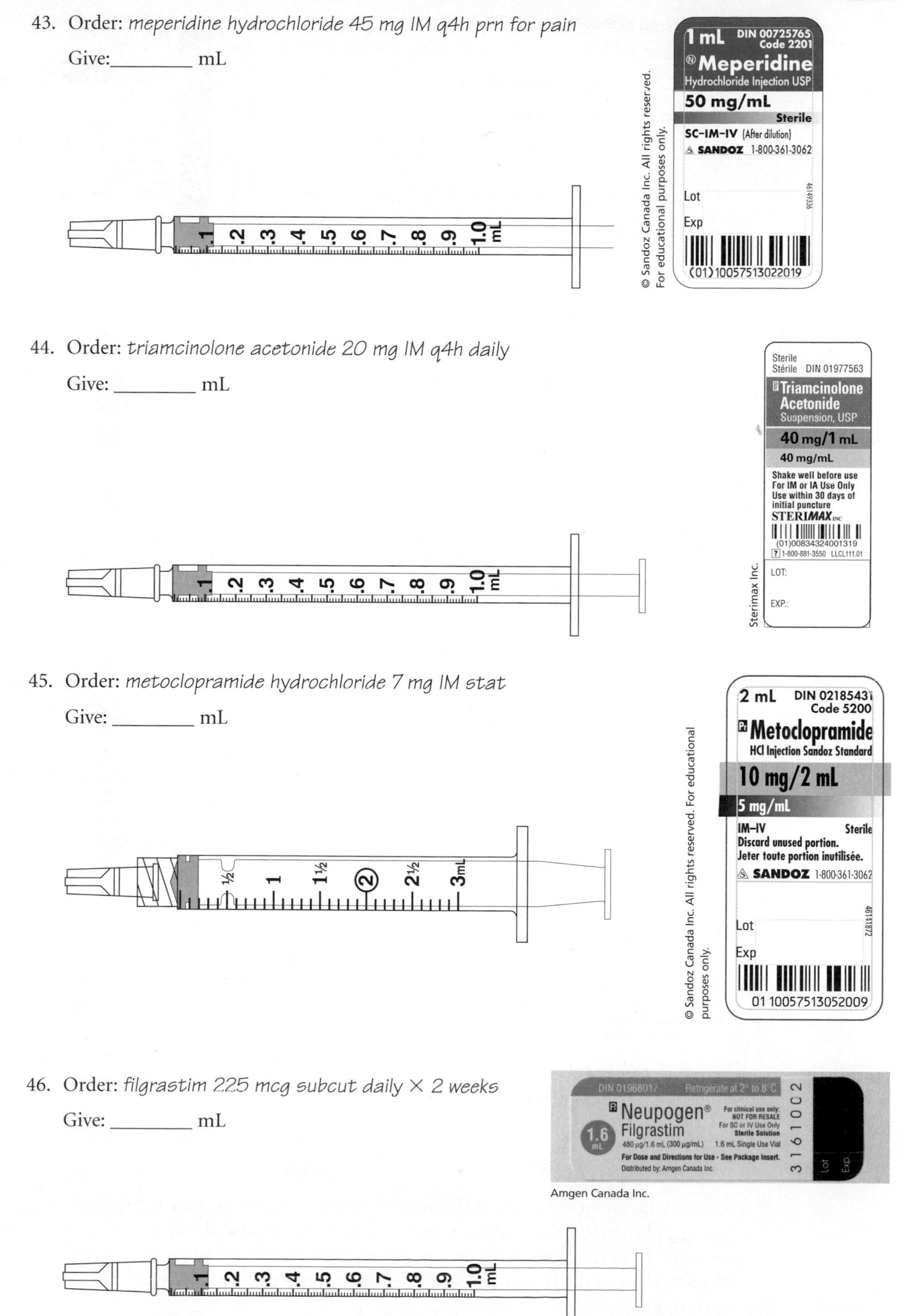

1 mL DIN 00725765 Code 2201
Meperidine
Hydrochloride Injection USP
50 mg/mL
Sterile
SC-IM-IV (After dilution)
SANDOZ 1-800-361-3062
Lot
Exp
(01)10057513022019
© Sandoz Canada Inc. All rights reserved. For educational purposes only.
.1 .2 .3 .4 .5 .6 .7 .8 .9 1.0 mL
Sterile
Stérile DIN 01977563
Triamcinolone Acetonide
Suspension, USP
40 mg/1 mL
40 mg/mL
Shake well before use
For IM or IA Use Only
Use within 30 days of initial puncture
STERIMAX INC
(01)00834324001319
1-800-881-3550 LLCL111.01
LOT:
EXP.:
Sterimax Inc.
.1 .2 .3 .4 .5 .6 .7 .8 .9 1.0 mL
2 mL DIN 02185431 Code 5200
Metoclopramide
HCl Injection Sandoz Standard
10 mg/2 mL
5 mg/mL
IM–IV Sterile
Discard unused portion.
Jeter toute portion inutilisée.
SANDOZ 1-800-361-3062
Lot
Exp
01 10057513052009
© Sandoz Canada Inc. All rights reserved. For educational purposes only.
½ 1 1½ 2 2½ 3mL
DIN 01968017 Refrigerate at 2° to 8°C
Neupogen®
Filgrastim
1.6 mL
480 µg/1.6 mL (300 µg/mL) 1.6 mL Single Use Vial
For clinical use only: NOT FOR RESALE
For SC or IV Use Only
Sterile Solution
For Dose and Directions for Use - See Package Insert.
Distributed by: Amgen Canada Inc.
3 1 6 1 0 C 2
Lot Exp
Amgen Canada Inc.
.1 .2 .3 .4 .5 .6 .7 .8 .9 1.0 mL

47. Order: *Novolin® ge Toronto insulin 32 units with Novolin® ge NPH insulin 54 units subcut before breakfast*

    Give: ________ total units

48. Order: *Novolin® ge 30/70 insulin 46 units subcut before dinner*

    Give: ________ units

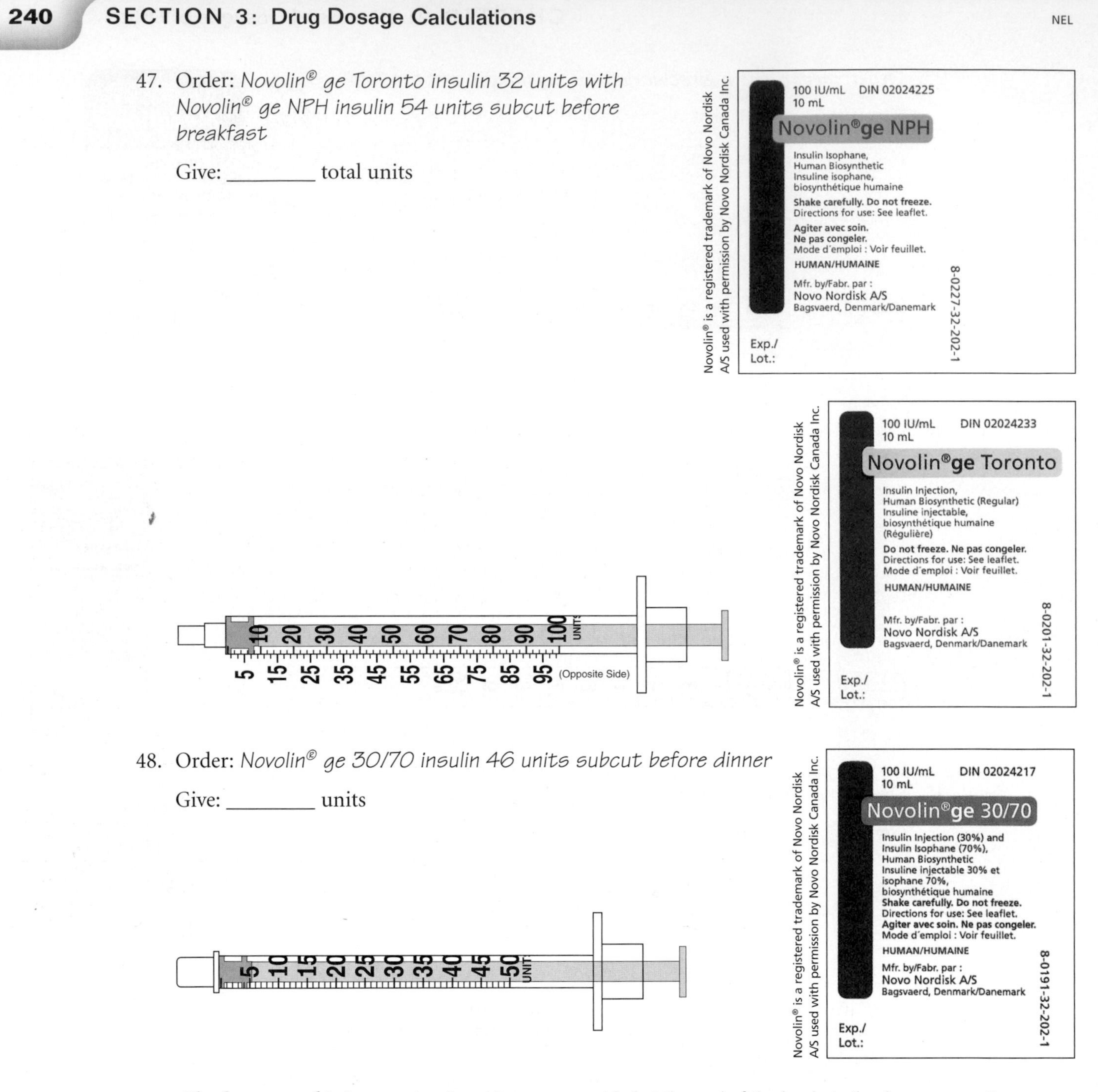

Check your work! Answers to all problems are provided at the end of the book, in the Answers section. Worked solutions for some Practice Problems are also provided there.

APPLICATION OF CLINICAL REASONING

9-1 Describe the clinical reasoning you would implement to prevent this patient safety incident.

Possible Scenario

Suppose the prescriber ordered Humulin R insulin 20 units mixed with Humulin N insulin 40 units to be administered subcut before breakfast. The nurse selected the vials of Humulin R and Humulin N insulin from the medication drawer and injected 20 units of air in the Humulin N vial and 40 units of air in the Humulin R vial, drew up 40 units of Humulin R, and then drew up 20 units of Humulin N.

Potential Outcome

The patient received the incorrect dosage of insulin because the nurse drew up 40 units of Humulin R and 20 units of Humulin N instead of the dosage that was ordered: 20 units of Humulin R and 40 units of Humulin N. Because the patient received too much short-acting insulin (twice the amount ordered), the patient would likely show signs of hypoglycemia, such as shakiness, confusion, and diaphoresis.

Prevention

____

____

9-2. Describe the clinical reasoning you would implement to prevent this patient safety incident.

Possible Scenario

Suppose the prescriber ordered *10 units of Novolin® ge Toronto insulin subcut stat* for a patient with a blood glucose of 17 mmol/L. The nurse selected the Novolin® ge Toronto insulin from the patient's medication drawer and selected a 1-mL syringe to administer the dose. The nurse looked at the syringe for the 10-unit mark and was confused over how much should have been drawn up. The nurse finally decided to draw up 1 mL of insulin into the syringe, administered the dose, and then began to question whether the correct dosage was administered. The nurse called the supervisor for advice.

Potential Outcome

The patient received 10 times the correct dosage of insulin. Because this was a short-acting insulin, the patient would likely show signs of severe hypoglycemia, such as loss of consciousness and seizures.

Prevention

____

____

Check your work! Answers to all Application of Clinical Reasoning problems are provided at the end of the book, in the Answers section.

ANSWERS TO REVIEW SETS

Review Set 9-1

1) 0.67

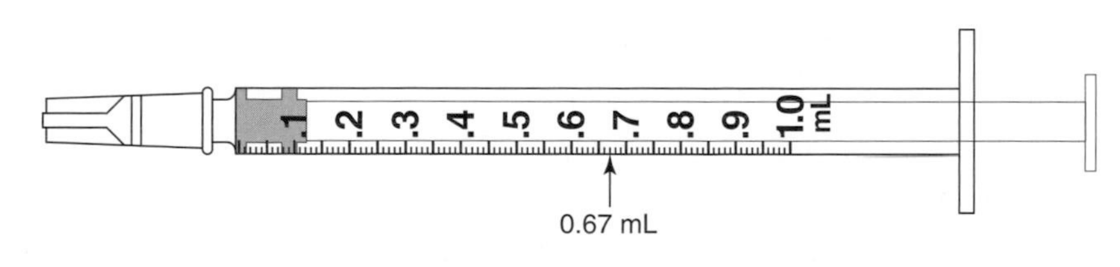

2) 1

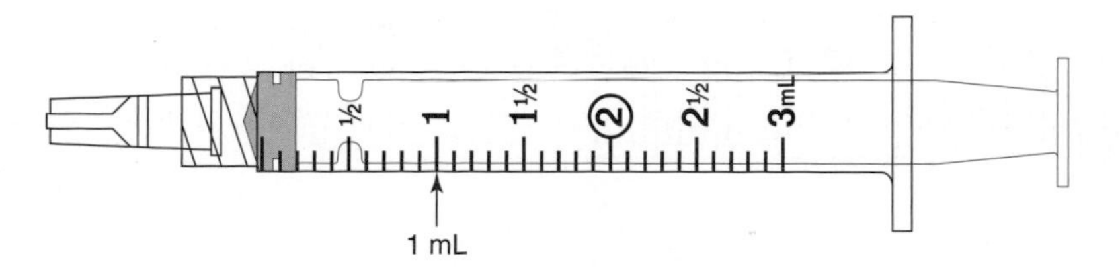

3) 0.4

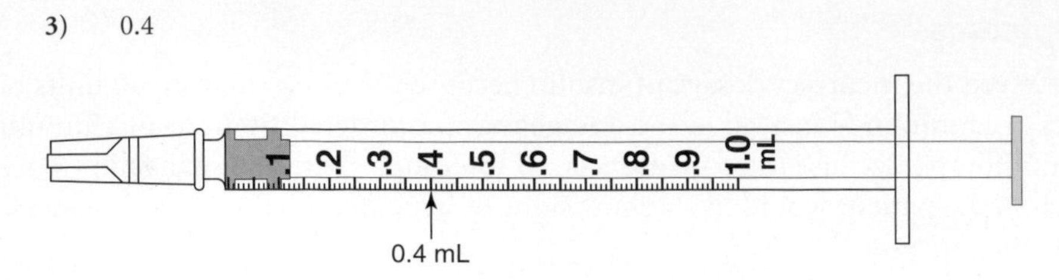

4) 0.15

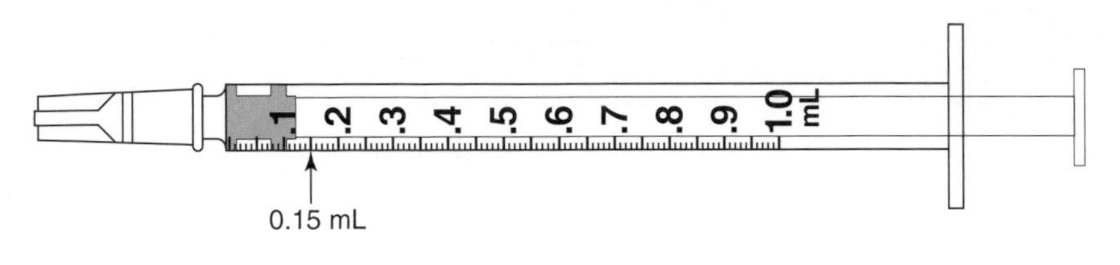

5) 2

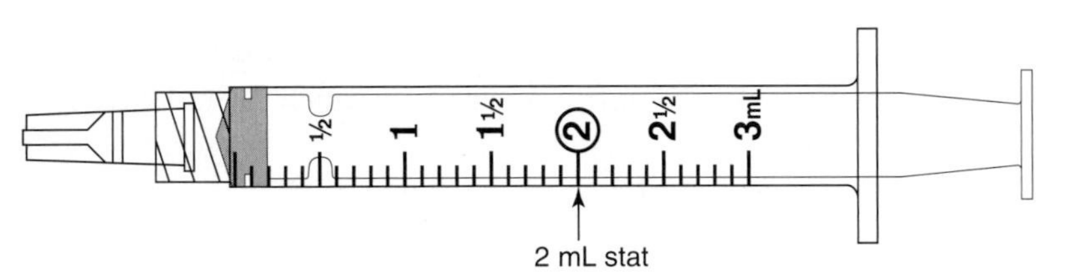

6) 0.35

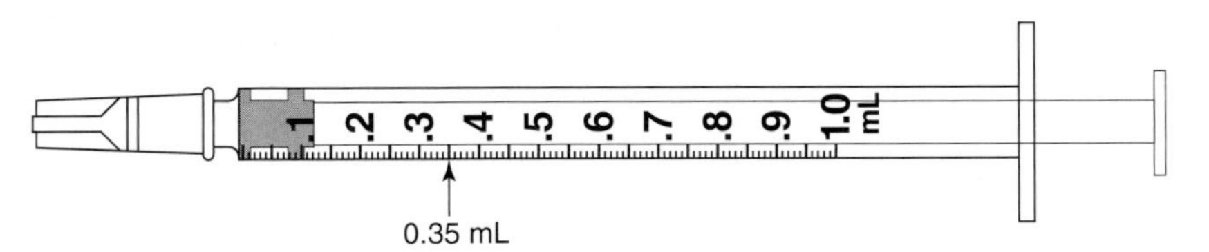

7) 1

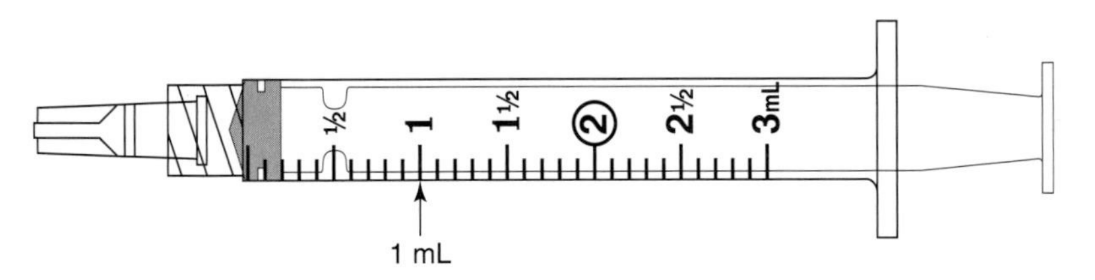

8) 0.7

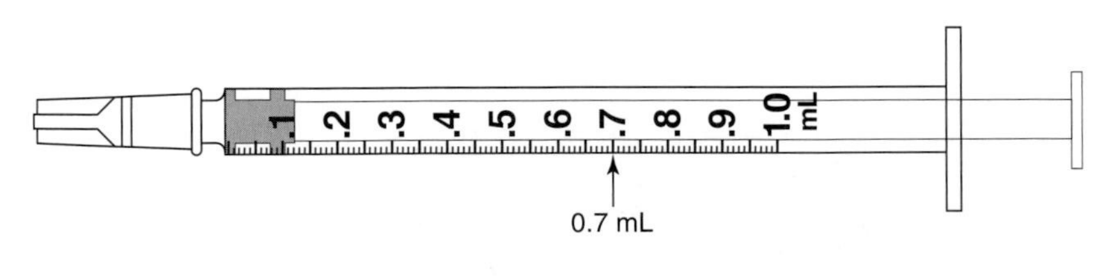

9) 4

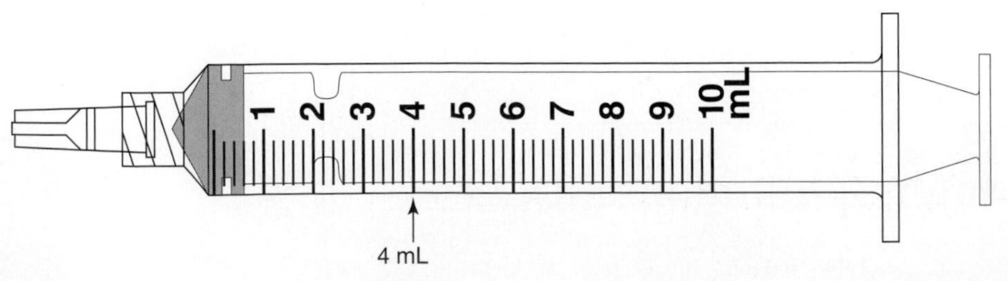

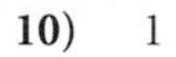

10) 1

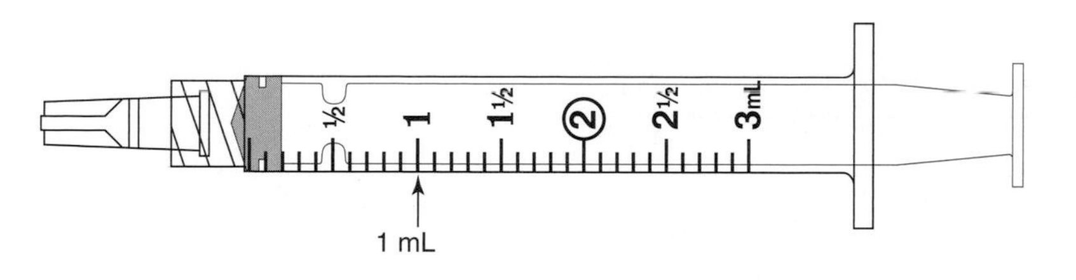

11) 0.75 mL

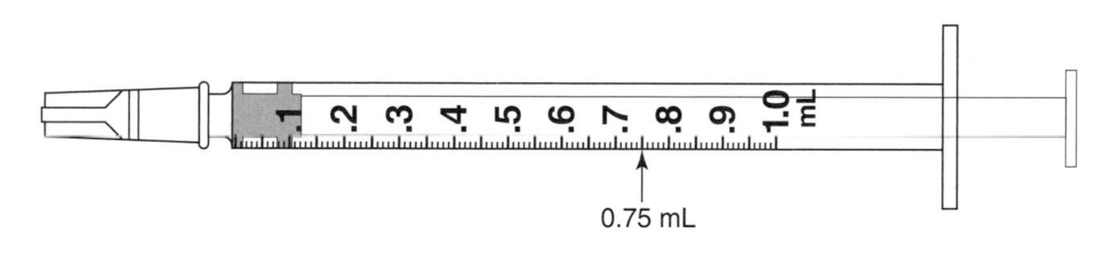

12) 0.4

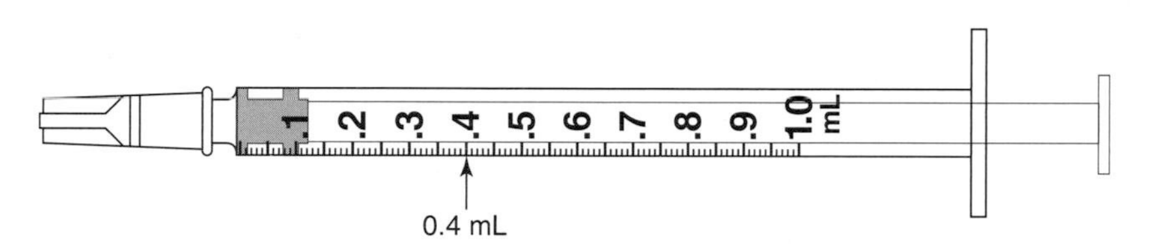

13) 2.5

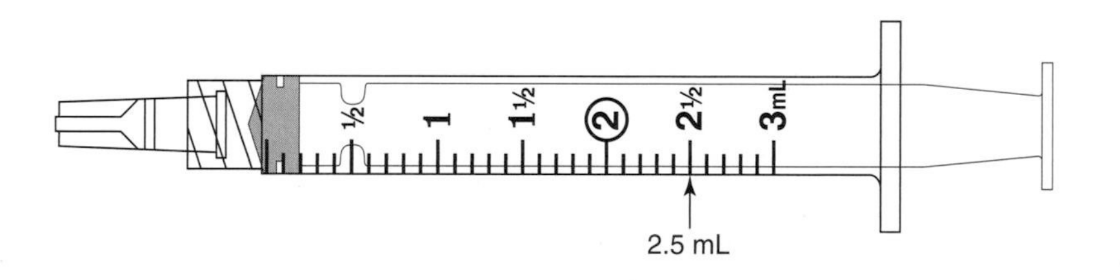

14) 0.5

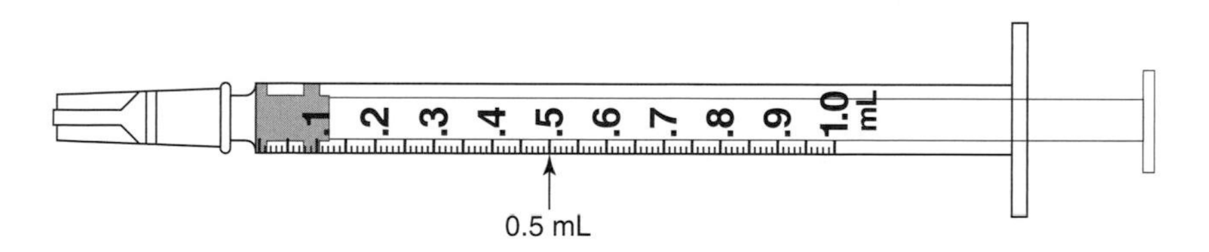

15) 0.5

16) 1.5

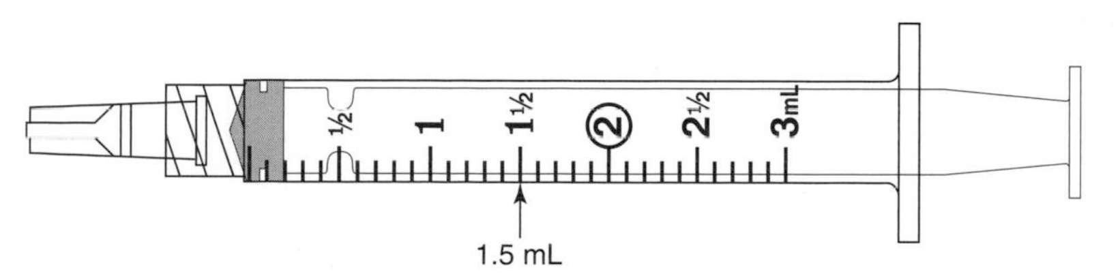

17) 0.5

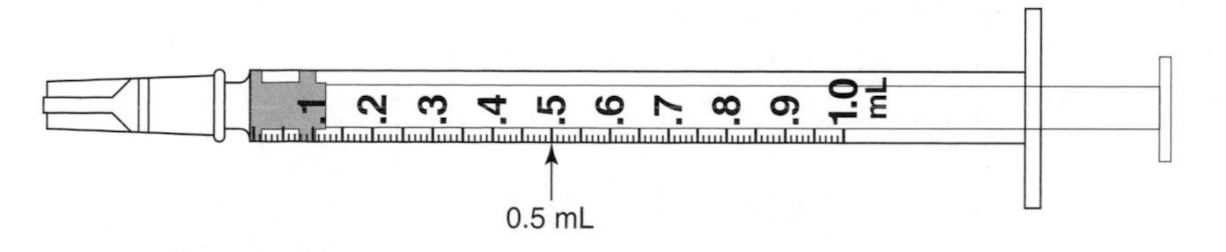

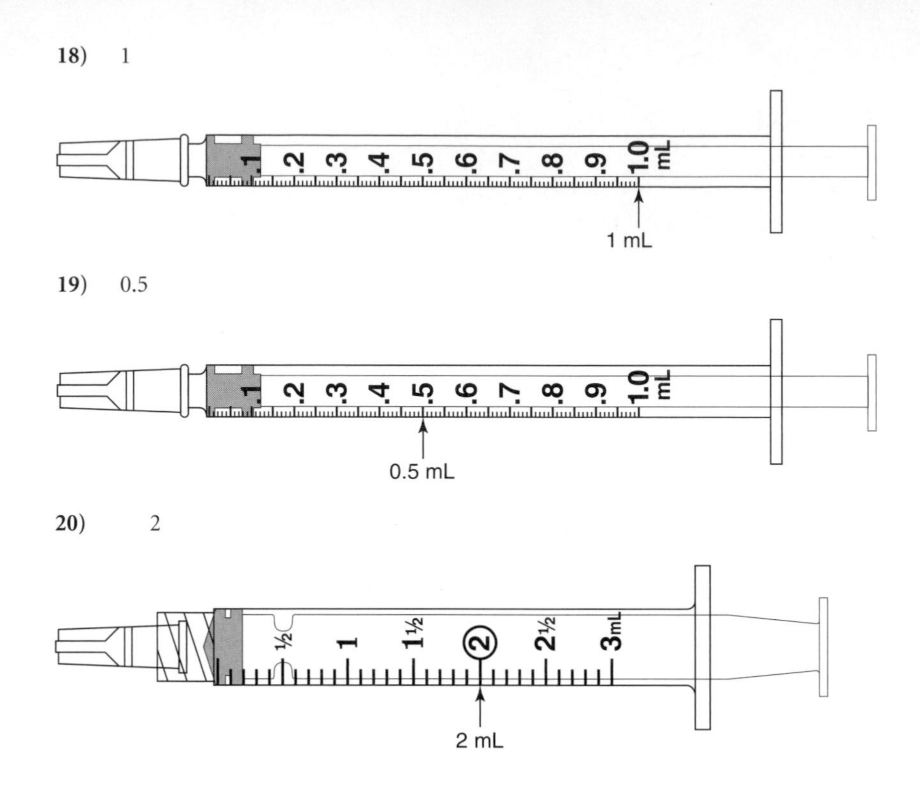

Review Set 9-2

1) C **2)** C **3)** B **4)** Humulin R, short-acting **5)** Novolin® ge NPH, intermediate-acting **6)** Levemir Penfill, long-acting **7)** Humalog, short-acting **8)** Humulin 30/70, short- and intermediate-acting **9)** Lo-dose 30, 30 units; lo-dose 50, 50 units; 100-unit syringe **10)** Lo-dose 30 **11)** Lo-dose 50 **12)** 100 units **13)** False **14)** A sliding insulin scale is the administration of a predetermined amount of short-acting insulin in response to hyperglycemia in a hospitalized patient; normal blood glucose level. **15)** An insulin pump or a continuous subcutaneous insulin infusion (CSII) is used to individualize insulin administration regimens based on the needs of the patient. It is considered to be a safe and effective way to deliver flexible insulin therapy using rapid-acting or short-acting insulins over a 24-hour period. **16)** 20 000 units **17)** 5000 units **18)** 7200 units **19)** No; the dose amount in the syringe is 68 units **20)** Yes; the dose amount in the syringe is 12 units **21)** No; the dose amount in the syringe is 32 units **22)** Yes; the dose amount in the syringe is 52 units **23)** 7.2 mL

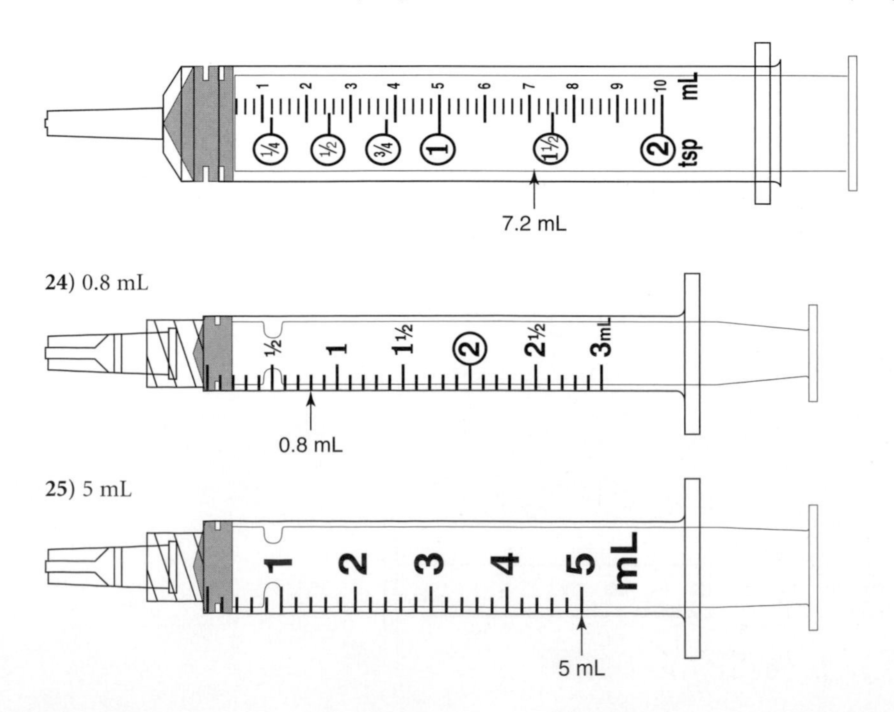

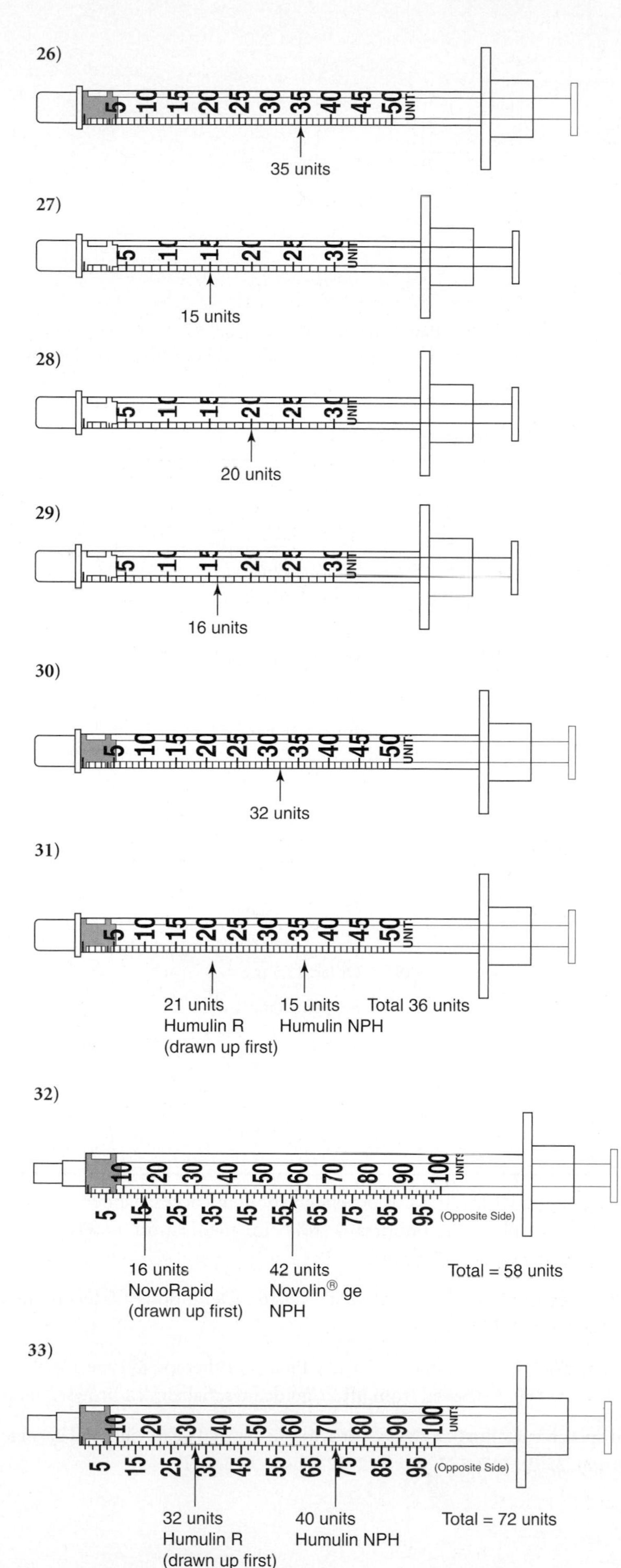
26)
35 units
27)
15 units
28)
20 units
29)
16 units
30)
32 units
31)
21 units
Humulin R
(drawn up first)
15 units
Humulin NPH
Total 36 units
32)
(Opposite Side)
16 units
NovoRapid
(drawn up first)
42 units
Novolin® ge
NPH
Total = 58 units
33)
(Opposite Side)
32 units
Humulin R
(drawn up first)
40 units
Humulin NPH
Total = 72 units

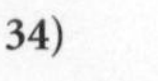

34)

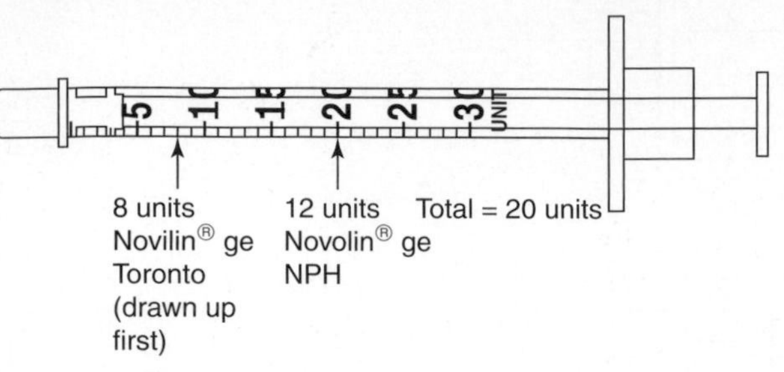

35) 5 units **36)** 39 units **37)** Before meals (before insulin administration) **38)** Blood glucose levels of 8 mmol to 19.9 mmol **39)** Give 4 units of Humulin R regular insulin **40)** None: do not administer insulin **41)** Give 10 units of insulin

SELECTED SOLUTIONS TO REVIEW SETS

Review Set 9-1

1) Order: 100 mg

Supply: 150 mg/mL

$$\frac{D}{H} \times Q = \frac{10\cancel{0}\ \text{mg}}{15\cancel{0}\ \text{mg}} \times 1\ \text{mL} = \frac{10}{15}\ \text{mL} = 0.67\ \text{mL}$$

2) Order: 10 units

Supply: 10 units/mL

$$\frac{D}{H} \times Q = \frac{10\ \text{units}}{10\ \text{units}} \times 1\ \text{mL} = 1\ \text{mL}$$

3) Order: 2 mg

Supply: 5 mg/mL

$$\frac{D}{H} \times Q = \frac{2\ \cancel{\text{mg}}}{5\ \cancel{\text{mg}}} \times 1\ \text{mL} = \frac{2}{5}\ \text{mL} = 0.4\ \text{mL}$$

6) Order: 3500 units

Supply: 10 000 units/mL

$$\frac{D}{H} \times Q = \frac{35\cancel{00}\ \cancel{\text{units}}}{10\ 0\cancel{00}\ \cancel{\text{units}}} \times 1\ \text{mL} = \frac{35}{100}\ \text{mL} = 0.35\ \text{mL}$$

9) Order: 40 mg

Supply: 10 mg/mL

$$\frac{D}{H} \times Q = \frac{40}{10} \times 1\ \text{mL} = 4\ \text{mL}$$

10) Order: 15 mg

Supply: 15 mg/mL

$$\frac{D}{H} \times Q = \frac{\cancel{15}\ \cancel{\text{mg}}}{\cancel{15}\ \cancel{\text{mg}}} \times 1\ \text{mL} = 1\ \text{mL}$$

11) Order: 15 mg

Supply: 20 mg/mL

$$\frac{D}{H} \times Q = \frac{\overset{3}{\cancel{15}}\ \cancel{\text{mg}}}{\underset{4}{\cancel{20}}\ \cancel{\text{mg}}} \times 1\ \text{mL} = \frac{3}{4}\ \text{mL} = 0.75\ \text{mL}$$

19) Order: 12.5 mg

Supply: 25 mg/1 mL

$$\frac{D}{H} \times Q = \frac{12.5\ \text{mg}}{25\ \text{mg}} \times 1\ \text{mL} = 0.5\ \text{mL}$$

REFERENCES

Institute for Safe Medication Practices. (ISMP). (2013). Independent double checks: Undervalued and misused: Selective use of this strategy can play an important role in medication safety. Retrieved from www.ismp.org/newsletters/acutecare/showarticle.aspx?id=51

Institute for Safe Medication Practices Canada. (ISMP Canada). (2016). Definitions of terms. Retrieved from www.ismp-canada.org/definitions.htm

McGibbon, A., Richardson, C., Hernandez, C., & Dornan, J. (2013). Pharmacotherapy in type 1 diabetes. *Canadian Journal of Diabetes, 37*(Suppl. 1), S56–S60. Retrieved from http://guidelines.diabetes.ca/browse/Chapter12

Spollett, G. R. (2012). Improved disposable insulin pen devices provide an alternative to vials and syringes for insulin administration. *Diabetes Spectrum*, 25(2), 117–122. doi:10.2337/diaspect.25.2.117

CHAPTER

10

Reconstitution of Solutions

OBJECTIVES

1. Define the terms *solvent/diluent*, *solute*, and *solution*.
2. Reconstitute and label medications supplied in powder or dry form.
3. Differentiate between alternative instructions for reconstitution, and select the correct set to prepare the dosage ordered.
4. Apply the Three-Step Approach to calculate accurate dosages.
5. Calculate the amount of solute and solvent needed to prepare a desired strength and quantity of an irrigating solution or enteral feeding.

Some parenteral and oral medications are supplied in powder form and must be mixed with water or some other liquid before administration. As more healthcare is provided in the home setting, nurses and other healthcare providers must dilute topical irrigants, soaks, and nutritional feedings. The process of mixing and diluting solutions is called *reconstitution.*

The process of reconstitution is comparable to the preparation of hot chocolate from a powdered mix. Adding the correct amount of hot water (called the *solvent* or *diluent*) to the package of powdered hot chocolate drink mix (called the *solute*) results in a tasty, hot beverage (the resulting *solution*).

The components of solutions are important concepts to learn. These concepts will be applied again with the administration of intravenous solutions.

SOLUTION COMPONENTS

Refer to Figures 10-1 and 10-2 and define the terms related to reconstitution.

- *Solute*—a substance to be dissolved or diluted. It can be in solid or liquid form.
- *Solvent*—a substance (liquid) that dissolves another substance to prepare a solution. *Diluent* is a synonymous term.
- *Solution*—the resulting mixture of a solute plus a solvent.

To prepare a therapeutic solution, it is necessary to add a solvent or diluent (usually normal saline or water) to a solute (solid substance or concentrated stock solution) to obtain the required strength of a stated volume of a solution. This means that the solid substance or concentrate, the solute, is diluted with a solvent to obtain a reconstituted solution of a weaker strength. However, the amount of the drug that is in the pure solute or concentrated stock solution still equals the amount of pure drug in the diluted solution. The solvent has simply been added to the solute, increasing the total volume.

In Figure 10-1, the amount of pure drug (solute) is the same in the concentrated form and in the resulting solution. However, in the solution, notice that the solute is dispersed throughout the resulting weaker solution.

The *strength* of a solution or *concentration* was briefly discussed in Chapters 7 and 8. The solution strength indicates the ratio of solute to solvent. Consider how each of these substances—solute and solvent—contributes a certain number of parts to the total solution.

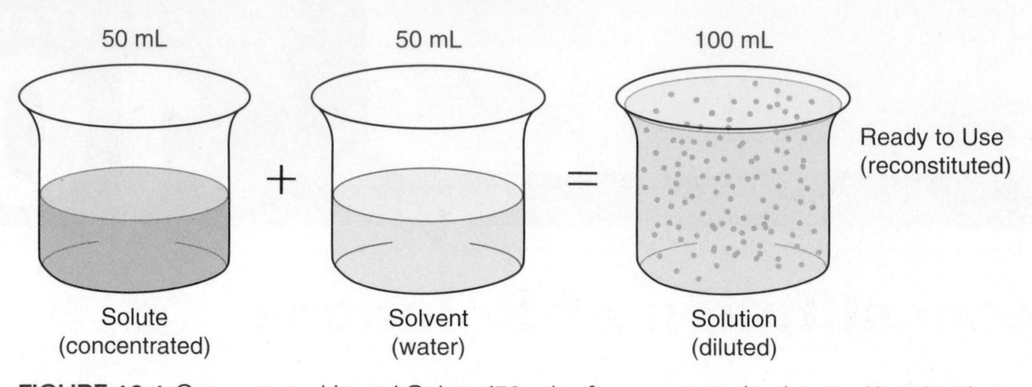

FIGURE 10-1 Concentrated Liquid Solute (50 mL of concentrated solute is diluted with 50 mL of solvent to make 100 mL of diluted solution.)

Examine the azithromycin dihydrate 500-mg label in Figure 10-2. Reconstitution directions may often be found on the label; however, the nurse may be referred to the package insert for detailed instructions for use, such as the insert shown here for azithromycin dihydrate. The insert directions advise that 4.8 mL of sterile water (solvent) should be added to the powder (solid solute) to prepare the reconstituted solution. As the insert indicates, the resulting supply dosage is 100 mg of azithromycin dihydrate per 1 mL of solution. It is also important to note that the prepared azithromycin must be further diluted in an appropriate diluent for intravenous administration. This step is usual for a medication that is given intermittently using a larger amount of fluid and administered over a longer period of time.

ZITHROMAX for Injection:

RECONSTITUTION OF ZITHROMAX FOR INJECTION				
Strength	Reconstitution Solution	Volume to be Added	Approximate Volume Available	Nominal Concentration
500 mg	Sterile Water for Injection	4.8 mL	5 mL	100 mg/mL

Prepare the initial solution of **ZITHROMAX** for Injection by adding 4.8 mL of Sterile Water for Injection to the 500 mg vial. Shake the vial until all of the drug is dissolved. Since the vial is evacuated, it is recommended that a standard 5 mL (non-automated) syringe be used to ensure that the exact volume of 4.8 mL is dispensed. Each mL of reconstituted solution contains azithromycin dihydrate equivalent to 100 mg azithromycin. Reconstituted solution is stable for 24 hours when stored below 30°C. **The reconstituted solution must be further diluted prior to administration.**

Dilution of reconstituted solution: To provide azithromycin over a concentration range of 1.0 - 2.0 mg/mL, transfer 5 mL of the 100 mg/mL azithromycin solution into the appropriate amount of the following diluents:

Final Infusion Concentration (mg/mL)	Amount of Diluent (mL)
1.0 mg/mL	500 mL
2.0 mg/mL	250 mL

Appropriate Diluents
0.9% Sodium Chloride Injection
5% Dextrose in Water for Injection
0.45% Sodium Chloride Injection
Lactated Ringer's Injection
5% Dextrose in 0.45% Sodium Chloride Injection with 20 mEq Potassium Chloride
5% Dextrose in Lactated Ringer's Injection
5% Dextrose in 0.3% Sodium Chloride Injection
5% Dextrose in 0.45% Sodium Chloride Injection
Normosol-M in 5% Dextrose

Diluted solutions prepared in this manner are stable for 24 hours at or below room temperature (30°C), or for 72 hours if stored under refrigeration (5°C). As with all parenteral drug products, intravenous admixtures should be inspected visually for clarity, particulate matter, precipitate, discoloration and leakage prior to administration, whenever solution and container permit. Solutions showing haziness, particulate matter, precipitate, discoloration or leakage should be discarded.

Only limited data are available on the compatibility of **ZITHROMAX** for Injection with other intravenous substances, therefore additives or other medications should not be added to **ZITHROMAX** for Injection or infused simultaneously through the same intravenous line. If the same intravenous line is used for sequential infusion of several different drugs, the line should be flushed before and after infusion of **ZITHROMAX** for Injection with an infusion solution compatible with **ZITHROMAX** for Injection and with any other drug(s) administered via the common line. If **ZITHROMAX** for Injection is to be given concomitantly with another drug, each drug should be given separately in accordance with the recommended dosage and route of administration for each drug.

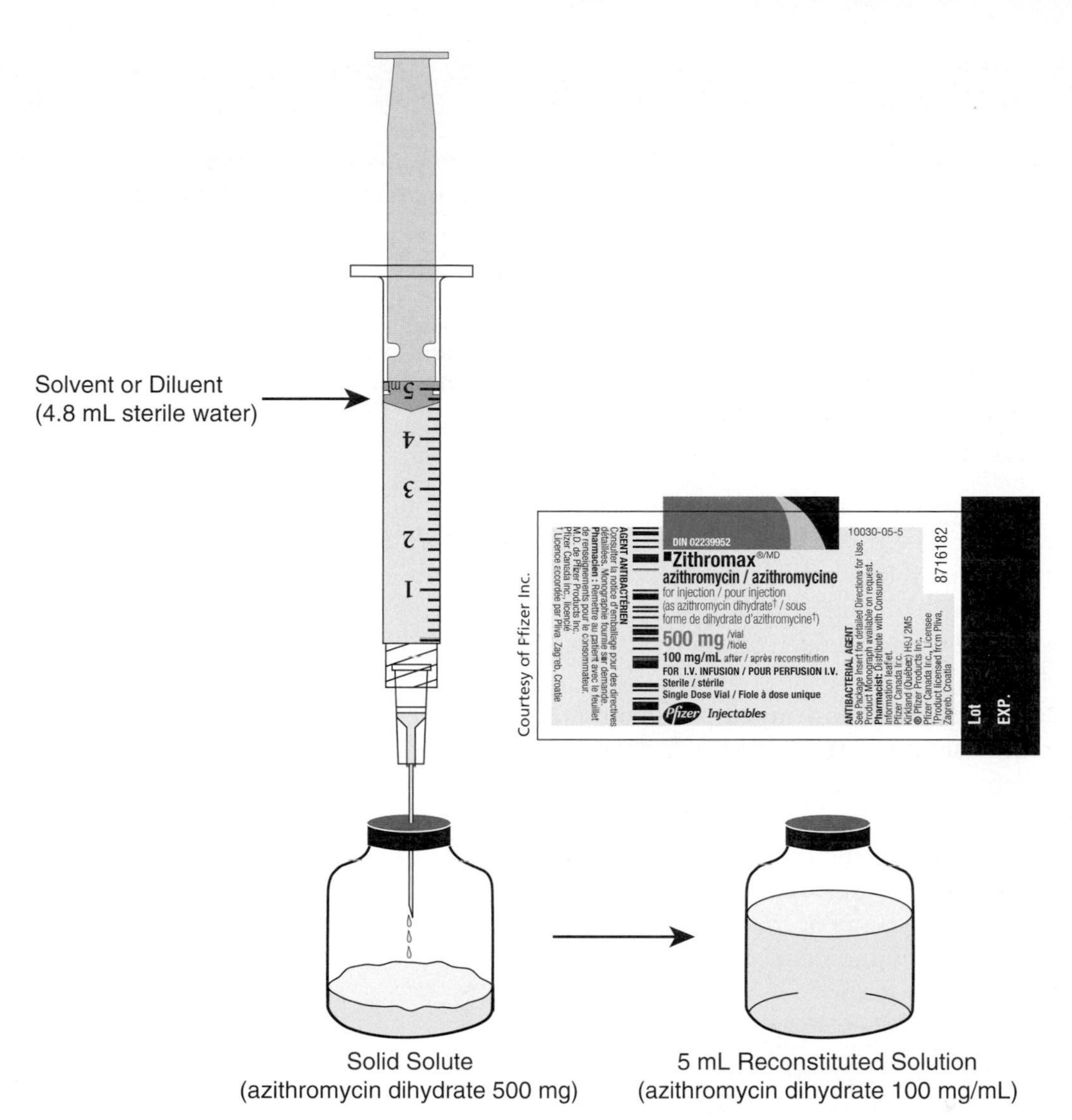

FIGURE 10-2 Solid Solute. The solid powder form of 500 mg of azithromycin dihydrate is reconstituted with 4.8 mL of sterile water as the diluent to make 5 mL of azithromycin dihydrate IV solution with the supply dosage of 100 mg/mL.

RECONSTITUTION OF INJECTABLE MEDICATIONS IN POWDER FORM

Some medications are unstable when stored in solution or liquid form. Thus, they are packaged in powdered form and must be dissolved or reconstituted by a liquid solvent or diluent and mixed thoroughly just prior to administration. Reconstitution is a necessary step in medication preparation to create a measurable and usable dosage form. The pharmacist often completes this step before dispensing liquid medications, for oral as well as parenteral routes. However, nurses must understand reconstitution and the steps to accomplish it.

CAUTION

Before reconstituting injectable drugs, read and follow the label or package insert directions carefully, including checking the drug and diluent expiry dates. Consult a pharmacist if you have any questions.

There are standard principles for reconstituting injectable medications from powder to liquid form. Follow these principles carefully to ensure that the patient receives the correct dosage of the intended solution.

RATIONALE FOR PRACTICE

When reconstituting injectable medications, determine both the *type* and *amount* of diluent to be used. Carefully read the instructions for reconstitution on either the drug label or the package insert. The manufacturer of the drug provides information about the amount of diluent or solvent to be added, as well as the type of diluent (see, e.g., the azithromycin dihydrate insert in Figure 10-2). The concentration of the reconstituted drug is also indicated on the label, as is the expiry date or the time the drug remains usable. Remember that the route of administration may dictate the amount of diluent to be used for reconstitution (e.g., a drug may have different concentrations depending on whether it is intended for intravenous or intramuscular use).

Some powdered medications are packaged by the manufacturer with special diluents for reconstitution. Sterile water and 0.9% sodium chloride (normal saline) prepared for injection are the most commonly used diluents in parenteral medications. Both sterile water (Figure 10-3) and normal saline are available *preservative-free* when intended for single use only, as well as in *bacteriostatic* form with preservative when intended for more than one use. Carefully check the instructions, expiry date, and vial label or drug insert for the appropriate diluent.

Because many reconstituted parenteral medications can be administered either intramuscularly or intravenously, it is essential to verify the route of administration before reconstituting the medication. Remember that the intramuscular volume per injection site is determined by the patient's age and condition and the intramuscular site selected. The directions take these factors into account by including the minimum volume or quantity of diluent that should be added to the powdered drug for intramuscular use. The powder displaces the liquid as it dissolves and increases the resulting total volume. This resulting volume of the reconstituted drug is usually provided on the label. The resulting volume determines the liquid's concentration or supply dosage.

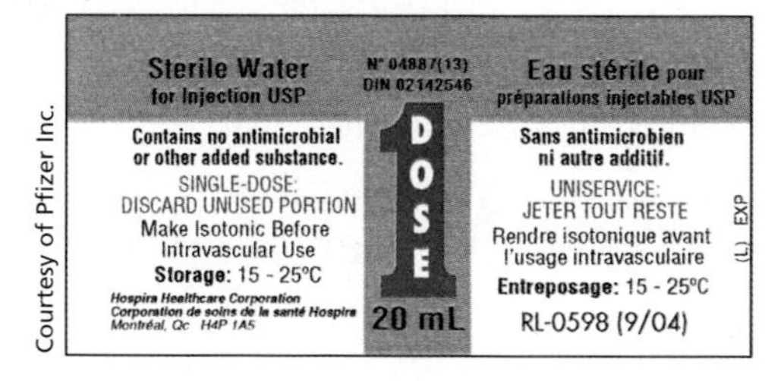

FIGURE 10-3 Reconstitution Diluent for Parenteral Powdered Drugs

RATIONALE FOR PRACTICE

When reconstituting injectable medications, determine the volume in mL of diluent to be used for the route as ordered, then reconstitute the drug and note the resulting supply dosage on the vial.

The drug label provides the amount of diluent for reconstitution but not the type of diluent; therefore, the package insert is consulted for the type of diluent. The instructions from the package insert for cefazolin reconstitution are as follows: "Reconstitution: IM: add 2 mL 0.9% Sodium Chloride Injection. Provides 225 mg/mL." The label provides the amount of diluent but not the type of diluent to be used, so be sure to consult the package insert. Note that when 2 mL of diluent is added and the powder is dissolved, the powder adds an additional 0.2 mL for a total solution volume of 2.2 mL. (The amount of diluent added will vary with each medication.) Thus, the supply dosage available after reconstitution is *225 mg of cefazolin per mL of solution.* Figure 10-4(b) illustrates the reconstitution procedure for cefazolin 500 mg, to fill the order for *cefazolin 225 mg IM q6h.*

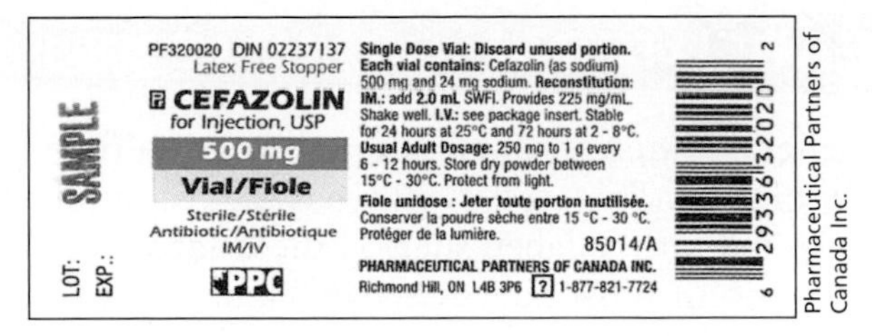

FIGURE 10-4(a) Cefazolin 500 mg Powder

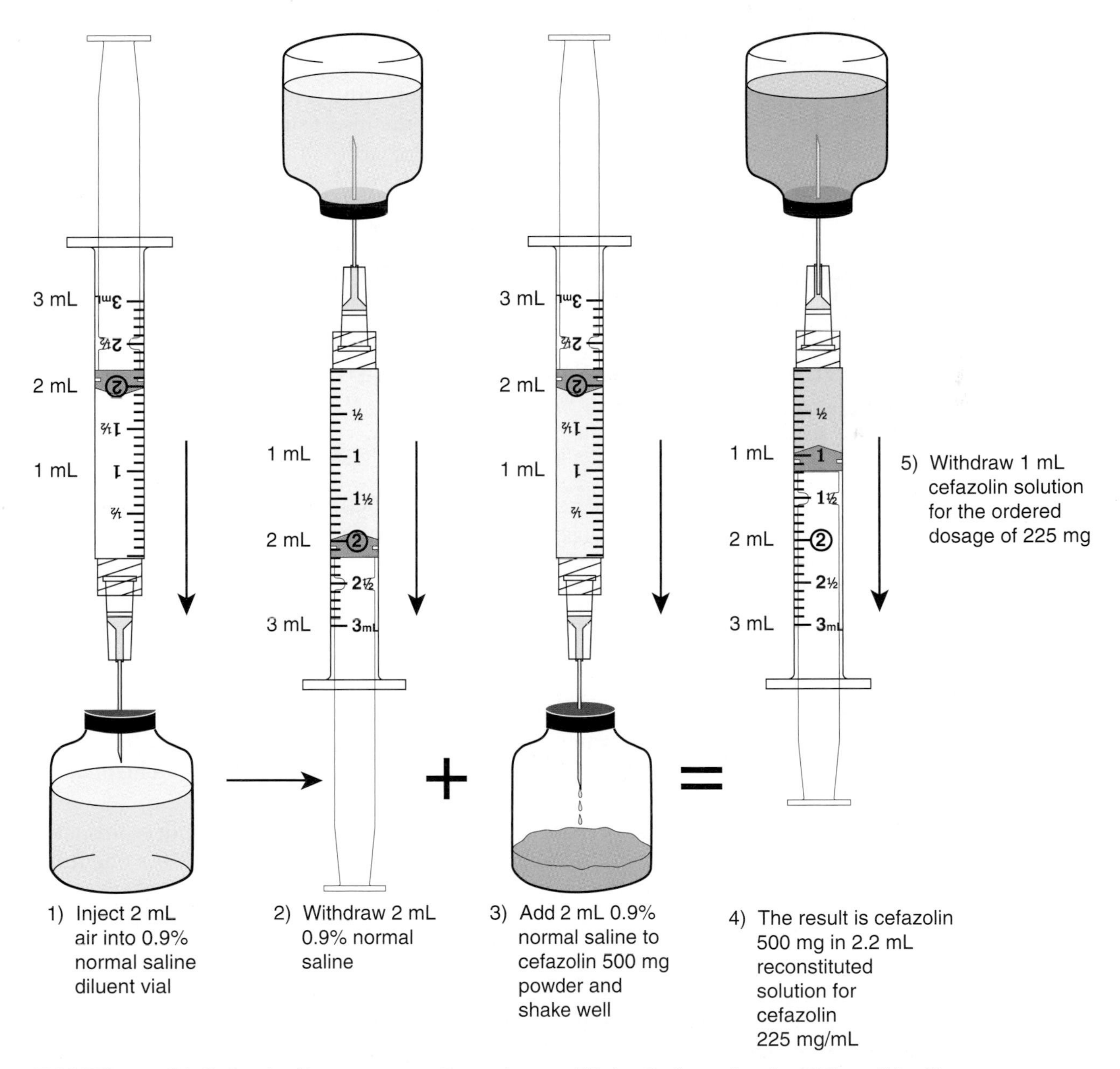

FIGURE 10-4(b) Cefazolin Reconstitution Procedure to Fill the Order *cefazolin 225 mg IM q6h*

Single-dose vials contain only enough medication for one dose, and the resulting contents are administered after the powder is diluted. In some cases, however, the nurse may also dilute a powdered medication in a multiple-dose vial that will yield more than one dose. In this case, it is important to check the package insert or label for drug stability and storage recommendations to clearly label the vial after reconstitution. Labelling is discussed in the next section.

TYPES OF RECONSTITUTED PARENTERAL SOLUTIONS

There are two types of reconstituted parenteral solutions: single strength and multiple strength. The simplest type to dilute is a *single-strength* solution. This type usually has the recommended dilution directions and resulting supply dosage printed on the label, such as the cefazolin 500 mg label in Figure 10-4(a) (page 251) and the azithromycin dihydrate insert in Figure 10-5. Single-dose or single-use vials are labelled as such by the manufacturer because they typically lack an antimicrobial preservative.

Some medications have several directions for dilution that allow the nurse to select the best supply dosage. This type of medication is called a *multiple-strength* solution and requires even more careful reading of the instructions. See, for example, the penicillin G sodium label shown in Figure 10-6 (page 255). Because these directions for reconstitution will not fit on the vial label, the nurse must consult the package insert or other printed instructions to ensure accurate dilution of the parenteral medication. When reading the insert or other instructions, the nurse must use clinical judgment to make a clinical decision regarding the relevant factors. For example, the nurse must consider the route of administration, the type of diluent, the dose ordered, the dosage amount required, the age of the patient, and the drug concentration and volume available that is close to the amount of the ordered dose for the route of administration.

Let us look at some examples to clarify what the healthcare provider needs to do to correctly reconstitute and calculate dosages of parenteral medications supplied in powder form.

Single-Strength Solution/Single-Dose Vial

Example 1:

Order: *azithromycin dihydrate 400 mg IV daily × 2 days*

Supply: The directions on the package insert of a 500-mg vial of powdered azithromycin dihydrate read, "Reconstitute to 100 mg/mL with 4.8 mL of sterile water for injection"; see Figure 10-5(b).

Carefully read and analyze the information provided on the insert.

- First, how much and what type of diluent must you add? The directions are to *add 4.8 mL of sterile water.*
- Second, what is the resulting supply dosage or concentration? When reconstituted, the *supply dosage is azithromycin dihydrate 100 mg/mL.*
- Third, what is the resulting total volume of the reconstituted solution? The *total volume is 5 mL.* The powder added 0.2 mL to the solution.
- Finally, to fill the order as prescribed, how many full doses are available in this vial? The order is for 400 mg and the single-dose vial contains 500 mg. This is enough for one full dose, but not enough for two full doses.

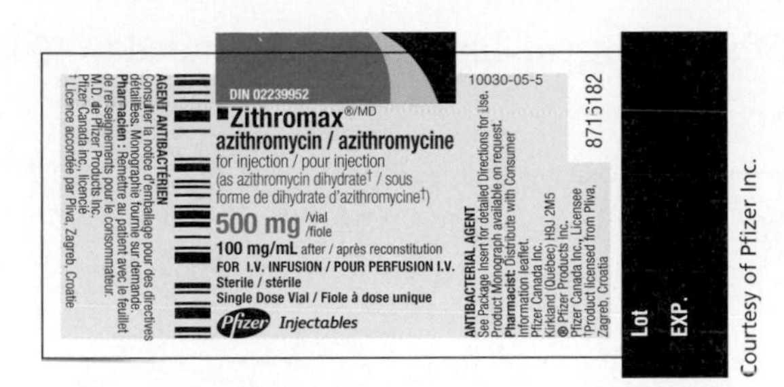

Courtesy of Pfizer Inc.

Now, put it all together.

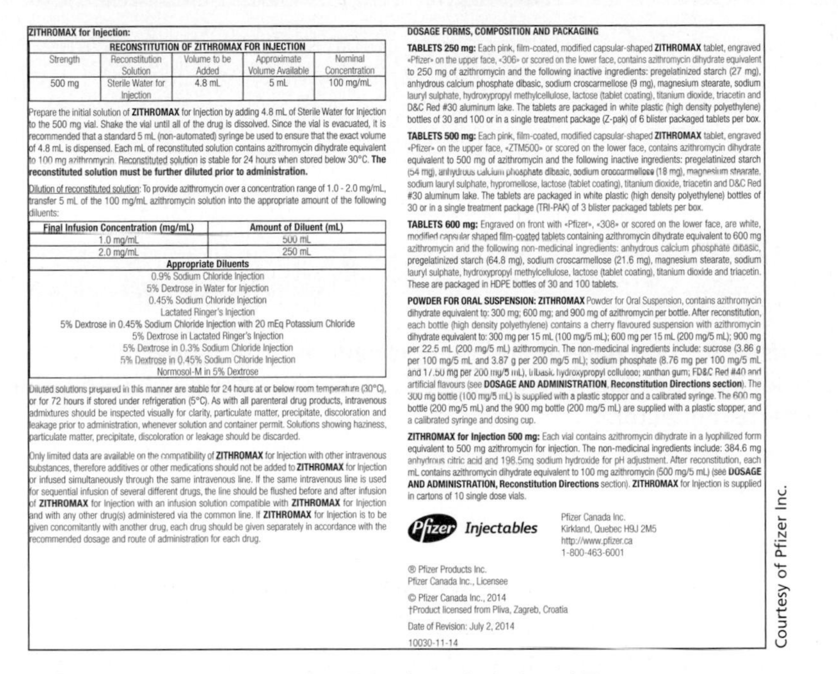

ZITHROMAX for Injection:

RECONSTITUTION OF ZITHROMAX FOR INJECTION				
Strength	Reconstitution Solution	Volume to be Added	Approximate Volume Available	Nominal Concentration
500 mg	Sterile Water for Injection	4.8 mL	5 mL	100 mg/mL

Prepare the initial solution of **ZITHROMAX** for Injection by adding 4.8 mL of Sterile Water for Injection to the 500 mg vial. Shake the vial until all of the drug is dissolved. Since the vial is evacuated, it is recommended that a standard 5 mL (non-automated) syringe be used to ensure that the exact volume of 4.8 mL is dispensed. Each mL of reconstituted solution contains azithromycin dihydrate equivalent to 100 mg azithromycin. Reconstituted solution is stable for 24 hours when stored below 30°C. **The reconstituted solution must be further diluted prior to administration.**

Dilution of reconstituted solution: To provide azithromycin over a concentration range of 1.0 - 2.0 mg/mL, transfer 5 mL of the 100 mg/mL azithromycin solution into the appropriate amount of the following diluents:

Final Infusion Concentration (mg/mL)	Amount of Diluent (mL)
1.0 mg/mL	500 mL
2.0 mg/mL	250 mL
Appropriate Diluents	
0.9% Sodium Chloride Injection	
5% Dextrose in Water for Injection	
0.45% Sodium Chloride Injection	
Lactated Ringer's Injection	
5% Dextrose in 0.45% Sodium Chloride Injection with 20 mEq Potassium Chloride	
5% Dextrose in Lactated Ringer's Injection	
5% Dextrose in 0.3% Sodium Chloride Injection	
5% Dextrose in 0.45% Sodium Chloride Injection	
Normosol-M in 5% Dextrose	

Diluted solutions prepared in this manner are stable for 24 hours at or below room temperature (30°C), or for 72 hours if stored under refrigeration (5°C). As with all parenteral drug products, intravenous admixtures should be inspected visually for clarity, particulate matter, precipitate, discoloration and leakage prior to administration, whenever solution and container permit. Solutions showing haziness, particulate matter, precipitate, discoloration or leakage should be discarded.

Only limited data are available on the compatibility of **ZITHROMAX** for Injection with other intravenous substances, therefore additives or other medications should not be added to **ZITHROMAX** for Injection or infused simultaneously through the same intravenous line. If the same intravenous line is used for sequential infusion of several different drugs, the line should be flushed before and after infusion of **ZITHROMAX** for Injection with an infusion solution compatible with **ZITHROMAX** for Injection and with any other drug(s) administered via the common line. If **ZITHROMAX** for Injection is to be given concomitantly with another drug, each drug should be given separately in accordance with the recommended dosage and route of administration for each drug.

DOSAGE FORMS, COMPOSITION AND PACKAGING

TABLETS 250 mg: Each pink, film-coated, modified capsular-shaped **ZITHROMAX** tablet, engraved «Pfizer» on the upper face, «306» or scored on the lower face, contains azithromycin dihydrate equivalent to 250 mg of azithromycin and the following inactive ingredients: pregelatinized starch (27 mg), anhydrous calcium phosphate dibasic, sodium croscarmellose (9 mg), magnesium stearate, sodium lauryl sulphate, hydroxypropyl methylcellulose, lactose (tablet coating), titanium dioxide, triacetin and D&C Red #30 aluminum lake. The tablets are packaged in white plastic (high density polyethylene) bottles of 30 and 100 or in a single treatment package (Z-pak) of 6 blister packaged tablets per box.

TABLETS 500 mg: Each pink, film-coated, modified capsular-shaped **ZITHROMAX** tablet, engraved «Pfizer» on the upper face, «ZTM500» or scored on the lower face, contains azithromycin dihydrate equivalent to 500 mg of azithromycin and the following inactive ingredients: pregelatinized starch (54 mg), anhydrous calcium phosphate dibasic, sodium croscarmellose (18 mg), magnesium stearate, sodium lauryl sulphate, hypromellose, lactose (tablet coating), titanium dioxide, triacetin and D&C Red #30 aluminum lake. The tablets are packaged in white plastic (high density polyethylene) bottles of 30 or in a single treatment package (TRI-PAK) of 3 blister packaged tablets per box.

TABLETS 600 mg: Engraved on front with «Pfizer», «308» or scored on the lower face, are white, modified capsular shaped film-coated tablets containing azithromycin dihydrate equivalent to 600 mg azithromycin and the following non-medicinal ingredients: anhydrous calcium phosphate dibasic, pregelatinized starch (64.8 mg), sodium croscarmellose (21.6 mg), magnesium stearate, sodium lauryl sulphate, hydroxypropyl methylcellulose, lactose (tablet coating), titanium dioxide and triacetin. These are packaged in HDPE bottles of 30 and 100 tablets.

POWDER FOR ORAL SUSPENSION: ZITHROMAX Powder for Oral Suspension, contains azithromycin dihydrate equivalent to: 300 mg; 600 mg; and 900 mg of azithromycin per bottle. After reconstitution, each bottle (high density polyethylene) contains a cherry flavoured suspension with azithromycin dihydrate equivalent to: 300 mg per 15 mL (100 mg/5 mL); 600 mg per 15 mL (200 mg/5 mL); 900 mg per 22.5 mL (200 mg/5 mL) azithromycin. The non-medicinal ingredients include: sucrose (3.86 g per 100 mg/5 mL and 3.87 g per 200 mg/5 mL); sodium phosphate (8.76 mg per 100 mg/5 mL and 17.50 mg per 200 mg/5 mL), tribasic hydroxypropyl cellulose; xanthan gum; FD&C Red #40 and artificial flavours (see **DOSAGE AND ADMINISTRATION**, **Reconstitution Directions section**). The 300 mg bottle (100 mg/5 mL) is supplied with a plastic stopper and a calibrated syringe. The 600 mg bottle (200 mg/5 mL) and the 900 mg bottle (200 mg/5 mL) are supplied with a plastic stopper, and a calibrated syringe and dosing cup.

ZITHROMAX for Injection 500 mg: Each vial contains azithromycin dihydrate in a lyophilized form equivalent to 500 mg azithromycin for injection. The non-medicinal ingredients include: 384.6 mg anhydrous citric acid and 198.5mg sodium hydroxide for pH adjustment. After reconstitution, each mL contains azithromycin dihydrate equivalent to 100 mg azithromycin (500 mg/5 mL) (see **DOSAGE AND ADMINISTRATION, Reconstitution Directions** section). **ZITHROMAX** for Injection is supplied in cartons of 10 single dose vials.

Pfizer Injectables

Pfizer Canada Inc.
Kirkland, Quebec H9J 2M5
http://www.pfizer.ca
1-800-463-6001

® Pfizer Products Inc.
Pfizer Canada Inc., Licensee

†Product licensed from Pliva, Zagreb, Croatia

Date of Revision: July 2, 2014

10030-11-14

Courtesy of Pfizer Inc.

FIGURE 10-5 Azithromycin Dihydrate Label and Reconstitution Instructions from the Package Insert. Single-Dose Vial

A vial of 500 mg of azithromycin dihydrate is available, to which 4.8 mL of sterile water is added as the diluent. The powdered drug displaces 0.2 mL. The resulting 5 mL of the solution contains 500 mg of the drug, and there are 100 mg of azithromycin dihydrate in each 1 mL of solution.

After reconstitution, you are ready to apply the Three-Step Approach to dosage calculation that you learned in Chapters 8 and 9.

Step 1 Convert No conversion is necessary.

Order: *azithromycin dihydrate 400 mg IV daily × 2 days*

Supply: 100 mg/mL

Step 2 Think You want to give more than 1 mL. In fact, you want to give 4 times 1 mL.

Step 3 Calculate $\frac{D}{H} \times Q = \frac{\overset{4}{\cancel{400\text{ mg}}}}{\underset{1}{\cancel{100\text{ mg}}}} \times 1\text{ mL} = \frac{4}{1}\text{ mL} = 4\text{ mL}$; give 4 mL azithromycin dihydrate reconstituted to 100 mg/mL intravenously each day for 2 days

This vial of azithromycin dihydrate 500 mg contains one full ordered dose of reconstituted drug. Any remaining medication is usually discarded. Because this vial provides only one dose, no label or storage of any of the reconstituted drug is required.

Select a 5-mL syringe and measure 4 mL of azithromycin dihydrate reconstituted to 100 mg/mL.

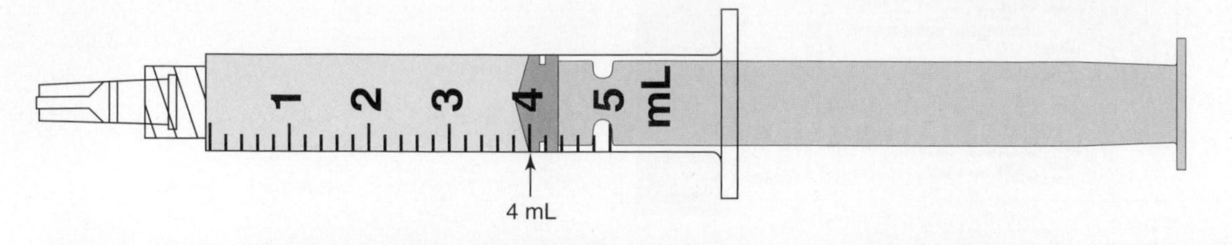

CAUTION

The reconstituted vial must be further diluted prior to administration. The 4 mL prescribed dosage can be withdrawn from the vial of 100 mg/mL azithromycin solution and injected into the appropriate amount (either 250 mL or 500 mL) of the appropriate diluent (see insert), and then infused into the patient over a specified time/rate once daily for 2 days.

RATIONALE FOR PRACTICE

Single-use vials are used for one patient and one procedure, with a new, clean needle and syringe. After the procedure has been completed, the vial and syringe should be discarded in the appropriate sharps collector.

Example 2:

Suppose the drug order reads *azithromycin dihydrate 250 mg IV daily*.

Using the same size vial of azithromycin dihydrate and the same dilution instructions as in Example 1, you now have two full doses of azithromycin dihydrate. However, this is not a multiple-dose vial. Because this particular drug is contained in a single-use vial, the remaining drug and vial are discarded.

$$\frac{D}{H} \times Q = \frac{25\not{0} \cancel{mg}}{10\not{0} \cancel{mg}} \times 1\,mL = 2.5\,mL$$

Select a 3-mL syringe and measure 2.5 mL of azithromycin dihydrate reconstituted to 100 mg/mL.

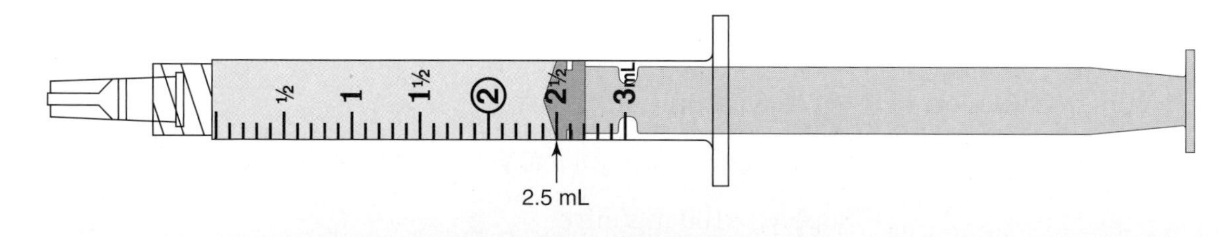

CAUTION

The reconstituted vial must be further diluted prior to administration. The 2.5 mL prescribed dosage can be withdrawn from the vial of 100 mg/mL azithromycin solution and injected into the appropriate amount (either 250 mL or 500 mL) of the appropriate diluent (see insert), then infused into the patient over a specified time/rate once daily. Also note that according to the insert, the reconstituted solution is stable for 24 hours at or below 30°C, or for 72 hours if refrigerated (5°C). This means before the vial has been punctured with a needle. Once punctured: **For single-use only. Discard any unused portion after use**.

The Multi-Dose Vial

A multi-dose vial is a vial of liquid medication intended for parenteral administration (by injection or intravenous infusion) that contains more than one dose of medication. Multi-dose vials typically contain an antimicrobial preservative to help prevent the growth of bacteria. This preservative has no effect on viruses and does not protect against contamination when safe injection practices are not followed.

Multi-dose vials are dedicated to a single patient whenever possible. If multiple doses result from the reconstitution of a powdered drug, the solution must be used in a timely manner. Because the drug potency (or stability) may be several hours to several days, check the drug label, package information sheet, or hospital formulary for the length of time that the drug may be used after reconstitution. Store the drug appropriately: at room temperature or refrigerate according to the manufacturer's instructions.

RATIONALE FOR PRACTICE

When reconstituting multiple-dose injectable medications, verify the length of drug potency. Store the reconstituted drug appropriately with a reconstitution label attached.

CAUTION

The length of potency is different from the expiry date. The expiry date is provided by the manufacturer on the label. It indicates the *last* date the drug may be reconstituted and used.

When you reconstitute or mix a multiple-dose vial of medication in powdered form, it is important that the vial be clearly labelled with the *date* and *time* of preparation, the strength or *supply dosage* you prepared, *length of potency*, *storage directions*, and your *initials*. Because the medication becomes unstable after storage for long periods, the date and time are especially important.

The Multiple-Strength Solution

Some parenteral powdered medications have directions for preparing several different solution strengths, to allow you to select a particular dosage strength (Figure 10-6). This results in a reasonable amount to be given to a particular patient.

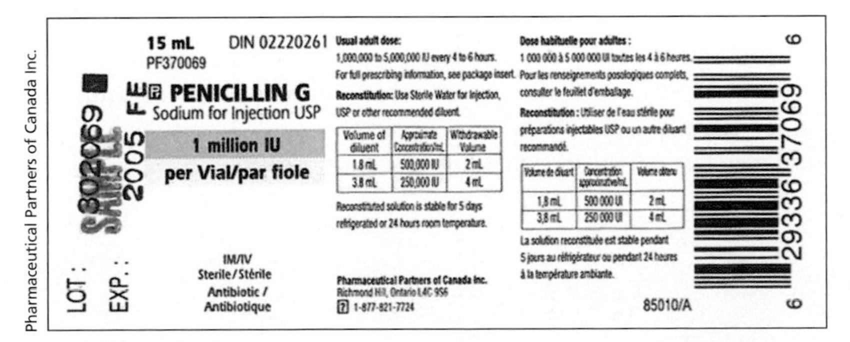

Pharmaceutical Partners of Canada Inc.

FIGURE 10-6 Penicillin G Sodium Label

Example:

Order: *penicillin G sodium 300 000 units IM QID*

Supply: penicillin G sodium 1 000 000-unit vial

This vial contains a total of 1 000 000 units of penicillin G sodium. The reconstitution instructions are shown on the right side of the label. The instructions detail two different parenteral solution supply dosages or concentrations that are determined by the added diluent volume. Examine each of the two instructions. Notice how these reconstituted concentrations differ and when each might be selected.

Add 1.8 mL of Diluent

The first set of directions instructs you to add 1.8 mL diluent for a solution concentration of 500 000 units/mL. Examine this information.

- First, how much and what type of diluent must be added? According to the directions, add 1.8 mL of diluent. (Check the package insert to determine the type of diluent because complete information is not stated on the label. Use sterile water for injection, isotonic sodium chloride injection, or dextrose injection.)
- Second, what is the supply dosage of the reconstituted penicillin G sodium? When adding 1.8 mL of diluent, the supply dosage is 500 000 units/mL.
- Third, what is the resulting total volume of this reconstituted solution? The total volume is 2 mL. This is because we are adding 1.8 mL of diluent and 0.2 mL of powder. The powder displaces 0.2 mL of the solution. (Notice that this solution is the most concentrated, or the strongest, of the 4 concentrations.)
- Finally, how many full doses of penicillin G sodium are available in this vial? The vial contains 1 000 000 units and the order is for 300 000 units. Regardless of the concentration, there are three full doses (plus some extra) in this vial.

This means that when you add 1.8 mL of diluent to this vial of powdered penicillin, the result is a concentration of 500 000 units of penicillin G sodium per mL.

Apply the Three-Step Approach to dosage calculation.

Step 1 Convert No conversion is necessary.

Order: *penicillin G sodium 300 000 units IM QID*

Supply: 500 000 units/mL

Step 2 Think You want to give less than 1 mL.

Step 3 Calculate

$$\frac{D}{H} \times Q = \frac{\overset{3}{\cancel{300\,000}}\ \cancel{\text{units}}}{\underset{5}{\cancel{500\,000}}\ \cancel{\text{units}}} \times 1\ \text{mL} = \frac{3}{5}\ \text{mL} = 0.6\ \text{mL}$$

Because each dose is 0.6 mL and the total volume is 2 mL, you would have enough for two additional full doses. This supply dosage will result in a reasonable volume for an intramuscular injection for an infant, a small child, or anyone with wasted muscle mass.

Select a *3-mL syringe, and measure 0.6 mL* of penicillin G sodium reconstituted to 500 000 units/mL.

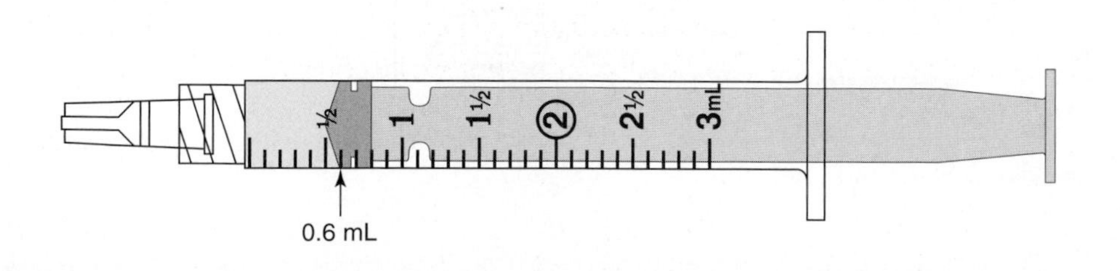

Finally, add a label to the reconstituted penicillin G sodium 500 000-unit/mL vial (Figure 10-7).

30/01/xx, 0800, reconstituted as 500 000 units/mL. Expires 06/02/xx, 0800, keep refrigerated. B.S.

FIGURE 10-7 Reconstitution Label for Penicillin G Sodium 1 000 000 Units with 1.8 mL Diluent

Add 3.8 mL of Diluent

Refer to the second set of directions on the penicillin label, which are to add 3.8 mL of diluent for 250 000 units per millilitre of solution. Would this set of directions prepare an appropriate concentration to fill the order?

What is different about this set of directions? Analyze the information provided on the label.

- First, how much and what type of diluent must be added? The directions are to add 3.8 mL of diluent. (Remember, check the package insert to determine the type of diluent because the only recommendation on the label is for sterile water for injection. Use isotonic sodium chloride injection or dextrose injection.)
- Second, what is the supply dosage of the reconstituted penicillin G sodium? When adding 3.8 mL of diluent, the supply dosage is 250 000 units/mL.
- Third, what is the resulting total volume of this reconstituted solution? The total volume is 4 mL. The powder adds 0.2 mL volume to the solution.
- Finally, how many full doses of penicillin are available in this vial? The vial contains 1 000 000 units and the order is for 300 000 units. Regardless of the concentration, there are still three full doses (plus some extra) in this vial. A reconstitution label is needed.

This means that when 3.8 mL of sterile diluent is added to the vial of powdered penicillin G sodium, the result is 4 mL of solution with 250 000 units of penicillin G sodium per millilitre.

Apply the Three-Step Approach to calculate one dose.

Step 1 Convert No conversion is necessary.

Order: *penicillin G sodium 300 000 units IM QID*

Supply: 250 000 units/mL

Step 2 Think You want to give more than 1 mL but less than 2 mL.

Step 3 Calculate $\frac{D}{H} \times Q = \frac{\overset{6}{\cancel{300\,000}}\ \cancel{\text{units}}}{\underset{5}{\cancel{250\,000}}\ \cancel{\text{units}}} \times 1\text{ mL} = \frac{6}{5}\text{ mL} = 1.2\text{ mL}$

Because each dose is 1.2 mL and the total volume is 4 mL, you would have enough for two additional full doses. As an intramuscular dose, 5 mL is the maximum volume for a large, adult muscle. This concentration would result in a reasonable volume that would be readily absorbed. This is a good choice of concentration instructions to use to prepare this order.

Select a *3-mL syringe, and measure 1.2 mL* of penicillin G sodium reconstituted to 250 000 units/mL.

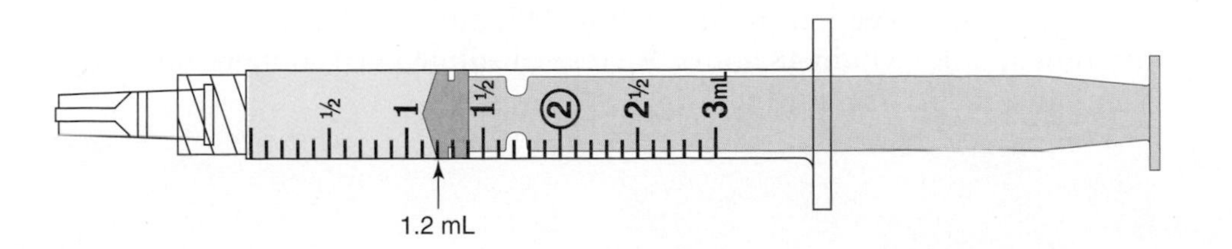

CAUTION

The supply dosage of a reconstituted drug is an essential detail that the preparer must write on the multiple-dose vial label. Once a powdered drug is reconstituted, there is no way to verify how much diluent was actually added, unless it is properly labelled. It is recommended that multi-dose vials be dedicated to a single patient whenever possible.

Add a label to the reconstituted penicillin G sodium 250 000-unit/mL vial (Figure 10-8).

30/01/xx, 0800, reconstituted as 250 000 units/mL. Expires 06/02/xx, 0800, keep refrigerated. B.S.

FIGURE 10-8 Reconstitution Label for Penicillin G Sodium 1 000 000 Units with 3.8 mL Diluent

It is evident from these possible reconstituted strengths that three full doses are available from this multiple-dose vial in each case. The added diluent volume is the key factor that determines the resulting concentration. The *supply dosage* ultimately determines the *injectable volume per dose.*

MATH TIP

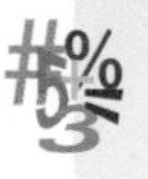

When multiple directions for diluting are given, the *smaller* the amount of diluent added, the *greater* or *stronger* the resulting solution concentration will be.

RECONSTITUTED PARENTERAL SOLUTIONS USED WITH VARIOUS ROUTES

A variety of drugs are labelled and packaged with reconstitution instructions for IM use only or for IV use only. Others may be used for either. Some are even suitable for subcutaneous, IM, or IV administration. Carefully check the route and appropriate reconstitution directions. The following material gives examples of several types of directions you will encounter.

Drugs with Injection Reconstitution Instructions for Either IM or IV

Example:

Order: *methylprednisolone sodium succinate 200 mg IV q6h*

Supply: The directions on the label of the 500-mg vial of powdered methylprednisolone sodium succinate for IM or IV injection shown in Figure 10-9 read, "Reconstitution: Add 7.8 mL Sterile Water for Injection and use within 24 hours or 7.8 mL of Bacteriostatic Water for Injection and use within 48 hours. Each reconstituted vial contains approximately 8 mL. Each mL contains 62.5 mg methylprednisolone."

Sterile/Stérile DIN 02231895
METHYLPREDNISOLONE Sodium Succinate for Injection, USP
Succinate sodique de MÉTHYLPREDNISOLONE pour injection, USP
500 mg
methylprednisolone per vial / de méthylprednisolone par fiole
IM or IV Use / Usage IM ou IV
Novopharm Limited

FIGURE 10-9 Methylprednisolone Sodium Succinate 500 mg Label

What is known?

- First, to fill the order, how much and what type of diluent must be added? The directions are to add 7.8 mL of sterile water for injection for use within 24 hours or bacteriostatic water for injection and use within 48 hours.
- Second, what is the supply dosage of the reconstituted methylprednisolone? When adding 7.8 mL of diluent, the supply dosage is 62.5 mg/mL.
- Third, what is the resulting total volume of this reconstituted solution? The total volume is 8 mL. This is because 62.5 mg/mL × 8 mL = 500 mg.
- Finally, how many full doses of methylprednisolone sodium succinate are available in this vial? The vial contains 500 mg and the order is for 200 mg. There are two full doses in the vial. A reconstitution label is needed.

This means that there is a vial of 500 mg of methylprednisolone sodium succinate available to which you will add 8 mL of diluent. The final yield of the solution is 62.5 mg per mL, which is the supply dosage.

Apply the Three-Step Approach to calculate one dose.

Step 1 Convert No conversion is necessary.

Order: *methylprednisolone sodium succinate 200 mg IV q6h*

Supply: 62.5 mg/mL

Step 2 Think You want to give more than 1 mL. In fact, you want to give more than 3 times 1 mL.

Step 3 Calculate $\frac{D}{H} \times Q = \frac{200 \text{ mg}}{62.5 \text{ mg}} \times 1 \text{ mL} = 3.2 \text{ mL}$; given intravenously every 6 hours

> *30/01/xx, 0800, reconstituted as 62.5 mg/mL. Expires 01/02/xx, 0800, store at room temperature 15–25°C. B.S.*

Select a 5-mL syringe and measure 3.2 mL of methylprednisolone sodium succinate.

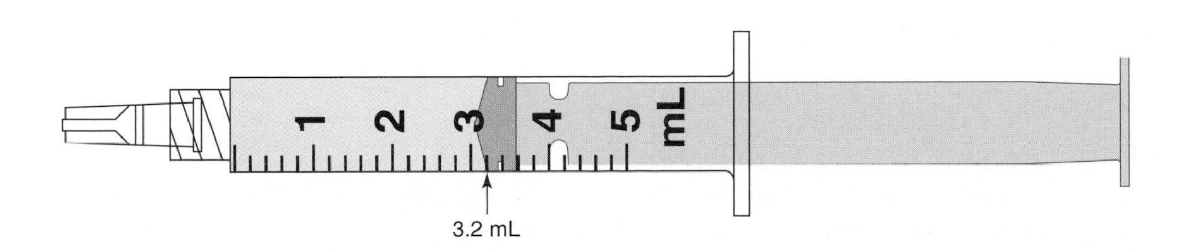

Drugs with Different IM and IV Reconstitution Instructions

The ceftazidime label in Figure 10-10 has one set of instructions for IM administration and another set of instructions for IV administration. The nurse must carefully check the route ordered, and then follow the directions that correspond to that route. In such cases, it is important not to interchange the dilution instructions for IM and IV administrations.

Example 1:

Order: *ceftazidime 250 mg IM q12h*

Supply: The IM reconstitution directions on the label of a 1-g 1000-mg vial of powdered ceftazidime (Figure 10-10) are "IM: Add 3 mL of Sterile Water for Injection or other approved diluent. SHAKE WELL. Provides ceftazidime approx. 280 mg per mL."

- First, to fill the order, how much and what type of diluent must be added? The directions are to add 3 mL of sterile water for injection or another approved diluent. (Bacteriostatic water for injection is also listed in the package insert as another possible diluent.)
- Second, what is the supply dosage of the reconstituted ceftazidime? When adding 3 mL of diluent, the resulting supply dosage is 280 mg/mL.
- Third, how many full doses of ceftazidime are available in this vial? The vial contains 1000 mg and the order is for 250 mg. There are four full doses in the vial. A reconstitution label is needed.
- Finally, what is the resulting total volume of this reconstituted solution? The total volume is 3.6 mL, as indicated on the insert (not shown) for IM reconstitution.

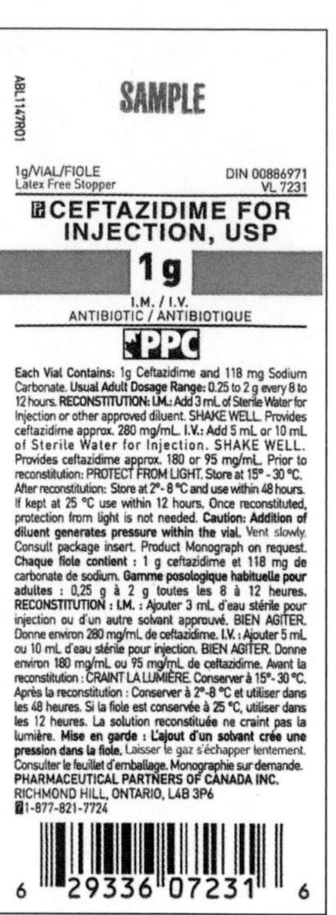

FIGURE 10-10
Ceftazidime Label

This means that you have a vial of 1 g of ceftazidime available to which you will add 3 mL of diluent. The final supply dosage is 280 mg/mL.

Apply the Three-Step Approach to calculate one dose.

Step 1 Convert No conversion is necessary.

Order: *ceftazidime 250 mg IM q12h*

Supply: 280 mg/mL

Step 2 Think You want to give less than 1 mL.

Step 3 Calculate $\frac{D}{H} \times Q = \frac{25\not{0}\ \cancel{mg}}{28\not{0}\ \cancel{mg}} \times 1\text{ mL} = 0.9\text{ mL};$ given intramuscularly every 12 hours

30/01/xx, 0800, reconstituted as 280 mg/mL for IM use. Expires 01/02/xx, 0800, store in refrigerator. B.S.

Select a 1-mL syringe and measure 0.9 mL of ceftazidime. A 3-mL syringe could also be used for administration.

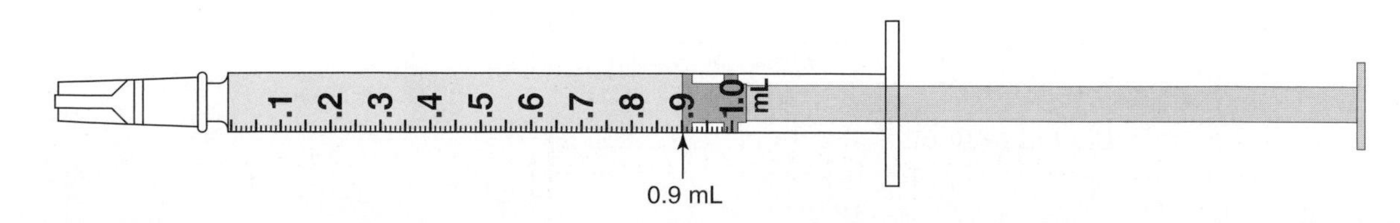

CAUTION

Because this is an intramuscular dose, it may be necessary to change needles. Choose the appropriate needle prior to drawing up medication. Changing needles after the medication has been measured may change the actual dose of medication injected.

Example 2:

Order: *ceftazidime 400 mg IV q8h*

Supply: The IV reconstitution directions on the label of a 1-g vial of powdered ceftazidime are "IV: Add 5 mL or 10 mL of Sterile Water for Injection. SHAKE WELL. Provides ceftazidime approx. 180 or 95 mg/mL."

- First, to prepare the order, how much and what type of diluent must be added? The directions are to add 5 mL or 10 mL of sterile water.
- Second, what is the supply dosage of the reconstituted ceftazidime? When adding 5 mL of diluent, the resulting dosage is 1000 mg/5.6 mL or 180 mg/mL.
- Third, what is the resulting total volume of this reconstituted solution? The total volume is 5.6 mL. In this scenario, the solution volume dilutes the powder, adding additional volume. Sometimes adding diluent does not add additional volume. Always check the instructions.
- Finally, how many full doses of ceftazidime are available in this vial? The vial contains 1 g and the order is for 400 mg. There are two full doses in the vial. A reconstitution label is needed.

This means that you have a vial of 1 g of ceftazidime available to which you will add 5 mL of diluent. The final yield of the solution is 5.6 mL with a supply dosage of 180 mg/mL. Most IV antibiotics are further diluted in an approved IV solution and infused over a specified time period. You will learn more about this in the next section and in Chapter 14.

Apply the Three-Step Approach to calculate one dose.

Step 1 Convert No conversion is necessary.

Order: *ceftazidime 400 mg IV q8h*

Supply: 180 mg/mL

Step 2 Think You want to give more than 1 mL.

Step 3 Calculate $\frac{D}{H} \times Q = \frac{\overset{20}{\cancel{400}\ \cancel{mg}}}{\underset{9}{\cancel{180}\ \cancel{mg}}} \times 1\text{ mL} = 2.2\text{ mL};$

given intravenously every 8 hours

Select a 5-mL syringe and measure 2.2 mL of ceftazidime. A 3-mL syringe could also be used.

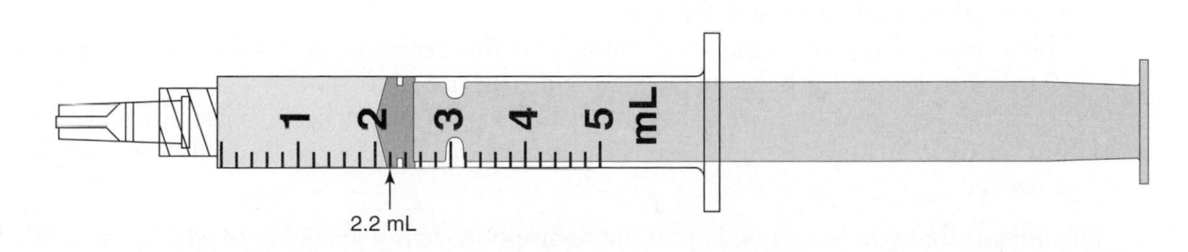

Drugs with Instructions to "See Package Insert" for Dilution and Administration

Some labels provide only the dosage strength contained in the vial and other minimal information that is insufficient to properly reconstitute or safely store the drug. To prepare the powdered medication, examine the package insert. Examine the amphotericin B label in Figure 10-11. There are no instructions for reconstitution on the label, so it is important to check the package insert for specific directions, also shown in Figure 10-11.

Example:

Order: *amphotericin B 37.5 mg IV daily*

Supply: amphotericin B 50 mg

For hospital use only.
Protect from light during administration.
Pour l'usage exclusif des hôpitaux.
Protéger de la lumière pendant l'administration.
*TM of/MC de Bristol-Myers Squibb Canada
1222136
For / Pour reconstitution
List/e 043780
DIN 00029149
FUNGIZONE*
INTRAVENOUS / INTRAVEINEUSE
Amphotericin B for Injection, U.S.P.
Injection d'amphotéricine B, U.S.P.
50 mg per vial / par fiole
Bristol-Myers Squibb Canada
Lot
Exp.

PREPARATION OF SOLUTIONS

Reconstitute as follows: An initial concentrate of 5 mg amphotericin B per mL is first prepared by rapidly expressing 10 mL sterile water for injection, USP without a bacteriostatic agent directly into the lyophilized cake, using a sterile needle (minimum diameter: 20 gauge) and syringe. Shake the vial immediately until the colloidal solution is clear. The infusion solution, providing 0.1 mg amphotericin B per mL, is then obtained by further dilution (1:50) with 5% Dextrose injection, USP of pH above 4.2 . The pH of each container of Dextrose injection should be ascertained before use. Commercial Dextrose Injection usually has a pH above 4.2; however, if it is below 4.2, then 1 or 2 mL of buffer should be added to the Dextrose injection before it is used to dilute the concentrated solution of amphotericin B. The recommended buffer has the following composition

Dibasic sodium phosphate (anhydrous)	1.59 g
Monobasic sodium phosphate (anhydrous)	0.96 g
Water for injection, USP	qs 100.0 mL

The buffer should be sterilized before it is added to the Dextrose injection, either by filtration through a bacterial retentive stone mat or membrane, or by autoclaving for 30 minutes at 15 lb pressure (121°C). **CAUTION: Aseptic technique must be strictly observed in all handling,** since no preservative or bacteriostatic agent is present in the antibiotic or in the materials used to prepare it for administration. **All entries into the vial or into the diluents must be made with a sterile needle. Do not reconstitute with saline solutions. The use of any diluent other than the ones recommended or the presence of a bacteriostatic agent** (e.g., benzyl alcohol) **in the diluent may cause precipitation of the antibiotic. Do not use the initial concentrate or the infusion solution if there is any evidence of precipitation or foreign matter in either one.**

An in-line membrane filter may be used for intravenous infusion of amphotericin B; **however, the mean pore diameter of the filter should not be less than 1.0 micron in order to assure passage of the antibiotic dispersion.**

FIGURE 10-11 Amphotericin B Label and Package Insert Instructions for Reconstitution

- First, to fill the order, how much and what type of diluent must you add? The directions advise the preparer, for initial reconstitution, to add 10 mL of sterile water for injection without a bacteriostatic agent. The reconstitution needs to be done first before diluting further.
- Second, what is the supply dosage of the reconstituted amphotericin B? When adding 10 mL of diluent, the supply dosage is 5 mg/mL.
- Third, what is the resulting total volume of this reconstituted solution? The total volume is 10 mL. You know this because the supply dosage is 5 mg/mL.
- Finally, how many full doses of amphotericin B are available in this vial? The vial contains 50 mg and the order is for 37.5 mg. There is enough for one full dose in the vial. No reconstitution label is needed.

This means that you have a vial of 50 mg of amphotericin B available to which you will add 10 mL of diluent using strict aseptic technique. The final yield of the solution is 5 mg/mL (50 mg/10 mL), which is your supply dosage.

Apply the Three-Step Approach to calculate one dose of the initial concentration (before further dilution).

Step 1 Convert No conversion is necessary.

Order: *amphotericin B 37.5 mg IV daily*

Supply: amphotericin B 5 mg/mL

Step 2 Think You want to give more than 1 mL, but less than 10 mL.

Step 3 Calculate 37.5 mg/5 mg × 1 mL = 7.5 mL; given intravenously

Select a 10-mL syringe and measure 7.5 mL of amphotericin B.

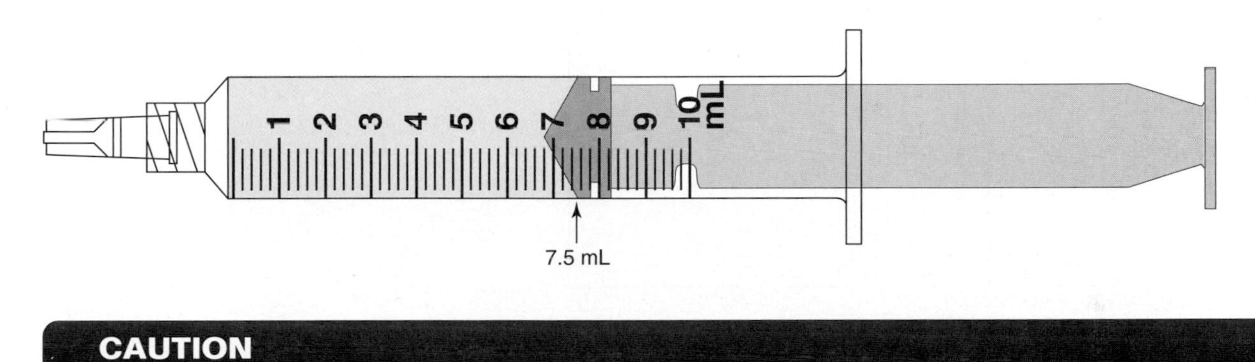

CAUTION

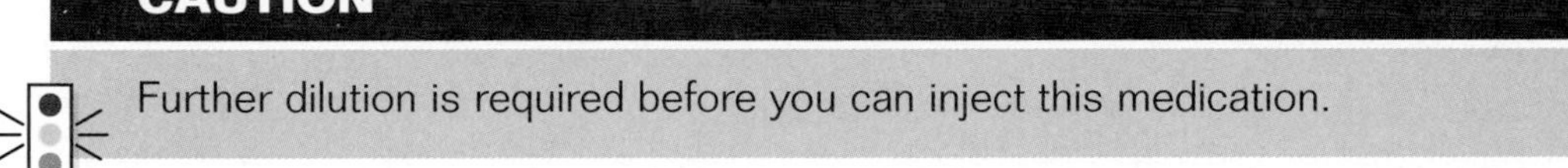

Further dilution is required before you can inject this medication.

Using strict aseptic technique, the preparer (usually the pharmacy technician in the hospital pharmacy) will withdraw 7.5 mL of amphotericin B from the reconstituted vial and inject it into a 500-mL IV bag of 5% dextrose solution. The IV bag will then be appropriately labelled as containing 37.5 mg amphotericin B in 500 mL of 5% dextrose (concentration of 37.5 mg/500 mL or 0.75 mg/mL). The IV bag would then be delivered to the appropriate nursing unit to be infused into the patient at a slow infusion rate (over 2 to 6 hours, i.e., 100 mL/h) once daily.

QUICK REVIEW

It is important to remember the following points when reconstituting drugs:

- Check the expiry dates of the drug and the diluent before beginning the reconstitution process.
- If any medicine remains for future use after reconstitution and can be stored for a future dose, clearly label it with the following information:
  1. Date and time of preparation;
  2. Strength or concentration per volume;
  3. Potency expiration;
  4. Recommended storage;
  5. Your initials.
- Read all instructions carefully. If no instructions accompany the vial, confer with the pharmacist before proceeding.
- When reconstituting multiple-strength parenteral powders, select the dosage strength that is appropriate for the patient's age, size, and condition.
- Carefully select the correct reconstitution directions for IM or IV administration.

REVIEW SET 10-1

Calculate the amount you will prepare for each dose. The labels provided are the drugs available. Draw an arrow to the syringe calibration to indicate the amount that you will draw up. Prepare a reconstitution label, if needed.

1. Order: *ceftazidime 200 mg IM q12h*

   Reconstitute with ________ mL diluent for a concentration of ________ mg/mL.

   Give: ________ mL

   How many full doses are available in this vial? ________ dose(s)

   Prepare a reconstitution label for the remaining solution.

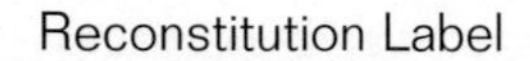

Reconstitution Label

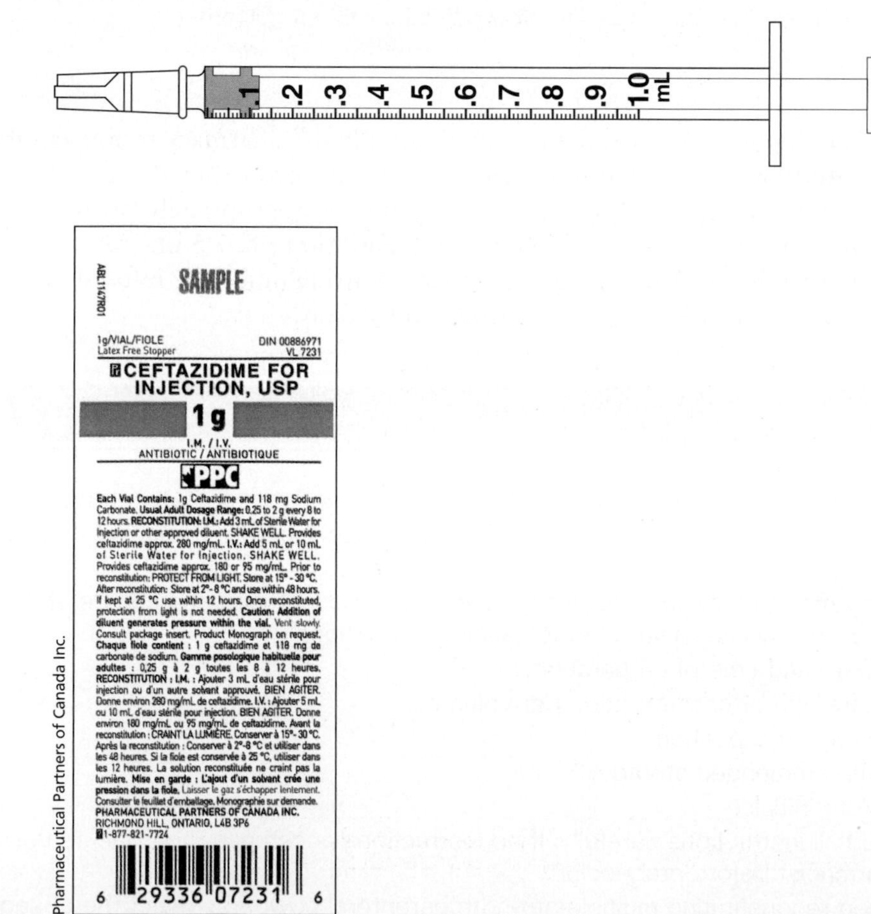

2. Order: *bacitracin 2500 units IM q12h*

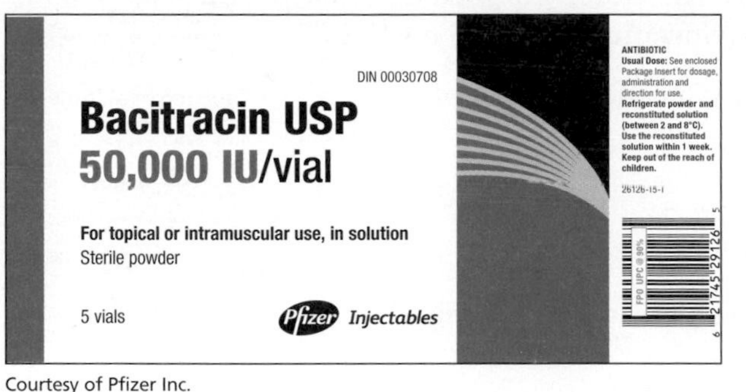

Courtesy of Pfizer Inc.

DOSAGE AND ADMINISTRATION

TO BE ADMINISTERED INTRAMUSCULARLY.

Infant dose:

For infants under 2500 grams – 900 units/kg/24 hours in 2 or 3 divided doses. For infants over 2500 grams – 1,000 units/kg/24 hours, in 2 or 3 divided doses. Intramuscular injections of the solution should be given in the upper outer quadrant of the buttocks, alternating right and left and avoiding multiple injections in the same region because of the transient pain following injection.

Preparation of Solutions:

Should be dissolved in Sodium Chloride Injection containing 2 percent procaine hydrochloride. The concentration of the antibiotic in the solution should not be less than 5,000 units per mL nor more than 10,000 units per mL.

Diluents containing parabens should not be used to reconstitute bacitracin; cloudy solutions and precipitate formation have occurred. Reconstitution of the 50,000 unit vial with 9.8 mL of diluent will result in a concentration of 5,000 units per mL.

TO BE ADMINISTERED TOPICALLY.

Preparation of Solution:

Solutions for topical application are prepared by dissolving bacitracin in Sterile Water for Injection or Sodium Chloride Injection in amounts to give the following concentrations:

Skin	500 units per mL
Ophthalmic Solutions	500 to 1,000 units per mL
Intranasal Therapy	250 units per mL
Aerosol	500 to 1,000 units per mL

Courtesy of Pfizer Inc.

Reconstitute with ________ mL diluent for a concentration of ________ units/mL.

Give: _________ mL

How many full doses are available in this vial? ________ dose(s)

Prepare a reconstitution label for the remaining solution.

Reconstitution Label

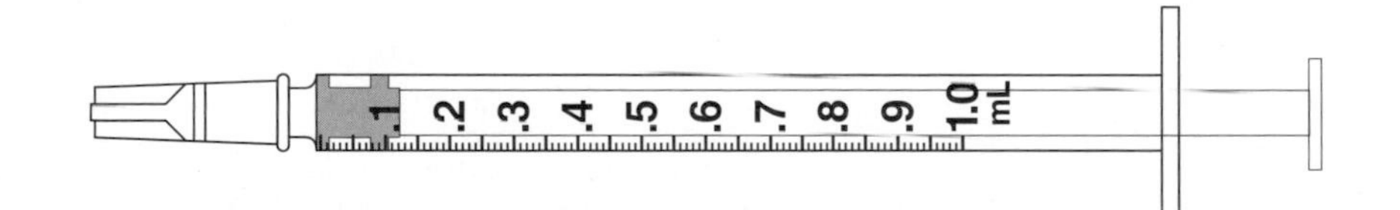

3. Order: *enfuvirtide 90 mg subcutaneously BID*

   Package insert directions: "Add 1.1 mL Sterile Water supplied diluent to make a total volume of 1.2 mL and a concentration of 90 mg/mL."

   Reconstitute with ________ mL diluent for a concentration of ________ mg/________ mL.

   Give: ________ mL

   How many full doses are available in this vial? ________ dose(s)

   Does this reconstituted medication require a reconstitution label? ________

   Explain: ____

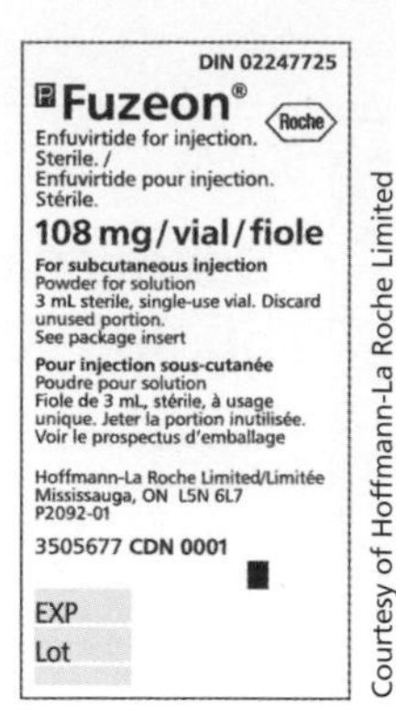

Courtesy of Hoffmann-La Roche Limited

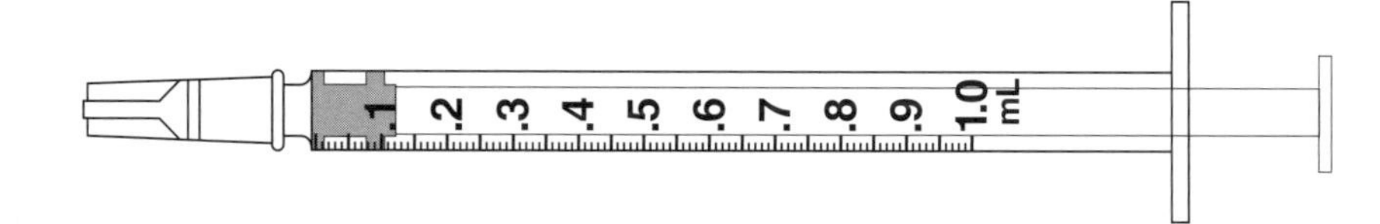

4. Order: *azithromycin dihydrate 0.5 g IV daily X 2 days, then 250 mg IV daily X 5 days. The nurse prepares to administer the first dose.*

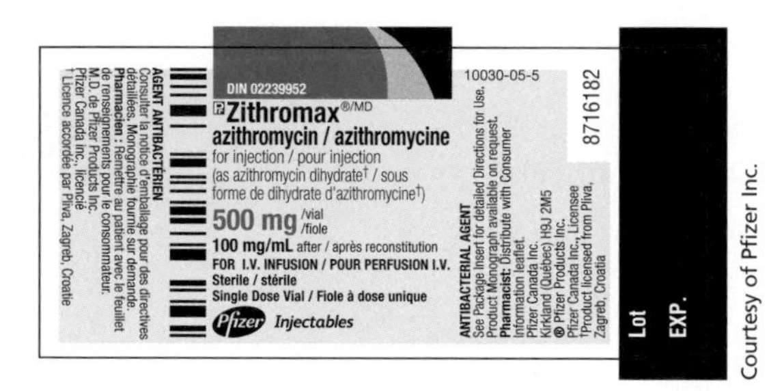

Courtesy of Pfizer Inc.

ZITHROMAX for Injection:

RECONSTITUTION OF ZITHROMAX FOR INJECTION				
Strength	Reconstitution Solution	Volume to be Added	Approximate Volume Available	Nominal Concentration
500 mg	Sterile Water for Injection	4.8 mL	5 mL	100 mg/mL

Prepare the initial solution of **ZITHROMAX** for Injection by adding 4.8 mL of Sterile Water for Injection to the 500 mg vial. Shake the vial until all of the drug is dissolved. Since the vial is evacuated, it is recommended that a standard 5 mL (non-automated) syringe be used to ensure that the exact volume of 4.8 mL is dispensed. Each mL of reconstituted solution contains azithromycin dihydrate equivalent to 100 mg azithromycin. Reconstituted solution is stable for 24 hours when stored below 30°C. **The reconstituted solution must be further diluted prior to administration.**

Dilution of reconstituted solution: To provide azithromycin over a concentration range of 1.0 - 2.0 mg/mL, transfer 5 mL of the 100 mg/mL azithromycin solution into the appropriate amount of the following diluents:

Final Infusion Concentration (mg/mL)	Amount of Diluent (mL)
1.0 mg/mL	500 mL
2.0 mg/mL	250 mL

Appropriate Diluents
0.9% Sodium Chloride Injection
5% Dextrose in Water for Injection
0.45% Sodium Chloride Injection
Lactated Ringer's Injection
5% Dextrose in 0.45% Sodium Chloride Injection with 20 mEq Potassium Chloride
5% Dextrose in Lactated Ringer's Injection
5% Dextrose in 0.3% Sodium Chloride Injection
5% Dextrose in 0.45% Sodium Chloride Injection
Normosol-M in 5% Dextrose

Diluted solutions prepared in this manner are stable for 24 hours at or below room temperature (30°C), or for 72 hours if stored under refrigeration (5°C). As with all parenteral drug products, intravenous admixtures should be inspected visually for clarity, particulate matter, precipitate, discoloration and leakage prior to administration, whenever solution and container permit. Solutions showing haziness, particulate matter, precipitate, discoloration or leakage should be discarded.

Only limited data are available on the compatibility of **ZITHROMAX** for Injection with other intravenous substances, therefore additives or other medications should not be added to **ZITHROMAX** for Injection or infused simultaneously through the same intravenous line. If the same intravenous line is used for sequential infusion of several different drugs, the line should be flushed before and after infusion of **ZITHROMAX** for Injection with an infusion solution compatible with **ZITHROMAX** for Injection and with any other drug(s) administered via the common line. If **ZITHROMAX** for Injection is to be given concomitantly with another drug, each drug should be given separately in accordance with the recommended dosage and route of administration for each drug.

Courtesy of Pfizer Inc.

Reconstitute with ________ mL diluent for a concentration of ________ mg/mL.

Withdraw: ________ mL of reconstituted azithromycin dihydrate and further dilute to appropriate volume with appropriate diluent (see package insert)

How many full doses are available in this vial? ________ dose(s)

Does this reconstituted medication require a reconstitution label? ________

Explain: ____

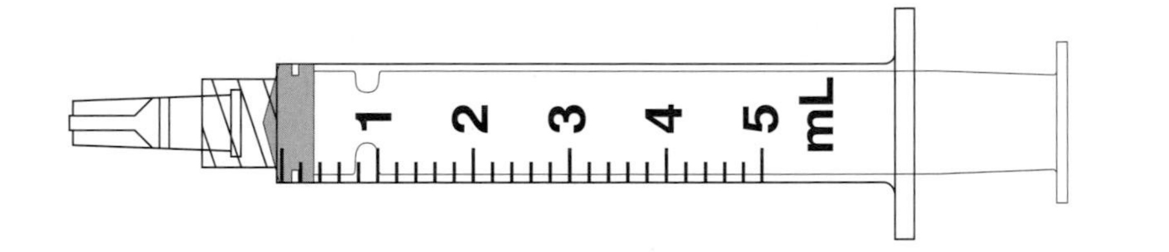

5. Order: *ceftriaxone 750 mg IM daily*

Reconstitute with ________ mL diluent for an initial concentration of ________ mg/mL.
Give: ________ mL

How many full doses are available in this vial?
________ dose(s)

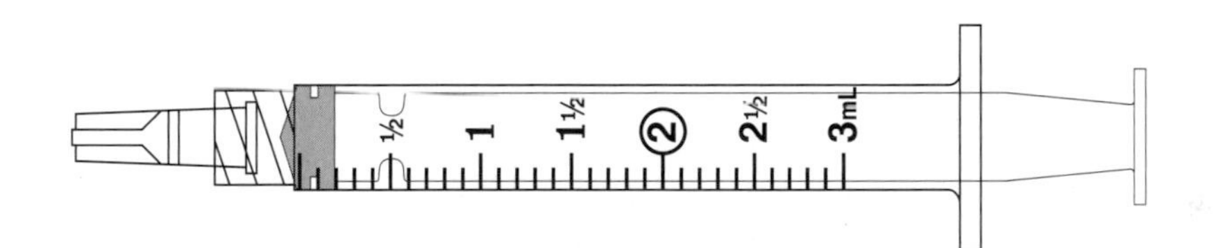

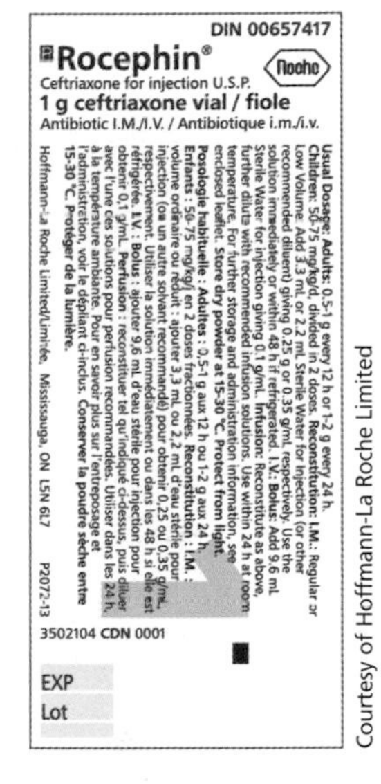

Courtesy of Hoffmann-La Roche Limited

6. Order: *penicillin G sodium 1 000 000 units IM q6h*

LOT : 302081
EXP. : 2005-FE
SAMPLE

15 mL DIN 02220288
PF370070

PENICILLIN G
Sodium for Injection USP

5 million IU
per Vial/par fiole

IM/IV
Sterile / Stérile
Antibiotic / Antibiotique

Usual adult dose:
1,000,000 to 5,000,000 IU every 4 to 6 hours.
For full prescribing information, see package insert.
Reconstitution: Use Sterile Water for Injection, USP or other recommended diluent.

Volume of diluent	Approximate Concentration/mL	Withdrawable Volume
3.1 mL	1,000,000 IU	5 mL
8.2 mL	500,000 IU	10 mL

Reconstituted solution is stable for 5 days refrigerated or 24 hours room temperature.

Pharmaceutical Partners of Canada Inc.
Richmond Hill, Ontario L4C 9S6
1-877-821-7724

Dose habituelle pour adultes :
1 000 000 à 5 000 000 UI toutes les 4 à 6 heures.
Pour les renseignements posologiques complets, consulter le feuillet d'emballage.
Reconstitution : Utiliser de l'eau stérile pour préparations injectables USP ou un autre diluant recommandé.

Volume de diluant	Concentration approximative/mL	Volume obtenu
3,1 mL	1 000 000 UI	5 mL
8,2 mL	500 000 UI	10 mL

La solution reconstituée est stable pendant 5 jours au réfrigérateur ou pendant 24 heures à la température ambiante.

85009/A

6 29336 37070 2

Pharmaceutical Partners of Canada Inc.

Describe the two concentrations, and calculate the amount to give for each supply dosage concentration.

Reconstitute with ________ mL diluent for a concentration of ________ units/mL, and give ________ mL.

Reconstitute with ________ mL diluent for a concentration of ________ units/mL, and give ________ mL.

Indicate the concentration you would choose, and explain the rationale for your selection.

Select ________ units/mL and give ________ mL. Rationale: ______________________

____

How many full doses are available in this vial? ________ dose(s)

Prepare a reconstitution label for the remaining solution.

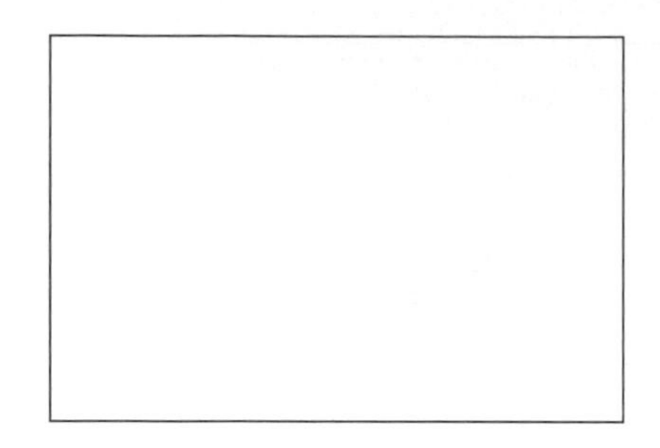

Reconstitution Label

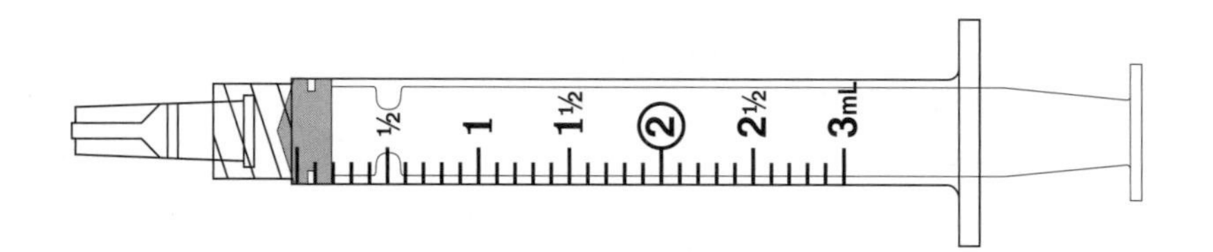

7. Order: *methylprednisolone sodium succinate 175 mg IM daily*

Sterile/Stérile DIN 02231895
METHYLPREDNISOLONE
Sodium Succinate
for Injection, USP
Succinate sodique de
MÉTHYLPREDNISOLONE
pour injection, USP
500 mg
methylprednisolone per vial /
de méthylprednisolone par fiole
IM or IV Use /
Usage IM ou IV

GLUCOCORTICOID / ANTI-INFLAMMATORY
Each vial contains methylprednisolone 500 mg (as methylprednisolone sodium succinate 663 mg).
Reconstitution: Add 7.8 mL Sterile Water for Injection and use within 24 hours or 7.8 mL Bacteriostatic Water for Injection and use within 48 hours. Each reconstituted vial contains approximately 8 mL. Each mL contains 62.5 mg methylprednisolone. **Discard unused solution.**
Store powder at room temperature (15°C – 25°C).
Protect from light. See enclosed Package Insert.
Product Monograph available upon request.
GLUCOCORTICOÏDE / ANTI-INFLAMMATOIRE
Chaque fiole contient 500 mg de méthylprednisolone (sous forme de 663 mg de succinate sodique de méthylprednisolone). **Reconstitution :** Ajouter 7,8 mL d'eau stérile pour injection et utiliser la solution dans les 24 heures, ou ajouter 7,8 mL d'eau bactériostatique pour injection et utiliser la solution dans les 48 heures. Une fois reconstituée, la fiole contient environ 8 mL de solution. Un mL renferme 62,5 mg de méthylprednisolone. **Jeter toute solution inutilisée.**
Conserver la poudre à la température ambiante (15 °C à 25 °C). Protéger de la lumière. Voir le dépliant de conditionnement. Monographie du produit fournie sur demande.
®-Reg'd Trademark of Novopharm Limited,
®-Marque déposée de Novopharm Limitée.
Toronto, Canada M1B 2K9
76573LA-0001 Rev. 02 N1-383200-902
Lot: Exp:

Novopharm Limited

Reconstitute with ________ mL diluent for a concentration of ________ mg/mL.

Give: ________ mL

How many full doses are available in this vial? ________ dose(s)

Prepare a reconstitution label for the remaining solution.

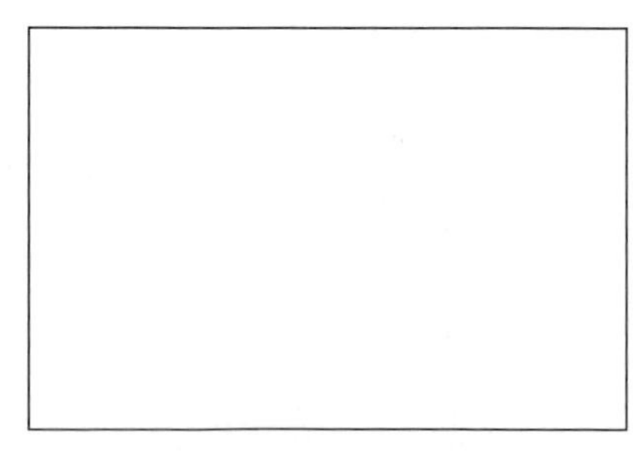

Reconstitution Label

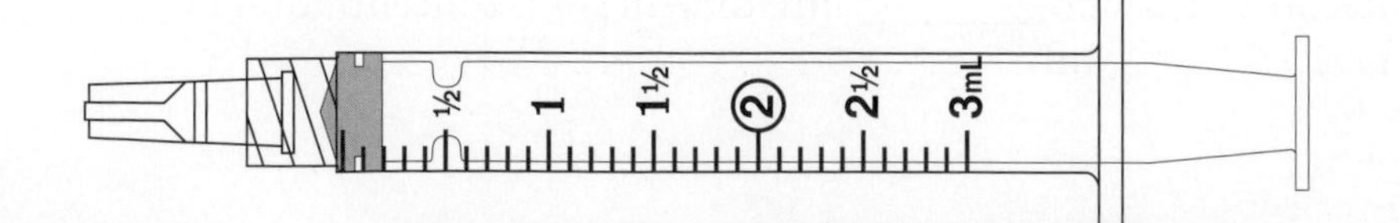

8. Order: *piperacillin 200 mg IM q6h*

Parenteral Products - Reconstitution
For Intramuscular Use (Solutions for Reconstitution)
Sterile water for injection or 0.5 to 1.0% lidocaine HCl (without epinephrine) in sterile water for injection. (Lidocaine is contraindicated in patients with a known history of hypersensitivity to local anesthetics of the amide type).

Reconstitution Table

Vial Size	Volume to be added	Approximate Available Volume	Approximate Available Concentration
2 g	4.0 mL	5.0 mL	0.4 g/mL
3 g	6.0 mL	7.5 mL	0.4 g/mL
4 g	8.0 mL	10.0 mL	0.4 g/mL

Shake well until dissolved.

Note: Intramuscular injections should be limited to 2 g per injection site. Injection should be given into the upper outer quadrant of the buttock (i.e. gluteus maximus).

For Intravenous Injection or Infusion
For intravenous injection or infusion, reconstitute Piperacillin for Injection with sterile water for injection.

Reconstitution Table

Vial Size	Volume of Diluent to be added	Approximate Available Volume	Approximate Average Concentration
2 g	10 mL	11 mL	0.18 g/mL
3 g	15 mL	17 mL	0.18 g/mL
4 g	20 mL	22 mL	0.18 g/mL

Shake well until dissolved.

The prepared solution may be further diluted to the desired volume (at least 15 mL/g for infusion) with any intravenous solutions or intravenous admixtures listed below.

Intravenous Solutions:
Dextrose 5% in water (D W)
0.9% sodium chloride (normal saline) [NS]
Dextrose 5% and 0.9% sodium chloride (D_5NS)
Lactated ringer's injection
Dextran 6% in 0.9% sodium chloride

Intravenous Admixtures:
Normal saline [+ KCl 40 mEq/500 mL]
5% dextrose in water (D_5W) [+ KCl 40 mEq/500 mL]
5% dextrose/normal saline (D_5NS) [+KCl 40 mEq/500 mL]
Ringer's injection [+KCl 40 mEq/500 mL]
Lactated ringer's injection [+KCl 40 mEq/500 mL]

Diluted Solutions
As with all parenteral drug products, intravenous admixtures should be inspected visually for clarity, particulate matter, precipitate, discolouration and leakage prior to administration, whenever solution and container permit. Solution showing haziness, particulate matter, precipitate, discolouration or leakage should not be used. Discard unused portion.

Courtesy of Pfizer Inc.

Reconstitute with ________ mL diluent for a concentration of ________ g/________ mL or ________ mg/________ mL.

Give: ________ mL

How many full doses are available in this vial? ________ dose(s)

½ 1 1½ 2 2½ 3mL

9. Order: *penicillin G sodium 500 000 units IM q6h*

15 mL DIN 02220261
PF370069
PENICILLIN G
Sodium for Injection USP
1 million IU
per Vial/par fiole
IM/IV
Sterile/Stérile
Antibiotic / Antibiotique
LOT : S302069
EXP. : 2005 FE

Usual adult dose:
1,000,000 to 5,000,000 IU every 4 to 6 hours.
For full prescribing information, see package insert.
Reconstitution: Use Sterile Water for Injection, USP or other recommended diluent.

Volume of diluent	Approximate Concentration/mL	Withdrawable Volume
1.8 mL	500,000 IU	2 mL
3.8 mL	250,000 IU	4 mL

Reconstituted solution is stable for 5 days refrigerated or 24 hours room temperature.

Pharmaceutical Partners of Canada Inc.
Richmond Hill, Ontario L4C 9S6
1-877-821-7724

Dose habituelle pour adultes :
1 000 000 à 5 000 000 UI toutes les 4 à 6 heures.
Pour les renseignements posologiques complets, consulter le feuillet d'emballage.
Reconstitution : Utiliser de l'eau stérile pour préparations injectables USP ou un autre diluant recommandé.

Volume de diluant	Concentration approximative/mL	Volume retirable
1,8 mL	500 000 UI	2 mL
3,8 mL	250 000 UI	4 mL

La solution reconstituée est stable pendant 5 jours au réfrigérateur ou pendant 24 heures à la température ambiante.

85010/A

6 29336 37069 6

Pharmaceutical Partners of Canada Inc.

Describe the two concentrations, and calculate the amount to give for each of the supply dosage concentrations.

Reconstitute with ________ mL diluent for a concentration of ________ units/mL, and give ________ mL.

Reconstitute with ________ mL diluent for a concentration of ________ units/mL, and give ________ mL.

Indicate the concentration you would choose, and explain the rationale for your selection.

Select ________ units/mL and give ________ mL. Rationale: ____________________

____

How many full doses are available in this vial? ________ dose(s)

Prepare a reconstitution label for the remaining solution.

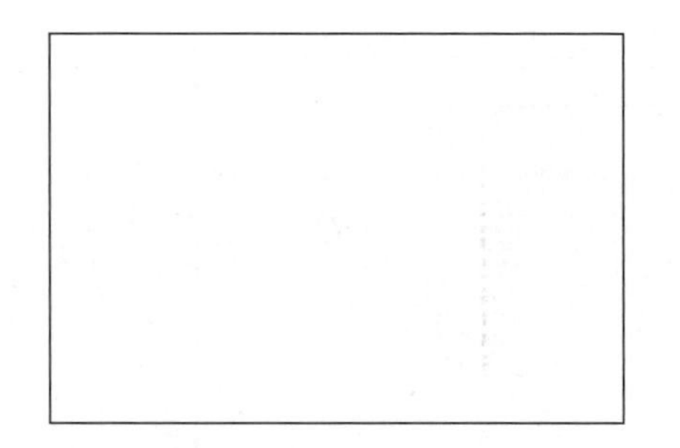

Reconstitution Label

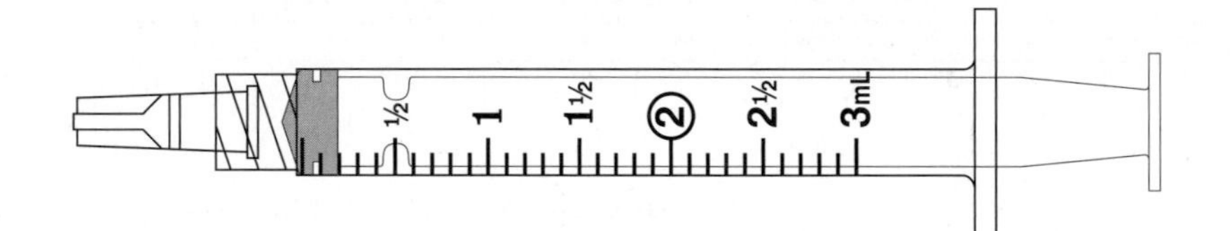

10. Order: *ampicillin sodium 500 mg IV q6h*

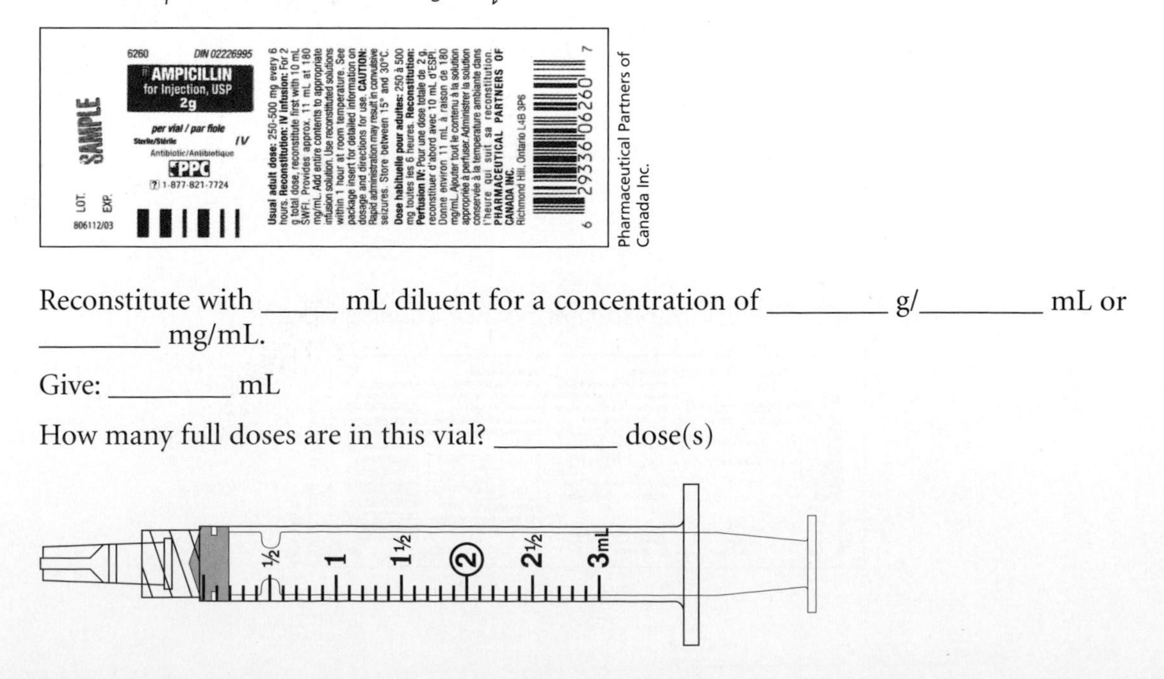

Pharmaceutical Partners of Canada Inc.

Reconstitute with _____ mL diluent for a concentration of ________ g/________ mL or ________ mg/mL.

Give: ________ mL

How many full doses are in this vial? ________ dose(s)

11. Order: *methylprednisolone sodium succinate 24 mg IM daily*

Sterile/Stérile DIN 02231893
METHYLPREDNISOLONE Sodium Succinate for Injection, USP
Succinate sodique de MÉTHYLPREDNISOLONE pour injection, USP
40 mg
methylprednisolone per vial
de méthylprednisolone par fiole
IM or IV Use
Usage IM ou IV
Novopharm Limited

Reconstitute with ________ mL diluent for a concentration of ________ mg/mL.

Give ________ mL

How many full doses are available in this vial? ________ dose(s)

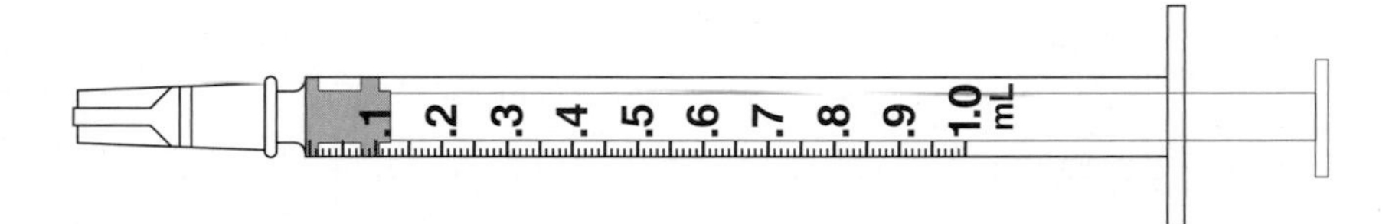

12. Order: *ceftazidime 250 mg IV q12h*

Reconstitute with ________ mL diluent for a concentration of ________ g/________ mL or ________ mg/mL.

Give: ________ mL

How many full doses are available in this vial? ________ dose(s)

Will the drug remain potent to use all available doses? ________ Explain: ________

Prepare a reconstitution label for the remaining solution.

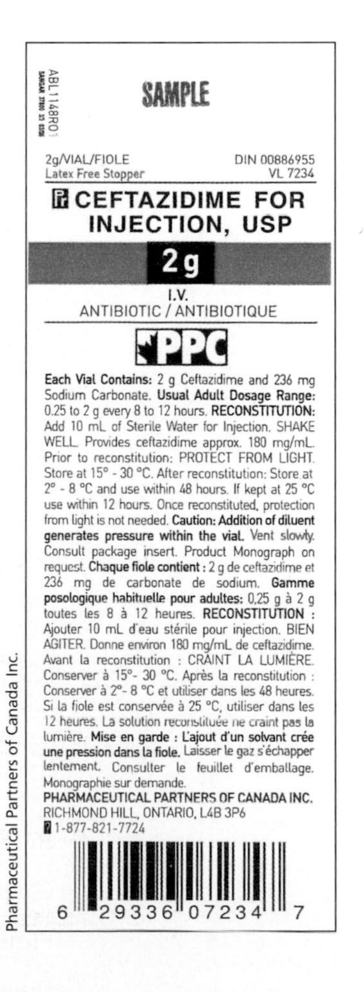

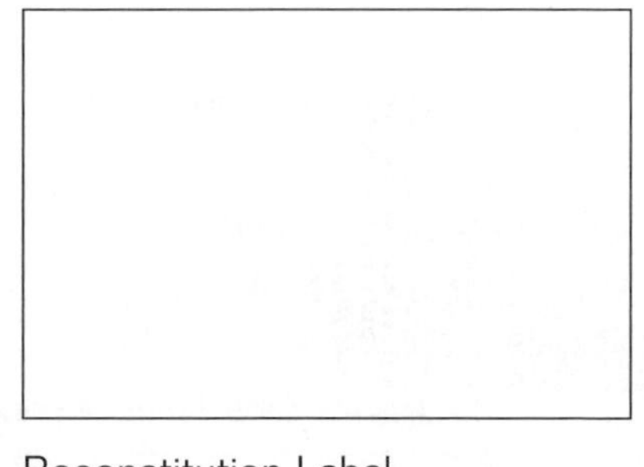

Reconstitution Label

½ 1 1½ 2 2½ 3mL

13. Order: *ceftriaxone 750 mg IV q6h in 50 mL D_5W (5% Dextrose & Water minibag administration solution)*

Reconstitute vial with ________ mL diluent for an initial concentration of ________ mg/mL. Withdraw: ________ mL and inject in 50 mL minibag of D_5W

How many full doses are available in this vial?
________ dose(s)

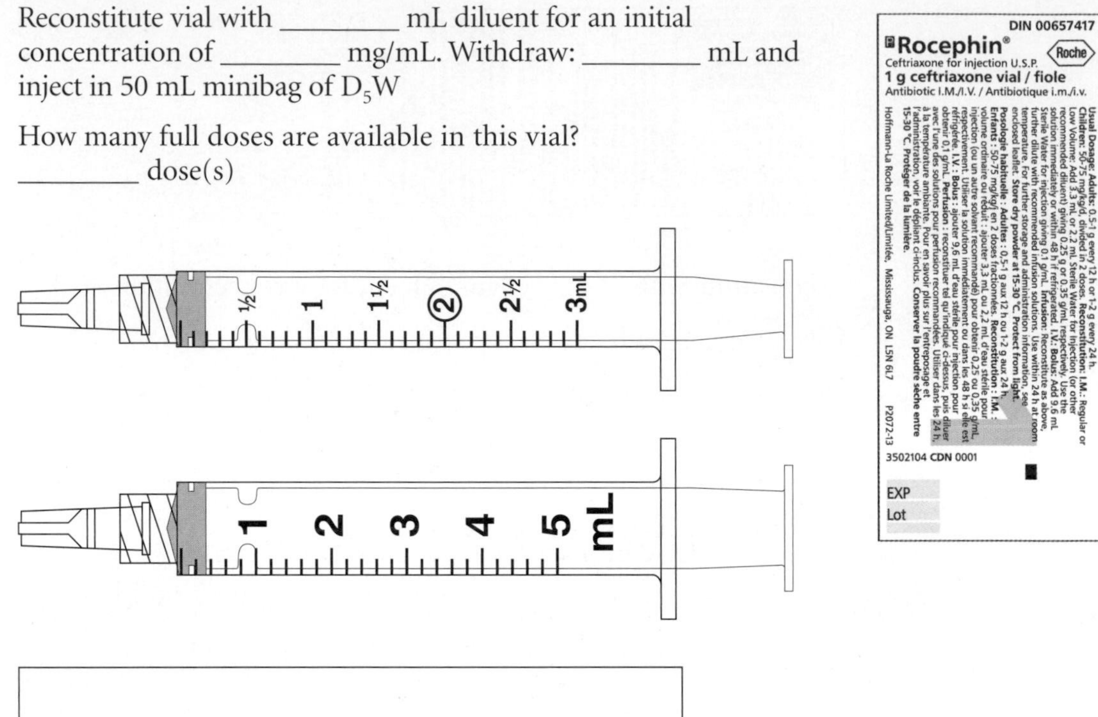

Courtesy of Hoffmann-La Roche Limited

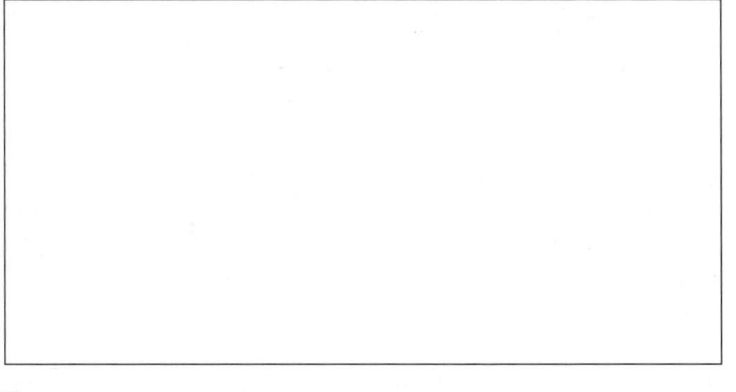

Reconstitution Label

14. Order: *tobramycin sulfate 80 mg IV q8h*

C300351 DIN 00533688
Latex Free Stopper
Tobramycin for Injection, USP
1.2 g Tobramycin/Vial/Fiole
For Hospital use only / Pharmacy Bulk Sterile Vial
For Intravenous infusion Only
Réservé à l'usage intrahospitalier
Fiole grand format stérile pour pharmacies
Pour perfusion intraveineuse seulement
PPC
equivalent to 1.2 g Tobramycin

ANTIBIOTIC
Each vial contains: tobramycin sulfate equivalent to 1.2 g tobramycin with no preservatives.
Usual Adult Dosage Range: 60 to 80 mg every 8 hours.
I.V. use: add 30 mL Sterile Water for Injection. Provides tobramycin 40 mg/mL. Shake to dissolve. Consult package insert.
Store at room temperature. The reconstituted solution should be dispensed and diluted for use within 8 hours. Discard unused portion.
Product Monograph available on request.
ANTIBIOTIQUE
Usage I.V. : ajouter 30 mL d'eau stérile pour injection. Donne 40 mg/mL de tobramycine. Bien agiter pour dissoudre.
Conserver à température ambiante. La solution reconstituée devrait être diluée et administrée dans les 8 heures. Jeter toute portion inutilisée.
Monographie du produit disponible sur demande.
VIAL ENTRY: Date ______ Time ______
TOBRAMYCIN FOR INJECTION, USP
PHARMACEUTICAL PARTNERS OF CANADA INC.
Richmond Hill, Ontario L4B 3P6
402177A
LIFT HERE
6 29336-303-51 9

Pharmaceutical Partners of Canada Inc.

Reconstitute with ________ mL diluent for a concentration of ________ mg/mL.

Give: ________ mL

How many full doses are available in this vial? ________ dose(s)

Prepare a reconstitution label for the remaining solution.

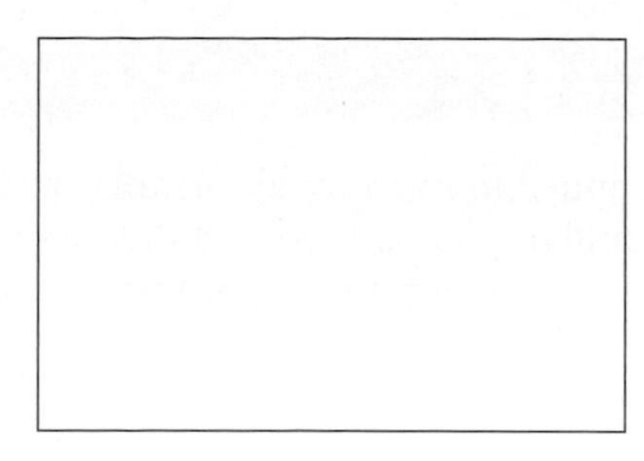

Reconstitution Label

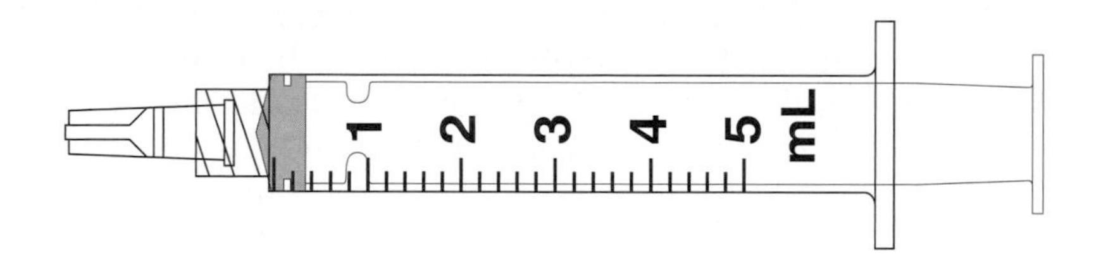

15. Order: *cefazolin 250 mg IM q6h*

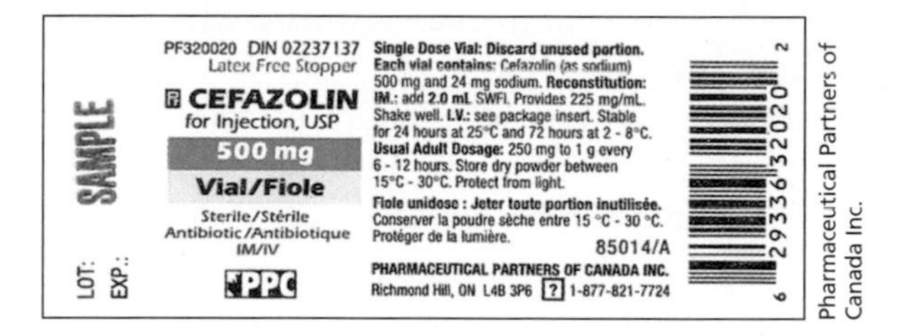

SAMPLE
LOT:
EXP.:
PF320020 DIN 02237137
Latex Free Stopper
CEFAZOLIN
for Injection, USP
500 mg
Vial/Fiole
Sterile/Stérile
Antibiotic/Antibiotique
IM/IV
PPC
Single Dose Vial: Discard unused portion.
Each vial contains: Cefazolin (as sodium) 500 mg and 24 mg sodium. Reconstitution: IM.: add 2.0 mL SWFI. Provides 225 mg/mL. Shake well. I.V.: see package insert. Stable for 24 hours at 25°C and 72 hours at 2 - 8°C.
Usual Adult Dosage: 250 mg to 1 g every 6 - 12 hours. Store dry powder between 15°C - 30°C. Protect from light.
Fiole unidose : Jeter toute portion inutilisée.
Conserver la poudre sèche entre 15 °C - 30 °C.
Protéger de la lumière.
85014/A
PHARMACEUTICAL PARTNERS OF CANADA INC.
Richmond Hill, ON L4B 3P6 ? 1-877-821-7724
6 29336 32020 2

Pharmaceutical Partners of Canada Inc.

Reconstitute with ________ mL diluent for a concentration of ________ mg/mL.

Give: ________ mL

How many full doses are available in this vial? ________ dose(s)

Prepare a reconstitution label for the remaining solution.

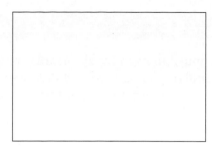

Reconstitution Label

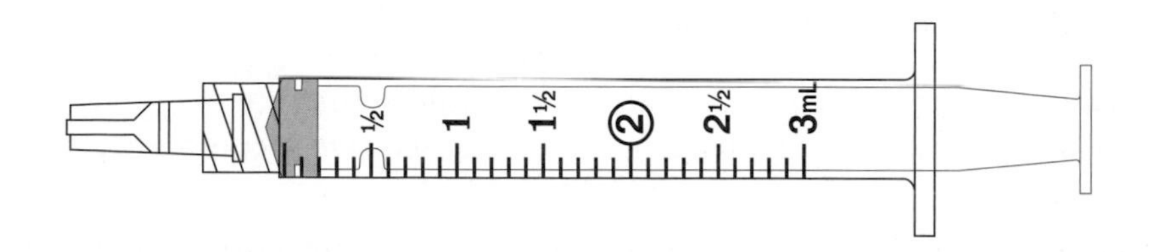

Check your work! Answers to all Review Sets are provided at the end of each chapter. Worked solutions for selected Review Sets are also provided there.

RECONSTITUTION OF NONINJECTABLE SOLUTIONS

The principles of reconstitution can also be applied to nutritional formulas and irrigating solutions. Although many solutions are specifically formulated to be used in full strength, in many cases the nurse or healthcare provider must dilute a liquid concentrate (solute) with water or saline (solvent) to make a weaker solution.

Solution Concentration

An important concept for understanding solution concentration or strength is that the amount of solvent used to decrease the total concentration is determined by the desired final strength of the solution. The *less* solvent added, the more concentrated the final solution strength; the *more* solvent added, the less concentrated the final solution strength. To illustrate this concept, think of orange juice concentrate. The directions require three cans of water to be added to one can of orange juice concentrate. The result is "reconstituted juice," a ready-to-drink beverage. If you like a stronger orange taste, you could add only two cans of water, making it a *more* concentrated juice, but you will have *less total volume* to drink. If you have several people wanting to drink orange juice, you might choose to add four cans of water to the final total volume. You will have *more* volume, but the orange juice will be *less* concentrated; therefore, it is more dilute because you have increased the water (solvent) content. Note that in each example, the amount of orange juice concentrate in the final solution is the same.

A ratio, percent, or fraction is used to express the strength of a solution. The fraction is the preferred form because it is easily applied in calculations and helps explain the ratio of solute to total solution. Recall that a ratio or percent can also be expressed as a fraction.

RATIONALE FOR PRACTICE

When the strength of a solution made from a liquid concentrate is expressed as a fraction,

- **The numerator of the fraction is the number of parts of solute;**
- **The denominator of the fraction is the total number of parts of total solution; and**
- **The difference between the denominator (final solution) and the numerator (parts of solute) is the number of parts of solvent.**

Some solutions made from liquid concentrates follow.

Example 1:

$\frac{1}{4}$ *strength reconstituted orange juice* made from canned frozen concentrate

$$\frac{1}{4}\text{ strength} = \frac{1\text{ part (can) of frozen orange juice concentrate}}{4\text{ parts (cans) of total reconstituted orange juice}}$$

- 1 part (can) frozen orange juice concentrate (*solute*, numerator)
- 4 parts (cans) of total reconstituted orange juice (*solution*, denominator)
- $4 - 1 = 3$ parts (cans) of water (*solvent*)

Three cans of water added to 1 can of frozen orange juice concentrate makes 4 cans of a final reconstituted orange juice solution. The resulting $\frac{1}{4}$ strength reconstituted orange juice is comparable to the strength of fresh juice.

Example 2:

$\frac{1}{3}$ *strength nutritional formula*

- 1 part concentrate formula as the solute
- 3 parts of total solution
- $3 - 1 = 2$ parts solvent (water)

Calculating Solutions

To prepare a prescribed solution of a certain strength from a solute, you can apply a similar formula to the one you learned for calculating dosages: $D \times Q = X$.

RATIONALE FOR PRACTICE

To prepare solutions,

1. D (desired solution strength) × Q (quantity of desired solution) = X (amount of solute)
2. Quantity of desired solution − Amount of solute = Amount of solvent

In this application, D is the strength of the desired solution, which is written as a fraction. Q is the amount of solution you want to prepare, usually expressed as millilitres or ounces. The unknown X you are solving for is the amount of solute you will add to the solvent to prepare the desired solution. Let us now examine how this rationale and formula are applied in healthcare.

TOPICAL SOLUTIONS/IRRIGANTS

Topical and irrigating solutions can be mixed from powders, salts, or liquid concentrates. Asepsis in the preparation, storage, and use is essential. Liquids can harbour microorganisms. Our focus is to review the essentials of reconstitution; however, nurses and other healthcare providers need to be alert at all times to the chain of infection.

Usually, healthcare providers will further dilute ready-to-use solutions, or *full-strength* or stock solutions, to create a less concentrated liquid. Consider both the desired solution strength and the final volume needed to complete the dilution.

Example:

Hydrogen peroxide, which is usually available full strength as a 3% solution, can be drying to the skin and should not be directly applied undiluted. For use as a topical antiseptic, the therapeutic protocol is to reconstitute hydrogen peroxide to $\frac{1}{2}$ strength with normal saline used as the solvent. You decide to make 120 mL that can be kept in a sterile container at the patient's bedside for traction pin care.

Apply the Three-Step Approach to the calculation.

Step 1 Convert No conversion is necessary.

Step 2 Think The fraction represents the desired solution strength: $\frac{1}{2}$ strength means 1 part solute (hydrogen peroxide) to 2 total parts solution. The amount of solvent is $2 - 1 = 1$ part saline. Because you need 120 mL of solution, you estimate that you will need $\frac{1}{2}$ of it as solute and $\frac{1}{2}$ of it as solvent, or 60 mL hydrogen peroxide and 60 mL saline to make a total of 120 mL of $\frac{1}{2}$ strength hydrogen peroxide.

Step 3 Calculate $D \times Q = X$

$\frac{1}{2}$ (strength of desired solution) $\times$ 120 mL (quantity desired) = X (amount of solute)

$$\frac{1}{2} \times 120 \text{ mL} = 60 \text{ mL}$$

X (60 mL) is the quantity of solute (full-strength hydrogen peroxide) you need to prepare the desired solution (120 mL of $\frac{1}{2}$ strength hydrogen peroxide). The amount of solvent is 120 mL − 60 mL = 60 mL. If you add 60 mL of full-strength hydrogen peroxide (solute) to 60 mL of normal saline (solvent), you will prepare 120 mL of a $\frac{1}{2}$ strength hydrogen peroxide topical antiseptic.

ORAL AND ENTERAL FEEDINGS

The principles of reconstitution are frequently applied to nutritional supplements for children and adults who have special needs. Premature infants require increased calories for growth but cannot take large volumes of fluid. Children with intestinal malabsorption require incremental changes as their bodies adjust to more concentrated formulas. Adults, especially older adults, also experience nutritional problems that can be treated with liquid nutrition. Prepared solutions that are taken orally or through feeding tubes are usually available and ready to use from manufacturers. Nutritional solutions may also be mixed from powders or liquid concentrates. Figure 10-12 shows examples of the three forms of one nutritional formula. Directions on the label detail how much water should be added to the powdered form or liquid concentrate. Nutritionists provide further expertise in creating complex solutions for special patient needs.

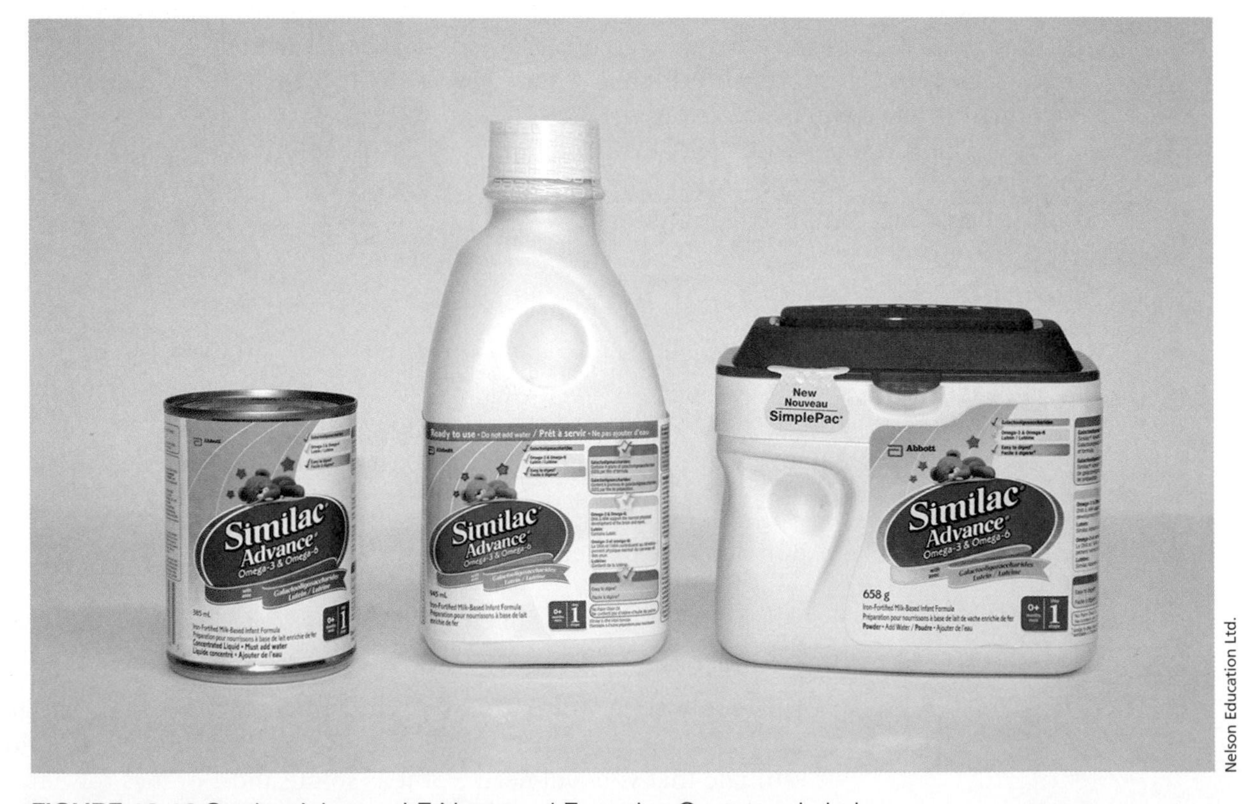

FIGURE 10-12 Similac Advance LF Nutritional Formulas Container Labels

Asepsis in the preparation, storage, and use of nutritional supplements is essential. Healthcare providers must be alert at all times to the potential for a break in the chain of infection. Because nutritional supplements contain sugars, they have an increased risk of contamination during preparation and of spoilage during storage and use. These are important concepts to teach a patient's family members.

Diluting Ready-to-Use Nutritional Supplements

Ready-to-use liquid nutritional supplements are normally administered directly from the container without any further dilution. A variety of ready-to-use supplements are available that contain various amounts of proteins, carbohydrates, and fats as well as other nutrients. They vary in calorie count (usually determined per 100 mL) and are given to both children and adults. The manufacturer balances the solute (nutrition) and solvent (water) to create a balanced, full-strength solution. However, some children and adults require less than full-strength supplement for a short period to normalize intestinal absorption. Nutritional supplements are diluted with sterile water or tap water for oral use. Consult the institution policy regarding the use of tap water to reconstitute nutritional supplements. A few typical examples follow.

Example 1:

The prescriber orders *Ensure $\frac{1}{4}$ strength 120 mL q2h via NG tube × 3 feedings* for a patient who is recovering from gastric surgery. A 235-mL can of Ensure ready-to-use product is available.

Apply the Three-Step Approach to dosage calculation.

Step 1 Convert No conversion is necessary.

Step 2 Think You need 120 mL total reconstituted meal replacement product for each of 3 feedings. This is a total of $120 \times 3 = 360$ mL. But you must dilute the full-strength Ensure to $\frac{1}{4}$ strength. You know that $\frac{1}{4}$ strength means 1 part Ensure to 4 parts solution. The solvent needed is $4 - 1 = 3$ parts water. You will need $\frac{1}{4}$ of the solution as solute ($\frac{1}{4} \times 360$ mL $= 90$ mL) and $\frac{3}{4}$ of the solution as solvent ($\frac{3}{4} \times 360$ mL $= 270$ mL). Therefore, if you mix 90 mL of full-strength Ensure with 270 mL of water, you will have 360 mL of $\frac{1}{4}$ strength Ensure.

Step 3 Calculate $D \times Q = \frac{1}{4} \times 360$ mL $= 90$ mL full-strength Ensure

You need 90 mL of Ensure (solute). Use 90 mL from the 235-mL can. The amount of solvent needed is 360 mL $-$ 90 mL $=$ 270 mL water. Add 270 mL water to 90 mL of full-strength Ensure to make a total of 360 mL of $\frac{1}{4}$ strength Ensure. There is now enough for 3 full feedings. Administer 120 mL to the patient for each feeding.

Example 2:

The prescriber orders *800 mL of $\frac{3}{4}$ strength Boost Plus through a gastrostomy tube over 8 h* to supplement a patient while he sleeps. Boost Plus ready-to-use product is available in 237-mL bottles.

Apply the Three-Step Approach to dosage calculation.

Step 1 Convert No conversion is necessary.

Step 2 Think The ordered solution strength is $\frac{3}{4}$. This means "3 parts solute to 4 total parts in solution." You know that $\frac{3}{4}$ of the 800 mL will be solute or full-strength Boost Plus ($\frac{3}{4} \times 800$ mL $= 600$ mL) and $\frac{1}{4}$ of the solution will be solvent or water ($\frac{1}{4} \times 800$ mL $= 200$ mL). This proportion of solute to solvent will reconstitute the Boost Plus to the required $\frac{3}{4}$ strength and total volume of 800 mL.

Step 3 Calculate $D \times Q = \frac{3}{4} \times 800$ mL $= 600$ mL of full-strength Boost Plus

You need 600 mL of Boost Plus (solute). Because the bottle contains 237 mL, you will need 2.6 bottles (600 mL) to prepare the $\frac{3}{4}$ strength Boost Plus as ordered. The amount of solvent needed is 800 mL $-$ 600 mL $=$ 200 mL water. Add 200 mL water to 600 mL (2.6 bottles) of full-strength Boost Plus to make a total of 800 mL of $\frac{3}{4}$ strength Boost Plus for the full feeding.

QUICK REVIEW

- *Solute*—a concentrated or solid substance to be dissolved or diluted.
- *Solvent*/Diluent—a liquid substance that dissolves another substance to prepare a solution.
- *Solution*—the resulting mixture of a solute plus a solvent.
- When a fraction expresses the strength of a desired solution to be made from a liquid concentrate,
  - The *numerator* of the fraction is the number of parts of *solute*;
  - The *denominator* of the fraction is the total number of parts of *solution*; and
  - The *difference between the denominator and the numerator* is the number of parts of *solvent*.
- To prepare solutions:

  1. D (Desired solution strength) $\times$ Q (Quantity of desired solution) $=$ X (Amount of solute)

  2. Quantity of desired solution $-$ Amount of solute $=$ Amount of solvent

REVIEW SET 10-2

Explain how you would prepare each of the following from ready-to-use nutritional formulas for the specified time period. Note which supply would require the least discard of unused product.

1. $\frac{1}{3}$ *strength Ensure 900 mL via NG tube over 9 h*

   Supply: Ensure 235-mL can ______________________

2. $\frac{1}{4}$ *strength Isomil 120 mL PO q4h for 24 h*

   Supply: Isomil 235-mL can ______________________

3. $\frac{2}{3}$ *strength Boost Plus 300 mL PO QID*

   Supply: Boost Plus 237-mL bottle ______________________

4. $\frac{1}{2}$ *strength Ensure 780 mL via gastrostomy tube over 5 h*

   Supply: Ensure 235-mL can ______________________

5. $\frac{1}{2}$ *strength Boost Plus 250 mL PO QID*

   Supply: Boost Plus 237-mL bottle ____________

6. $\frac{3}{4}$ *strength Isomil 240 mL PO q4h for 24 h*

   Supply: Isomil 235-mL can ____________

7. $\frac{2}{3}$ *strength Ensure 180 mL via gastrostomy tube over 2 h*

   Supply: Ensure 235-mL can ____________

8. $\frac{1}{4}$ *strength Ensure 480 mL via NG tube over 6 h*

   Supply: Ensure 235-mL can ____________

Prepare the following solutions using the same principles used for preparing enteral feeding solutions with water as the diluent.

9. *70% solution from 50 mL of mouthwash* ____________
10. *20% solution from 80 mL of skin cleanser* ____________
11. *2% solution from 5 mL of sodium bicarbonate* ____________
12. *50% solution from 240 mL of hydrogen peroxide* ____________

Check your work! Answers to all Review Sets are provided at the end of each chapter. Worked solutions for selected Review Sets are also available there.

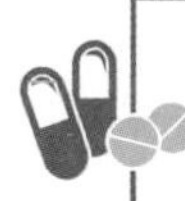

UNDERSTANDING NCLEX QUESTIONS

Here's an example of a standard question used in textbooks:

Cefotaxime sodium 800 mg IV QID is ordered. Available is a 2-g vial. The drug when reconstituted with 10 mL of sterile water for injection provides 180 mg/mL. Each dose will contain:

a. 2.4 mL
b. 3.4 mL
c. 4.4 mL
d. 5.4 mL

Here's how the question would look in an NCLEX examination:

The nurse is to administer cefotaxime sodium 800 mg IV QID. Available is a 2-g vial. The drug insert states to reconstitute with 10 mL of sterile water for injection to provide 180 mg/mL. How many mL of the drug should the nurse administer for each dose?

a. 2.4 mL
b. 3.4 mL
c. 4.4 mL
d. 5.4 mL

Answer: c

$$\frac{D}{H} \times Q = \frac{800 \text{ mg}}{180 \text{ mg}} \times 1 \text{ mL} = 4.444 = 4.4 \text{ mL}$$

APPLICATION OF CLINICAL REASONING

Errors in formula dilution occur when the nurse fails to correctly calculate the amount of solute and solvent needed for the required solution strength.

Potential Patient Safety Incident

Incorrect calculation of solute and solvent.

Possible Scenario

Suppose the prescriber orders *$\frac{1}{3}$ strength Isomil 90 mL PO q3h for four feedings* for an infant recovering from gastroenteritis. The concentration will be increased after these feedings. The nurse knows she will give all four feedings during her 12-hour shift, so she requires 360 mL of product. She takes a 235-mL can of ready-to-use Isomil, removes 120 mL, and adds 360 mL of water for oral use. She thinks, "One-third means 120 mL of formula and 360 mL of water. This is easy!"

Potential Outcome

What the nurse has actually mixed is a $\frac{1}{4}$ strength solution. Because the infant is getting a more dilute solution than intended, the amount of water to solute is increased and the incremental tolerance of more concentrated product could be jeopardized. Thinking the infant is tolerating $\frac{1}{3}$ strength, the physician might increase it to $\frac{2}{3}$ strength, and the infant may have problems digesting this more concentrated product. The infant's progress could be jeopardized.

Prevention

The nurse should have thought through the meaning of the terms of a solution. If so, she would have recognized that $\frac{1}{3}$ strength means 1 part solute (formula) to 3 total parts of solution with 2 parts water, not 1 part formula to 3 parts water. She should have applied the calculation formula to determine the amount of solute (full-strength Isomil) needed and the amount of solvent (water) to add. If she did not know how to prepare the product, she should have consulted another nurse or called the pharmacy or dietary services for assistance. Never guess. Think and calculate with accuracy.

Application of Critical Reasoning Additional application problems are provided at the end of the chapter. Answers are provided at the end of the book.

PRACTICE PROBLEMS—CHAPTER 10

Calculate the amount you will prepare for one dose. Indicate the syringe you will select to measure the medication.

1. Order: *piperacillin sodium/tazobactam sodium 2.5 g IV q8h*

   Supply: 3.375-g vial of powdered piperacillin sodium/tazobactam sodium

   Directions: Reconstitute piperacillin sodium/tazobactam sodium with 15 mL of a compatible diluent for a total solution volume of 17.36 mL at 0.194 g/mL.

   The concentration is ________ g/ ________ mL.

   Give: ________ mL

   Select: ________ syringe

2. Order: *ampicillin sodium 500 mg IM q4h*

   Supply: ampicillin sodium 500 mg

   Directions: Reconstitute with 1.8 mL diluent for a concentration of 250 mg/mL.

   Give: ________ mL

   Select: ________ syringe

3. Order: *cefazolin sodium 500 mg IV q6h*

   Supply: cefazolin sodium 1 g

   Directions: Reconstitute with 2.5 mL diluent to yield 3 mL with concentration of 330 mg/mL.

   Give: ________ mL

   Select: ________ syringe

4. Order: *ceftriaxone sodium 750 mg IV q6h in 50 mL 5% Dextrose & Water IV solution*

   Supply: See label and package insert below for ceftriaxone sodium IV vial.

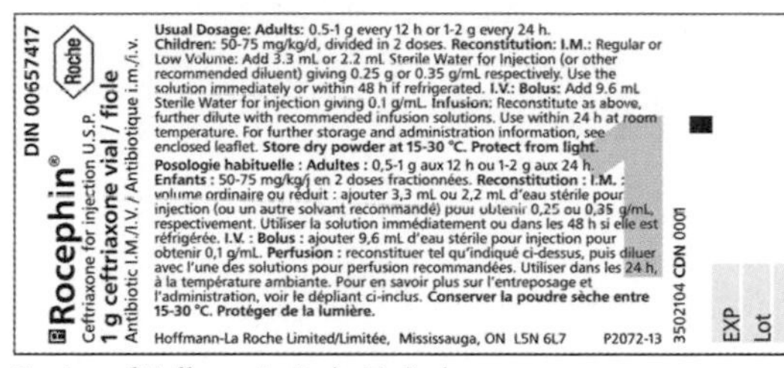

Courtesy of Hoffmann-La Roche Limited

3599043 CDN
0504.1075

Rocephin®
Ceftriaxone for injection

Please refer to product monograph for full product information

Dosage and administration

ROCEPHIN (ceftriaxone sodium) may be administered intravenously or intramuscularly after reconstitution.

Dosage and route of administration should be determined by the severity of infection, susceptibility of the causative organisms, and condition of the patient. The intravenous route is preferable for patients with septicemia or other severe or life threatening infections.

Dosage

Adults

Type of infection	Route	Dose	Frequency	Total daily dose
Moderate and severe infections	I.V. or I.M.	1 or 2 g	q24 h	1 or 2 g
		0.5 or 1 g	q12 h	1 or 2 g

There is limited experience with daily doses of 3–4 g administered as single dose or two equally divided doses. The total daily dose should not exceed 4 g.

Uncomplicated gonorrhea	I.M.	0.25 g	Single dose	–

Infants and children (one month to 12 years of age)

Type of infection	Route	Dose	Frequency	Total daily dose
Serious miscellaneous infections	I.V. or I.M.	25 or 37.5 mg per kg	q12 h	50 or 75 mg per kg

The total daily dose should not exceed 2 g. If body weight is 50 kg or more the adult dose should be used.

Meningitis	I.V. or I.M.	50 mg/kg*	q12 h	100 mg/kg

* With or without a loading dose of 75 mg/kg.
The total daily dose should not exceed 4 g.

With the exception of gonorrhea, which is treated with a single dose, the administration of ROCEPHIN should be continued for a minimum of 48–72 hours after the patient defervesces or after evidence of bacterial eradication has been obtained, usually 4–14 days. In bone and joint infections the average duration of treatment during clinical trials was 6 weeks, with a range of 1–13 weeks, depending on the severity of the infection.

When treating infections caused by beta hemolytic streptococcus, it is recommended that therapy be continued for at least 10 days. The average duration of therapy for infections associated with beta hemolytic streptococcus during clinical trials was 2 weeks, with a range of 1–5 weeks, depending on the site and severity of the infection.

Prophylaxis
(vaginal or abdominal hysterectomy, coronary artery bypass surgery, biliary tract surgery)
For preoperative use as prophylaxis before vaginal or abdominal hysterectomy or coronary artery bypass surgery or biliary tract surgery in patients at risk of infection, a single

Impairment of renal and/or hepatic function
In patients with mild to moderate renal impairment, changes in the dosage regimen are not required, provided liver function is intact. In cases of preterminal renal failure (creatinine clearance less than 10 mL per min), periodic monitoring of serum ceftriaxone concentrations is recommended. The daily dosage should be limited to 2 g or less. In patients with liver damage, there is no need for the dosage to be reduced provided renal function is intact. In cases of coexistent renal and clinically significant hepatic insufficiency, close monitoring of serum ceftriaxone concentrations, at regular intervals, is recommended. If there is evidence of accumulation, dosage should be decreased accordingly.

Administration

Intramuscular
The reconstituted solution of ROCEPHIN should be administered by deep intragluteal injection. It is recommended that not more than 1 g be injected at a single site. Pain on intramuscular injection is usually mild and less frequent when ROCEPHIN is administered in sterile 1% lidocaine solution.

Intravenous (bolus) injection
The reconstituted solution should be administered over approximately 5 minutes. If the distal port of an intravenous administration set is used, stop the primary flow, inject the reconstituted ROCEPHIN solution and then restart the primary flow. This will prevent mixing with the primary fluid and possible incompatibilities.

Short intravenous infusion
The further diluted intravenous solution should be given over a period of 10–15 minutes in infants and children and 20–30 minutes in adults.

Note: ROCEPHIN solution should not be physically mixed with aminoglycoside antibiotics nor administered at the same site because of possible chemical incompatibility. There have also been literature reports of physical incompatibilities between ceftriaxone and vancomycin, amsacrine, or fluconazole.

Reconstitution

For intramuscular use
Reconstitute ROCEPHIN powder with the appropriate diluent:
- Sterile Water for Injection
- 0.9% Sodium Chloride Injection
- 5% Dextrose Injection
- Bacteriostatic Water for Injection
- 1% Lidocaine Solution

Reconstitute as follows:

Regular volume reconstitution table (I.M.)*

Vial size	Volume to be added to vial mL	Approximate available volume mL	Approximate average concentration g/mL
0.25 g	0.9	1.0	0.25
1.0 g	3.3	4.0	0.25
2.0 g	6.6	8.0	0.25

*Shake well until dissolved.

Low volume reconstitution table (I.M.)*

Vial size	Volume to be added to vial mL	Approximate available volume mL	Approximate average concentration g/mL
0.25 g	Not recommended for this vial size		
1.0 g	2.2	2.8	0.35
2.0 g	4.4	5.6	0.35

*Shake well until dissolved.

Note: solutions prepared for intramuscular use or any solution containing lidocaine or bacteriostatic

For intravenous use
Reconstitute only with Sterile Water for Injection.

Reconstitute as follows:

Reconstitution table (I.V.)**

Vial size	Volume to be added to vial mL	Approximate available volume mL	Approximate average concentration g/mL
0.25 g	2.4	2.5	0.1
1.0 g	9.6	10.1	0.1
2.0 g	19.2	20.5	0.1

**Shake well until dissolved. The prepared solution may be further diluted to the desired volume with any of the "Solutions for I.V. Infusion" listed below.

Solutions for I.V. infusion
- 0.9% Sodium Chloride Injection
- 5% Dextrose Injection
- Dextrose and Sodium Chloride Injection

Pharmacy bulk vial reconstitution for preparation of intravenous infusion solutions
The closure of the pharmacy bulk vial shall be penetrated only one time after reconstitution, using a suitable sterile transfer device or dispensing set which allows measured dispensing for the contents.

Reconstitution table for bulk pharmacy vial***

Vial size	Volume to be added to vial mL	Approximate available volume mL	Approximate average concentration g/mL
10 g	95	101	0.1

***Shake well until dissolved. Withdraw the required amount and dilute with one of the "Solutions for I.V. infusion". Any unused solution remaining within a period of 8 hours should be discarded.

Stability and storage recommendations

ROCEPHIN sterile powder should be stored at a controlled room temperature (between 15 and 30 °C) and protected from light.

Reconstituted solutions –
Stability and storage recommendations
1. *For intramuscular use:* Solutions should be reconstituted immediately before use. If storage is required, these solutions may be stored under refrigeration and should be used within 48 hours.
2. *For I.V. bolus injection (without further dilution):* Reconstituted solutions should be administered within 24 hours when stored at room temperature and within 72 hours when refrigerated (2–8 °C).
3. *For I.V. infusion:* Further diluted reconstituted solutions should be administered within 24 hours when stored at room temperature.
   a) Solutions further diluted with 0.9% Sodium Chloride Injection, or with 5% Dextrose Injection should be administered within 72 hours when stored under refrigeration (2–8 °C).
   b) Solutions further diluted with Dextrose and Sodium Chloride Injection as diluent should not be refrigerated. These solutions are not physically compatible when refrigerated.
4. *Extended use of intravenous admixtures:* Although intravenous admixtures may often be physically and chemically stable for longer periods, **due to microbiological considerations, they are usually recommended for use within a maximum of 24 hours at room temperature or 72 hours when refrigerated (2–8 °C).** Hospitals and institutions that have recognized admixture programs and use validated aseptic techniques for preparation of intravenous solutions may extend the storage times for ROCEPHIN admixtures with 0.9% Sodium Chloride Injection or 5% Dextrose Injection in glass or polyvinyl chloride

Warning
As with all parenteral drug products, intravenous admixtures should be visually inspected prior to administration, whenever solution and container permit. Solutions showing any evidence of haziness or cloudiness, particulate matter, precipitation, discolouration or leakage should not be used.

5. *Frozen I.V. infusion solutions:* Hospitals and institutions that have recognized admixture programs and use validated aseptic techniques for preparation of intravenous solutions may freeze and store ROCEPHIN I.V. infusion solutions when prepared in accordance with the following instructions.
   I.V. infusion solutions prepared from reconstituted ROCEPHIN (ceftriaxone sodium) further diluted with 5% Dextrose Injection or 0.9% Sodium Chloride Injection, in flexible polyvinyl chloride infusion containers, in concentrations up to 40 mg ceftriaxone per mL, may be stored at –10 to –20 °C for periods up to three months.
   The frozen solutions should be thawed in a refrigerator (2–8 °C) overnight and should subsequently be used within 24 hours when stored at room temperature or seven days when stored under refrigeration (2–8 °C).
   After thawing, check for leaks by squeezing the bag firmly. If leaks are found, discard the container as sterility may be impaired. Do not use unless the solution is clear and seals/outlet ports are intact. Ceftriaxone solutions range from light yellow to amber in colour. Parenteral drug products should be inspected visually for particulate matter and discolouration prior to administration whenever the solution and container permit.
   DO NOT REFREEZE the previously frozen ceftriaxone I.V. infusion solutions.

Incompatibility
ROCEPHIN should not be physically mixed with other antimicrobial agents, vancomycin, amsacrine, or fluconazole.
ROCEPHIN should not be added to blood products, protein hydrolysates or amino acids.
ROCEPHIN should not be added to solutions containing calcium.

Availability of dosage forms
1. ROCEPHIN vials containing sterile ceftriaxone sodium powder equivalent to 0.25 g, 1 g and 2 g of ceftriaxone.
2. ROCEPHIN Pharmacy Bulk vials containing sterile ceftriaxone sodium powder equivalent to 10 g ceftriaxone (not for direct administration). The availability of the pharmacy bulk vial is restricted to hospitals with a recognized intravenous admixture programme.

Product monograph dated March 5, 2004
This leaflet issued May 2005

Hoffmann-La Roche Limited
Mississauga, ON L5N 6L7

Courtesy of Hoffmann-La Roche Limited

Add ________ mL diluent to the vial.

The concentration is ________ mg/mL.

Give: ________ mL

How many full doses are available in this vial? ________ dose(s)

Select: ________ syringe

5. Order: *cefepime hydrochloride 500 mg IM q12h*

   Supply: cefepime hydrochloride 1 g

   Directions: Reconstitute with 2.4 mL diluent for an approximate available volume of 3.6 mL and a concentration of 280 mg/mL.

   Give: ________ mL

   Select: ________ syringe

   How many full doses are available in this vial? ________ dose(s)

   Prepare a reconstitution label for the remaining solution. The drug is stable for up to 72 hours refrigerated.

Reconstitution Label

6. Order: *tigecycline 100 mg IV X 1 dose followed by 50 mg IV q12h administered over 30 to 60 min*

   Supply: 50 mg/vial

   Directions: Reconstitute with 5.3 mL of 0.9% Sodium Chloride Injection, 5% Dextrose Injection, or Lactated Ringer's Injection to yield a concentration of 10 mg/mL of tigecycline.The vial should be gently swirled until the drug dissolves

   Give: ________ mL for the initial dose followed by ________ q12h

   Select: ________ syringe for the initial dose and a ________ syringe for the following doses

Calculate one dose of each of the drug orders numbered 7 through 15. The labels show the medications you have available. Indicate which syringe you would select to measure the dose to be administered. Specify whether a reconstitution label is required for multiple-dose vials.

7. Order: *cefazolin sodium 300 mg IM q8h*

   Reconstitute with ________ mL diluent for a concentration of ________ mg/mL and give ________ mL.

   Select: ________ syringe

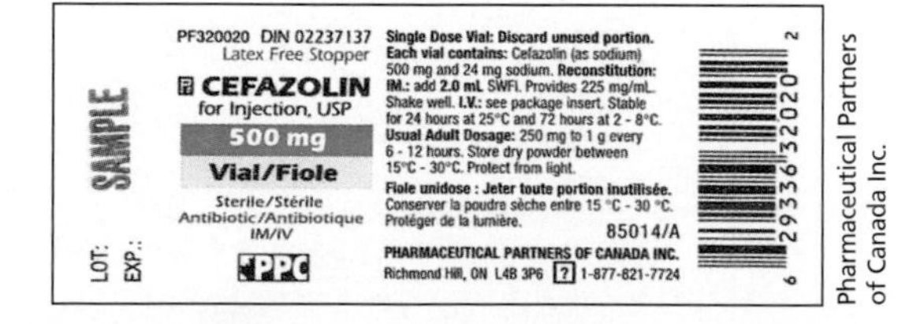

Pharmaceutical Partners of Canada Inc.

   How many full doses are available in this vial? ________ dose(s)

   Is a reconstitution label required? ________

8. Order: *methylprednisolone sodium succinate 200 mg IV q6h*

   Reconstitute with ________ mL diluent for a concentration of ________ mg/mL and give ________ mL.

   Select: ________ syringe

   How many full doses are available in this vial? ________ dose(s)

   Is a reconstitution label required? ________

Sterile/Stérile DIN 02241229
METHYLPREDNISOLONE Sodium Succinate for Injection, USP
Succinate sodique de MÉTHYLPREDNISOLONE pour injection, USP
1 g
methylprednisolone per vial / de méthylprednisolone par fiole
IM or IV Use / Usage IM ou IV

Novopharm Limited, Toronto, ON

9. Order: *cefazolin sodium 350 mg IM q12h*

   Reconstitute with ________ mL diluent for a concentration of ________ mg/mL and give ________ mL.

   Select: ________ syringe

   How many full doses are available in this vial? ________ dose(s)

   Is a reconstitution label required? ________

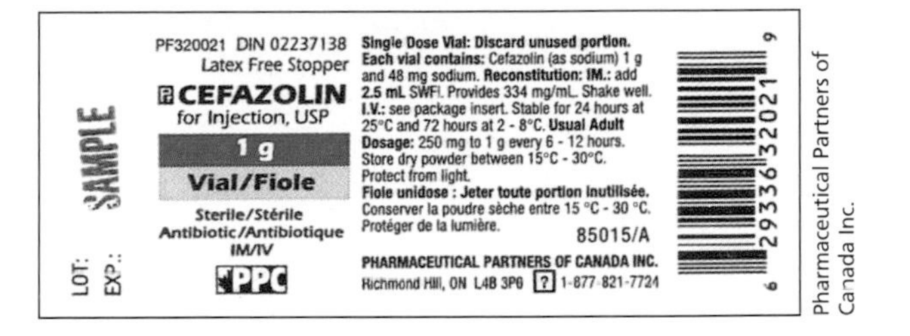

Pharmaceutical Partners of Canada Inc.

10. Order: *bacitracin 7500 units IM q12h*

    Reconstitution of the 50 000-unit vial with 9.8 mL of diluent will result in a concentration of 5000 units per mL. Solutions are stable for 1 week when refrigerated.

    Reconstitute with ________ mL diluent for a concentration of ________ units/mL and give ________ mL.

    Select: ________ syringe

    How many full doses are available in this vial? ________ dose(s)

    Is a reconstitution label required? ________

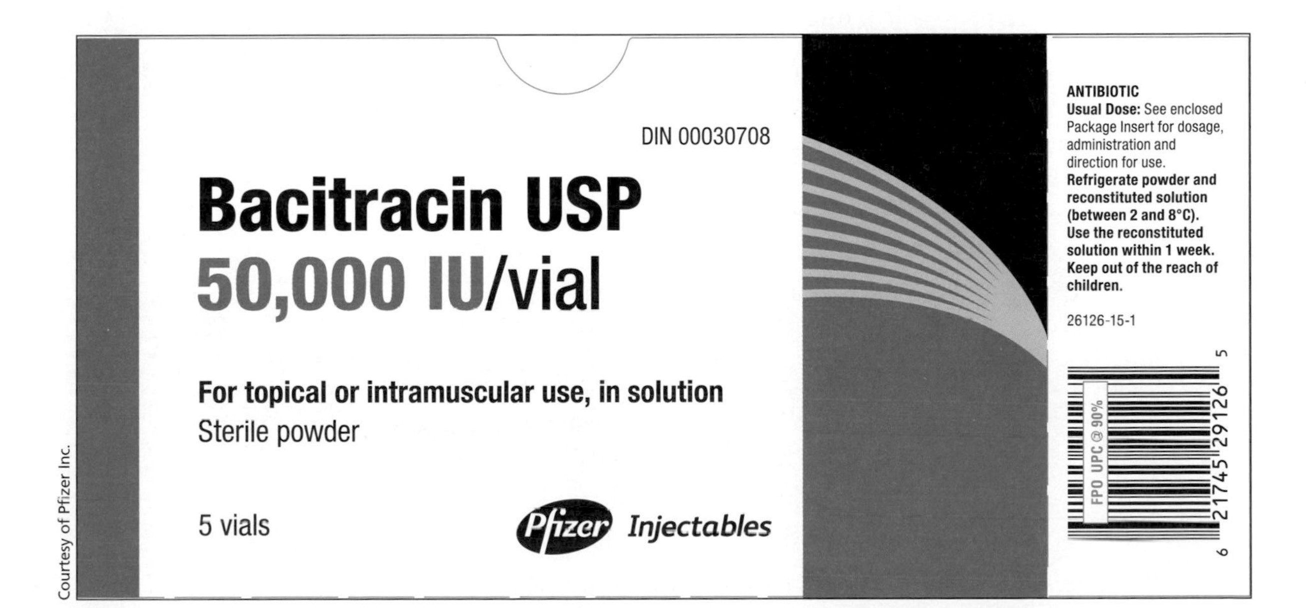

Courtesy of Pfizer Inc.

11. Order: *ceftazidime 1.25 g IV q12h*

    Reconstitute with ________ mL diluent for a concentration of ________ mg/mL and give ________ mL.

    Select: ________ syringe

    How many full doses are available in this vial? ________ dose(s)

    Is a reconstitution label required? ________

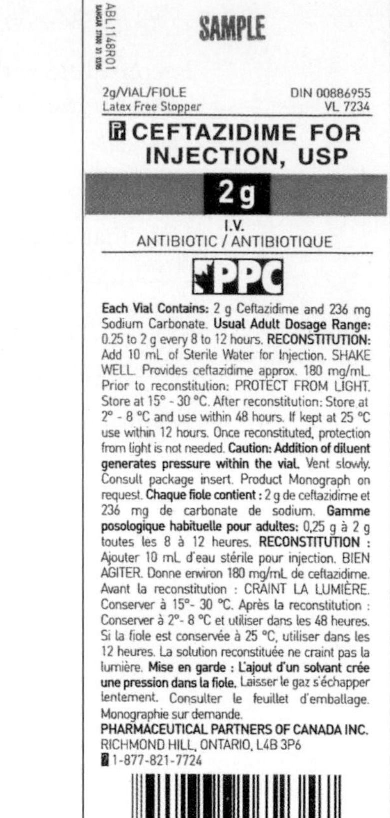

Pharmaceutical Partners of Canada Inc.

12. Order: *tobramycin sulfate 60 mg IV q8h*

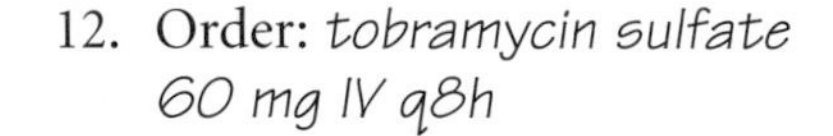

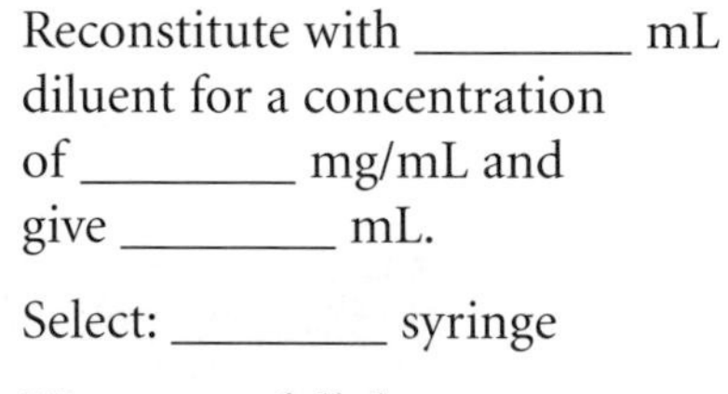

    Reconstitute with ________ mL diluent for a concentration of ________ mg/mL and give ________ mL.

    Select: ________ syringe

    How many full doses are available in this vial? ________ dose(s)

    Is a reconstitution label required? ________

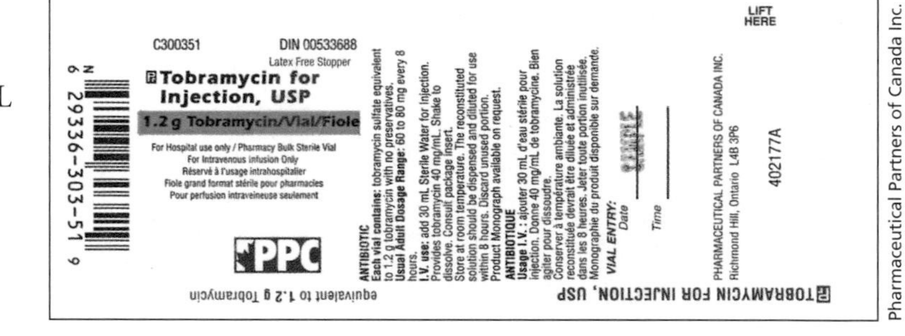

Pharmaceutical Partners of Canada Inc.

13. Order: *penicillin G sodium 2 000 000 units IM q8h*

    Reconstitute with ________ mL diluent for a concentration of ________ units/mL and give ________ mL.

    Select: ________ syringe

    How many full doses are available in this vial? ________ dose(s)

    Is a reconstitution label required? ________

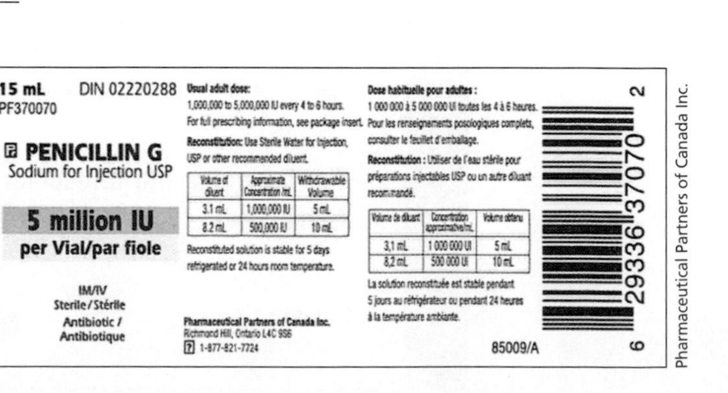

Pharmaceutical Partners of Canada Inc.

14. Order: *penicillin G sodium 1 000 000 units IM q8h*

    Reconstitute with ________ mL diluent for a concentration of ________ units/mL and give ________ mL.

    Select: ________ syringe

    How many full doses are available in this vial? ________ dose(s)

    Is a reconstitution label required? ________

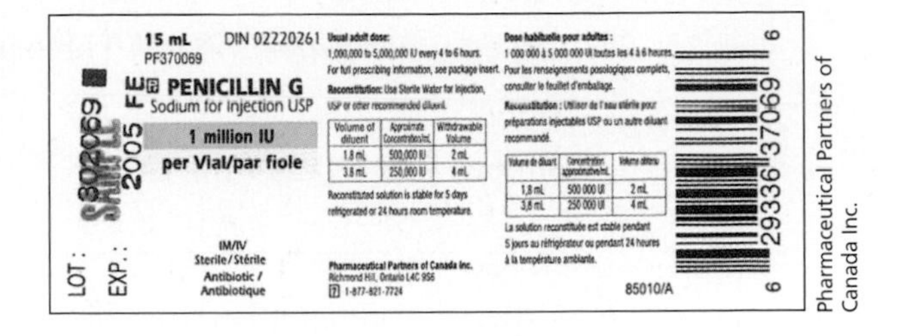

Pharmaceutical Partners of Canada Inc.

15. Order: *cefazolin sodium 400mg IM q8h*

    Reconstitute with ________ mL diluent for a concentration of ________ mg/mL and give _____ mL.

    Select: ________ syringe

    How many full doses are available in this vial? ________ dose(s)

    Is a reconstitution label required? ________

Pharmaceutical Partners of Canada Inc.

Explain how you would prepare each of the hydrogen peroxide (solute) and normal saline (solvent) irrigation orders in questions 16 through 21.

16. *480 mL of $\frac{1}{8}$ strength solution* ________________

17. *320 mL of $\frac{3}{8}$ strength solution* ________________

18. *80 mL of $\frac{5}{8}$ strength solution* ________________

19. *540 mL of $\frac{2}{3}$ strength solution* ________________

20. *500 mL of $\frac{7}{8}$ strength solution* ________________

21. *1 L of $\frac{1}{4}$ strength solution* ________________

Explain how you would prepare each of the following from ready-to-use nutritional formulas for the specified time period. Note how many cans or bottles of supply are needed and how much unused formula would remain from the used supply.

22. Order: *$\frac{1}{4}$ strength Enfamil 12 mL via NG tube hourly for 10 h*

    Supply: Enfamil 235-mL can

    ____

23. Order: *$\frac{3}{4}$ strength Boost Plus 360 mL over 4 h via gastrostomy*

    Supply: Boost Plus 237-mL bottles

    ____

24. Order: *$\frac{2}{3}$ strength Ensure. Give 90 mL hourly for 5 h via NG tube*

    Supply: Ensure 235-mL can

    ____

25. Order: $\frac{3}{8}$ *strength Enfamil.* Three patients need 960 mL of the $\frac{3}{8}$ strength Enfamil for one feeding each.

    Supply: Enfamil 235-mL can

    ____

26. Order: $\frac{1}{8}$ *strength Ensure. Give 160 mL stat via NG tube*

    Supply: Ensure 235-mL can

    ____

27. Order: $\frac{1}{2}$ *strength Ensure 55 mL hourly for 10 h via gastrostomy tube*

    Supply: Ensure 235-mL can

    ____

The nurse is making up $\frac{1}{4}$ strength Enfamil formula for several infants in the nursery.

28. If 235-mL cans of ready-to-use Enfamil are available, how many cans of formula will be needed to make 1.4 L of reconstituted $\frac{1}{4}$ strength Enfamil? ________ can(s)

29. How many mL of water will be added to the Enfamil in question 28 to correctly reconstitute the $\frac{1}{4}$ strength Enfamil? ________ mL

Check your work! Answers to all problems are provided at the end of the book, in the Answers section. Worked solutions for some Practice Problems are also provided there.

APPLICATION OF CLINICAL REASONING

10-1 Describe the patient safety incident that took place and the strategy that you would implement to prevent the patient safety incident.

Possible Scenario

The order for your patient is *ceftazidime 250 mg IM stat and q8h.*

The nurse reconstituted the vial with 10 mL of sterile water for injection as diluent. Next, the nurse calculated the dosage using the $\frac{D}{H} \times Q = X$ formula.

$$\frac{D}{H} \times Q = \frac{250 \cancel{mg}}{95 \cancel{mg}} \times 1 \text{ mL} = 2.62 \text{ or } 2.6 \text{ mL}$$

The nurse administered 2.6 mL of ceftazidime IM.

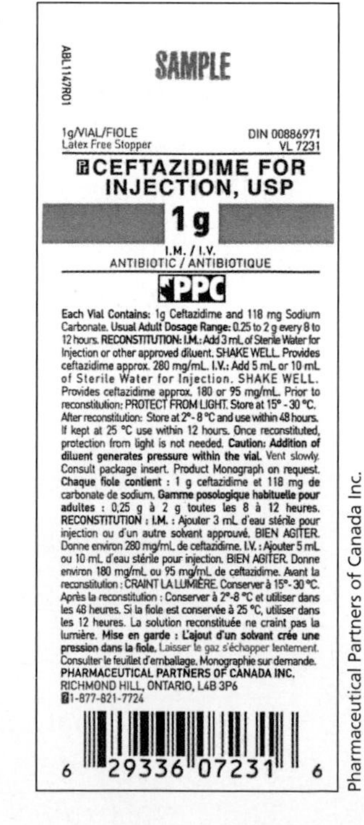

Pharmaceutical Partners of Canada Inc.

Potential Outcome

The nurse has administered a solution that is indicated for IV injection not IM. The total solution would not be used, so the vial would also be labelled incorrectly, resulting in the dosage strength for any further doses taken from this vial being incorrect.

Prevention

____

____

Check your work! Answers to all Application of Clinical Reasoning problems are provided at the end of the book, in the Answers section.

ANSWERS TO REVIEW SETS

Review Set 10-1

1) 3; 280; 0.7; 5

Reconstitution Label

06/02/XX, 0800, reconstituted as 280 mg/mL. Expires 08/02/XX, 0800. Keep refrigerated. G.D.P.

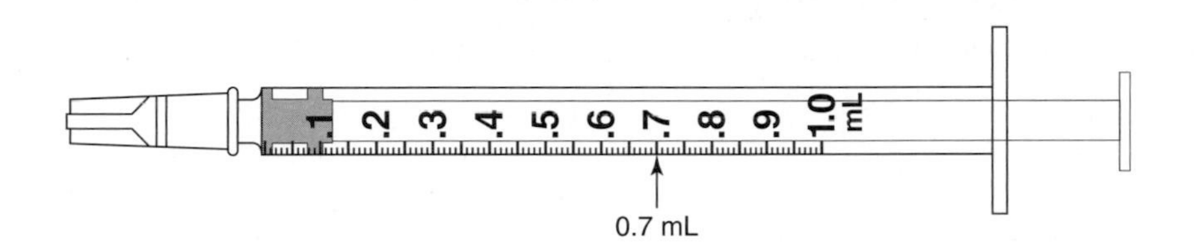

(**Note**: Reconstituted solutions are to be used within 48 hours when refrigerated.)

2) 9.8; 5000; 0.5; 20

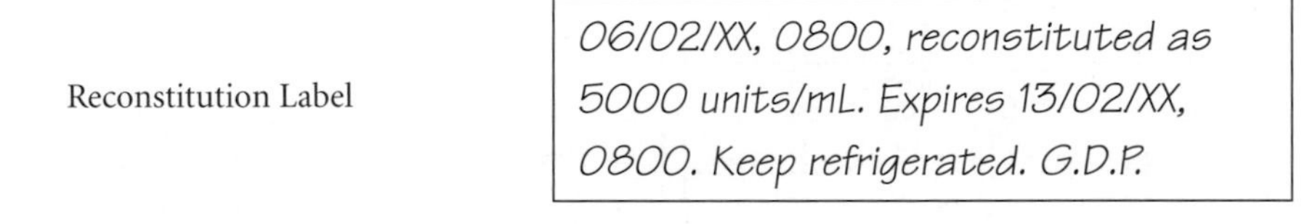
Reconstitution Label

06/02/XX, 0800, reconstituted as 5000 units/mL. Expires 13/02/XX, 0800. Keep refrigerated. G.D.P.

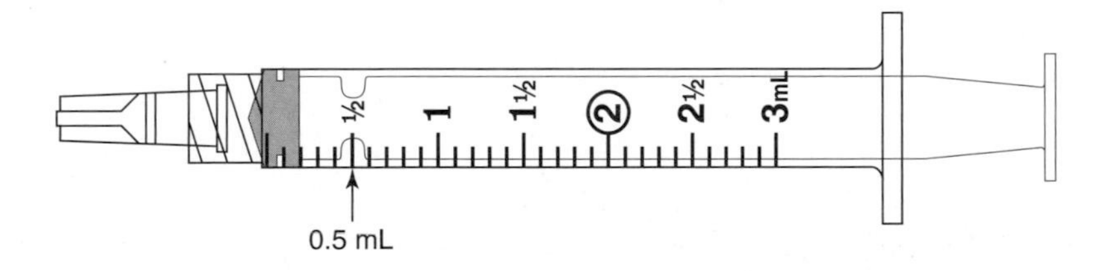

3) 1.1 mL

The vial contains 108 mg of enfuvirtide for delivery of 90 mg/mL when reconstituted. The vial is for single use. No reconstitution label is needed.

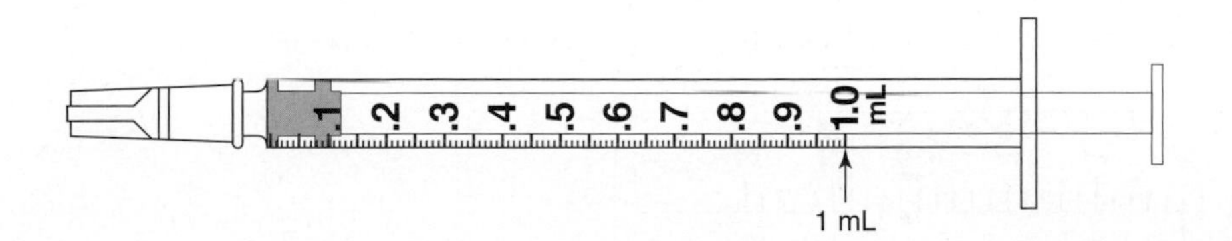

4) 4.8; 100; 5

No reconstitution label is required; all the medication will be used for one dose.

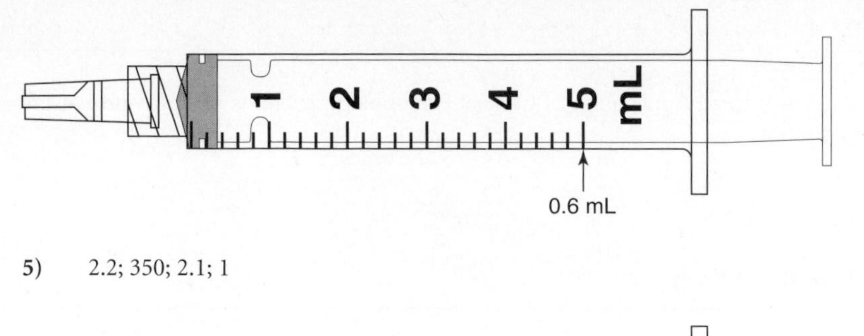

5) 2.2; 350; 2.1; 1

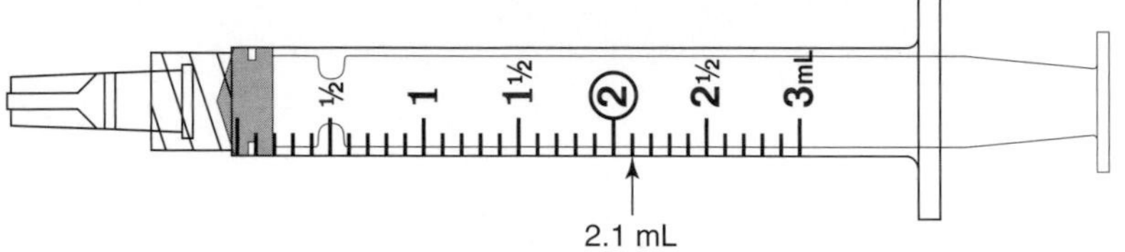

6) 8.2; 500 000; 2

3.1; 1 000 000; 1

Select 500 000 units/mL and give 2 mL. Either 1 mL or 2 mL is an appropriate amount to give IM depending on reconstitution, but 500 000 units/mL is less concentrated than 1 000 000 units/mL and is therefore less irritating to the muscle.

Five doses available in vial.

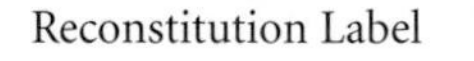
Reconstitution Label

06/02/XX, 0800, reconstituted as 500 000 units/mL. Expires 11/02/XX, 0800. Keep refrigerated. G.D.P.

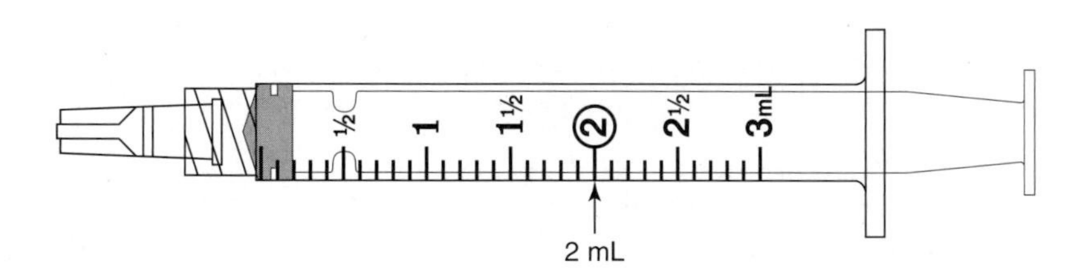

7) 7.8; 62.5; 2.8; 2

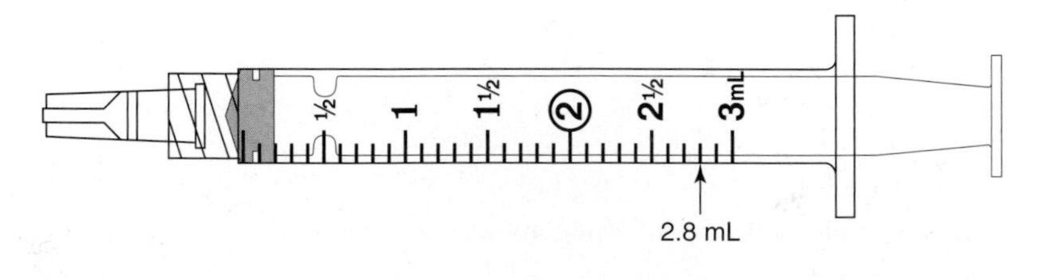

8) 4; 2 g/5 mL or 400 mg/mL; 0.5; single-dose vial, discard unused portion

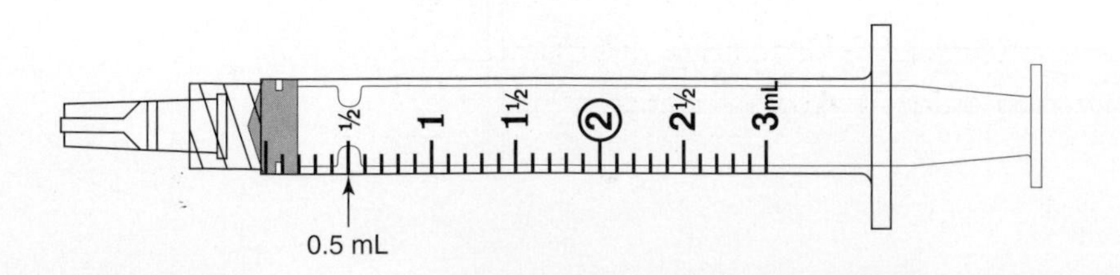

9) 1.8; 500 000; 2

3.8; 250 000; 4

Select 500 000 units/mL and give 1.8 mL. The 3.8 mL volume would require 2 injections and would be more painful as a result.

Two doses available.

Reconstitution Label

06/02/XX, 0800, reconstituted as 500 000 units/mL. Expires 11/02/XX, 0800. Keep refrigerated. G.D.P.

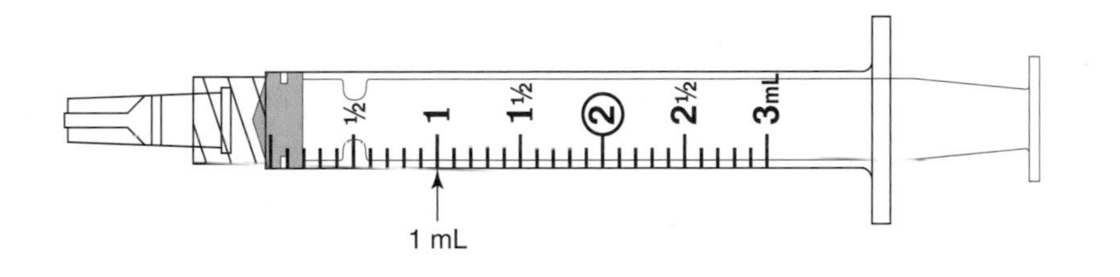

10) 10; 1.8; 180; 2.8; 4

(reconstituted, ampicillin is stable for 72 h)

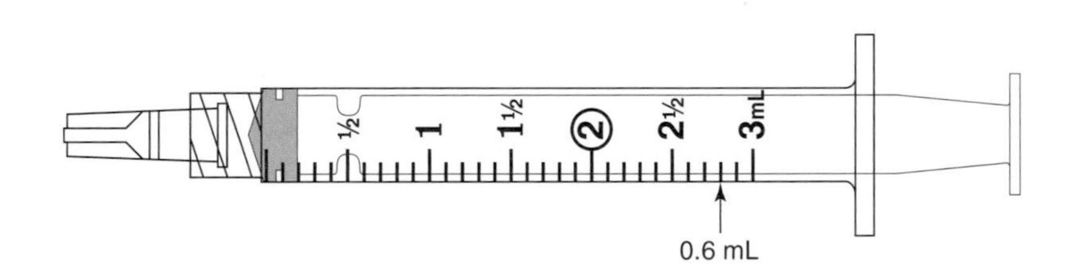

11) 1; 40; 0.6; 1

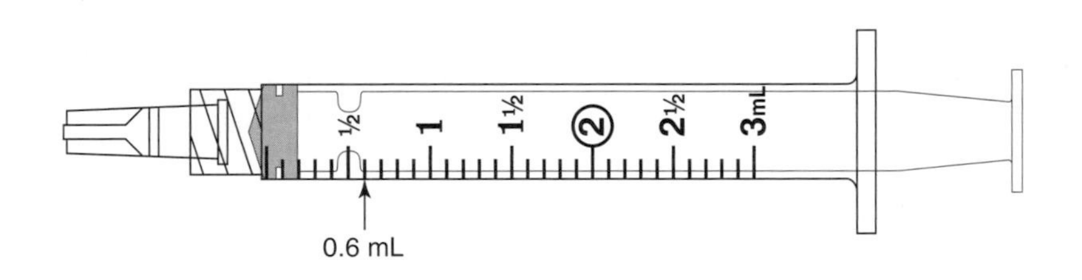

12) 10, 1800 mg/10 mL; 180; 1.4

Seven full doses of 1.4 mL are available.

No; the drug is ordered for administration twice a day; however, the solution is good for 48 hours under refrigeration. Therefore, only four doses can be used from this vial.

Reconstitution Label

06/02/XX, 0800, reconstituted as 180 mg/mL. Expires 08/02/XX, 0800. Keep refrigerated. G.D.P.

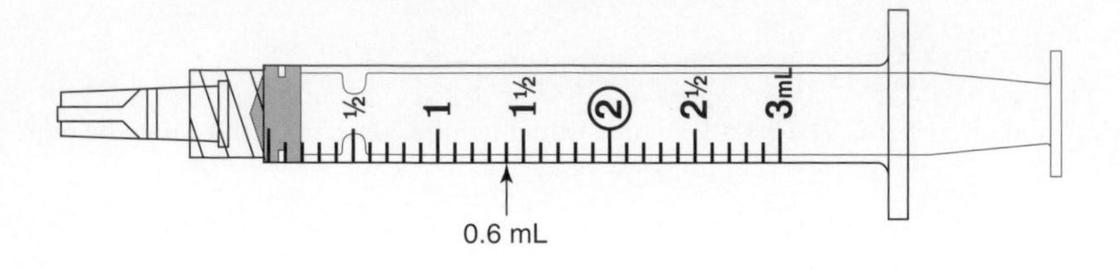

13) 9.6; 100; 7.5; 1; no label is necessary because one dose is available for use

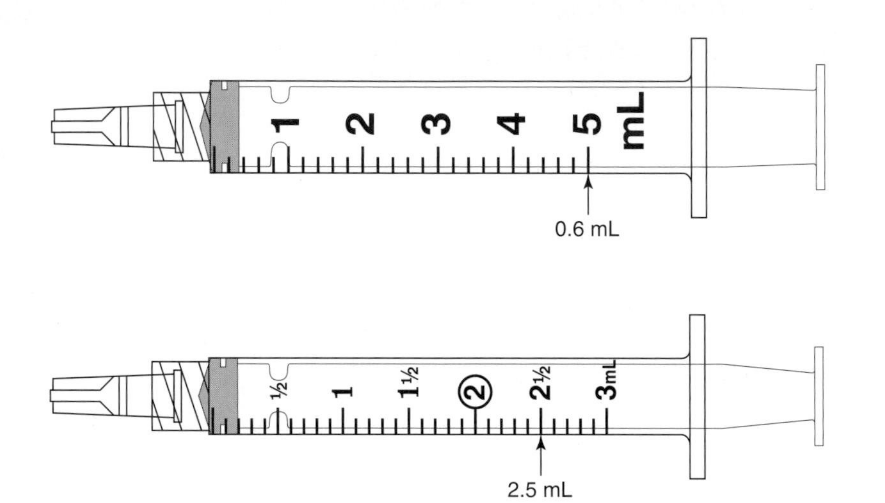

14) 30; 40; 2; 1; the solution should be used within 8 hours and the remaining unused portion discarded. No reconstitution label.

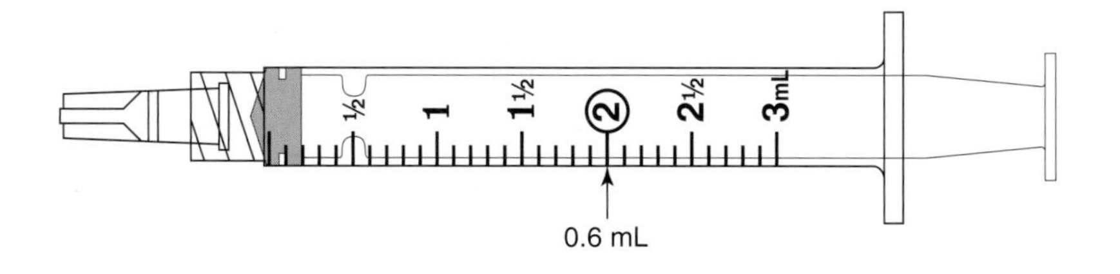

15) 2; 225; 1.1; 2

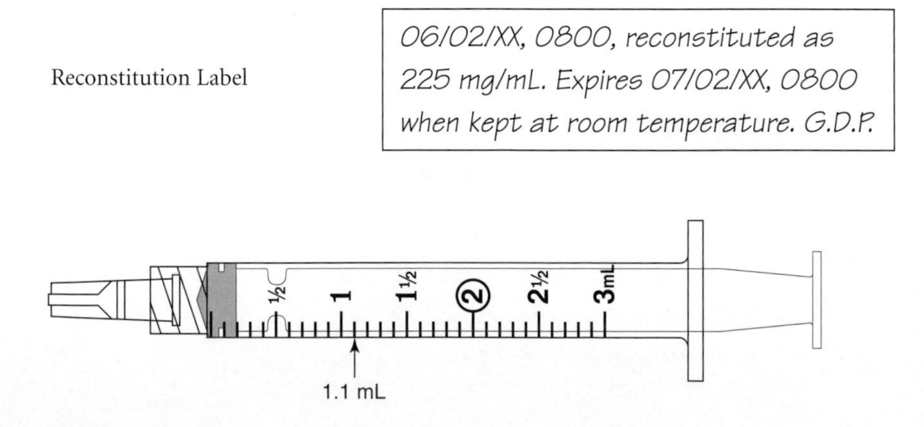
Reconstitution Label

Review Set 10-2

1) 300 mL Ensure + 600 mL water = 900 mL $\frac{1}{3}$-strength Ensure; 2 cans; discard 170 mL.

2) 180 mL Isomil + 540 mL water = 720 mL $\frac{1}{4}$-strength Isomil; one 235-mL can; discard 55 mL.

3) 800 mL Boost Plus + 400 mL water = 1200 mL $\frac{2}{3}$-strength Boost Plus; 4 bottles; discard 148 mL.

4) 390 mL Ensure + 390 mL water = 780 mL $\frac{1}{2}$-strength Ensure; 2 cans; discard 80 mL.

5) 500 mL Boost Plus + 500 mL water = 1000 mL $\frac{1}{2}$-strength Boost Plus three 237-mL bottles. Discard 211 mL.

6) 1080 mL Isomil + 360 mL water = 1440 $\frac{3}{4}$-strength Isomil; use 5 cans. Discard 95 mL.

7) 120 mL Ensure + 60 water = 180 $\frac{2}{3}$-strength Ensure; use one 235-mL can. Discard 115 mL.

8) 120 mL Ensure + 360 mL water = 480 mL $\frac{1}{4}$-strength Ensure; use one can. Discard 115 mL.

9) 35 mL mouthwash + 15 mL water

10) 16 mL skin cleanser + 64 mL water

11) 0.1 mL sodium bicarbonate + 4.9 mL water

12) 120 mL hydrogen peroxide + 120 mL water

SELECTED SOLUTIONS TO REVIEW SETS

Review Set 10-1

1) Order: 200 mg

Supply: 280 mg/mL

$$\frac{D}{H} \times Q = \frac{200 \cancel{mg}}{280 \cancel{mg}} \times 1 \text{ mL} = 0.714 \text{ mL} = 0.7 \text{ mL}$$

1000 $\cancel{mg}$/vial ÷ 200 $\cancel{mg}$/dose = 5 doses/vial

2) Order: 2500 units

Supply: 5000 units/mL

$$\frac{D}{H} \times Q = \frac{\overset{1}{\cancel{2500}} \cancel{units}}{\underset{2}{\cancel{5000}} \cancel{units}} \times 1 \text{ mL} = 0.5 \text{ mL}$$

50 000 $\cancel{units}$/vial ÷ 2500 $\cancel{units}$/dose = 20 doses/vial

6) Order: 1 000 000 units

Supply: 250 000 units/mL

$$\frac{D}{H} \times Q = \frac{\overset{4}{\cancel{1\,000\,000}} \cancel{units}}{\underset{1}{\cancel{250\,000}} \cancel{units}} \times 1 \text{ mL} = 4 \text{ mL}$$

Order: 1 000 000 units

Supply: 500 000 units/mL

$$\frac{D}{H} \times Q = \frac{\overset{2}{\cancel{1\,000\,000}} \cancel{units}}{\underset{1}{\cancel{500\,000}} \cancel{units}} \times 1 \text{ mL} = 2 \text{ mL}$$

Order: 1 000 000 units

Supply: 1 000 000 units/mL

$$\frac{D}{H} \times Q = \frac{\overset{1}{\cancel{1\,000\,000}} \cancel{units}}{\underset{1}{\cancel{1\,000\,000}} \cancel{units}} \times 1 \text{ mL} = 1 \text{ mL}$$

5 000 000 $\cancel{units}$/vial ÷ 1 000 000 $\cancel{units}$/dose = 5 doses (available per vial)

8) Order: 200 mg

Supply: 400 mg/2.5 mL

$$\frac{D}{H} \times Q = \frac{\overset{1}{\cancel{200}} \cancel{mg}}{\underset{2}{\cancel{400}} \cancel{mg}} \times 1 \text{ mL} = 0.5 \text{ mL}$$

12) Order: 250 mg

Supply: 180 mg/mL

$$\frac{D}{H} \times Q = \frac{25\cancel{0} \cancel{mg}}{18\cancel{0} \cancel{mg}} \times 1 \text{ mL} = \frac{25}{18} \text{ mL} = 1.38 \text{ mL} = 1.4 \text{ mL}$$

If looking at weight, there would be potentially 11 doses available—2000 $\cancel{mg}$/vial ÷ 180 $\cancel{mg}$/dose = 11 doses/vial. However, because the solution can be refrigerated for 48 hours, only 4 doses would be obtained from this vial.

Review Set 10-2

1) $D \times Q = \frac{1}{\cancel{3}_1} \times \cancel{900}^{300} \text{ mL} = 300 \text{ mL Ensure}$

900 mL (total solution) − 300 mL (Ensure) =

600 mL (water)

one can = 235 mL

470 mL (two full cans) − 300 mL (Ensure needed)

= 170 mL (discarded)

2) 120 mL q4h = 120 mL/feeding × 6 feedings =

720 mL total

$D \times Q = \frac{1}{\cancel{4}_1} \times \cancel{720}^{180} = 180 \text{ mL (Isomil)}$

720 mL (solution) − 180 mL (Isomil) = 540 mL;

use one 235-mL can; discard 55 mL.

8) $D \times Q = \frac{1}{4} \times 480 \text{ mL} = 120 \text{ mL Ensure}$

480 mL (solution) − 120 mL (Ensure) = 360 mL

water; use one 235-mL can Ensure. Discard 115 mL.

CHAPTER 11

Pediatric and Adult Dosages Based on Body Weight

OBJECTIVES

1. Convert pounds to kilograms.
2. Consult a reputable drug resource to calculate the recommended safe dosage per kilogram of body weight.
3. Compare the ordered dosage with the recommended safe dosage.
4. Determine whether the ordered dosage is safe to administer.
5. Apply body weight dosage calculations to patients across the life span.

The prescriber is responsible for ordering the dosage of medications; however, before administering a drug, the nurse must know whether the ordered dosage is accurate and safe. This is important for all patients, but it is especially important for infants, children, frail older adults, and critically ill adults.

CAUTION

Those who administer drugs to patients are legally responsible for recognizing incorrect and unsafe dosages and for alerting the prescriber when incorrect and unsafe dosages are discovered.

The individual who administers a drug is just as responsible for the safety of the patient as the individual who prescribes the drug. For both the nurse's and patient's protection, the nurse must be familiar with the recommended dosage of drugs or consult a reputable drug reference or the hospital formulary. The drug insert (often now available on the Internet or on the Health Canada Drug Database) is also a reliable source of current information about the drug.

Standard adult dosage is determined by the drug manufacturer. Dosage is usually recommended based on the requirements of an adult of average weight. Frequently, an adult dosage range is given, listing a minimum and maximum safe dosage, allowing the nurse to simply compare what is ordered to what is recommended.

Dosages for infants and children are based on their unique and changing body differences. The prescriber must consider the weight, height, body surface area, age, and condition of the child as contributing factors to safe and effective medication dosages. The two methods currently used for calculating safe pediatric dosages are *body weight* (such as milligrams of dosage per kilogram of body weight) and *body surface area* (BSA, measured in square metres, m^2). The body weight method is more common in pediatric situations and is emphasized in this chapter. The BSA method is based on both weight and height. It is used primarily in oncology and critical care situations. BSA is discussed in Chapter 13. Although the body weight and BSA methods are used most frequently in pediatrics, both methods are also used for adults, especially for adults in critical care situations. The calculations are the same.

ADMINISTERING MEDICATIONS TO CHILDREN

Numerically, the infant's or child's dosage appears smaller, but pediatric dosages are frequently much larger proportionally per kilogram of body weight than the usual adult dosage. Compared with larger persons, infants (birth to 1 year) have a greater percentage of body water and a diminished ability to absorb water-soluble drugs, which may necessitate higher dosages of oral and parenteral drugs. Children (ages 1 to 12 years) metabolize drugs more readily than adults, which necessitates higher dosages. Both infants and children are growing, and their organ systems are still maturing. Immature physiological processes related to drug pharmacokinetics (absorption, distribution, metabolism, and excretion) place them at risk of overdose, toxic reactions, and even death. Adolescents (ages 13 to 18 years) are often erroneously thought of as adults because of their body weight (greater than 50 kg) and mature physical appearance. In fact, they should still be regarded as physiologically immature, with unpredictable growth spurts and hormonal surges. Drug therapy for the pediatric population is further complicated because limited detailed pharmacological research has been carried out on children and adolescents. The infant or child, therefore, must be frequently evaluated for the desired clinical responses to medications, and serum drug levels may be needed to help adjust some drug dosages. It is important to remember that administration of an incorrect dosage to adult patients is dangerous, but with a child, the risk is even greater.

A reputable drug reference developed specifically for pediatric clinicians is the *Pediatric & Neonatal Dosage Handbook* (2015–2016). Another classic pediatric handbook is *The Harriet Lane Handbook* (Engorn & Flerlage, 2015).

CONVERTING POUNDS TO KILOGRAMS

The body weight method uses calculations based on the patient's weight in kilograms. However, it may sometimes be necessary to convert pounds to kilograms to accurately calculate medication doses.

RULE

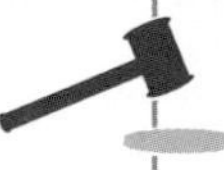

1 kg = 2.2 lb

Simply stated, weight in pounds is approximately twice (slightly more) the metric weight in kilograms; or weight in kilograms is approximately $\frac{1}{2}$ (slightly less) the weight in pounds. Kilograms can be estimated by halving the weight in pounds.

MATH TIP

When converting pounds to kilograms, round the kilogram weight to one decimal place (tenths).

Example 1:

Convert 45 lb to kg.

Approximate equivalent: 1 kg = 2.2 lb

Think: $\frac{1}{2}$ of 45 = approximately 23 (answer will be slightly less)

Smaller ↑ Larger → Divide (÷)

$45 \text{ lb} \div 2.2 \text{ lb/kg} = 45 \cancel{\text{lb}} \times 1 \text{ kg}/2.2 \cancel{\text{lb}} \div 2.2 = 20.45 \text{ kg} = 20.5 \text{ kg}$

Example 2:

Convert 10 lb 12 oz to kg.

Approximate equivalents: 1 kg = 2.2 lb

1 lb = 16 oz

Smaller ↑ Larger → Divide (÷)

$$12 \text{ oz} \div 16 \text{ oz/lb} = 12 \not{oz} \times 1 \text{ lb}/16 \not{oz} = \frac{\overset{3}{\not{12}}}{\underset{4}{\not{16}}} \text{ lb} = \frac{3}{4} \text{ lb; so } 10 \text{ lb } 12 \text{ oz} = 10\frac{3}{4} \text{ lb}$$

Now, you are ready to convert $10\frac{3}{4}$ lb to kg. Because you are converting to the metric system, the answer must be in decimals.

Think: $\frac{1}{2}$ of $10\frac{3}{4}$ = approximately 5

Smaller ↑ Larger → Divide (÷)

$$10\frac{3}{4} \text{ lb} = 10.75 \text{ lb} \div 2.2 \text{ lb/kg} = 10.75 \not{lb} \times 1 \text{ kg}/2.2 \not{lb} = 4.88 \text{ kg} = 4.9 \text{ kg}$$

BODY WEIGHT METHOD FOR CALCULATING SAFE PEDIATRIC DOSAGES

The most common method of prescribing and administering the therapeutic amount of medication for a child is to calculate the amount of drug according to the child's body weight in **kilograms**. The nurse then compares the child's ordered dosage to the recommended safe dosage from a reputable drug resource before administering the medication. The intent is to ensure that the ordered dosage is safe before calculating the amount to give and administering the dose to the patient.

RATIONALE FOR PRACTICE

To verify safe pediatric dosage,

1. Convert the child's weight from pounds to kilograms (rounded to tenths);
2. Calculate the safe dosage in mg/kg or mcg/kg (rounded to tenths) for a child of this weight, as recommended by a reputable drug reference: **multiply mg/kg by the child's weight in kg;**
3. Compare the ordered dosage to the recommended dosage, and decide whether the dosage is safe; and
4. If safe, calculate the amount to give and administer the dose; if the dosage seems unsafe, consult with the ordering practitioner before administering the drug.

Note: The dosage per kg may be mg/kg, mcg/kg, g/kg, mEq/kg, units/kg, and so on.

For each pediatric medication order, it is important to question whether the dosage is safe. Following are some examples to work through.

Single-Dose Drugs

Single-dosage drugs are intended to be given either once or when necessary. Dosage ordered by the body weight method is based on **mg/kg/dose, and calculated by multiplying the recommended mg by the patient's weight in kg for each dose.**

Example:

The prescriber orders *morphine sulfate 1.8 mg IM stat*. The child weighs 79 lb. Is this dosage safe?

1. **Convert lb to kg.** Approximate equivalent: 1 kg = 2.2 lb

   Think: $\frac{1}{2}$ of 79 = approximately 40

   Smaller ↑ Larger → Divide (÷)

   $79 \text{ lb} \div 2.2 \text{ lb/kg} = 79 \cancel{\text{lb}} \times 1 \text{ kg}/2.2 \cancel{\text{lb}} = 35.90 \text{ kg} = 35.9 \text{ kg}$

2. **Calculate the mg/kg/dose as recommended by a reputable drug resource.** According to a reputable drug resource, the usual intramuscular or subcutaneous dosage may begin at 0.05 mg/kg/dose.

   Multiply mg/kg/dose by the child's weight in kg.

   $0.05 \text{ mg}/\cancel{\text{kg}}/\text{doses} \times 35.9 \cancel{\text{kg}} = 1.79 \text{ mg/dose} = 1.8 \text{ mg/dose}$

MATH TIP

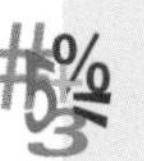

Notice that the kg unit of measurement cancels out, leaving the unit as mg/dose.

$$\frac{\text{mg}}{\cancel{\text{kg}}/\text{dose}} \times \cancel{\text{kg}} = \text{mg/dose}$$

Or

$\text{mg}/\cancel{\text{kg}}/\text{dose} \times \cancel{\text{kg}} = \text{mg/dose}$

3. **Decide whether the dosage is safe by comparing the ordered and the recommended dosages.** For this child's weight, 1.8 mg is the recommended dosage and 1.8 mg is the ordered dosage. Yes, the dosage is safe.

4. **Calculate one dose.** Apply the Three-Step Approach to dosage calculation.

   Order: *morphine sulfate 1.8 mg IM stat*

   Supply: morphine sulfate 5 mg/mL (Figure 11-1)

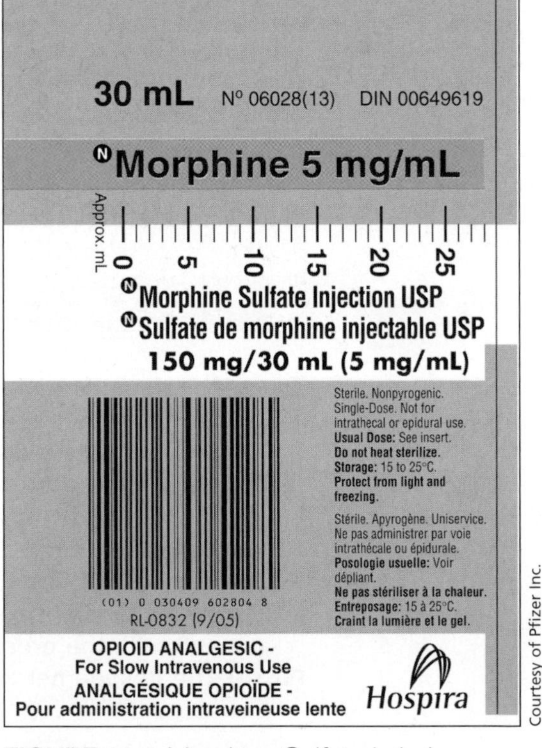

30 mL
N° 06028(13)
DIN 00649619
Morphine 5 mg/mL
Approx. mL
0 5 10 15 20 25
Morphine Sulfate Injection USP
Sulfate de morphine injectable USP
150 mg/30 mL (5 mg/mL)
Sterile. Nonpyrogenic. Single-Dose. Not for intrathecal or epidural use.
Usual Dose: See insert.
Do not heat sterilize.
Storage: 15 to 25°C.
Protect from light and freezing.
Stérile. Apyrogène. Uniservice. Ne pas administrer par voie intrathécale ou épidurale.
Posologie usuelle: Voir dépliant.
Ne pas stériliser à la chaleur.
Entreposage: 15 à 25°C.
Craint la lumière et le gel.
(01) 0 030409 602804 8
RL-0832 (9/05)
OPIOID ANALGESIC - For Slow Intravenous Use
ANALGÉSIQUE OPIOÏDE - Pour administration intraveineuse lente
Hospira
Courtesy of Pfizer Inc.

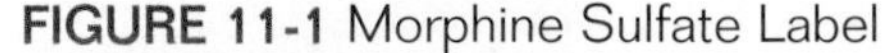

FIGURE 11-1 Morphine Sulfate Label

Step 1 Convert No conversion is necessary.

Step 2 Think You want to give less than 1 mL. Estimate that you want to give less than 0.5 mL.

Step 3 Calculate $\frac{D}{H} \times Q = \frac{1.8 \cancel{\text{mg}}}{5 \cancel{\text{mg}}} \times 1 \text{ mL}$

$= 0.36 \text{ mL}$

This is a small, child's dose. Measure 0.36 mL in a 1-mL syringe. Route is IM. Select the appropriate injection needle.

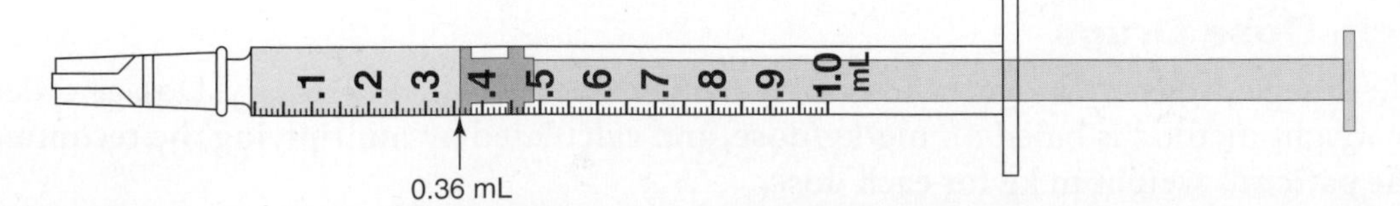

Single-Dose-Range Drugs

The manufacturers of some single-dosage medications provide a minimum and maximum range, or a safe dosage range.

Example:

The prescriber orders *hydroxyzine hydrochloride 20 mg IM q4h, prn for nausea*. The child weighs 44 lb. Is this a safe dosage?

1. **Convert lb to kg.** Approximate equivalent: 1 kg = 2.2 lb

   Think: $\frac{1}{2}$ of 44 = 22

   44 lb ÷ 2.2 lb/kg = 44 ~~lb~~ × 1 kg/2.2 ~~lb~~ = 20 kg

2. **Calculate the recommended dosage.** According to a reputable drug resource, the usual IM dosage is 0.5 mg to 1 mg/kg/dose every 4 hours as needed. The recommended dosage is represented as a range of "0.5–1 mg/kg/dose" for dosing flexibility. Calculate the minimum and maximum safe dosage range.

   Multiply mg/kg/dose times the child's weight in kg.

   Minimum mg per dose: 0.5 mg/~~kg~~/dose × 20 ~~kg~~ = 10 mg/dose

   Maximum mg per dose: 1 mg/~~kg~~/dose × 20 ~~kg~~ = 20 mg/dose

3. **Decide whether the ordered dosage is safe.** The recommended dosage range is 10 mg/dose to 20 mg/dose, and the ordered dosage of 20 mg is within this range. Yes, the ordered dosage is safe.

4. **Calculate one dose.** Apply the Three-Step Approach to dosage calculation.

   Order: *hydroxyzine hydrochloride 20 mg IM q4h, prn for nausea*

   Supply: hydroxyzine hydrochloride 50 mg/mL (Figure 11-2)

Step 1 Convert No conversion is necessary.

Step 2 Think Estimate that you want to give less than 1 mL; in fact, you want to give less than 0.5 mL.

Step 3 Calculate $\frac{D}{H} \times Q = \frac{2\cancel{0}\ \cancel{mg}}{5\cancel{0}\ \cancel{mg}} \times 1\ mL = \frac{2}{5}\ mL = 0.4\ mL$

This is a small, child's dose. Measure it in a 1-mL syringe. Route is IM. Select the appropriate injection needle.

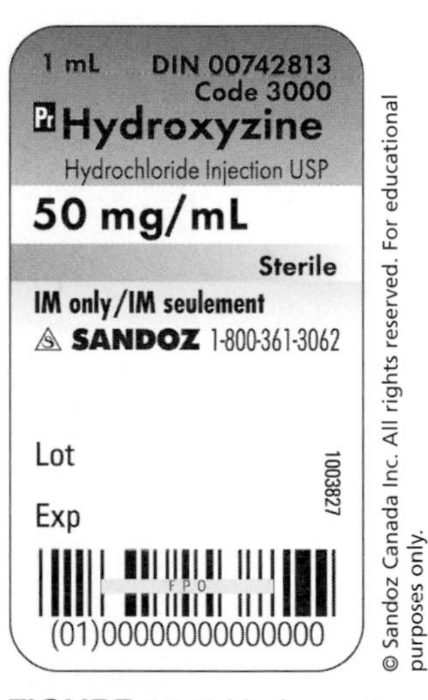

1 mL
DIN 00742813
Code 3000
Hydroxyzine
Hydrochloride Injection USP
50 mg/mL
Sterile
IM only/IM seulement
SANDOZ 1-800-361-3062
Lot
Exp
1003827
(01)00000000000000

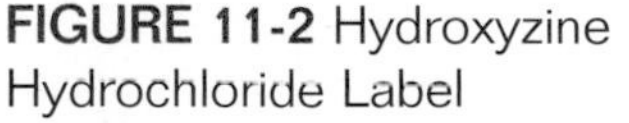
FIGURE 11-2 Hydroxyzine Hydrochloride Label

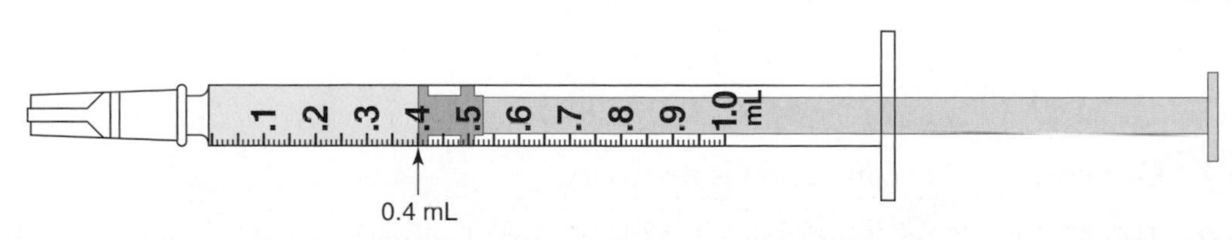

Routine or Round-the-Clock Drugs

Routine or round-the-clock drugs are intended to produce a continuous therapeutic effect over 24 hours. They are recommended as a *total daily dosage:* **mg/kg/day to be divided into some number of individual doses,** such as "three divided doses," "four divided doses," and "divided doses every 8 hours." "Three divided doses" means the drug total daily dosage is divided equally and is administered 3 times per day, either TID or q8h. Likewise, "four divided doses" means the total daily drug dosage is divided equally and administered 4 times per day either QID or q6h. Recommendations such as "divided doses every 8 hours" specify that the total daily drug dosage should be divided equally and administered q8h.

Example:

The prescriber orders *clarithromycin 115 mg PO BID*. The child weighs $33\frac{1}{2}$ lb. Is this dosage safe?

1. **Convert lb to kg.** Approximate equivalent: 1 kg = 2.2 lb

   Think: $\frac{1}{2}$ of 33 = approximately 17 (answer will be slightly less)

   $33\frac{1}{2}\text{ lb} = 33.5\text{ lb} \div 2.2\text{ lb/kg} = 33.5\ \cancel{\text{lb}} \times 1\text{ kg}/2.2\ \cancel{\text{lb}} = 15.22\text{ kg} = 15.2\text{ kg}$

   Note: Represent $33\frac{1}{2}$ as 33.5 because you are converting lb to kg, which is a metric unit and must be in decimals.

2. **Calculate the recommended dosage.** The recommended dosage on the drug label (Figure 11-3) reads, "Usual dose—Children, 15 mg per kg a day . . . in divided doses every 12 hours." First, calculate the total daily dosage: $15\text{ mg}/\cancel{\text{kg}}/\text{day} \times 15.2\ \cancel{\text{kg}} = 228\text{ mg/day}$. Then, divide this total daily dosage into 2 doses: 228 mg ÷ 2 doses = 114 mg/dose.

3. **Decide whether the ordered dosage is safe.** Yes, the ordered dosage is safe because this is an *oral* dose and 115 mg is a *reasonably safe* dosage for a 114 mg recommended single dosage.

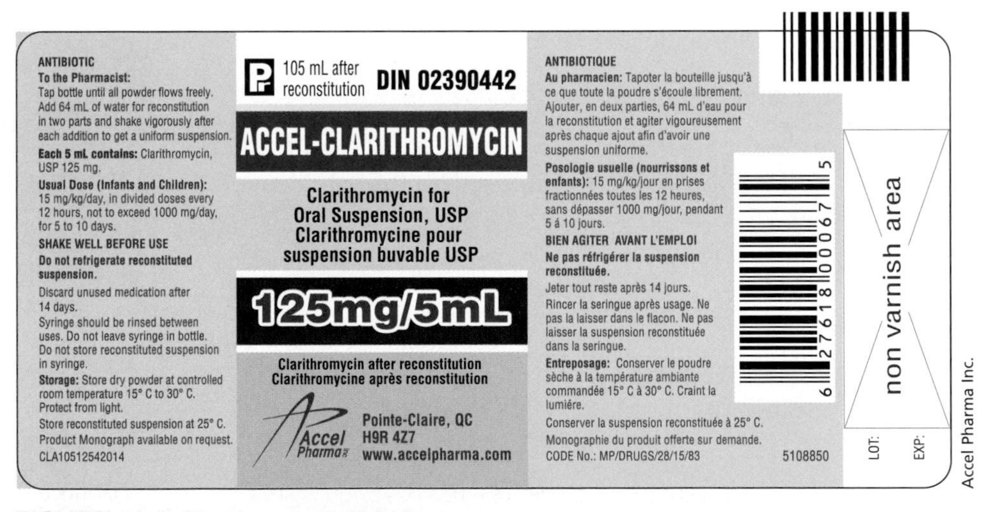

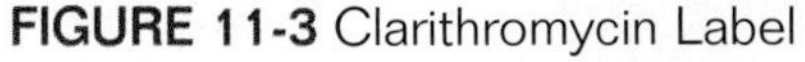

FIGURE 11-3 Clarithromycin Label

4. **Calculate one dose.** Apply the Three-Step Approach to dosage calculation.

   Order: *clarithromycin 115 mg PO BID*

   Supply: clarithromycin 125 mg/5 mL

Step 1 Convert No conversion is necessary.

Step 2 Think You want to give less than 5 mL. Estimate that you want to give between 2.5 mL and 5 mL.

Step 3 Calculate $\frac{D}{H} \times Q = \frac{\overset{23}{\cancel{115\text{ mg}}}}{\underset{25}{\cancel{125\text{ mg}}}} \times 5\text{ mL} = \frac{23}{25} \times 5\text{ mL} = 4.6\text{ mL}$

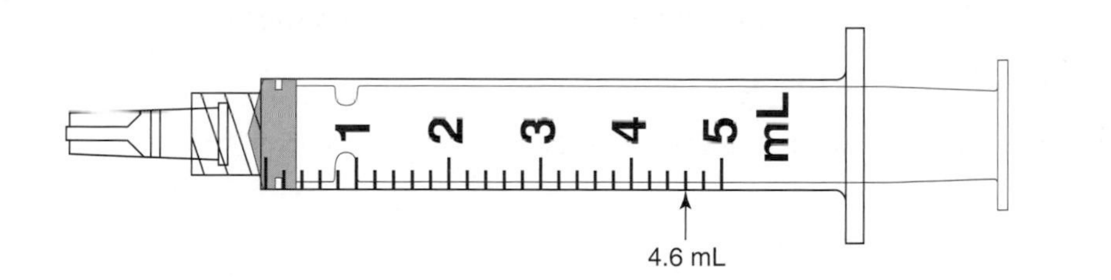

1
2
3
4
5
mL
4.6 mL

Daily-Dose-Range Drugs

Many medications have a minimum and maximum recommended mg/kg range per day to be divided into some number of doses. Amoxicillin is an antibiotic that is used to treat a variety of infections in adults and children. It is often given in divided doses round the clock for a total daily dosage.

Example:

The prescriber orders *amoxicillin 200 mg PO q8h* for a child who weighs 22 lb. Is this dosage safe?

1. **Convert lb to kg.** Approximate equivalent: 1 kg = 2.2 lb

   Think: $\frac{1}{2}$ of 22 = 11 (answer will be slightly less)

   $22\text{ lb} \div 2.2\text{ lb/kg} = 22\ \cancel{\text{lb}} \times 1\text{ kg}/2.2\ \cancel{\text{lb}} = 10\text{ kg}$

2. **Calculate recommended dosage.** Examine the label for amoxicillin in Figure 11-4. The label provides the recommended dosage: "20 to 40 mg/kg/day in divided doses every 8 hours," which results in 3 doses in 24 hours.

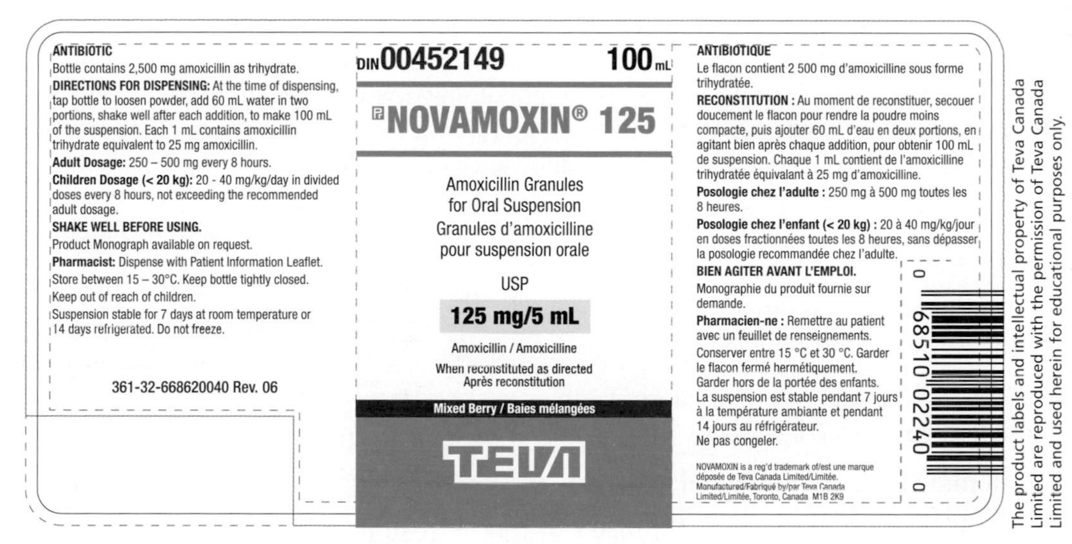

ANTIBIOTIC
Bottle contains 2,500 mg amoxicillin as trihydrate.
DIRECTIONS FOR DISPENSING: At the time of dispensing, tap bottle to loosen powder, add 60 mL water in two portions, shake well after each addition, to make 100 mL of the suspension. Each 1 mL contains amoxicillin trihydrate equivalent to 25 mg amoxicillin.
Adult Dosage: 250 – 500 mg every 8 hours.
Children Dosage (< 20 kg): 20 - 40 mg/kg/day in divided doses every 8 hours, not exceeding the recommended adult dosage.
SHAKE WELL BEFORE USING.
Product Monograph available on request.
Pharmacist: Dispense with Patient Information Leaflet.
Store between 15 – 30°C. Keep bottle tightly closed.
Keep out of reach of children.
Suspension stable for 7 days at room temperature or 14 days refrigerated. Do not freeze.
361-32-668620040 Rev. 06
DIN 00452149
100 mL
NOVAMOXIN® 125
Amoxicillin Granules for Oral Suspension
Granules d'amoxicilline pour suspension orale
USP
125 mg/5 mL
Amoxicillin / Amoxicilline
When reconstituted as directed
Après reconstitution
Mixed Berry / Baies mélangées
TEVA
ANTIBIOTIQUE
Le flacon contient 2 500 mg d'amoxicilline sous forme trihydratée.
RECONSTITUTION : Au moment de reconstituer, secouer doucement le flacon pour rendre la poudre moins compacte, puis ajouter 60 mL d'eau en deux portions, en agitant bien après chaque addition, pour obtenir 100 mL de suspension. Chaque 1 mL contient de l'amoxicilline trihydratée équivalant à 25 mg d'amoxicilline.
Posologie chez l'adulte : 250 mg à 500 mg toutes les 8 heures.
Posologie chez l'enfant (< 20 kg) : 20 à 40 mg/kg/jour en doses fractionnées toutes les 8 heures, sans dépasser la posologie recommandée chez l'adulte.
BIEN AGITER AVANT L'EMPLOI.
Monographie du produit fournie sur demande.
Pharmacien-ne : Remettre au patient avec un feuillet de renseignements.
Conserver entre 15 °C et 30 °C. Garder le flacon fermé hermétiquement.
Garder hors de la portée des enfants.
La suspension est stable pendant 7 jours à la température ambiante et pendant 14 jours au réfrigérateur.
Ne pas congeler.
NOVAMOXIN is a reg'd trademark of/est une marque déposée de Teva Canada Limited/Limitée.
Manufactured/Fabriqué by/par Teva Canada Limited/Limitée, Toronto, Canada M1B 2K9
0 68510 02240 0

FIGURE 11-4 Novamoxin Label

Calculate the minimum and maximum dosage for each single dose. According to the label, the recommendations are for the total daily dosage to be divided and administered every 8 hours, resulting in 3 doses in 24 hours.

Minimum total daily dosage: 20 mg/kg/day × 10 kg = 200 mg/day

Minimum dosage for each single dose: 200 mg ÷ 3 doses = 66.7 mg/dose

Maximum total daily dosage: 40 mg/kg/day × 10 kg = 400 mg/day

Maximum dosage for each single dose: 400 mg ÷ 3 doses = 133.3 mg/dose

The single dosage range is 66.7 to 133.3 mg/dose.

3. **Decide whether the ordered dosage is safe.** The ordered dosage is 200 mg, and the allowable, safe dosage is 66.7 to 133.3 mg/dose. No, this dosage is too high and is not safe.
4. **Contact the prescriber to discuss the order.**
   You can save yourself a calculation step with the following shortcut, based on the total daily dosage.

   Calculate recommended minimum and maximum daily dosage range for *this* child.

   You know the total daily dosage is divided into 3 doses in 24 hours.

   Minimum total daily dosage: 20 mg/kg/day × 10 kg = 200 mg/day

   Maximum total daily dosage: 40 mg/kg/day × 10 kg = 400 mg/day

   Daily dosage for this order: 200 mg/dose × 3 doses/day = 600 mg/day

   Decide whether the ordered daily dosage is safe. The ordered daily dosage is 600 mg, and the allowable safe daily dosage is 200 to 400 mg/day. No, the dosage ordered is too high and is not safe. Although an antibiotic overdose can occur, it rarely causes serious adverse effects. Adverse effects are usually gastric distress and diarrhea.

Daily-Dose-Range Drugs with Maximum Daily Allowance

The manufacturers of some medications provide a recommended a range of mg/kg/day, and specify a maximum allowable total amount per day.

Example:

The prescriber orders *cefazolin sodium 2.1 g IV q8h* for a child with a serious joint infection. The child weighs 95 lb. The usual intramuscular or intravenous dosage of cefazolin sodium for infants older than 1 month and children is 25 to 50 mg/kg/day divided into three or four divided doses; for severe infections the dosage may be increased to 100 mg/kg/day. This means that regardless of how much the child weighs, the maximum safe allowance of this drug is 100 mg/kg per 24 hours.

1. **Convert lb to kg.** Approximate equivalent: 1 kg = 2.2 lb

   Think: $\frac{1}{2}$ of 95 = approximately 48 (answer will be slightly less)

   95 lb ÷ 2.2 lb/kg = 95 lb ÷ 1 kg/2.2 lb = 43.18 kg = 43.2 kg

SAMPLE
LOT:
EXP.:
PF320021 DIN 02237138
Latex Free Stopper
CEFAZOLIN
for Injection, USP
1 g
Vial/Fiole
Sterile/Stérile
Antibiotic/Antibiotique
IM/IV
PPC
Single Dose Vial: Discard unused portion. Each vial contains: Cefazolin (as sodium) 1 g and 48 mg sodium. **Reconstitution: IM.:** add **2.5 mL** SWFI. Provides 334 mg/mL. Shake well. **I.V.:** see package insert. Stable for 24 hours at 25°C and 72 hours at 2 - 8°C. **Usual Adult Dosage:** 250 mg to 1 g every 6 - 12 hours. Store dry powder between 15°C - 30°C. Protect from light.
Fiole unidose : Jeter toute portion inutilisée. Conserver la poudre sèche entre 15 °C - 30 °C. Protéger de la lumière.
85015/A
PHARMACEUTICAL PARTNERS OF CANADA INC.
Richmond Hill, ON L4B 3P6 ? 1-877-821-7724
6 29336 32021 9

Pharmaceutical Partners of Canada Inc.

2. **Calculate the recommended dosage.**

   Minimum mg/kg/day: 25 mg/kg/day × 43.2 kg = 1080 mg/day

   Minimum mg/dose: 1080 mg ÷ 3 doses = 360 mg/dose or 0.36 g/dose

   (360 mg/dose = 360 mg/dose ÷ 1000 $\frac{\text{mg}}{1\text{ g}}$ = 0.36 g/dose)

   Maximum mg/kg/day: 100 mg/kg/day × 43.2 kg = 4320 mg/day

Maximum mg/dose: 4320 mg ÷ 3 doses = 1440 mg/dose or 1.44 g/dose

(1440 mg/dose = 1440 ~~mg~~/dose ÷ 1000 $\frac{\cancel{mg}}{1\text{ g}}$ = 1.44 g/dose)

3. **Decide whether the dosage is safe.** No, the dosage is too high. It exceeds both the highest mg/kg/dose extreme of the range (1440 mg/dose) and the maximum allowable dosage. At 4.32 g/day, no more than 1.44 g/dose would be allowed. The ordered dosage of 2.1 g is not safe because 3 doses/day would deliver 6.3 g of the drug (2.1 g × 3 = 6.3 g). This example points out the importance of carefully reading all dosage recommendations.
4. **Contact the prescriber to discuss the order.**

Underdosage

Underdosage can also be unsafe. If the medication is necessary for the treatment or comfort of the patient, then giving too little can be just as dangerous as giving too much. Dosage that is less than the recommended therapeutic amount is also considered unsafe because it may be ineffective.

Example:

The nurse notices that a baby's fever has not decreased to less than 39.2°C in spite of several doses of ibuprofen that the prescriber ordered as an antipyretic. The order is *ibuprofen 40 mg PO q6h prn, temp 38.7°C and above*. The 7-month-old baby weighs $17\frac{1}{2}$ lb.

1. **Convert lb to kg.** Approximate equivalent: 1 kg = 2.2 lb

   Think: $\frac{1}{2}$ of $17\frac{1}{2}$ = approximately 9 (answer will be slightly less)

   Represent $17\frac{1}{2}$ as 17.5 because you are converting lb to kg; kg is metric so it is measured in decimals.

   $17\frac{1}{2}$ lb = 17.5 lb ÷ 2.2 lb/kg = 17.5 ~~lb~~ × 1 kg/2.2 ~~lb~~ = 7.95 kg = 8 kg
2. **Calculate the recommended dosage.** According to the drug reference, "Usual dosage . . . oral: Children: . . . Antipyretic: 6 months to 12 years for a temperature less than 39.1°C: 5 mg/kg/dose; for a temperature more than or equal to 39.1°C: 10 mg/kg/dose, given every 6 hr; Maximum daily dose: 40 mg/kg/day."

   The recommended safe mg/kg dosage to treat this child's fever of 39.2°C is based on 10 mg/kg/dose. For the 8-kg child, per dose, 10 mg/~~kg~~/dose × 8 ~~kg~~ = 80 mg/dose.
3. **Decide whether the dosage is safe.** The nurse realizes that the dosage as ordered is insufficient to lower the child's fever. Because it is below the recommended therapeutic dosage, it is unsafe.
4. **Contact the prescriber.** Upon discussion with the prescriber, the prescriber agrees and revises the order to *ibuprofen 80 mg PO q6h prn, Temp more than 39.1°C* and *ibuprofen 40 mg PO q6h prn, Temp less than 39.1°C*. Underdosage with an antipyretic may result in serious complications of hyperthermia. Likewise, consider how underdosage of an antibiotic may lead to a lack of therapeutic response and the potential for antimicrobial resistance, and underdosage of a pain reliever may be inadequate to effectively treat the patient's pain, delaying recovery. Remember, the information in the drug reference provides important details related to the specific use of medications and the appropriate dosages for certain age groups to provide safe, therapeutic dosing. Both the physician and nurse must work together to ensure accurate and safe dosages that are within the recommended parameters as stated by the manufacturer on the label, in a drug insert, or in a reputable drug reference.

CAUTION

Once an adolescent reaches a weight of 50 kg (110 lb) or greater, the standard adult dosage is frequently prescribed instead of a dosage calculated by weight. The prescriber must ensure that the order for a child's dosage does not exceed the maximum adult dosage recommended by the manufacturer.

COMBINATION DRUGS

Some medications contain two drugs combined into one solution or suspension. To calculate the safe dosage of these medications, the nurse should consult a pediatric drug reference. Often, the nurse will need to calculate the safe dosage for each of the medications combined in the solution or suspension. Combination drugs are usually ordered by the amount to give or dose volume.

Example 1:

The prescriber orders *sulfamethoxazole/trimethoprim suspension 7.5 mL PO q12h* for a child who weighs 22 lb. According to the drug label, this combination drug contains trimethoprim 40 mg and sulfamethoxazole 200 mg in 5 mL oral suspension. The usual dose is based on the trimethoprim component, which is 6 to 12 mg/kg/day PO in divided doses q12h for a mild to moderate infection. Is this dose volume safe?

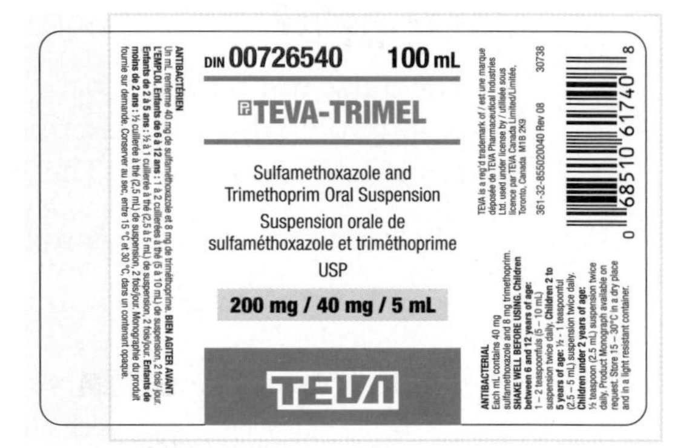

The product labels and intellectual property of Teva Canada Limited are reproduced with the permission of Teva Canada Limited and used herein for educational purposes only.

1. **Convert lb to kg.** Approximate equivalent: 1 kg = 2.2 lb

   Think: $\frac{1}{2}$ of 22 = 11 (answer will be slightly less)

   $22 \text{ lb} \div 2.2 \text{ lb/kg} = 22 \cancel{\text{lb}} \times 1 \text{ kg}/2.2 \cancel{\text{lb}} = 10 \text{ kg}$

2. **Calculate the safe dose for the trimethoprim range.**

   Trimethoprim minimum daily dosage: $6 \text{ mg}/\cancel{\text{kg}}/\text{day} \times 10 \cancel{\text{kg}} = 60 \text{ mg/day}$

   Divided into 2 doses/day: $60 \text{ mg} \div 2 \text{ doses} = 30 \text{ mg/dose}$

   Trimethoprim maximum daily dosage: $12 \text{ mg}/\cancel{\text{kg}}/\text{day} \times 10 \cancel{\text{kg}} = 120 \text{ mg/day}$

   Divided into 2 doses/day: $120 \text{ mg} \div 2 \text{ doses} = 60 \text{ mg/dose}$

3. **Calculate the volume of medication for the dosage range.**

   Minimum dose volume: $$\frac{D}{H} \times Q = \frac{\overset{3}{\cancel{30}} \cancel{\text{mg}}}{\underset{4}{\cancel{40}} \cancel{\text{mg}}} \times 5 \text{ mL} = \frac{15}{4} \text{ mL} = 3.75 \text{ mL, minimum per dose}$$

   Maximum dose volume: $$\frac{D}{H} \times Q = \frac{\overset{3}{\cancel{60}} \cancel{\text{mg}}}{\underset{2}{\cancel{40}} \cancel{\text{mg}}} \times 5 \text{ mL} = \frac{15}{2} \text{ mL} = 7.5 \text{ mL, maximum per dose}$$

4. **Decide whether the dose volume is safe.** Because the prescriber ordered 7.5 mL, the dosage is within the safe range and is safe.

   What dosage of trimethoprim did the prescriber actually order per dose for this child?

   Using the formula $\frac{D}{H} \times Q = X$, write in the quantities you already know.

$\frac{D\ \cancel{mg}}{40\ \cancel{mg}} \times 5\ mL = 7.5\ mL$ Solve for the unknown D, desired dosage.

$\frac{5D}{40} \times \frac{7.5}{1}$ Notice you now have a ratio-proportion.

$5D = 300$

$\frac{5D}{5} = \frac{300}{5}$

$D = 60\ mg$ This is the dosage of trimethoprim you would give in one 7.5-mL dose, which matches the upper limit of the safe dosage range.

Be sure to take the time to double-check pediatric dosages. The healthcare provider who administers the medication has the last opportunity to ensure safe drug administration.

Example 2:

The prescriber orders *amoxicillin trihydrate/clavulanic acid 5.6 mL PO BID* for a child weighing 44 lb. According to the pediatric drug reference, this combination drug contains 400 mg of amoxicillin trihydrate with 57 mg of clavulanic acid in every 5 mL oral suspension. The usual dosage for this drug to treat patients aged 3 months or older is 45 mg/kg/day BID based on the amoxicillin trihydrate component. Is the order safe?

Because this is a combination drug, notice that the order is for the dose volume (5.6 mL). To verify that the dose is safe, you must calculate the recommended dosage and the recommended quantity to give to supply that dosage for the amoxicillin trihydrate drug component.

1. **Convert lb to kg.** Approximate equivalent: 1 kg = 2.2 lb

   Think: $\frac{1}{2}$ of 44 = 22 (answer will be slightly less)

   $44\ lb \div 2.2\ lb/kg = 44\ \cancel{lb} \times 1\ kg/2.2\ \cancel{lb} = 20\ kg$

2. **Calculate the safe dosage for the amoxicillin trihydrate.**

   amoxicillin trihydrate per day: $45\ mg/\cancel{kg}/day \times 20\ \cancel{kg} = 900\ mg/day$; divided into 2 doses/day: $900\ mg \div 2\ doses = 450\ mg/dose$

3. **Calculate the volume of medication recommended for 1 dose for amoxicillin trihydrate.**

   amoxicillin trihydrate: 450 mg is the recommended dosage; the supply has 400 mg/5 mL.

   $\frac{D}{H} \times Q = \frac{\overset{5}{\cancel{450}}\ \cancel{mg}}{\underset{4}{\cancel{400}}\ \cancel{mg}} \times 5\ mL = \frac{45}{8}\ mL = 5.625\ mL = 5.6\ mL$ recommended to deliver 450 mg

   Because this is an oral dosage, it is safely and reasonably rounded to 5.6 mL.

4. **Decide whether the dose volume ordered is safe.** The ordered dose volume is 5.6 mL, and the appropriate dose based on the recommended dosage for the amoxicillin trihydrate is 5.6 mL. The dose is safe. **Because this is a combination product, 5.6 mL contains *both* medications delivered in this suspension.**

In some drug combinations, although the two drugs are combined into one solution or suspension, the dosage is determined based on one drug. One example is amoxicillin trihydrate/clavulanic acid. Amoxicillin trihydrate is the major drug component of the combination. The clavulanic acid is a β-lactamase inhibitor added to the β-lactam antibiotic amoxicillin trihydrate (at a much lower dose) to make the drug more powerful against β-lactamase-producing bacterial strains.

ADULT DOSAGES BASED ON BODY WEIGHT

Some adult dosage recommendations are also based on body weight, although less frequently than for children. The information learned about calculating and verifying children's body weight dosages can be applied to adults. It is important that the nurse become familiar and comfortable with reading labels, drug inserts, and drug reference books to check any order that appears questionable.

Figure 11-5 shows reconstitution instructions in the drug label for piperacillin sodium/tazobactam sodium. Adult dosage recommendations are often found on the label as well, but may be found in the insert. It is always important to refer to the insert when the information is not found on the label. The adult dosage information taken from the drug insert is based on the type of systemic and/or local infection. Depending on the drug prescribed, the recommended adult dosage form is often based on body weight.

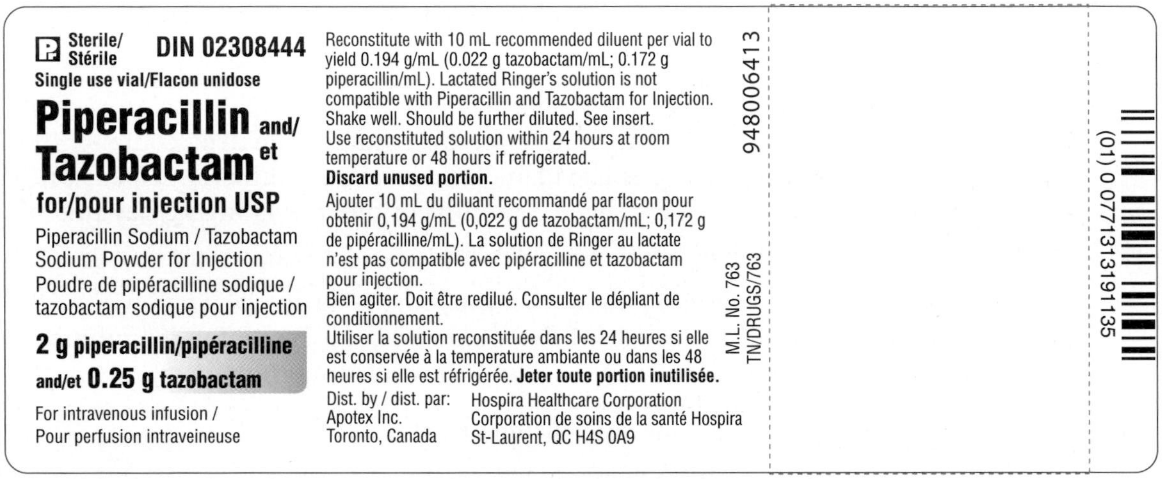

FIGURE 11-5 Piperacillin Sodium/Tazobactam Sodium Label

BODY WEIGHT DOSAGE CALCULATION

Some students find the following table helpful when calculating dosage ranges based on body weight for either adults or children. First convert the weight in lb to kg.

Example:

Order: *piperacillin sodium 3 g IV q6h* for a patient with bacterial septicemia

Supply: piperacillin sodium 180 mg/mL (2 g vial)

Recommended adult dosage from the package insert: 200–300 mg/kg/day q4 to q6h for serious infections

Patient's weight: 120 lb

Convert lb to kg. Approximate equivalent: 1 kg = 2.2 lb

Think: $\frac{1}{2}$ of 120 = 60 (answer will be slightly less)

$120 \text{ lb} \div 2.2 \text{ lb/kg} = 120 \cancel{\text{lb}} \times 1 \text{ kg}/2.2 \cancel{\text{lb}} = 54.54 \text{ kg} = 54.5 \text{ kg}$

	Minimum Dosage	Maximum Dosage
Body Weight (kg)	54.5 kg	54.5 kg
× Recommended Dosage	× 200 mg/kg/day	× 300 mg/kg/day
Total Daily Dosage	10 900 mg/kg/day	16 350 mg/kg/day
÷ Number of Doses/Day	÷ 4 doses/day	÷ 4 doses/day
Dosage Range/Dose	2725 mg/dose q6h to	4087.5 mg/dose q6h

The ordered dosage of piperacillin sodium 3 g (or 3000 mg) is between the recommended minimum (2.7 g or 2725 mg) and maximum (4.1 g or 4088 mg) doses. Therefore, it is safe.

QUICK REVIEW

To use the body weight method to verify the safety of pediatric and adult dosages,

- Convert body weight from pounds and ounces to kilograms: 1 kg = 2.2 lb; 1 lb = 16 oz;
- Calculate the recommended safe dosage in mg/kg;
- Compare the ordered dosage with the recommended dosage to decide whether the dosage is safe;
- If the dosage is safe, calculate the amount to give for one dose; if not, notify the prescriber; and
- Combination drugs are ordered by dose volume. Check a reputable drug reference to be sure the dose ordered contains the safe amount of each drug as recommended.

REVIEW SET 11-1

Calculate one safe pediatric dose for questions 1 through 10.

1. Order: *cloxacillin sodium 125 mg PO q6h* for a child who weighs 36 lb. The recommended dosage of cloxacillin sodium for children weighing less than 20 kg is 50 to 100 mg/kg/day PO in equally divided doses q6h for moderate to severe infections to a maximum of 4 g/day.

   Child's weight: ________ kg

   Recommended minimum daily dosage for this child: ________ mg/day

   Recommended minimum single dosage for this child: ________ mg/dose

   Recommended maximum daily dosage for this child: ________ mg/day

   Recommended maximum single dosage for this child: ________ mg/dose

   Is the dosage ordered safe? ________

2. Cloxacillin sodium is available as an oral suspension of 125 mg/5 mL. If the dosage ordered in question 1 is safe, give ________ mL. If not safe, explain why not and describe what the nurse should do. ____

   ____

3. Order: *chloramphenicol sodium succinate 55 mg IV q12h* for an 8-day-old infant who weighs 2200 g. The recommended dosage of chloramphenicol sodium succinate for neonates under 2 weeks of age is 25 mg/kg/day divided q6h; and for neonates over 14 days to 4 weeks of age the recommended dosage is 50 mg/kg/day divided q6h.

   Infant's weight: ________ kg

   Recommended daily dosage for this infant: ________ mg/day

   Recommended single dosage for this infant: ________ mg/dose

   Is the dosage ordered safe? ________

4. Chloramphenicol sodium succinate is available as a solution for injection of 1 g/10 mL. If the dosage ordered in question 3 is safe, give ________ mL. If not safe, explain why not and describe what the nurse should do. ____

____

5. Order: *cefixime 120 mg PO daily* for a child who weighs 33 lb. The recommended dosage of cefixime for children under 50 kg is 8 mg/kg PO once daily or 4 mg/kg PO q12h.

   Child's weight: ________ kg

   Recommended single dosage for this child: ________ mg/dose

   Is the dosage ordered safe? ________

6. Cefixime is available as a suspension of 100 mg/5 mL in a 50-mL bottle. If the dosage ordered in question 5 is safe, give ________ mL. If not safe, explain why not and describe what the nurse should do. ____

   ____

   How many doses are available in the bottle of cefixime? ________ dose(s)

7. Order: *acetaminophen 480 mg PO q4h prn for temperature more than or equal to 38.3°C*. The child's weight is 32 kg. The recommended child's dosage of acetaminophen is 10 to 15 mg/kg/dose PO q4h for fever. No more than 65 mg/kg/day for a maximum of 5 days is recommended.

   Recommended minimum single dosage for this child: ________ mg/dose

   Recommended maximum single dosage for this child: ________ mg/dose

   Is the dosage ordered safe? ________

8. Acetaminophen is available as a suspension of 160 mg/5 mL. If the dosage ordered in question 7 is safe, give ________ mL. If not safe, explain why not and describe what the nurse should do. ____

   ____

9. Order: *cephalexin 125 mg PO q6h* for a child who weighs 44 lb. The recommended pediatric dosage of cephalexin is 25 to 50 mg/kg/day in 4 equally divided doses.

   Child's weight: ________ kg

   Recommended minimum daily dosage for this child: ________ mg/day

   Recommended minimum single dosage for this child: ________ mg/dose

   Recommended maximum daily dosage for this child: ________ mg/day

   Recommended maximum single dosage for this child: ________ mg/dose

   Is the dosage ordered safe? ________

10. Cephalexin is available in an oral suspension of 125 mg/5 mL. If the dosage ordered in question 9 is safe, give ________ mL. If not safe, explain why not and describe what the nurse should do. ____

    ____

The labels below represent the drugs available to answer questions 11 through 25. Verify safe dosages, indicate the amount to give, and draw an arrow on the accompanying syringe. Explain unsafe dosages, and describe the appropriate action to take.

11. Order: *tobramycin sulfate 8 mg IV q12h* for an infant who weighs 5000 g and is 1 week old. The recommended pediatric dosage of tobramycin sulfate is up to 4 mg/kg/day administered q12h.

    Infant's weight: ________ kg

    Recommended total daily dosage for this infant: ________ mg/day

    Recommended daily single dosage for this infant: ________ mg/dose

    Is the dosage ordered safe? ________

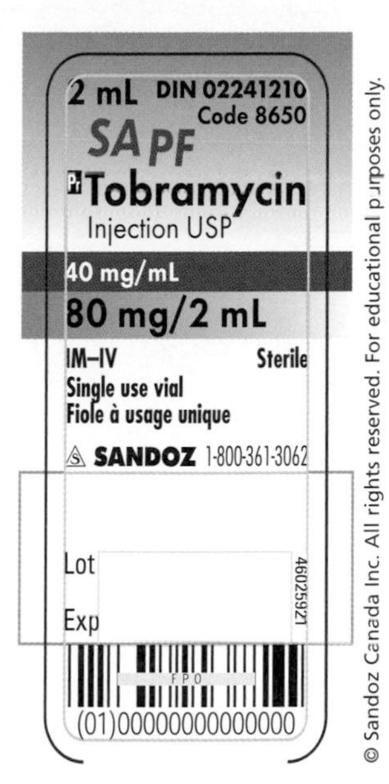

12. If the dosage ordered in question 11 is safe, give ________ mL. If not safe, explain why not and describe what the nurse should do.

    ____

    ____

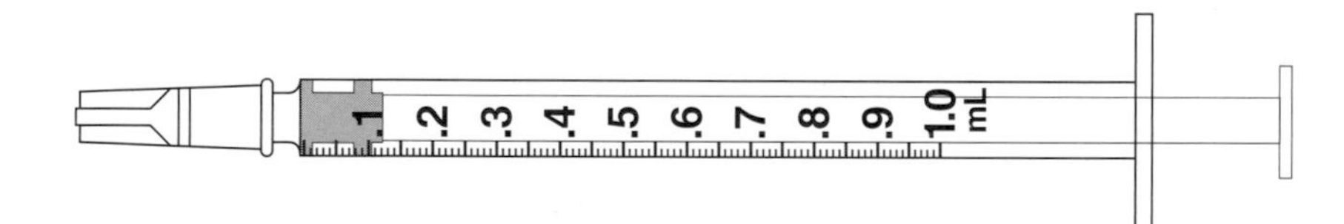

13. Order: *ceftazidime 34 mg IV q12h* for an infant who is 1 month old and weighs 7 lb 8 oz. The recommended daily dosage of ceftazidime for infants and children is as follows: 1–2 months is 12.5–25 mg/kg administered q12h (maximum 6 g/day); 2 months–12 years is 10–33 mg/kg administered q8h (maximum 6 g/day).

    Infant's weight: ________ kg

    Recommended minimum single dosage for this infant: ________ mg

    Recommended maximum single dosage for this infant: ________ mg

    Is the dosage ordered safe? ________

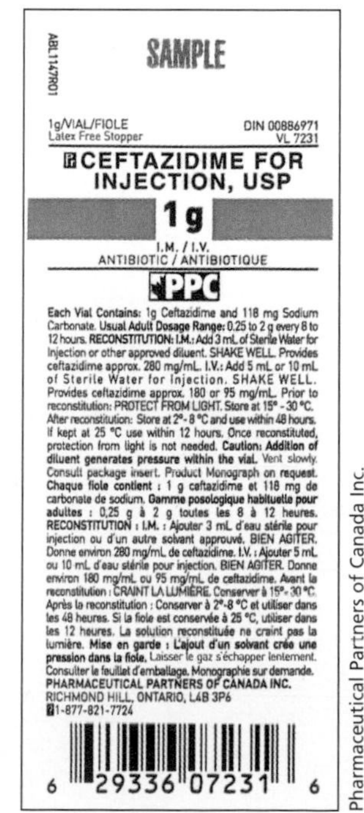

14. If the dosage ordered in question 13 is safe, give ________ mL. If not safe, explain why not and describe what the nurse should do. ____

____

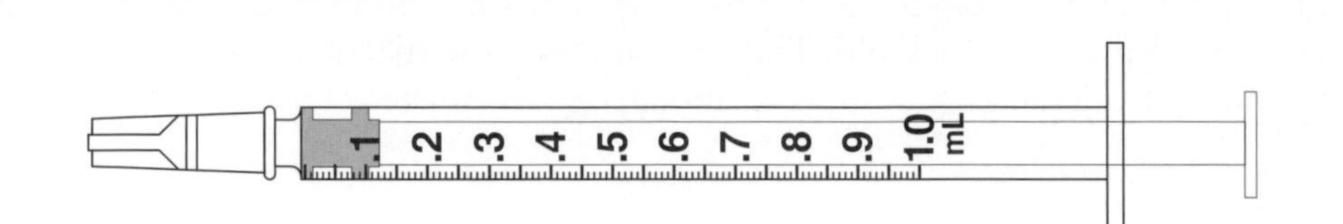

15. Order: *sulfamethoxazole/trimethoprim pediatric suspension 2.8 mL PO q12h* for a child who weighs 15 kg and has a bacterial infection. The recommended dosage of sulfamethoxazole and trimethoprim for such infections in children is based on the trimethoprim dosage at 3 mg/kg/day administered in 2 equal doses.

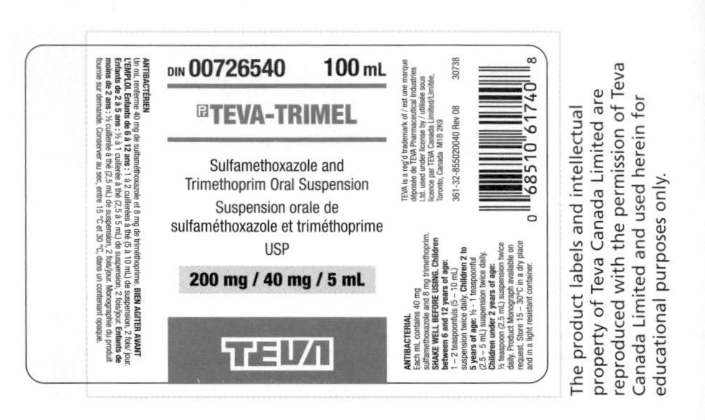

Recommended daily trimethoprim dosage for this child: ________ mg/day

Recommended single trimethoprim dosage for this child: ________ mg/dose

Recommended single dose for this child: ________ mL/dose

Is the dose ordered safe? ________

16. If the dose ordered in question 15 is safe, give ________ mL. If not safe, explain why not and describe what the nurse should do. ____

____

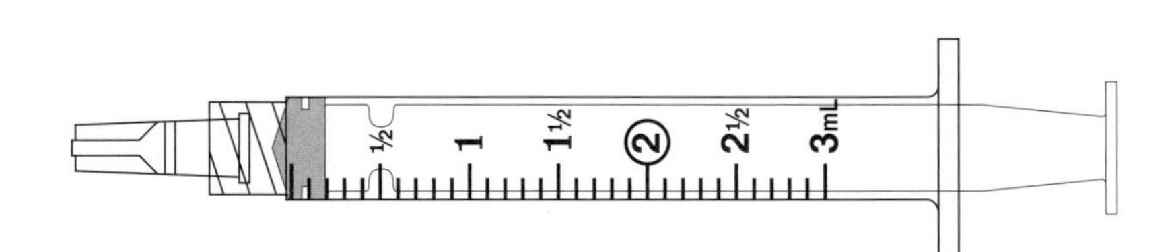

17. Order: *gentamicin sulfate 40 mg IV q8h* for a premature neonate who is 5 days old and weighs 1800 g. The recommended dosage of gentamicin sulfate for premature and full-term neonates 1 week of age or less is 6 mg/kg/day administered q12h; and for infants older than 1 week 6 mg/kg/day administered q8h.

Neonate's weight: ________ kg

Recommended single dosage for this neonate: ________ mg/dose

Is the ordered dosage safe? ________

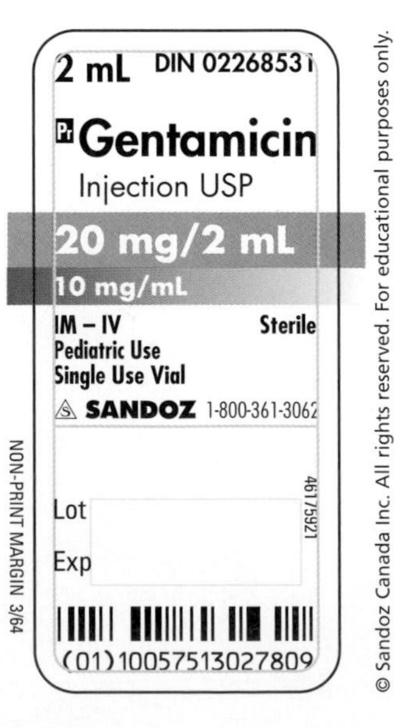

18. If the dosage ordered in question 17 is safe, give ________ mL. If not safe, explain why not and describe what the nurse should do. ____

____

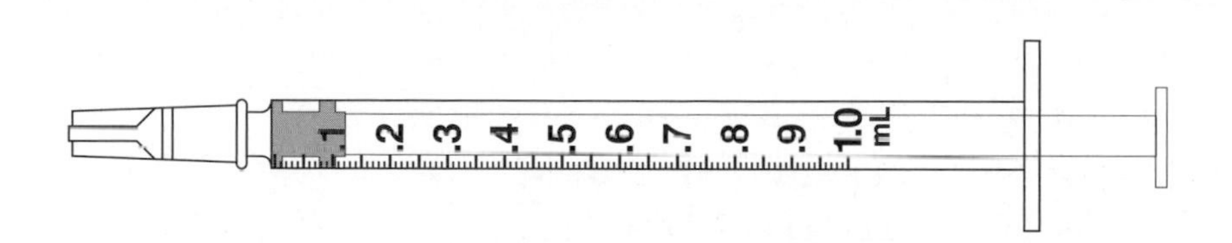

19. Order: *digoxin 0.15 mg PO q12h* for a maintenance dose for a 9-year-old child who weighs 70 lb. The recommended maintenance pediatric dosage of digoxin tablets (0.0625 mg) and oral solution (0.05 mg/mL) for children ages 5 to 10 years is 7 to 10 mcg/kg/day divided, and given in 2 equal doses per day.

    Child's weight: ________ kg

    Recommended minimum daily dosage for this child: ________ mg/day

    Recommended minimum single dosage for this child: ________ mg/dose

    Recommended maximum daily dosage for this child: ________ mg/day

    Recommended maximum single dosage for this child: ________ mg/dose

    Is the dosage ordered safe? ________

20. If the dosage ordered in question 19 is safe, give ________ mL. If not safe, explain why not and describe what the nurse should do. ____

____

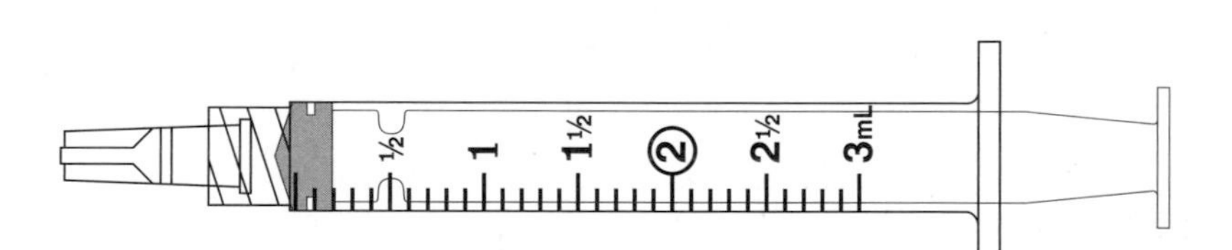

21. Order: *amoxicillin oral suspension 100 mg PO q8h* for a child who weighs 39 lb. Recommended dosage: See label.

ANTIBIOTIC
Bottle contains 2,500 mg amoxicillin as trihydrate.
DIRECTIONS FOR DISPENSING: At the time of dispensing, tap bottle to loosen powder, add 60 mL water in two portions, shake well after each addition, to make 100 mL of the suspension. Each 1 mL contains amoxicillin trihydrate equivalent to 25 mg amoxicillin.
Adult Dosage: 250 – 500 mg every 8 hours.
Children Dosage (< 20 kg): 20 - 40 mg/kg/day in divided doses every 8 hours, not exceeding the recommended adult dosage.
SHAKE WELL BEFORE USING.
Product Monograph available on request.
Pharmacist: Dispense with Patient Information Leaflet.
Store between 15 – 30°C. Keep bottle tightly closed.
Keep out of reach of children.
Suspension stable for 7 days at room temperature or 14 days refrigerated. Do not freeze.
361-32-668620040 Rev. 06

DIN 00452149 100 mL
NOVAMOXIN® 125
Amoxicillin Granules for Oral Suspension
Granules d'amoxicilline pour suspension orale
USP
125 mg/5 mL
Amoxicillin / Amoxicilline
When reconstituted as directed
Après reconstitution
Mixed Berry / Baies mélangées
TEVA

ANTIBIOTIQUE
Le flacon contient 2 500 mg d'amoxicilline sous forme trihydratée.
RECONSTITUTION : Au moment de reconstituer, secouer doucement le flacon pour rendre la poudre moins compacte, puis ajouter 60 mL d'eau en deux portions, en agitant bien après chaque addition, pour obtenir 100 mL de suspension. Chaque 1 mL contient de l'amoxicilline trihydratée équivalant à 25 mg d'amoxicilline.
Posologie chez l'adulte : 250 mg à 500 mg toutes les 8 heures.
Posologie chez l'enfant (< 20 kg) : 20 à 40 mg/kg/jour en doses fractionnées toutes les 8 heures, sans dépasser la posologie recommandée chez l'adulte.
BIEN AGITER AVANT L'EMPLOI.
Monographie du produit fournie sur demande.
Pharmacien-ne : Remettre au patient avec un feuillet de renseignements.
Conserver entre 15 °C et 30 °C. Garder le flacon fermé hermétiquement.
Garder hors de la portée des enfants.
La suspension est stable pendant 7 jours à la température ambiante et pendant 14 jours au réfrigérateur.
Ne pas congeler.
NOVAMOXIN is a reg'd trademark of/est une marque déposée de Teva Canada Limited/Limitée. Manufactured/Fabriqué by/par Teva Canada Limited/Limitée, Toronto, Canada M1B 2K9
0 68510 02240 0

    Child's weight: ________ kg

    Recommended minimum daily dosage for this child: ________ mg/day

    Recommended minimum single dosage for this child: ________ mg/dose

    Recommended maximum daily dosage for this child: ________ mg/day

    Recommended maximum single dosage for this child: ________ mg/dose

    Is the dosage ordered safe? ________

22. If the dosage ordered in question 21 is safe, give ________ mL. If not safe, explain why not and describe what the nurse should do. ____________________

____

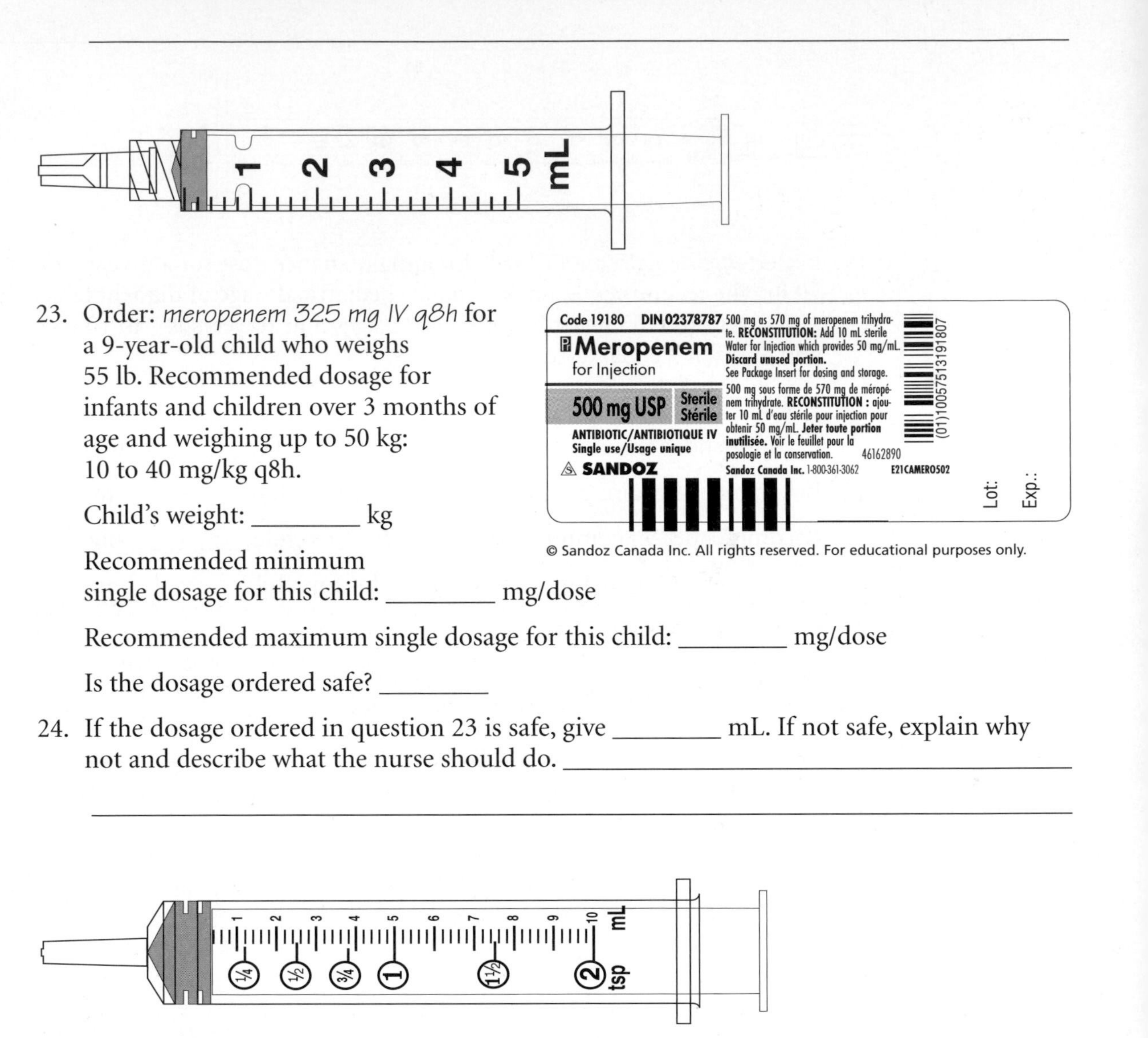

23. Order: *meropenem 325 mg IV q8h* for a 9-year-old child who weighs 55 lb. Recommended dosage for infants and children over 3 months of age and weighing up to 50 kg: 10 to 40 mg/kg q8h.

    Child's weight: ________ kg

    Recommended minimum single dosage for this child: ________ mg/dose

    Recommended maximum single dosage for this child: ________ mg/dose

    Is the dosage ordered safe? ________

24. If the dosage ordered in question 23 is safe, give ________ mL. If not safe, explain why not and describe what the nurse should do. ____________________

____

25. Order: *meropenem 275 mg IV daily* for a 7-year-old child who weighs 21 kg. Recommended dosage: See question 23.

    Is the ordered dosage safe? ________ Explain: ____________________

____

Check your work! Answers to all Review Sets are provided at the end of each chapter. Worked solutions for selected Review Sets are also available there.

APPLICATION OF CLINICAL REASONING

Patient safety incidents in pediatrics often occur when the nurse fails to properly identify the child before administering the dose.

Potential Patient Safety Incident

Failing to identify the child before administering a medication.

Possible Scenario

Suppose the prescriber ordered *ampicillin 500 mg IV q6h* for a child diagnosed with pneumonia. The nurse calculated the dosage to be safe, confirmed that the child had no allergies, and prepared the medication. The child had been assigned to a semi-private room. The nurse entered the room and noted only one child in the room and administered the IV ampicillin to that child, without checking the child's identification. Within an hour of the administered ampicillin, the child began to break out in hives and had signs of respiratory distress. The nurse asked the child's mother, "Does Johnny have any known allergies?" The mother replied, "This is James, not Johnny, and yes, James is allergic to penicillin. His roommate, Johnny, is in the playroom." At this point the nurse realized the ampicillin was given to the wrong child, who was allergic to penicillin.

Potential Outcome

James's prescriber would have been notified, and she would likely have ordered epinephrine subcutaneously stat (given for anaphylactic reactions), followed by close monitoring of the child. Anaphylactic reactions can range from mild to severe. Ampicillin is a derivative of penicillin and would not have been prescribed for a child such as James.

Prevention

This patient safety incident could easily have been avoided had the nurse remembered the cardinal rule of *identifying the child* before administering *any* medication. Children are mobile, and the identity of a child should not be assumed simply because the child is in a particular room. The correct method of identifying the child is to check the wrist or ankle band and compare it to the medication administration record with the child's name, room number, prescriber, and patient identification number. Finally, remember that the first of the *ten rights* of medication administration is the *right patient.*

Application of Critical Reasoning Additional application problems are provided at the end of the chapter. Answers are provided at the end of the book.

APPLICATION OF CLINICAL REASONING

When the recommended dosage of a medication is given with a high and low range, the minimum and maximum doses must be calculated to determine the safety of a drug order. This is the only way to ensure that the drug to be administered is not an overdose or an underdose.

Potential Patient Safety Incident

Calculating only the maximum recommended dose of an ordered medication to determine safety.

(continues)

(continued)

Possible Scenario

The prescriber ordered *tobramycin 9.5 mg IV q8h* for a 2-week-old infant who weighed 11 lb and had a serious infection. The recommended dosage for children and infants greater than 1 week old is 1.5 to 1.9 mg/kg q6h or 2 to 2.5 mg/kg q8h. The nurse calculated a safe dosage range prior to administering what would be the third dose of this medication, although it was administered 2 previous times by other nurses. First, the nurse correctly converted the infant's weight from pounds to kilograms by dividing 11 by 2.2 to equal 5 kg. Then the nurse correctly calculated the minimum and maximum recommended doses by multiplying the recommended dosage by the infant's weight.

Minimum single q8h dose: $2 \text{ mg}/\cancel{\text{kg}} \times 5 \cancel{\text{kg}} = 10 \text{ mg}$

Maximum single q8h dose: $2.5 \text{ mg}/\cancel{\text{kg}} \times 5 \cancel{\text{kg}} = 12.5 \text{ mg}$

The nurse recognized that the ordered dose fell below the minimum recommended dose for tobramycin to be administered every 8 hours. Considering the serious infection the infant had, the nurse doubted that the prescriber planned to give such a low dose and notified the prescriber. The prescriber realized that the dose was mistakenly calculated according to the q6h recommendation and wrote a new order.

Potential Outcome

The first two dosages of tobramycin fell slightly below the minimum recommended dose for the frequency ordered. This situation was discussed with the nurse manager of the pediatric unit along with the other two staff nurses involved. One staff nurse admitted to administering medication occasionally without actually calculating a safe dose if it looked like it was the correct dose. The other nurse always checked to see that ordered medications were not overdoses but did not usually worry about checking for underdoses. The nurse manager emphasized the importance of always verifying doses on pediatric patients, especially infants. In this situation, the mistake was caught early and corrected but could have caused significant harm to the infant by inadequately treating a severe infection.

Prevention

When reading drug reference guides, make sure you read all the dosage recommendations thoroughly. It is easy to see how, when in a hurry, a prescriber or nurse might have misinterpreted the drug reference information and thought that it read 1.5 to 1.9 mg/kg q8h. Do not hurry or take shortcuts when administering medications. Always calculate the minimum and maximum recommended doses when a dosage range is given.

Application of Critical Reasoning Additional application problems are provided at the end of the chapter. Answers are provided at the end of the book.

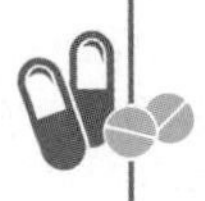

UNDERSTANDING NCLEX QUESTIONS

Here's an example of a standard question used in textbooks:

Cefaclor 35 mg/kg/day PO in 3 divided doses is ordered for Pina who weighs 30 kg. Available is cefaclor 375 mg/5 mL. Each dose will contain:

a. 1.5 mL
b. 3.6 mL
c. 4 mL
d. 4.7 mL

Here's how the question would look in an NCLEX examination:

The nurse is to administer cefaclor 35 mg/kg/day PO in 3 divided doses for a patient who weighs 30 kg. Available is cefaclor 375 mg/5 mL. What amount would the nurse administer per dose?

a. 1.5 mL
b. 3.6 mL
c. 4 mL
d. 4.7 mL

Answer: d

35 mg/kg/day × 30 kg = 1050 mg/day ÷ 3 doses = 350 mg/dose

$\frac{D}{H} \times Q = \frac{350}{375} \times 5 = 4.67 = 4.7\text{ mL}$

PRACTICE PROBLEMS—CHAPTER 11

For questions 1 through 8, convert the weights to kilograms. Round to one decimal place.

1. 12 lb = ________ kg
2. 8 lb 4 oz = ________ kg
3. 1570 g = ________ kg
4. 2300 g = ________ kg
5. 34 lb = ________ kg
6. 6 lb 10 oz = ________ kg
7. 52 lb = ________ kg
8. 890 g = ________ kg
9. The recommended dosage of tobramycin sulfate for adults with serious, non–life-threatening infections is 3 mg/kg/day in 3 equally divided doses or q8h. What should you expect the total daily dosage of tobramycin sulfate to be for an 80-kg adult with a serious infection? ________ mg/day
10. What should you expect the single dosage of tobramycin sulfate to be for the adult described in question 9? ________ mg/dose

The labels provided are the drugs available to answer questions 11 through 42. Verify safe dosages, indicate the amount to give, and draw an arrow on the accompanying syringe. Explain unsafe dosages, and describe the appropriate action to take.

2 mL DIN 0226853i
Gentamicin
Injection USP
20 mg/2 mL
10 mg/mL
IM – IV Sterile
Pediatric Use
Single Use Vial
SANDOZ 1-800-361-3062
Lot
Exp
4617921
(01)10057513027809
NON-PRINT MARGIN 3/64

11. Order: *gentamicin sulfate 40 mg IV q8h* for a child who weighs 43 lb. The recommended dosage for children is 3 to 6 mg/kg/day administered q8h.

    Child's weight: ________ kg

    Recommended minimum single dosage for this child: ________ mg/dose

    Recommended maximum single dosage for this child: ________ mg/dose

    Is the ordered dosage safe? ________

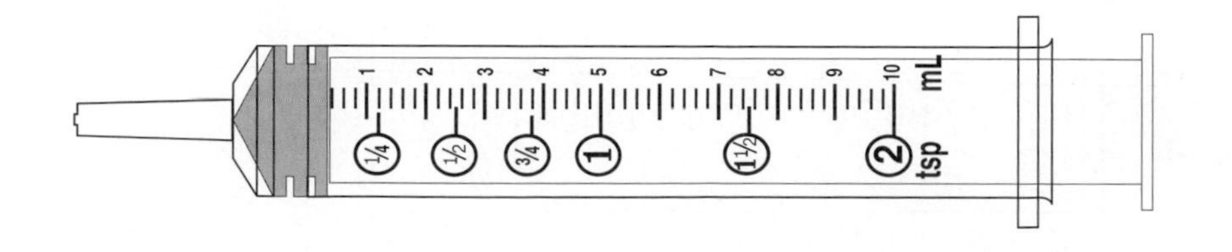

12. If the dosage ordered in question 11 is safe, give ________ mL. If not safe, explain why not and describe what the nurse should do. ______________________________

____

13. Order: *furosemide oral solution 5 mg PO BID* for a child who weighs 16 lb. The recommended pediatric dosage is 0.5 to 1 mg/kg/day BID. The maximum total daily dose should not exceed 2 mg/kg.

Lasix® Oral Solution / Solution orale
Furosemide Oral Solution, Mfr. Std.
Solution orale de furosémide, Norme-fabricant
10 mg/mL
Diuretic / Diurétique
120 mL
DIN 02224720
SANOFI

Child's weight: ________ kg

Recommended minimum single dosage for this child: ________ mg/dose

Recommended maximum single dosage for this child: ________ mg/dose

Is the ordered dosage safe? ________

14. If the dosage ordered in question 13 is safe, give ________ mL. If not safe, explain why not and describe what the nurse should do. ______________________________

____

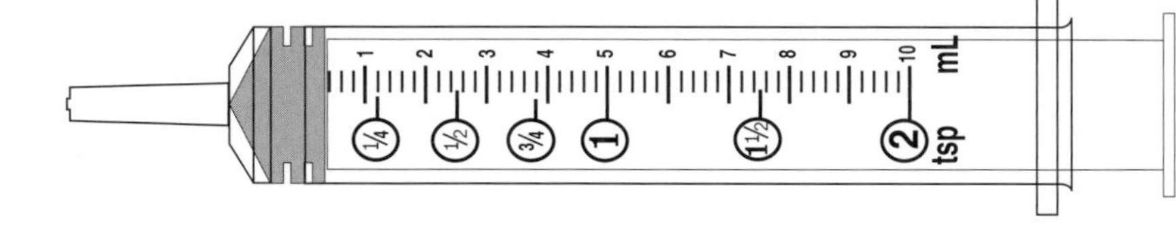

15. Order: *phenytoin oral suspension 250 mg PO BID* for a child who is 7 years old and weighs 50 lb. The recommended daily maintenance dosage for children is 4 to 8 mg/kg/day in 2 divided doses per day, not to exceed 300 mg/day.

Dilantin*-125 Suspension
Phenytoin Oral Suspension USP
Suspension orale de phénytoïne, USP
Not for parenteral use
Ne pas administrer par voie parentérale
125 mg/5 mL
250 mL
DIN 00023450
Pfizer

Child's weight: ________ kg

Recommended minimum daily dosage for this child: ________ mg/day

Recommended minimum single dosage for this child: ________ mg/dose

Recommended maximum daily dosage for this child: ________ mg/day

Recommended maximum single dosage for this child: ________ mg/dose

Is the dosage ordered safe? ________

16. If the dosage ordered in question 15 is safe, give ________ mL. If not safe, explain why not and describe what the nurse should do. ______________________________

____

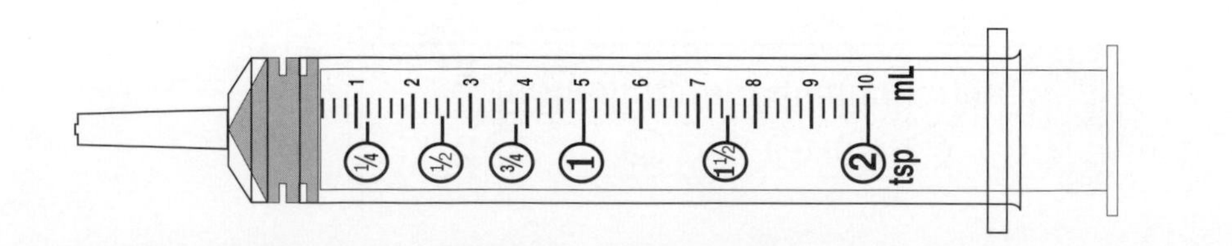

17. Order: *valproic acid 150 mg PO BID* for a child who is 10 years old and weighs 64 lb. The recommended dosage for adults and children 10 years and older is 10 to 15 mg/kg/day up to a maximum of 60 mg/kg/day. If the total daily dosage exceeds 250 mg, divide the dose.

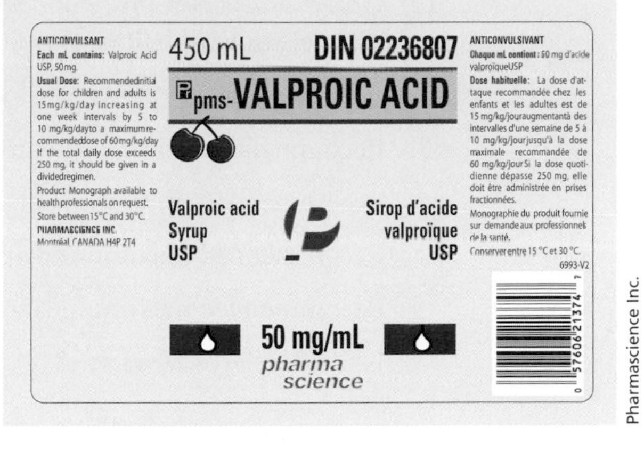

Pharmascience Inc.

Child's weight: ________ kg

Recommended minimum daily dosage for this child: ________ mg/day

Recommended minimum single dosage for this child: ________ mg/dose

Recommended maximum daily dosage for this child: ________ mg/day

Recommended maximum single dosage for this child: ________ mg/dose

Is the dosage ordered safe? ________

18. If the dosage ordered in question 17 is safe, give ________ mL. If not safe, explain why not and describe what the nurse should do. ________________

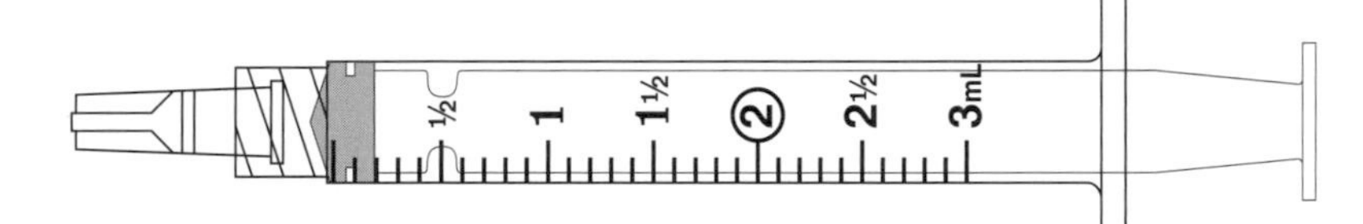

19. Order: *bacitracin 750 units IM q8h* for an infant who weighs 2500 g. The recommended dosage for infants 2.5 kg and below: 900 units/kg/day in 2 to 3 divided doses; infants over 2.5 kg: 1000 units/kg/day in 2 to 3 divided doses. Reconstitute the 50 000-unit vial with 9.8 mL of diluent for a concentration of 5000 units/mL.

DIN 00030708
Bacitracin USP
50,000 IU/vial
For topical or intramuscular use, in solution
Sterile powder
5 vials
Pfizer Injectables
ANTIBIOTIC
Usual Dose: See enclosed Package Insert for dosage, administration and direction for use.
Refrigerate powder and reconstituted solution (between 2 and 8°C).
Use the reconstituted solution within 1 week.
Keep out of the reach of children.
26126-15-1

Courtesy of Pfizer Inc.

Infant's weight: ________ kg

Recommended daily dosage for this infant: ________ units/day

Recommended single dosage for this infant: ________ units/dose

Is the ordered dosage safe? ________

20. If the dosage ordered in question 19 is safe, reconstitute with ________ mL diluent for a concentration of ________ units/mL. Give ________ mL. If not safe, explain why not and describe what the nurse should do. ________________

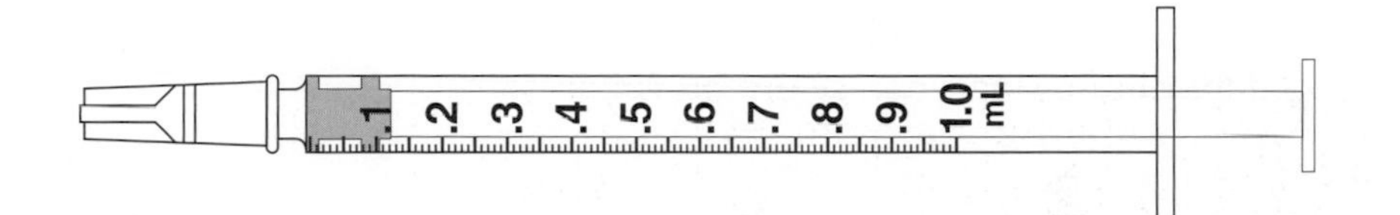

21. Order: *amoxicillin oral suspension 150 mg PO q8h* for a child who weighs 41 lb. Recommended dosage: See label below.

    Child's weight: ________ kg

    Recommended minimum daily dosage for this child: ________ mg/day

    Recommended minimum single dosage for this child: ________ mg/dose

    Recommended maximum daily dosage for this child: ________ mg/day

    Recommended maximum single dosage for this child: ________ mg/dose

    Is the dosage ordered safe? ________

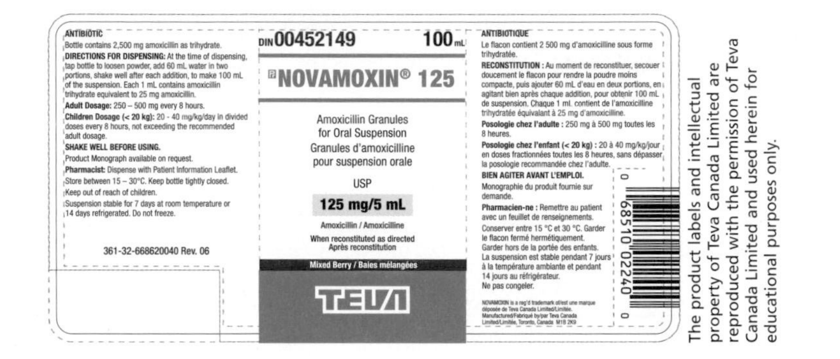

22. If the dosage ordered in question 21 is safe, give ________ mL. If not safe, explain why not and describe what the nurse should do. ____

    ____

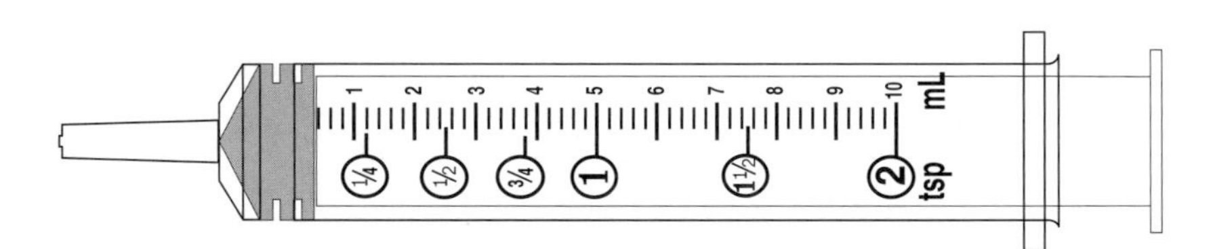

23. Order: *amoxicillin oral suspension 185 mg PO TID* for a child with otitis media and who weighs $20\frac{1}{2}$ lb. Recommended dosage: 2016 Canadian Paediatric Association recommendations are for 45 mg/kg/day–60 mg/kg/day divided 3 times per day.

    Child's weight: ________ kg

    Recommended minimum daily dosage for this child: ________ mg/day

    Recommended minimum single dosage for this child: ________ mg/dose

    Is the dosage ordered safe? ________

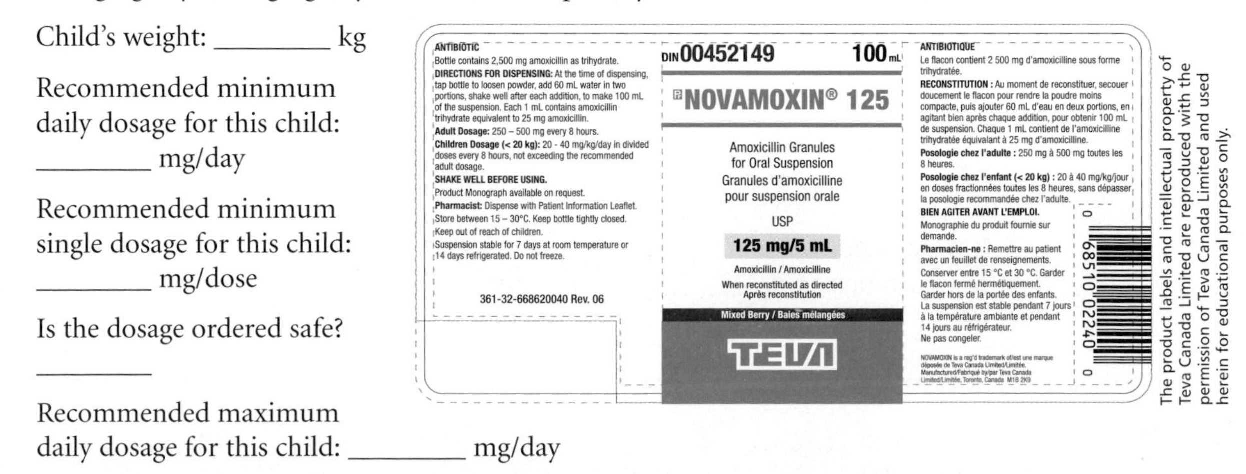

    Recommended maximum daily dosage for this child: ________ mg/day

    Recommended maximum single dosage for this child: ________ mg/ dose

24. If the dosage ordered in question 23 is safe, give ________ mL. If not safe, explain why not and describe what the nurse should do. ____

____

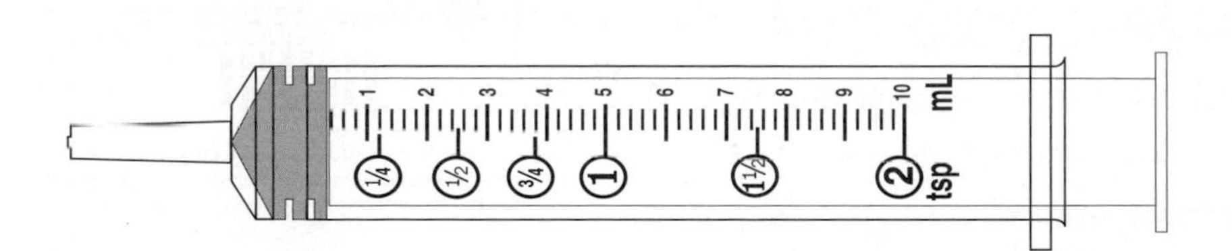

25. Order: *naloxone hydrochloride 100 mcg subcutaneously stat* for a child who weighs 22 lb. Recommended pediatric dosage: 0.01 mg/kg/dose.

    Child's weight: ________ kg

    Recommended single dosage for this child: ________ mg/dose

    Is the dosage ordered safe? ________

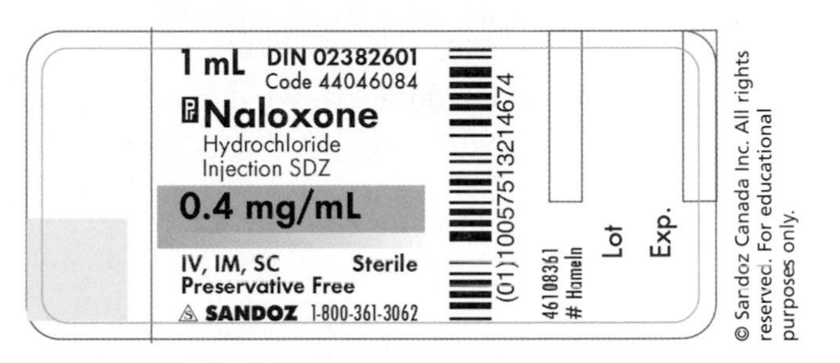

26. If the dosage ordered in question 25 is safe, give ________ mL. If not safe, explain why not and describe what the nurse should do.

____

____

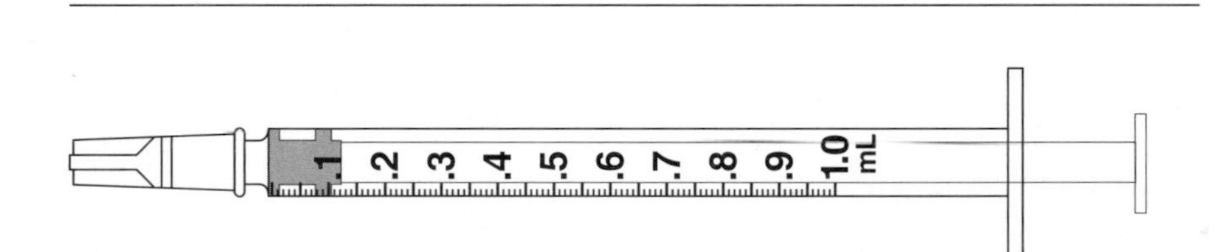

27. Order: *tobramycin sulfate 35 mg IV q8h* for a child who weighs 14 kg. The recommended pediatric dosage of tobramycin sulfate is 6 to 7.5 mg/kg/day in 3 or 4 equally divided doses.

    Recommended minimum single dosage for this child: ________ mg/dose

    Recommended maximum single dosage for this child: ________ mg/dose

    Is the dosage ordered safe? ________

28. If the dosage ordered in question 27 is safe, give ________ mL. If not safe, explain why not and describe what the nurse should do.

____

____

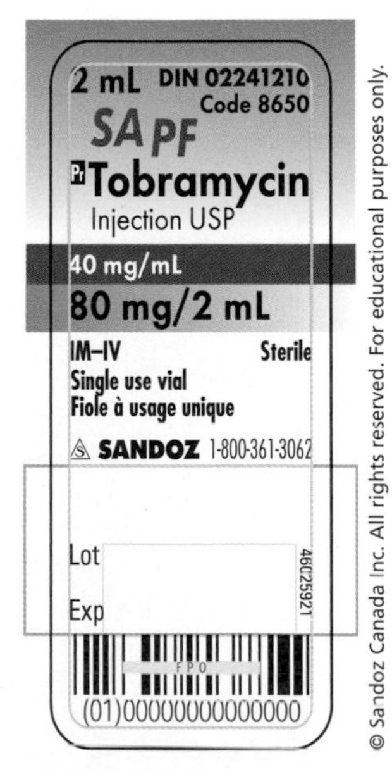

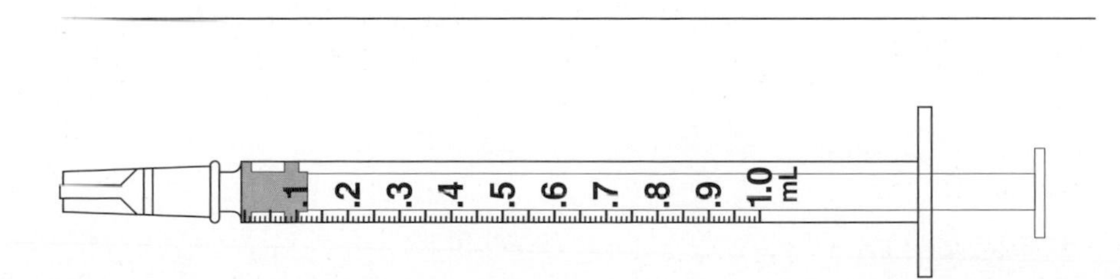

29. Order: *ceftriaxone sodium 1 g IV q12h* for a child who weighs 20 lb and has a serious infection. The recommended pediatric dosage of ceftriaxone sodium is 25 or 37.5 mg/kg.

    Child's weight: ________ kg

    Recommended minimum single dosage for this child: ________ mg/dose

    Recommended maximum single dosage for this child: ________ mg/dose

    Is the dosage ordered safe? ________

DIN 02287633
Sterile/Stérile
Ceftriaxone Sodium
For Injection
BP
1 g
Ceftriaxone per vial
Antibiotic / Antibiotique
IM / IV
Each vial contains 1 g of ceftriaxone in the form of the sodium salt. For **Dosage and Administration**, storage under refrigeration, see enclosed package insert. Reconstitute before use. Use reconstituted solutions within 24 hours if stored at room temperature. Product Monograph available on request. Store dry powder at 15-30°C. Protect from light.
Une fiole contient 1 g de ceftriaxone sous forme de sel sodique. Pour **la posologie et l'administration**, le mode de reconstitution (avant l'emploi) et l'entreposage au réfrigérateur, consulter le dépliant ci-inclus. Monographie fournie sur demande. Conserver la poudre sèche à 15° - 30 °C, à l'abri de la lumière.
Novopharm Limited / Limitée Toronto, Canada M1B 2K9 361-32-695120110 Rev 03
(01)00068510694102
E33CACTRX101
Lot:
Exp.:

30. If the dosage ordered in question 29 is safe, give ________ mL. If not safe, explain why not and describe what the nurse should do. ____

    ____

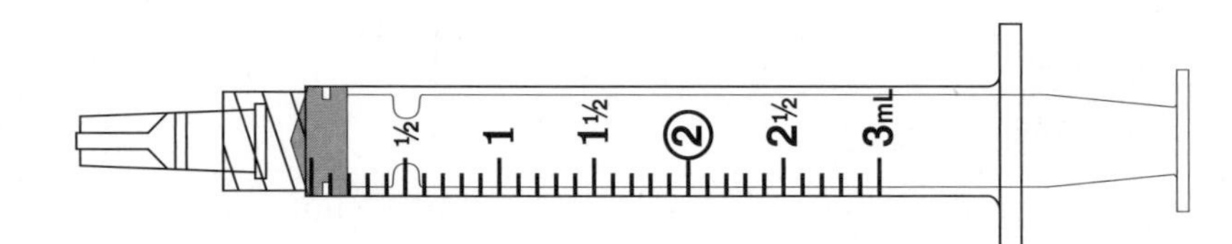

31. Order: *glycopyrrolate 50 mcg IM 60 min pre-op* for a child who weighs 11.4 kg. The recommended pre-anesthesia dosage of glycopyrrolate for a child is 0.005 mg/kg of body weight given intramuscularly, not to exceed 0.01 mg in a single dose.

    Recommended single dosage for this child: ________ mg/dose

    Is the dosage ordered safe? ________

32. If the dosage ordered in question 31 is safe, give ________ mL. If not safe, explain why not and describe what the nurse should do.

    ____

    ____

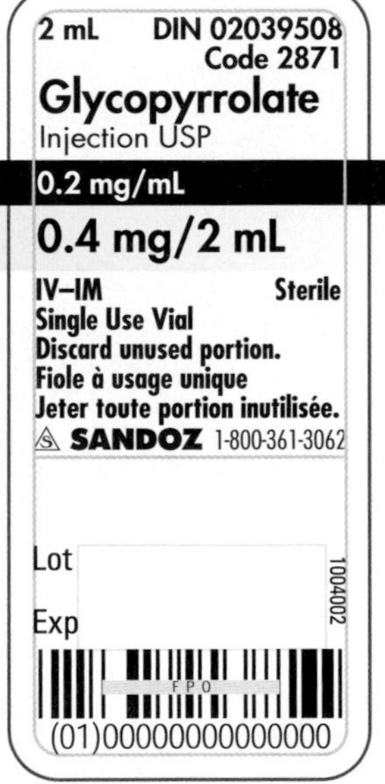

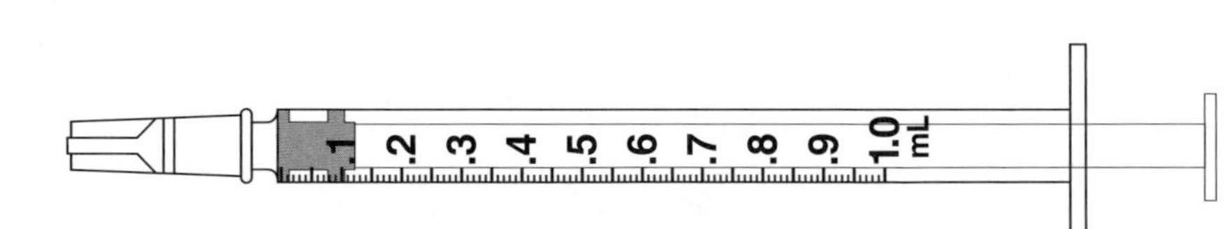

33. Order: *ceftazidime 400 mg IV q8h* for a 6-month-old infant who weighs 18 lb and has a serious infection. The recommended dosage of ceftazidime for infants and children 2 months to 12 years is 10 to 33 mg/kg q8h.

    Infant's weight: ________ kg

    Recommended minimum single dosage for this infant: ________ mg/dose

    Recommended maximum single dosage for this infant: ________ mg/dose

    Is the dosage ordered safe? ________

34. If the dosage ordered in question 33 is safe, reconstitute with ________ mL diluent for a total solution volume of ________ mL with a concentration of ________ mg/mL. Give ________ mL. If not safe, explain why not and describe what the nurse should do.

    ____

    ____

ABL1147R01

SAMPLE

1g/VIAL/FIOLE
Latex Free Stopper

DIN 00886971
VL 7231

CEFTAZIDIME FOR INJECTION, USP

1 g

I.M. / I.V.
ANTIBIOTIC / ANTIBIOTIQUE

PPC

Each Vial Contains: 1g Ceftazidime and 118 mg Sodium Carbonate. **Usual Adult Dosage Range:** 0.25 to 2 g every 8 to 12 hours. **RECONSTITUTION: I.M.:** Add 3 mL of Sterile Water for Injection or other approved diluent. SHAKE WELL. Provides ceftazidime approx. 280 mg/mL. **I.V.:** Add 5 mL or 10 mL of Sterile Water for Injection. SHAKE WELL. Provides ceftazidime approx. 180 or 95 mg/mL. Prior to reconstitution: PROTECT FROM LIGHT. Store at 15° - 30 °C. After reconstitution: Store at 2°- 8 °C and use within 48 hours. If kept at 25 °C use within 12 hours. Once reconstituted, protection from light is not needed. **Caution: Addition of diluent generates pressure within the vial.** Vent slowly. Consult package insert. Product Monograph on request.
Chaque fiole contient : 1 g ceftazidime et 118 mg de carbonate de sodium. **Gamme posologique habituelle pour adultes :** 0,25 g à 2 g toutes les 8 à 12 heures. **RECONSTITUTION : I.M. :** Ajouter 3 mL d'eau stérile pour injection ou d'un autre solvant approuvé. BIEN AGITER. Donne environ 280 mg/mL de ceftazidime. **I.V. :** Ajouter 5 mL ou 10 mL d'eau stérile pour injection. BIEN AGITER. Donne environ 180 mg/mL ou 95 mg/mL de ceftazidime. Avant la reconstitution : CRAINT LA LUMIÈRE. Conserver à 15°- 30 °C. Après la reconstitution : Conserver à 2°-8 °C et utiliser dans les 48 heures. Si la fiole est conservée à 25 °C, utiliser dans les 12 heures. La solution reconstituée ne craint pas la lumière. **Mise en garde : L'ajout d'un solvant crée une pression dans la fiole.** Laisser le gaz s'échapper lentement. Consulter le feuillet d'emballage. Monographie sur demande.
PHARMACEUTICAL PARTNERS OF CANADA INC.
RICHMOND HILL, ONTARIO, L4B 3P6
1-877-821-7724

6 29336 07231 6

1 2 3 4 5 mL

35. Order: *amoxicillin trihydrate/clavulanate potassium 200 mg PO q8h* for a 5-year-old child who weighs 45 lb. Recommended dosage: See label.

    Child's weight: ________ kg

    Recommended daily dosage for this child: ________ mg/day to ________ mg/day

    Recommended single dosage for this child: ________ mg/dose to ________ mg/dose

    Is the dosage ordered safe? ________

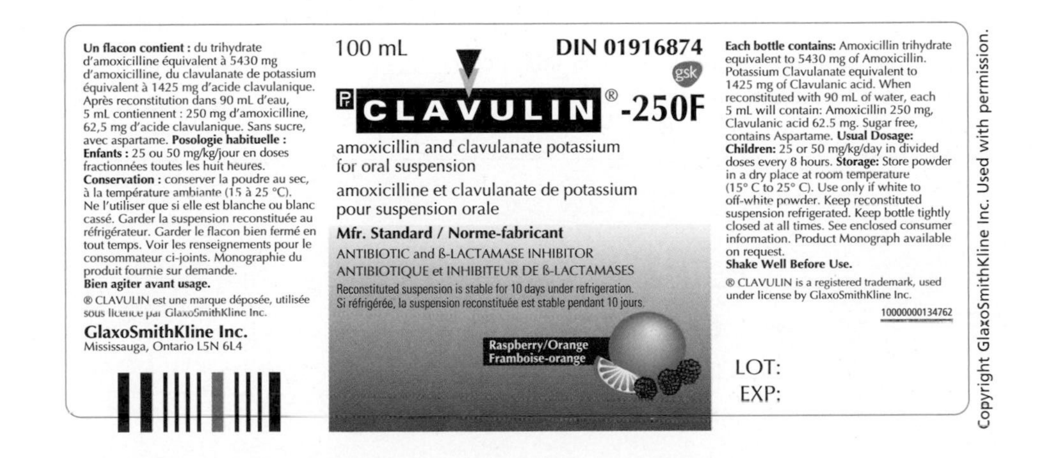

36. If the dosage ordered in question 35 is safe, give ________ mL. If not safe, explain why not and describe what the nurse should do. ____

____

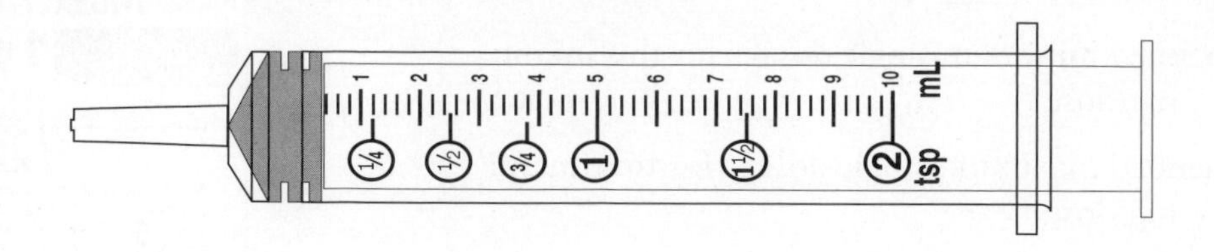

37. Order: *clarithromycin oral suspension 75 mg PO q12h* for a child with an upper respiratory tract infection who weighs 18 lb. Recommended dosage: See label.

    Child's weight: ________ kg

    Recommended daily dosage for this child: ________ mg/day

    Recommended single dosage for this child: ________ mg/dose

    Is the dosage ordered safe? ________

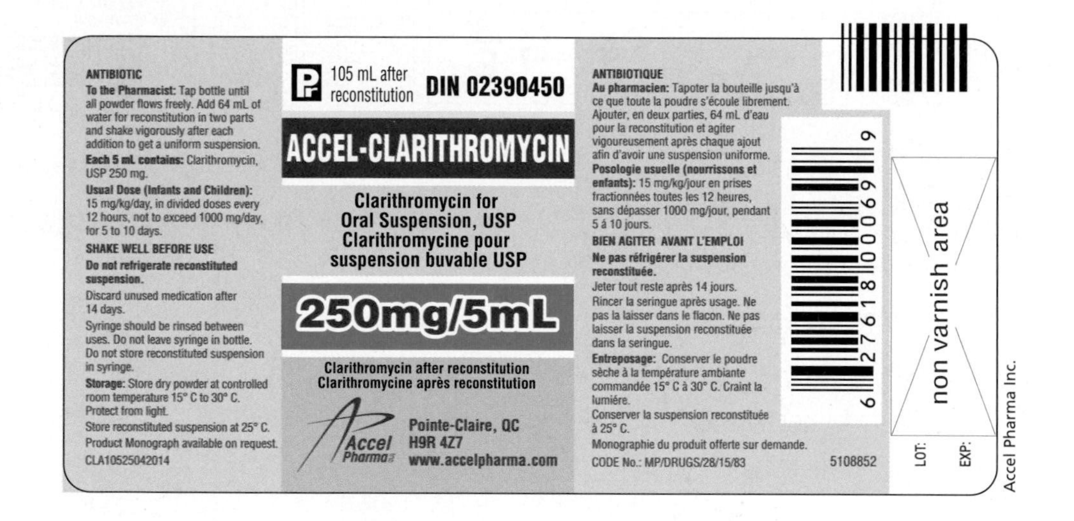

38. If the dosage ordered in question 37 is safe, give ________ mL. If not safe, explain why not and describe what the nurse should do. ____

____

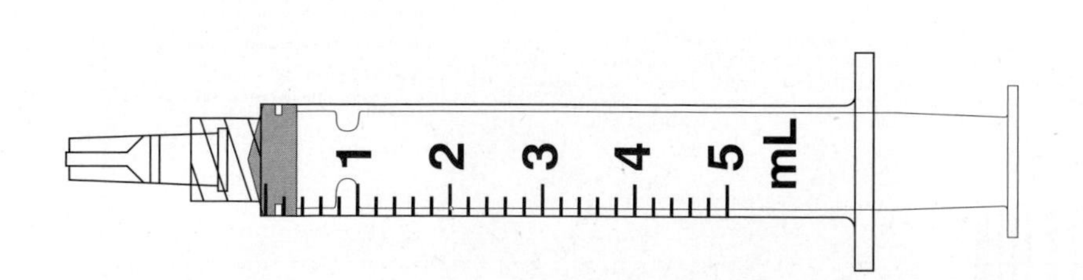

39. Order: *cephalexin oral suspension 125 mg PO QID × 10 days* for a 4-year-old child who weighs 45 lb and has tonsillitis. Recommended dosage: See label.

    Child's weight: ________ kg

    Recommended minimum daily dosage for this child: ________ mg/day

    Recommended single minimum dose: ________ mg/dose

    Recommended maximum daily dosage for this child: ________ mg/day

    Recommended single maximum dose: ________ mg/dose

    Is the dosage ordered safe? ________

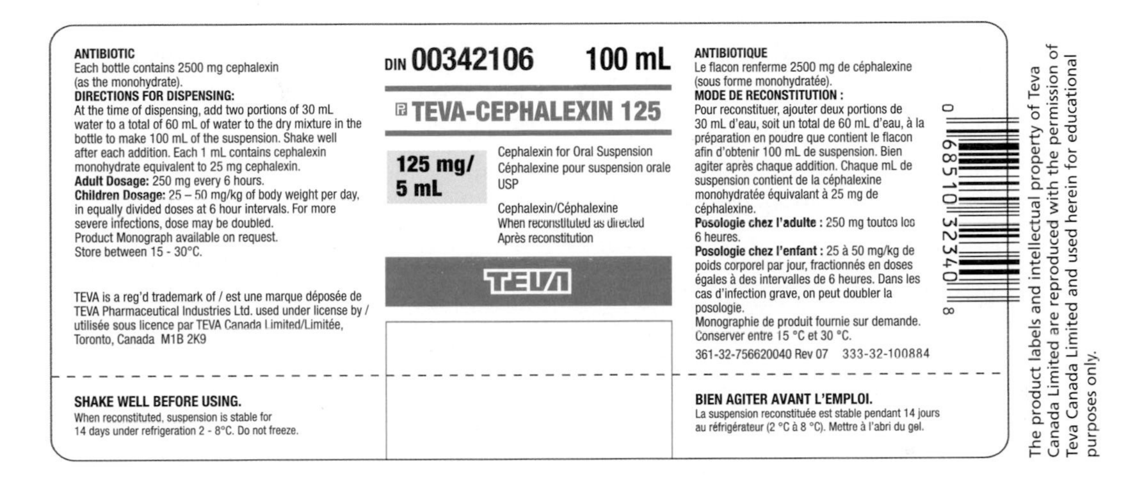

40. If the dosage ordered in question 39 is safe, give ________ mL. If not safe, explain why not and describe what the nurse should do. ____

    ____

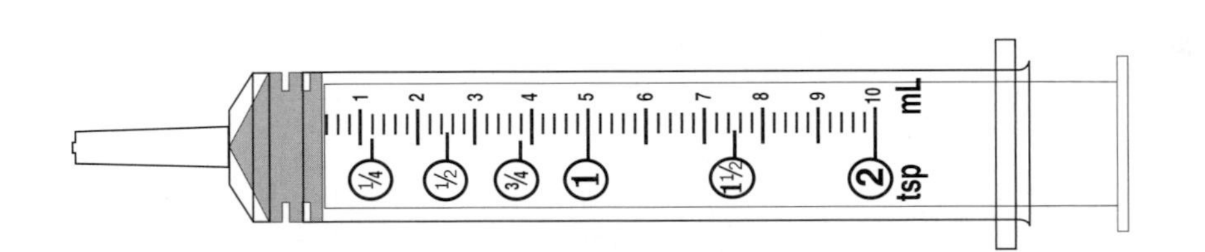

41. Order: *clarithromycin 175 mg PO q12h* for a child who weighs 51 lb. Recommended dosage for children: See label.

    Child's weight: ________ kg

    Recommended daily dosage for this child: ________ mg/day

    Recommended single dosage for this child: ________ mg/dose

    Is the dosage ordered safe? ________

ANTIBIOTIC
To the Pharmacist:
Tap bottle until all powder flows freely. Add 64 mL of water for reconstitution in two parts and shake vigorously after each addition to get a uniform suspension.
Each 5 mL contains: Clarithromycin, USP 125 mg.
Usual Dose (Infants and Children): 15 mg/kg/day, in divided doses every 12 hours, not to exceed 1000 mg/day, for 5 to 10 days.
SHAKE WELL BEFORE USE
Do not refrigerate reconstituted suspension.
Discard unused medication after 14 days.
Syringe should be rinsed between uses. Do not leave syringe in bottle. Do not store reconstituted suspension in syringe.
Storage: Store dry powder at controlled room temperature 15° C to 30° C. Protect from light.
Store reconstituted suspension at 25° C.
Product Monograph available on request.
CLA10512542014
Pr 105 mL after reconstitution DIN 02390442
ACCEL-CLARITHROMYCIN
Clarithromycin for Oral Suspension, USP
Clarithromycine pour suspension buvable USP
125mg/5mL
Clarithromycin after reconstitution
Clarithromycine après reconstitution
Accel Pharma Pointe-Claire, QC H9R 4Z7 www.accelpharma.com
ANTIBIOTIQUE
Au pharmacien: Tapoter la bouteille jusqu'à ce que toute la poudre s'écoule librement. Ajouter, en deux parties, 64 mL d'eau pour la reconstitution et agiter vigoureusement après chaque ajout afin d'avoir une suspension uniforme.
Posologie usuelle (nourrissons et enfants): 15 mg/kg/jour en prises fractionnées toutes les 12 heures, sans dépasser 1000 mg/jour, pendant 5 à 10 jours.
BIEN AGITER AVANT L'EMPLOI
Ne pas réfrigérer la suspension reconstituée.
Jeter tout reste après 14 jours.
Rincer la seringue après usage. Ne pas la laisser dans le flacon. Ne pas laisser la suspension reconstituée dans la seringue.
Entreposage: Conserver le poudre sèche à la température ambiante commandée 15° C à 30° C. Craint la lumiére.
Conserver la suspension reconstituée à 25° C.
Monographie du produit offerte sur demande.
CODE No.: MP/DRUGS/28/15/83
5108850
6 27618 00067 5
non varnish area
LOT:
EXP:

42. If the dosage ordered in question 41 is safe, give ________ mL. If not safe, explain why not and describe what the nurse should do. ____

____

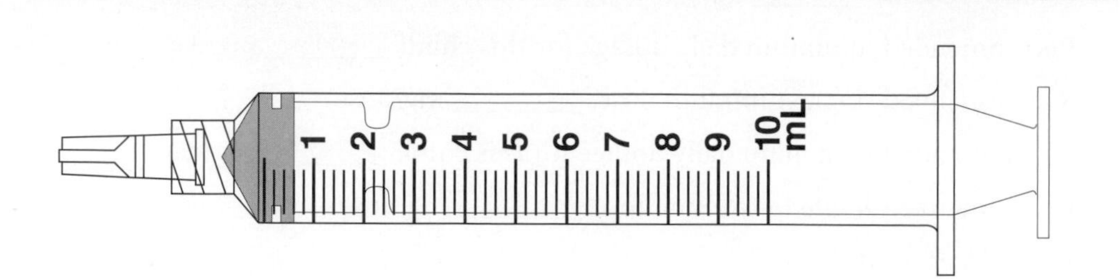

Questions 43 through 48 ask you to apply the steps on your own to determine safe dosages, just as you would do in the clinical setting. Calculate the amount to give and mark an arrow on the syringe, or explain unsafe dosages and describe the appropriate action.

43. Order: *methylprednisolone 10 mg IM q6h* for a child who weighs 95 lb. Recommended pediatric dosage: Not less than 0.5 mg/kg/day

If the dosage ordered is safe, give ________ mL. If not safe, explain why not and describe what the nurse should do. ____

____

____

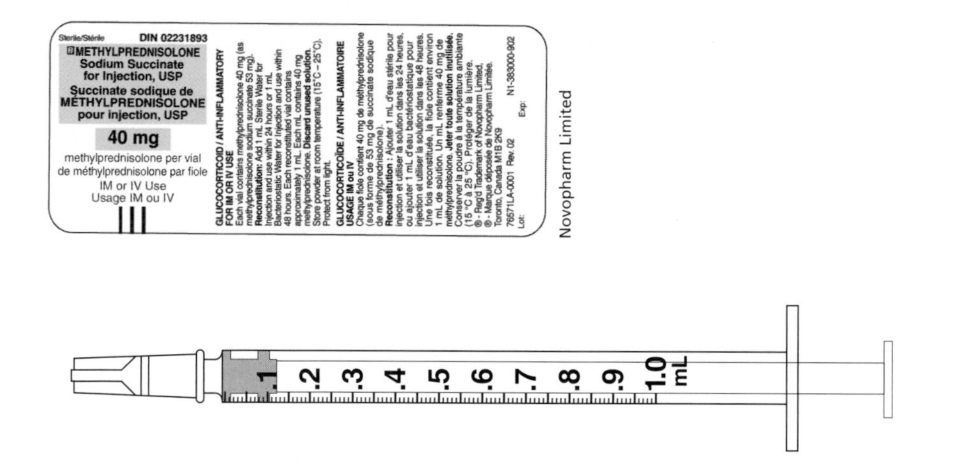

44. Order: *salbutamol 1.4 mg PO TID* for a 2-year-old child who weighs 31 lb. Recommended dosage: 0.1 mg/kg, not to exceed 2 mg TID.

If the dosage ordered is safe, give ________ mL. If not safe, explain why not and describe what the nurse should do. ____

____

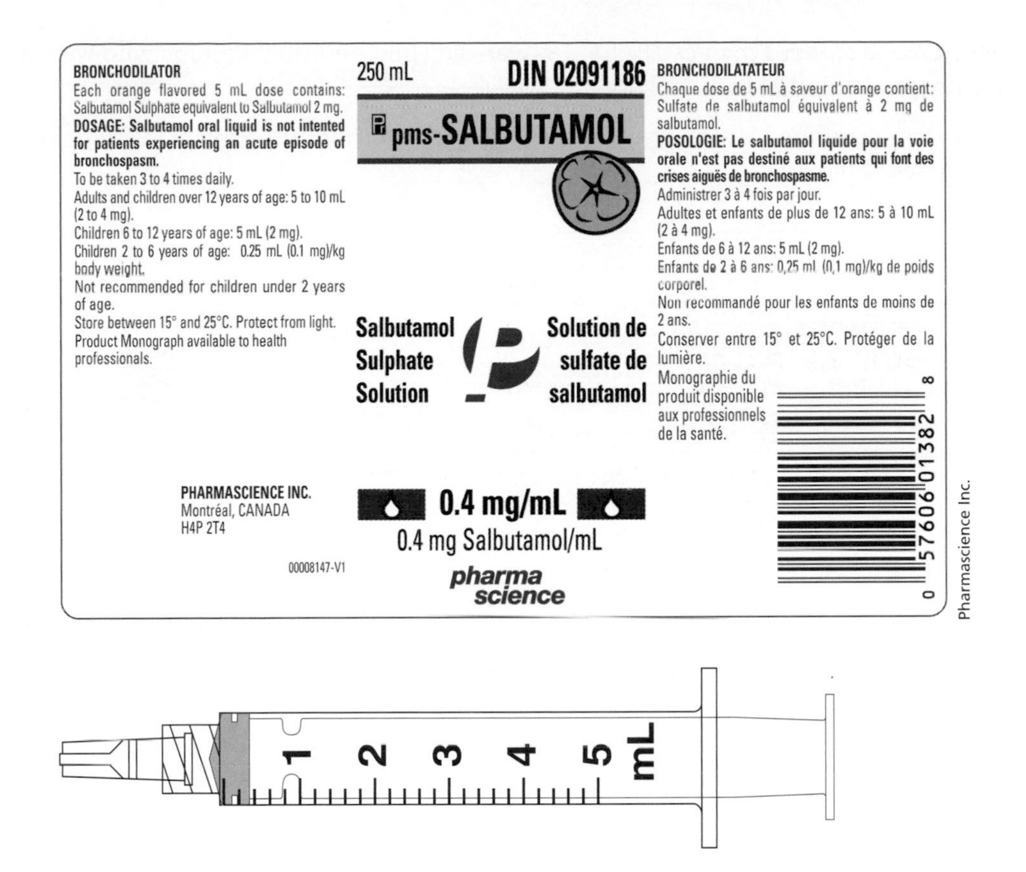

45. Order: *penicillin G sodium 450 000 units IM q6h* for a child who weighs 12 kg and has a streptococcal infection. Recommended pediatric dosage for streptococcal infections is 150 000 units/kg/day given in equal doses divided q4 to 6h.

If the dosage ordered is safe, reconstitute to a dosage supply of ________ units/mL and give ________ mL. If not safe, explain why not and describe what the nurse should do.

____

____

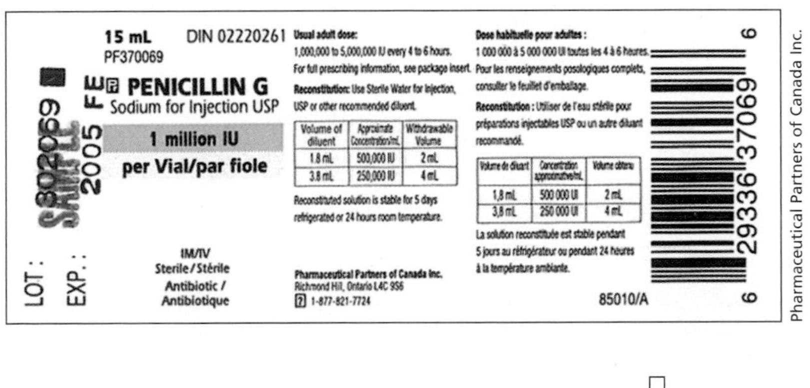

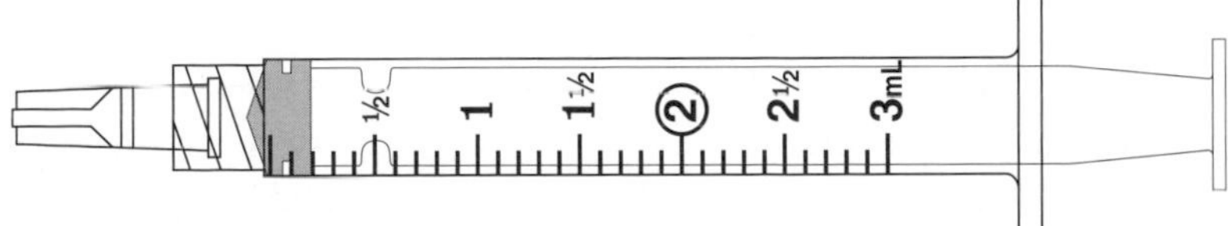

46. Order: *clonazepam 1 mg PO BID* for a 9-year-old child on initial therapy who weighs 56 lb. Recommended initial pediatric dosage: See label.

    If the dosage ordered is safe, give ________ tablet(s). If not safe, explain why not and describe what the nurse should do. ____

    ____

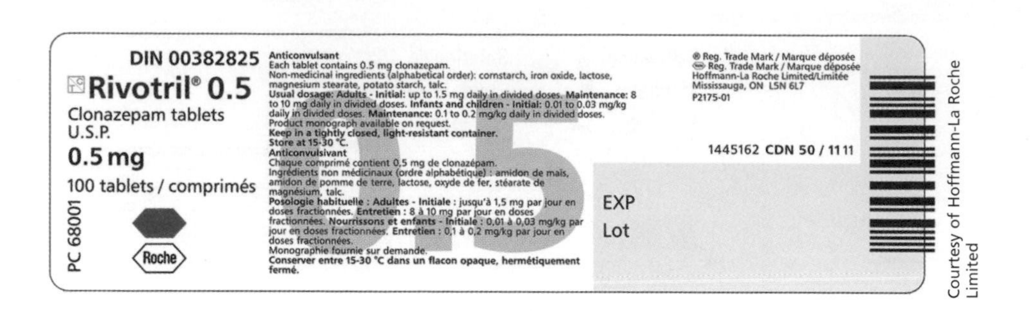

Courtesy of Hoffmann-La Roche Limited

47. Order: *meperidine hydrochloride 20 mg subcutaneously q3–4h prn for pain* for a child who weighs 18 lb. Recommended pediatric dosage: 1.1 to 1.8 mg/kg q3 to 4h prn; do not exceed adult dosage of 50 to 100 mg/dose.

    If the dosage ordered is safe, give ________ mL. If not safe, explain why not and describe what the nurse should do. ____

    ____

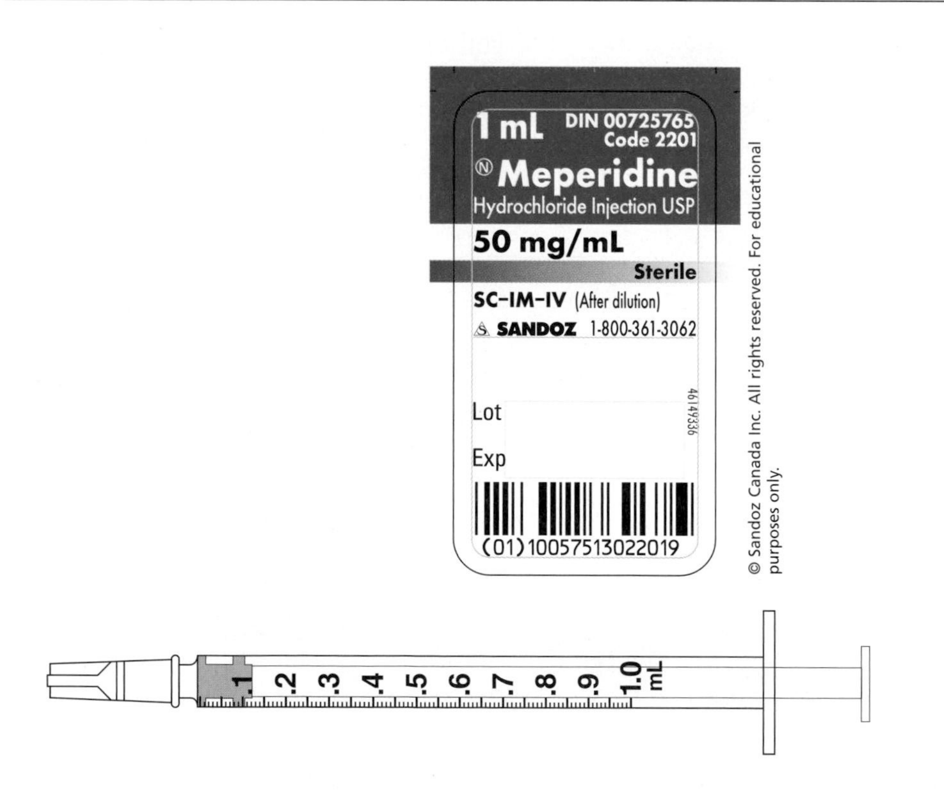

48. Order: *cefazolin sodium 250 mg IM q8h* for a 3-year-old child who weighs 35 lb. The recommended pediatric dosage of cefazolin sodium for children over 1 month: 25 to 50 mg/kg/day in 3 to 4 divided doses.

    If the dosage ordered is safe, give ________ mL. If not safe, explain why not and describe what the nurse should do. ____

    ____

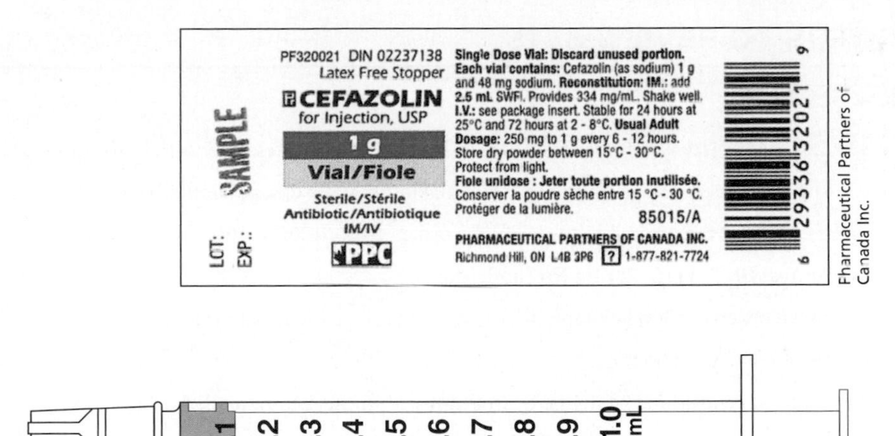

Pharmaceutical Partners of Canada Inc.

.1 .2 .3 .4 .5 .6 .7 .8 .9 1.0 mL

49. Refer back to questions 43 through 48. Identify which drugs require a reconstitution label.

____

____

Check your work! Answers to all problems are provided at the end of the book, in the Answers section. Worked solutions for some Practice Problems are also provided there.

APPLICATION OF CLINICAL REASONING

11-1 Describe the clinical reasoning you would implement to prevent this patient safety incident.

Possible Scenario

Suppose the family practice resident ordered *tobramycin sulfate 110 mg IV q8h* for a child with cystic fibrosis who weighs 10 kg. The pediatric reference guide states that the safe dosage of tobramycin sulfate for a child with severe infections is 7.5 mg/kg/day in 3 equally divided doses. The nurse received five admissions the evening of this order and thought, "I'm too busy to calculate the safe dosage this time." The pharmacist prepared and labelled the medication in a syringe and the nurse administered the first dose of the medication. An hour later, the resident arrived on the pediatric unit and inquired whether the nurse had given the first dose. When the nurse replied "yes," the resident became pale and stated, "I just realized that I ordered an adult dose of tobramycin sulfate. I hoped that the medication had not yet been given."

Potential Outcome

The resident's next step would likely have been to discontinue the tobramycin sulfate and order a stat tobramycin sulfate level. The level would most likely have been elevated, and the child would have required close monitoring for kidney damage and hearing loss.

Prevention

____

____

Check your work! Answers to all Application of Clinical Reasoning problems are provided at the end of the book, in the Answers section.

ANSWERS TO REVIEW SETS

Review Set 11-1

1) 16.4; 820; 205; 1640; 410; No (underdose) **2)** Underdose; contact prescriber for clarification **3)** 2.2; 55; 13.8; No (overdose) **4)** The ordered dosage is too high. The maximum daily dosage should be 55 mg. The child was ordered 55 mg every 12 hours. Contact the prescriber to clarify the order. **5)** 15; 120; Yes **6)** 6; 8 **7)** 32; 320; 480; Yes **8)** 15 **9)** 20; 500; 125; 1000; 250; Yes **10)** 5 **11)** 5; 20; 10; No (underdose)

12) The dosage ordered is too low (an underdose). Since the patient is an infant, contact the prescriber for clarification.

13) 3.4; 42.5, 85; No (an underdose)

14) The dosage of ceftazidime 34 mg IV q12h is not within the recommended dosage of 85 to 170 mg (an underdose). Contact the prescriber for clarification.

15) 45; 22.5; 2.8; Yes

16) 2.8

17) 1.8; 5.4; No (an overdose)

18) The ordered dosage of 40 mg is excessively high (8 times the recommended dose) and it is ordered to be given too frequently (q8h); total daily dose would be 120 mg (22 times the recommended dose!). The recommended dosage is 5.4 mg q12h. The prescriber should be notified and the order questioned.

19) 31.8; 0.22; 0.11; 0.32; 0.16; Yes

20) 3

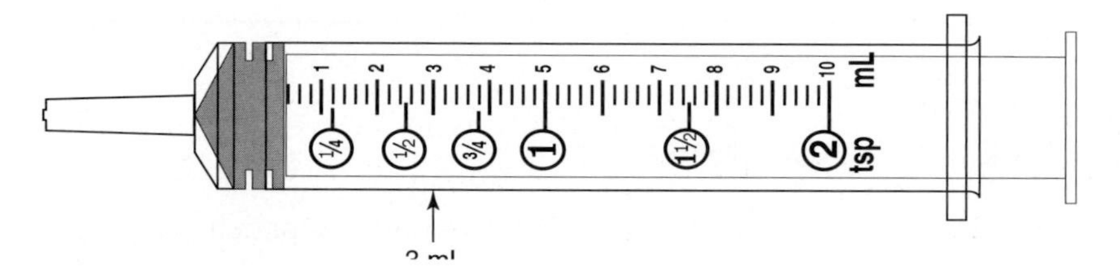

21) 17.7; 354; 118; 708; 236; No (an underdose)

22) No, the dosage is less than the recommended dosage for this child. Contact the prescriber for instructions.

23) 25; 250; 1000; Yes

24) 6.5 mL

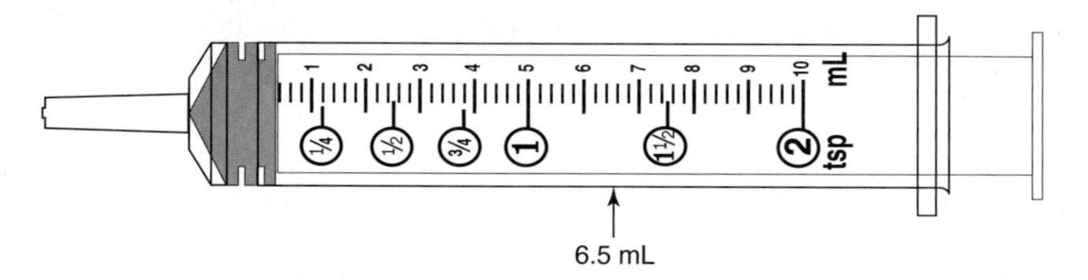

25) No, the ordered dosage is *not* safe. The recommended range is 210 to 840 mg q8h. The amount prescribed is 275 mg, but it is prescribed daily instead of every 8 hours. The prescriber should be contacted to clarify the order. This child is 7 years old, and the order is less than the minimum recommended dosage.

SELECTED SOLUTIONS TO REVIEW SETS

Review Set 11-1

1) 1 kg = 2.2 lb; smaller → larger: (÷)

36 lb = 36 ÷ 2.2 = 16.4 kg

Minimum daily dosage:

50 mg $\cancel{kg}$/day × 16.4 $\cancel{kg}$ = 820 mg/day

820 mg ÷ 4 doses = 205 mg/dose

Maximum daily dosage:

100 mg $\cancel{kg}$/day × 16.4 $\cancel{kg}$ = 1640 mg/day

1640 mg ÷ 4 doses = 410 mg/dose

No, the dose is *not* safe; it is too low. Contact the prescriber to clarify the order.

3) Convert g to kg: 2200 g = 2200 ÷ 1000 = 2.2 kg

25 mg/kg/day × 2.2 kg = 55 mg/day

55 mg ÷ 4 doses = 13.8 mg/dose; no, the dosage is *not* safe.

4) The ordered dosage is too high. The maximum daily dosage should be 55 mg. The child was ordered 55 mg every 12 hours rather than the frequency of every 6 hours. Contact the physician to clarify the order.

13) 1 lb = 16 oz; 8 oz = 8 ÷ 16 = $\frac{1}{2}$ lb

7 lb 8 oz = $7\frac{1}{2}$ lb = 7.5 ÷ 2.2 = 3.4 kg

12.5 mg/$\cancel{kg}$ × 3.4 $\cancel{kg}$ = 42.5 mg

25 mg $\cancel{kg}$ × 3.4 $\cancel{kg}$ = 85 mg/dose

Ordered dosage of 34 mg q12h is *not* within the safe range of 42.5 mg to 85 mg; therefore, it is *not* safe (underdose). Contact the prescriber for clarification of the order.

19) 70 lb = 70 ÷ 2.2 = 31.8 kg

Minimum daily dosage:

7 mcg/$\cancel{kg}$/day × 31.8 $\cancel{kg}$ = 222.6 mcg/day

Convert mcg to mg; 222.6 mcg/day =

222.6 ÷ 1000 = 0.2226 mg/day = 0.22 mg/day

Minimum single dosage:

0.22 mg ÷ 2 doses = 0.11 mg/dose

Maximum daily dosage:

10 mcg/$\cancel{kg}$ /day × 31.8 $\cancel{kg}$ = 318 mcg/day

Convert mcg to mg; 318 mcg/day =

318 ÷ 1000 = 0.318 mg/day = 0.32 mg/day

Maximum single dosage:

0.32 mg ÷ 2 doses = 0.16 mg/dose

Yes, dosage ordered is safe.

21) 39 lb = 39 ÷ 2.2 = 17.72 kg = 17.7 kg

Minimum daily dosage:

20 mg/$\cancel{kg}$/day × 17.7 $\cancel{kg}$ = 354 mg/day

Minimum single dosage:

354 mg ÷ 3 doses = 118 mg/dose

Maximum daily dosage:

40 mg/$\cancel{kg}$/day × 17.7 $\cancel{kg}$ = 708 mg/day

Maximum single dosage:

708 mg ÷ 3 doses = 236 mg/dose

The dosage of 100 mg q8h is *not* safe. It is an underdosage and would not produce a therapeutic effect because the recommended dosage range is 118 to 236 mg/dose.

REFERENCES

Le Saux, N. & Robinson, J. L. (2016). Management of acute otitis media in children 6 months of age and older. *Canadian Paediatric Society, 21*(1), 39–44. Retrieved from www.cps.ca/documents/position/acute-otitis-media.

Chapter 8: Oral Dosages of Drugs

The following labels A through N are the drugs you have available on your medication cart for the patient care orders in questions 1 through 10. Select the correct label, and identify the label letter that corresponds to each medication order. Calculate the amount to give.

1. Order: *allopurinol 0.2 g PO daily*
   Select label ________ and give ________ tablet(s)
2. Order: *clonazepam 1 mg daily*
   Select label ________ and give ________ tablet(s)
3. Order: *lorazepam 1 mg*
   Select label ________ and give ________ tablet(s)
4. Order: *cephalexin 187.5 mg PO q6h × 5 days*
   Select label ________ and give ________ mL
5. Order: *fluconazole 90 mg daily*
   Select label ________ and give ________ mL
6. Order: *ciprofloxacin 250 mg q12h*
   Select label ________ and give ________ mL
7. Order: *spironolactone 75 mg PO daily*
   Select label ________ and give ________ tablet(s)
8. Order: *lisinopril 7.5 mg PO daily*
   Select label ________ and give ________ tablet(s)
9. Order: *furosemide 12.5 mg PO BID*
   Select label ________ and give ________ mL
10. Order: *cefixime 70 mg BID*
    Select label ________ and give ________ mL

DIN 00382825
Rivotril® 0.5
Clonazepam tablets
U.S.P.
0.5 mg
100 tablets / comprimés
PC 68001
Roche

Anticonvulsant
Each tablet contains 0.5 mg clonazepam.
Non-medicinal ingredients (alphabetical order): cornstarch, iron oxide, lactose, magnesium stearate, potato starch, talc.
Usual dosage: Adults - Initial: up to 1.5 mg daily in divided doses. **Maintenance:** 8 to 10 mg daily in divided doses. **Infants and children** - Initial: 0.01 to 0.03 mg/kg daily in divided doses. **Maintenance:** 0.1 to 0.2 mg/kg daily in divided doses.
Product monograph available on request.
Keep in a tightly closed, light-resistant container.
Store at 15-30 °C.
Anticonvulsivant
Chaque comprimé contient 0,5 mg de clonazépam.
Ingrédients non médicinaux (ordre alphabétique) : amidon de maïs, amidon de pomme de terre, lactose, oxyde de fer, stéarate de magnésium, talc.
Posologie habituelle : Adultes - Initiale : jusqu'à 1,5 mg par jour en doses fractionnées. **Entretien :** 8 à 10 mg par jour en doses fractionnées. **Nourrissons et enfants** - Initiale : 0,01 à 0,03 mg/kg par jour en doses fractionnées. **Entretien :** 0,1 à 0,2 mg/kg par jour en doses fractionnées.
Monographie fournie sur demande.
Conserver entre 15-30 °C dans un flacon opaque, hermétiquement fermé.

® Reg. Trade Mark / Marque déposée
Reg. Trade Mark / Marque déposée
Hoffmann-La Roche Limited/Limitée
Mississauga, ON L5N 6L7
P2175-01

1445162 CDN 50 / 11 11

EXP
Lot

Courtesy of Hoffmann-La Roche Limited

A

ANTIBIOTIC
Each bottle contains 2500 mg cephalexin (as the monohydrate).
DIRECTIONS FOR DISPENSING:
At the time of dispensing, add two portions of 30 mL water to a total of 60 mL of water to the dry mixture in the bottle to make 100 mL of the suspension. Shake well after each addition. Each 1 mL contains cephalexin monohydrate equivalent to 25 mg cephalexin.
Adult Dosage: 250 mg every 6 hours.
Children Dosage: 25 – 50 mg/kg of body weight per day, in equally divided doses at 6 hour intervals. For more severe infections, dose may be doubled.
Product Monograph available on request.
Store between 15 - 30°C.

TEVA is a reg'd trademark of / est une marque déposée de TEVA Pharmaceutical Industries Ltd. used under license by / utilisée sous licence par TEVA Canada Limited/Limitée, Toronto, Canada M1B 2K9

SHAKE WELL BEFORE USING.
When reconstituted, suspension is stable for 14 days under refrigeration 2 - 8°C. Do not freeze.

DIN 00342106 100 mL
TEVA-CEPHALEXIN 125
125 mg/ 5 mL
Cephalexin for Oral Suspension
Céphalexine pour suspension orale
USP
Cephalexin/Céphalexine
When reconstituted as directed
Après reconstitution
TEVA

ANTIBIOTIQUE
Le flacon renferme 2500 mg de céphalexine (sous forme monohydratée).
MODE DE RECONSTITUTION :
Pour reconstituer, ajouter deux portions de 30 mL d'eau, soit un total de 60 mL d'eau, à la préparation en poudre que contient le flacon afin d'obtenir 100 mL de suspension. Bien agiter après chaque addition. Chaque mL de suspension contient de la céphalexine monohydratée équivalant à 25 mg de céphalexine.
Posologie chez l'adulte : 250 mg toutes les 6 heures.
Posologie chez l'enfant : 25 à 50 mg/kg de poids corporel par jour, fractionnés en doses égales à des intervalles de 6 heures. Dans les cas d'infection grave, on peut doubler la posologie.
Monographie de produit fournie sur demande.
Conserver entre 15 °C et 30 °C.
361-32-756620040 Rev 07 333-32-100884

0 68510 32340 8

BIEN AGITER AVANT L'EMPLOI.
La suspension reconstituée est stable pendant 14 jours au réfrigérateur (2 °C à 8 °C). Mettre à l'abri du gel.

B

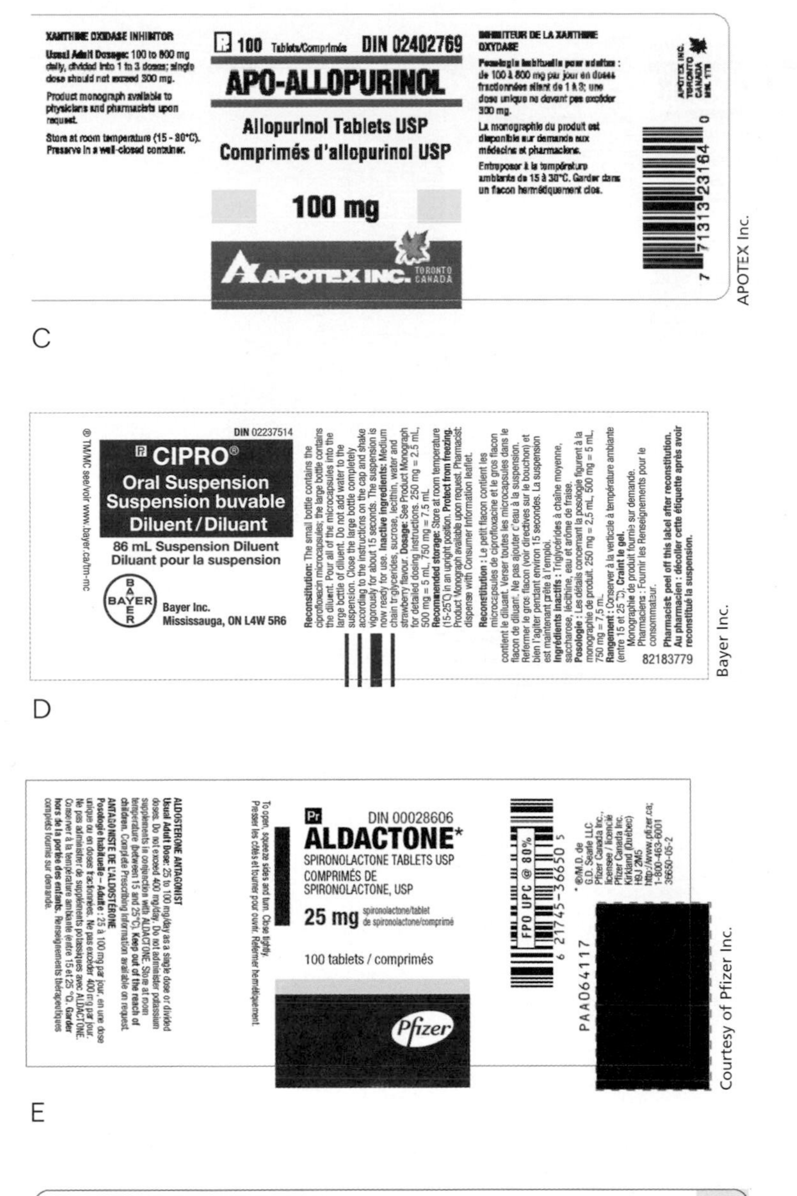

XANTHINE OXIDASE INHIBITOR
Usual Adult Dosage: 100 to 800 mg daily, divided into 1 to 3 doses; single dose should not exceed 300 mg.
Product monograph available to physicians and pharmacists upon request.
Store at room temperature (15 - 30°C). Preserve in a well-closed container.
100 Tablets/Comprimés DIN 02402769
APO-ALLOPURINOL
Allopurinol Tablets USP
Comprimés d'allopurinol USP
100 mg
APOTEX INC. TORONTO CANADA
INHIBITEUR DE LA XANTHINE OXYDASE
Posologie habituelle pour adultes : de 100 à 800 mg par jour en doses fractionnées allant de 1 à 3; une dose unique ne devant pas excéder 300 mg.
La monographie du produit est disponible sur demande aux médecins et pharmaciens.
Entreposer à la température ambiante de 15 à 30°C. Garder dans un flacon hermétiquement clos.
APOTEX INC. TORONTO CANADA
7 71313 23164 0
APOTEX Inc.
DIN 02237514
CIPRO®
Oral Suspension
Suspension buvable
Diluent / Diluant
86 mL Suspension Diluent
Diluant pour la suspension
Bayer Inc.
Mississauga, ON L4W 5R6
® TM/MC see/voir www.bayer.ca/tm-mc
Pharmacist peel off this label after reconstitution.
Au pharmacien : décoller cette étiquette après avoir reconstitué la suspension.
82183779
Bayer Inc.
DIN 00028606
ALDACTONE*
SPIRONOLACTONE TABLETS USP
COMPRIMÉS DE SPIRONOLACTONE, USP
25 mg spironolactone/tablet de spironolactone/comprimé
100 tablets / comprimés
Pfizer
ALDOSTERONE ANTAGONIST
To open, squeeze sides and turn. Close tightly.
Pressez les côtés et tournez pour ouvrir. Refermer hermétiquement.
FPO UPC @ 80%
6 21745-36650 5
PAA064117
Courtesy of Pfizer Inc.

C

D

E

DIN 00382841

Rivotril® 2

Clonazepam tablets U.S.P.

2 mg

100 tablets / comprimés

PC 68101

Roche

Anticonvulsant
Each tablet contains 2 mg clonazepam.
Non-medicinal ingredients (alphabetical order): cornstarch, lactose, magnesium stearate, microcrystalline cellulose.
Usual dosage: Adults - Initial: up to 1.5 mg daily in divided doses. Maintenance: 8 to 10 mg daily in divided doses. Infants and children - Initial: 0.01 to 0.03 mg/kg daily in divided doses. Maintenance: 0.1 to 0.2 mg/kg daily in divided doses.
Product monograph available on request.
Keep in a tightly closed, light-resistant container.
Store at 15-30 °C.

Anticonvulsivant
Chaque comprimé contient 2 mg de clonazépam.
Ingrédients non médicinaux (ordre alphabétique) : amidon de maïs, cellulose microcristalline, lactose, stéarate de magnésium.
Posologie habituelle : Adultes - Initiale : jusqu'à 1,5 mg par jour en doses fractionnées. Entretien : 8 à 10 mg par jour en doses fractionnées. Nourrissons et enfants - Initiale : 0,01 à 0,03 mg/kg par jour en doses fractionnées. Entretien : 0,1 à 0,2 mg/kg par jour en doses fractionnées.
Monographie fournie sur demande.
Conserver entre 15-30 °C dans un flacon opaque, hermétiquement fermé.

® Reg. Trade Mark / Marque déposée
Reg. Trade Mark / Marque déposée Hoffmann-La Roche Limited/Limitée
Mississauga, ON L5N 6L7
P2332-01

1445200 CDN 50 / 1111

EXP

Lot

Courtesy of Hoffmann-La Roche Limited

F

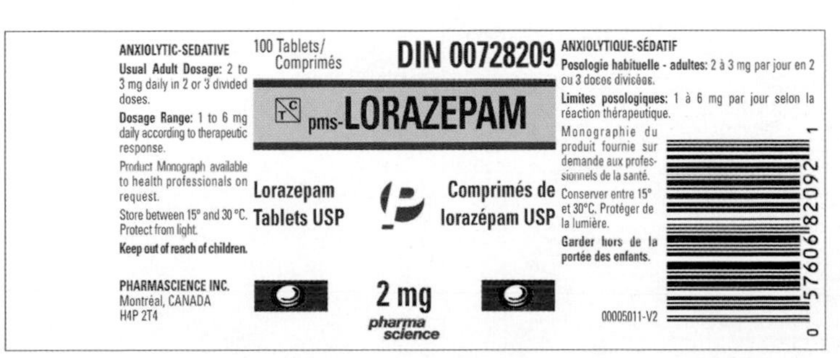

ANXIOLYTIC-SEDATIVE
Usual Adult Dosage: 2 to 3 mg daily in 2 or 3 divided doses.
Dosage Range: 1 to 6 mg daily according to therapeutic response.
Product Monograph available to health professionals on request.
Store between 15° and 30°C. Protect from light.
Keep out of reach of children.
PHARMASCIENCE INC.
Montréal, CANADA
H4P 2T4
100 Tablets/ Comprimés
DIN 00728209
pms-LORAZEPAM
Lorazepam Tablets USP
Comprimés de lorazépam USP
2 mg
pharma science
ANXIOLYTIQUE-SÉDATIF
Posologie habituelle - adultes: 2 à 3 mg par jour en 2 ou 3 doses divisées.
Limites posologiques: 1 à 6 mg par jour selon la réaction thérapeutique.
Monographie du produit fournie sur demande aux professionnels de la santé.
Conserver entre 15° et 30°C. Protéger de la lumière.
Garder hors de la portée des enfants.
00005011-V2
0 57606 82092 1
Pharmascience Inc.

G

DIN 02024152

DIFLUCAN®

FLUCONAZOLE FOR ORAL SUSPENSION

FLUCONAZOLE POUR SUSPENSION ORALE

50 mg/5 mL (10 mg/mL)

WHEN RECONSTITUTED

APRÈS RECONSTITUTION

35 mL of / de suspension

Pfizer

6 21027 07008 3

LOT

EXP

Courtesy of Pfizer Inc.

H

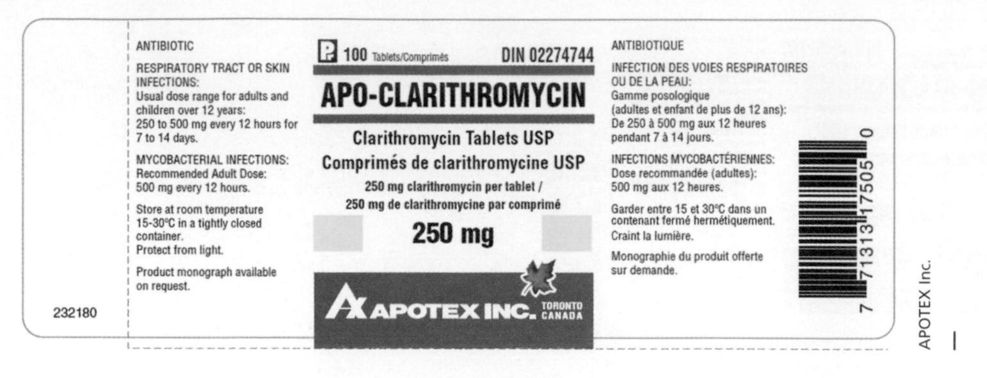

ANTIBIOTIC
RESPIRATORY TRACT OR SKIN INFECTIONS:
Usual dose range for adults and children over 12 years:
250 to 500 mg every 12 hours for 7 to 14 days.
MYCOBACTERIAL INFECTIONS:
Recommended Adult Dose:
500 mg every 12 hours.
Store at room temperature 15-30°C in a tightly closed container.
Protect from light.
Product monograph available on request.
232180
100 Tablets/Comprimés
DIN 02274744
APO-CLARITHROMYCIN
Clarithromycin Tablets USP
Comprimés de clarithromycine USP
250 mg clarithromycin per tablet /
250 mg de clarithromycine par comprimé
250 mg
APOTEX INC. TORONTO CANADA
ANTIBIOTIQUE
INFECTION DES VOIES RESPIRATOIRES OU DE LA PEAU:
Gamme posologique (adultes et enfant de plus de 12 ans):
De 250 à 500 mg aux 12 heures pendant 7 à 14 jours.
INFECTIONS MYCOBACTÉRIENNES:
Dose recommandée (adultes):
500 mg aux 12 heures.
Garder entre 15 et 30°C dans un contenant fermé hermétiquement.
Craint la lumière.
Monographie du produit offerte sur demande.
7 71313 17505 0

APOTEX Inc.

I

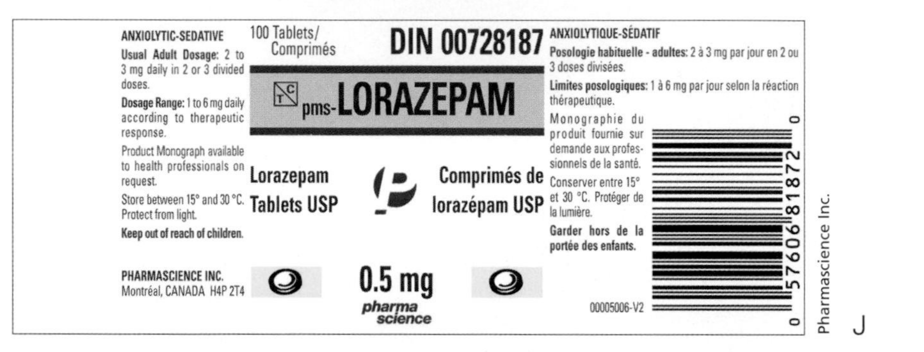

Pharmascience Inc.

J

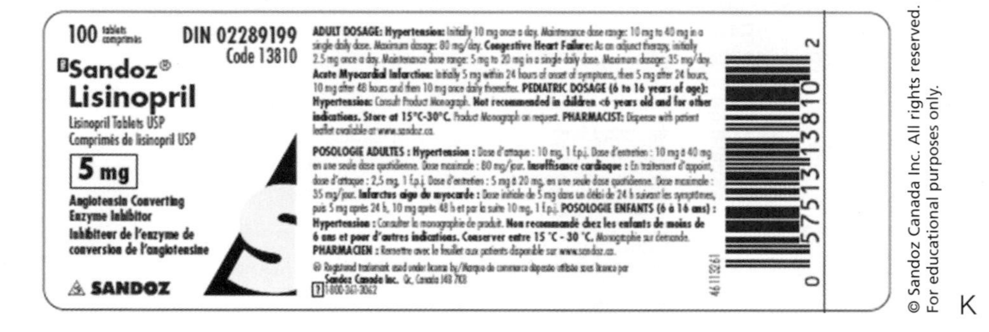

100 tablets comprimés
DIN 02289199
Code 13810
Sandoz®
Lisinopril
Lisinopril Tablets USP
Comprimés de lisinopril USP
5 mg
Angiotensin Converting Enzyme Inhibitor
Inhibiteur de l'enzyme de conversion de l'angiotensine
SANDOZ
ADULT DOSAGE: Hypertension: Initially 10 mg once a day. Maintenance dose range: 10 mg to 40 mg in a single daily dose. Maximum dosage: 80 mg/day. Congestive Heart Failure: As an adjunct therapy, initially 2.5 mg once a day. Maintenance dose range: 5 mg to 20 mg in a single daily dose. Maximum dosage: 35 mg/day. Acute Myocardial Infarction: Initially 5 mg within 24 hours of onset of symptoms, then 5 mg after 24 hours, 10 mg after 48 hours and then 10 mg once daily thereafter. PEDIATRIC DOSAGE (6 to 16 years of age): Hypertension: Consult Product Monograph. Not recommended in children <6 years old and for other indications. Store at 15°C-30°C. Product Monograph on request. PHARMACIST: Dispense with patient leaflet available at www.sandoz.ca.
0 57513 13810 2

© Sandoz Canada Inc. All rights reserved. For educational purposes only.

K

BIEN AGITER AVANT L'EMPLOI.
Le flacon contient de la céfixime sous forme de trihydrate correspondant à 1 g de céfixime anhydre.
POSOLOGIE – ADULTE : 400 mg, 1 fois par jour. Si nécessaire, 200 mg, 2 fois par jour.
Infections urinaires : 400 mg, 1 fois par jour.
ENFANT : 8 mg/kg/jour, 1 fois par jour. Si nécessaire, 4 mg/kg, 2 fois par jour.
Infections urinaires : 8 mg/kg/jour, 1 fois par jour.
RECONSTITUTION : Secouer légèrement le flacon plusieurs fois pour ameublir la poudre avant la reconstitution. Ajouter un volume total de 33 mL d'eau divisé en DEUX PORTIONS. Bien mélanger après chaque addition. Donne 20 mg/mL. La suspension peut être conservée pendant 14 jours à la température ambiante ou réfrigérée. Jeter la portion non utilisée.
Monographie du produit fournie sur demande ou disponible au www.sanofi.ca. Conserver la poudre à une température ambiante contrôlée se situant entre 15 et 30 °C.

(01)20065914106686

E50069005E

DIN 00868965

Suprax®

Cefixime for oral suspension, Mfr. Std. / Céfixime pour suspension orale, Norme-fabricant

100 mg / 5 mL*

Antibiotic / Antibiotique

50 mL

*when reconstituted / lorsque reconstitué

SANOFI

SHAKE WELL BEFORE USE.
The bottle contains cefixime as trihydrate, corresponding to 1 g cefixime anhydrous.
DOSAGE – ADULTS: 400 mg once daily. If necessary, 200 mg twice daily. Urinary tract infections: 400 mg once daily.
CHILDREN: 8 mg/kg/day once daily. If necessary, 4 mg/kg twice daily. Urinary tract infections: 8 mg/kg/day once daily.
RECONSTITUTION: Tap the bottle several times to loosen powder contents prior to reconstitution. Add a total volume of 33 mL of water split in TWO PORTIONS. Mix well after each addition. Provides 20 mg/mL. Suspension may be kept for 14 days at room temperature or under refrigeration. Discard unused portion. 1230421-E
Product Monograph available upon request or at www.sanofi.ca. Store powder at controlled room temperature between 15 and 30°C.

® Registered trade-mark of / Marque déposée de Astellas Pharma Inc., Osaka, Japan (Japon).
Mfd by / Fabr. par sanofi-aventis Canada Inc., Laval, Québec, Canada H7V 0A3
1 800 265-7927

Lot

Exp.

© sanofi-aventis Canada Inc. Used under licence. For educational purposes only.

L

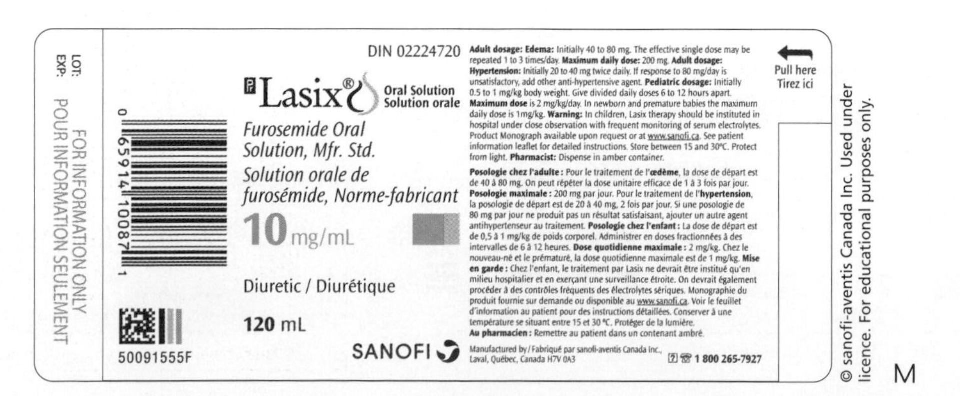

LOT:
EXP:
FOR INFORMATION ONLY
POUR INFORMATION SEULEMENT
0 65914 10087 1
50091555F
DIN 02224720
Lasix® Oral Solution Solution orale
Furosemide Oral Solution, Mfr. Std.
Solution orale de furosémide, Norme-fabricant
10 mg/mL
Diuretic / Diurétique
120 mL
SANOFI
Pull here
Tirez ici
1 800 265-7927

© sanofi-aventis Canada Inc. Used under licence. For educational purposes only.

M

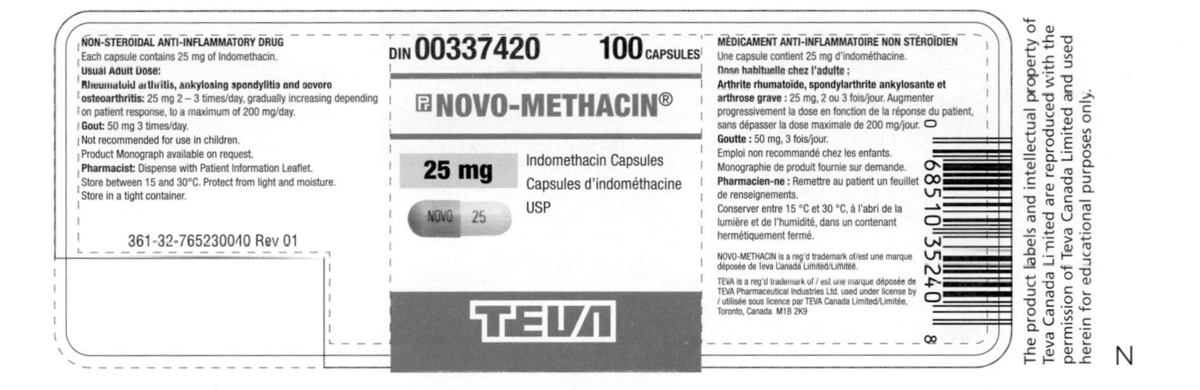

NON-STEROIDAL ANTI-INFLAMMATORY DRUG
Each capsule contains 25 mg of Indomethacin.
Not recommended for use in children.
Product Monograph available on request.
Pharmacist: Dispense with Patient Information Leaflet.
Store between 15 and 30°C. Protect from light and moisture.
Store in a tight container.
361-32-765230040 Rev 01
DIN 00337420
100 CAPSULES
NOVO-METHACIN®
25 mg
Indomethacin Capsules
Capsules d'indométhacine
USP
NOVO 25
TEVA
MÉDICAMENT ANTI-INFLAMMATOIRE NON STÉROÏDIEN
Une capsule contient 25 mg d'indométhacine.
0 68510 35240 8

N

Chapter 9: Parenteral Dosages of Drugs

The following labels A through H are the drugs that are available on your medication cart for the patient care orders in questions 11 through 18. Select the correct label, and identify the letter that corresponds to each parenteral medication order. Calculate the amount to give.

A

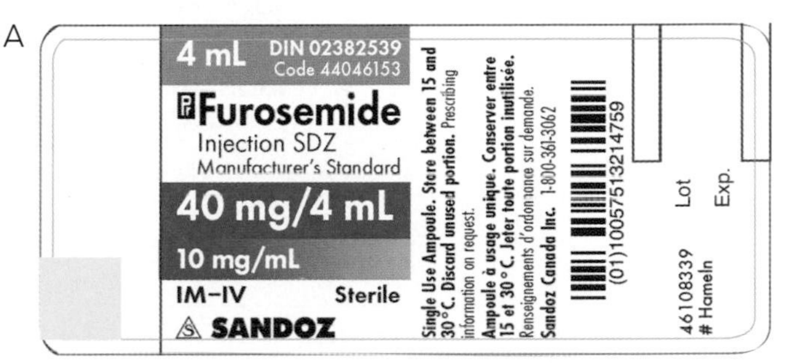

4 mL
DIN 02382539
Code 44046153
Furosemide
Injection SDZ
Manufacturer's Standard
40 mg/4 mL
10 mg/mL
IM–IV
Sterile
SANDOZ
Single Use Ampoule. Store between 15 and 30°C. Discard unused portion.
Ampoule à usage unique. Conserver entre 15 et 30°C. Jeter toute portion inutilisée.
Sandoz Canada Inc. 1-800-361-3062
(01)10057513214759
46108339
Hameln
Lot
Exp.

11. Order: *vitamin B_{12} 0.2 mg subcutaneously daily × 10 days*

    Select label ________ and give ________ mL

12. Order: *diazepam 2.5 mg IV stat*

    Select label ________ and give ________ mL

13. Order: *epinephrine 200 mcg subcutaneously stat*

    Select label ________ and give ________ mL

14. Order: *furosemide 40 mg IV daily*

    Select label ________ and give ________ mL

15. Order: *gentamicin sodium 60 mg IV q8h*

    Select label ________ and give ________ mL

16. Order: *heparin sodium 7500 units subcutaneously stat*

    Select label ________ and give ________ mL

17. Order: *morphine sulfate 7.5 mg subcutaneously q4h, prn for pain*

    Select label ________ and give ________ mL

18. Order: *naloxone hydrochloride 0.3 mg IM stat*

    Select label ________ and give ________ mL

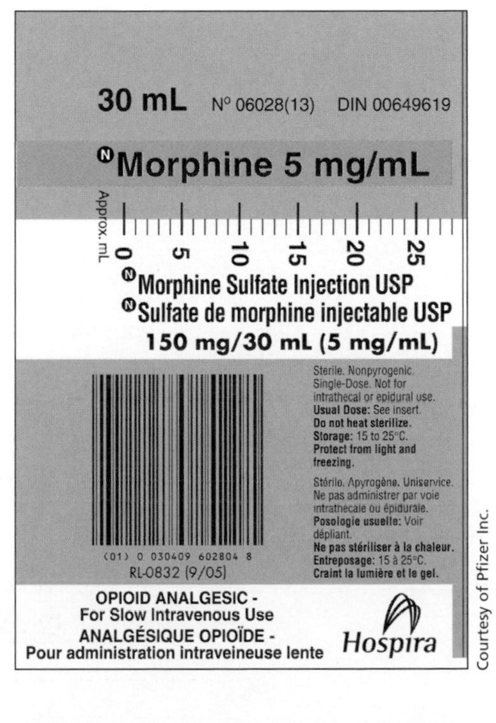

30 mL
Nº 06028(13)
DIN 00649619
Morphine 5 mg/mL
Approx. mL
0 5 10 15 20 25
Morphine Sulfate Injection USP
Sulfate de morphine injectable USP
150 mg/30 mL (5 mg/mL)
Sterile. Nonpyrogenic. Single-Dose. Not for intrathecal or epidural use.
Usual Dose: See insert.
Do not heat sterilize.
Storage: 15 to 25°C.
Protect from light and freezing.
Stérile. Apyrogène. Uniservice. Ne pas administrer par voie intrathécale ou épidurale.
Posologie usuelle: Voir dépliant.
Ne pas stériliser à la chaleur.
Entreposage: 15 à 25°C.
Craint la lumière et le gel.
(01) 0 030409 602804 8
RL-0832 (9/05)
OPIOID ANALGESIC - For Slow Intravenous Use
ANALGÉSIQUE OPIOÏDE - Pour administration intraveineuse lente
Hospira

B

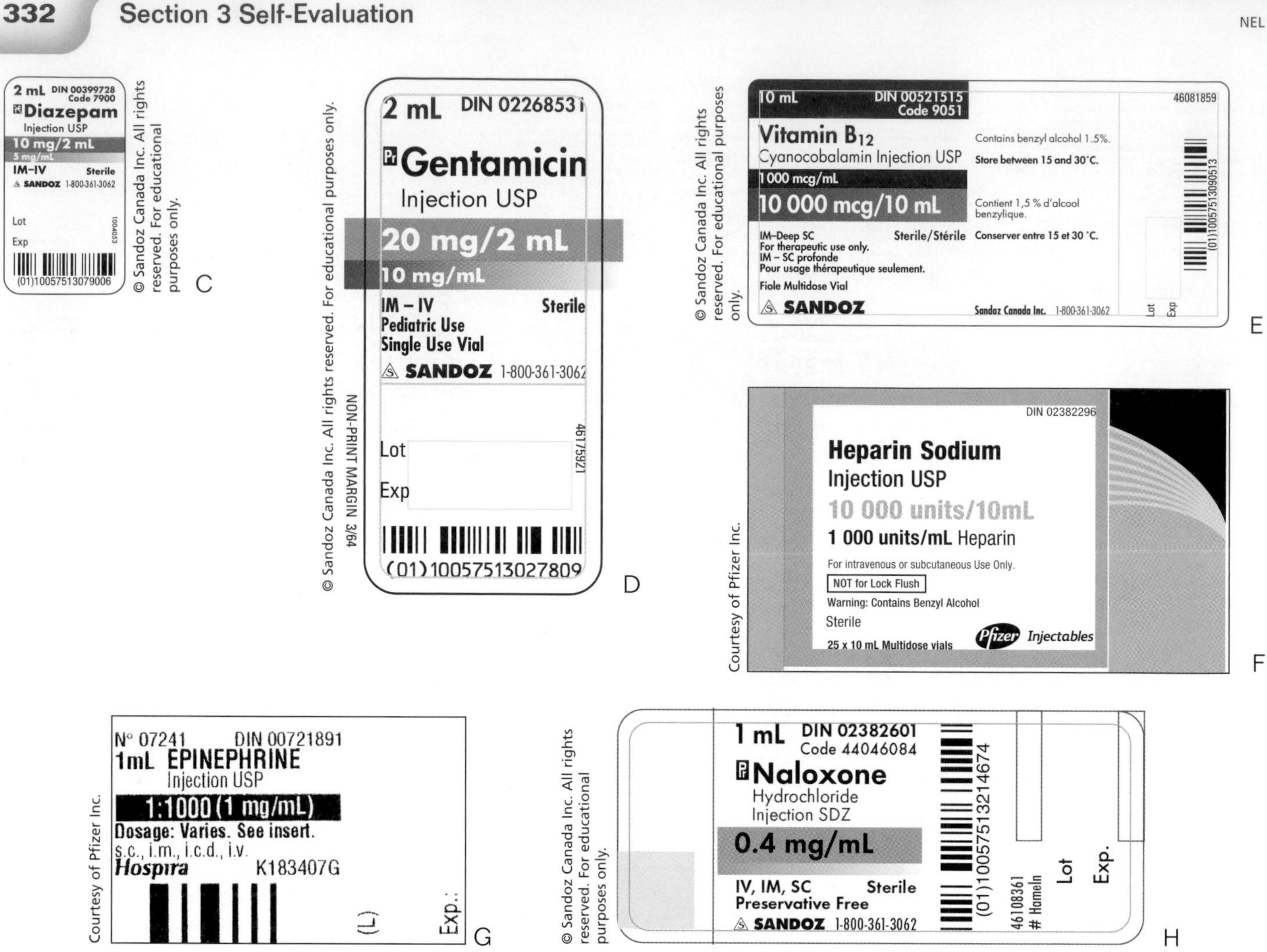

2 mL DIN 00399728 Code 7900
Diazepam
Injection USP
10 mg/2 mL
5 mg/mL
IM-IV Sterile
SANDOZ 1-800-361-3062
Lot
Exp
(01)10057513079006
© Sandoz Canada Inc. All rights reserved. For educational purposes only.
C
2 mL DIN 02268531
Gentamicin
Injection USP
20 mg/2 mL
10 mg/mL
IM – IV Sterile
Pediatric Use
Single Use Vial
SANDOZ 1-800-361-3062
Lot
Exp
(01)10057513027809
NON-PRINT MARGIN 3/64
© Sandoz Canada Inc. All rights reserved. For educational purposes only.
D
10 mL DIN 00521515 Code 9051
Vitamin B12
Cyanocobalamin Injection USP
1000 mcg/mL
10 000 mcg/10 mL
IM-Deep SC
For therapeutic use only.
IM – SC profonde
Pour usage thérapeutique seulement.
Sterile/Stérile
Fiole Multidose Vial
SANDOZ
Contains benzyl alcohol 1.5%.
Store between 15 and 30°C.
Contient 1,5 % d'alcool benzylique.
Conserver entre 15 et 30 °C.
Sandoz Canada Inc. 1-800-361-3062
46081859
Lot
Exp
© Sandoz Canada Inc. All rights reserved. For educational purposes only.
E
DIN 02382296
Heparin Sodium
Injection USP
10 000 units/10mL
1 000 units/mL Heparin
For intravenous or subcutaneous Use Only.
NOT for Lock Flush
Warning: Contains Benzyl Alcohol
Sterile
25 x 10 mL Multidose vials
Pfizer Injectables
Courtesy of Pfizer Inc.
F
N° 07241 DIN 00721891
1mL EPINEPHRINE
Injection USP
1:1000 (1 mg/mL)
Dosage: Varies. See insert.
s.c., i.m., i.c.d., i.v.
Hospira K183407G
(L)
Exp.:
Courtesy of Pfizer Inc.
G
1 mL DIN 02382601
Code 44046084
Naloxone
Hydrochloride
Injection SDZ
0.4 mg/mL
IV, IM, SC Sterile
Preservative Free
SANDOZ 1-800-361-3062
(01)10057513214674
46108361
Hameln
Lot
Exp.
© Sandoz Canada Inc. All rights reserved. For educational purposes only.
H

For questions 19 and 20, mark the amount to give on the correct syringe.

19. Order: *Humulin N insulin 48 units subcutaneously 15 min before breakfast*

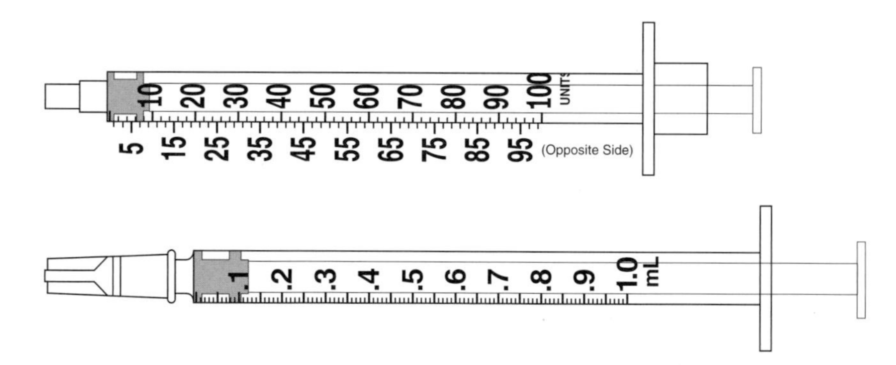

20. Order: *Humulin R insulin 12 units with Humulin N 100-unit insulin 28 units subcutaneously 15 min before dinner*

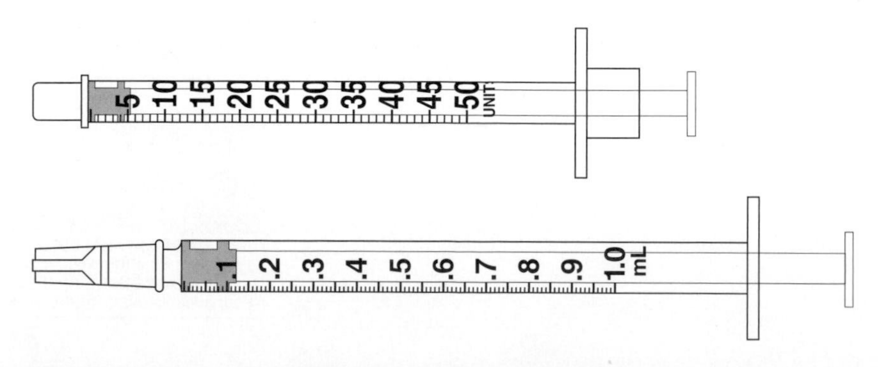

Chapter 10: Reconstitution of Solutions

For questions 21 through 28, specify the amount of diluent to add and the resulting solution concentration. Calculate the amount to give, and indicate the dose with an arrow on the accompanying syringe. Finally, make a reconstitution label, if required.

21. Order: *azithromycin dihydrate 400 mg IV daily*

    See package insert for instructions on dilution.

    Reconstitute with ________ mL diluent for a total solution volume of ________ mL with a concentration of ________ mg/mL.

    Withdraw: ________ mL and further dilute prior to administration

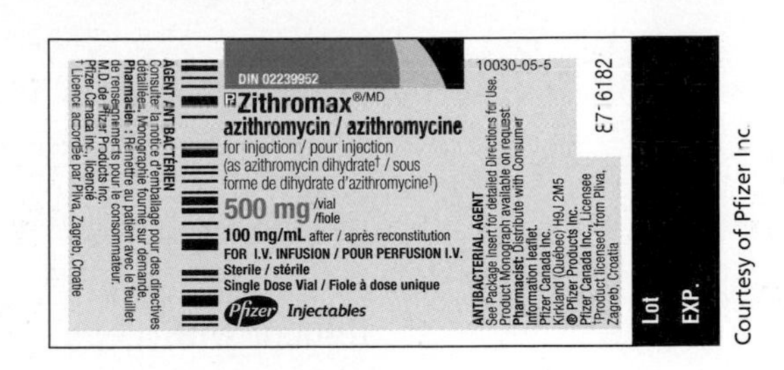

Courtesy of Pfizer Inc

ZITHROMAX for Injection:

	RECONSTITUTION OF ZITHROMAX FOR INJECTION			
Strength	Reconstitution Solution	Volume to be Added	Approximate Volume Available	Nominal Concentration
500 mg	Sterile Water for Injection	4.8 mL	5 mL	100 mg/mL

Prepare the initial solution of **ZITHROMAX** for Injection by adding 4.8 mL of Sterile Water for Injection to the 500 mg vial. Shake the vial until all of the drug is dissolved. Since the vial is evacuated, it is recommended that a standard 5 mL (non-automated) syringe be used to ensure that the exact volume of 4.8 mL is dispensed. Each mL of reconstituted solution contains azithromycin dihydrate equivalent to 100 mg azithromycin. Reconstituted solution is stable for 24 hours when stored below 30°C. **The reconstituted solution must be further diluted prior to administration.**

Dilution of reconstituted solution: To provide azithromycin over a concentration range of 1.0 - 2.0 mg/mL, transfer 5 mL of the 100 mg/mL azithromycin solution into the appropriate amount of the following diluents:

Final Infusion Concentration (mg/mL)	Amount of Diluent (mL)
1.0 mg/mL	500 mL
2.0 mg/mL	250 mL

Appropriate Diluents

0.9% Sodium Chloride Injection
5% Dextrose in Water for Injection
0.45% Sodium Chloride Injection
Lactated Ringer's Injection
5% Dextrose in 0.45% Sodium Chloride Injection with 20 mEq Potassium Chloride
5% Dextrose in Lactated Ringer's Injection
5% Dextrose in 0.3% Sodium Chloride Injection
5% Dextrose in 0.45% Sodium Chloride Injection
Normosol-M in 5% Dextrose

Diluted solutions prepared in this manner are stable for 24 hours at or below room temperature (30°C), or for 72 hours if stored under refrigeration (5°C). As with all parenteral drug products, intravenous admixtures should be inspected visually for clarity, particulate matter, precipitate, discoloration and leakage prior to administration, whenever solution and container permit. Solutions showing haziness, particulate matter, precipitate, discoloration or leakage should be discarded.

Only limited data are available on the compatibility of **ZITHROMAX** for Injection with other intravenous substances, therefore additives or other medications should not be added to **ZITHROMAX** for Injection or infused simultaneously through the same intravenous line. If the same intravenous line is used for sequential infusion of several different drugs, the line should be flushed before and after infusion of **ZITHROMAX** for Injection with an infusion solution compatible with **ZITHROMAX** for Injection and with any other drug(s) administered via the common line. If **ZITHROMAX** for Injection is to be given concomitantly with another drug, each drug should be given separately in accordance with the recommended dosage and route of administration for each drug.

Courtesy of Pfizer Inc.

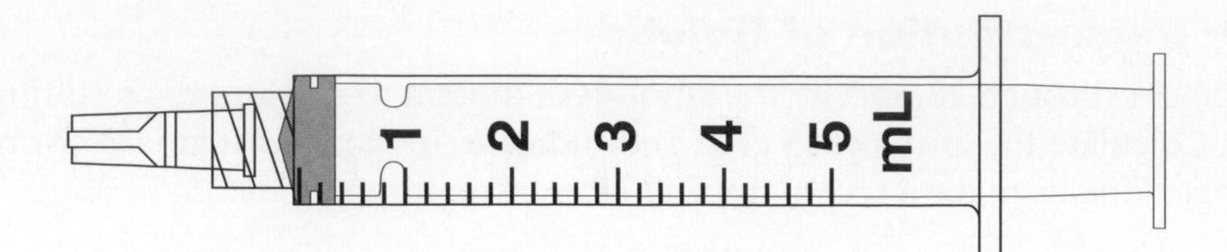

22. Order: *vancomycin hydrochloride 500 mg IV q6h*

See package instructions for dilution.

Reconstitute with ________ mL diluent with a concentration of ________ mg/mL.

Withdraw: ________ mL and further dilute prior to administration

There is/are ________ full dose(s) available in this vial.

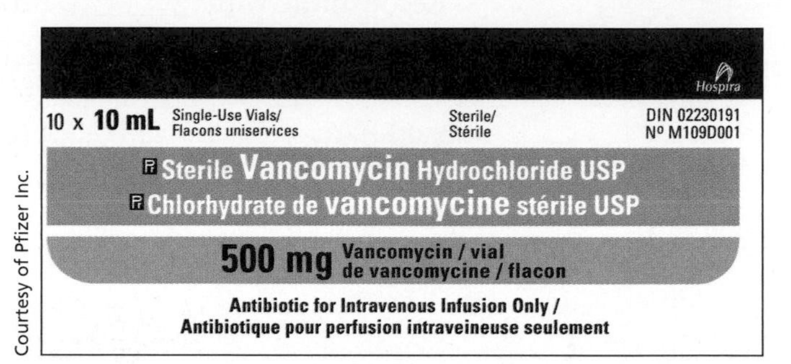

Hospira
10 x 10 mL Single-Use Vials/ Flacons uniservices
Sterile/ Stérile
DIN 02230191
Nº M109D001
Sterile Vancomycin Hydrochloride USP
Chlorhydrate de vancomycine stérile USP
500 mg Vancomycin / vial de vancomycine / flacon
Antibiotic for Intravenous Infusion Only /
Antibiotique pour perfusion intraveineuse seulement

Courtesy of Pfizer Inc.

Reconstitution
Flip-Top Vial

Solution for Reconstitution: Sterile Water for Injection USP
Reconstitute as follows:

Reconstitution Table

Flip-Top Vial Size	Volume to Be Added to Vial	Approx. Available Volume	Vancomycin in Concentration
500 mg	10 mL	10.3 mL	50 mg/mL
1 g	20 mL	20.6 mL	50 mg/mL

NOTE: FURTHER DILUTION IS REQUIRED
For Intermittent Intravenous Infusion

500 mg vial Reconstituted solutions must be diluted with at least 100 mL of 0.9% Sodium Chloride Injection or 5% Dextrose in Sterile Water for Injection USP.

1 g vial: Reconstituted solutions must be diluted with at least 200 mL of 0.9% Sodium Chloride Injection or 5% Dextrose in Sterile Water for Injection USP.

For Continuous Intravenous Infusion

The vials reconstituted according to the above table should be further diluted to the desired volume with one of the following intravenous solutions:

- 5% Dextrose Injection
- 3.3% Dextrose Injection and 0.3% Sodium Chloride Injection Lootated Ringer's Injection
- 0.9% Sodium Chloride Injection

A concentration of no greater than 5 mg/mL is recommended.

Stability and Storage Recommendations
Dry Powder

Vancomycin hydrochloride powder should be stored between 20 and 25°C (see "Controlled Room Temperature" in USP). Protect from freezing.

Solutions

Reconstituted solutions and further diluted infusion mixtures should be used within 24 hours if kept at room temperature or within 72 hours if stored under refrigeration (2 to 8°C). If prepared in a facility with a recognized parenteral intravenous admixture program, such mixtures may be kept up to 96 hours if stored under refrigeration (2 to 8°C).

NOTE: As with all parenteral drug products, intravenous admixtures should be inspected visually for clarity, particulate matter, precipitation, discolouration and leakage prior to administration whenever solution and container permit. Solutions showing haziness, particulate matter, precipitate, discolouration or leakage should not be used. Discard unused portion.

Courtesy of Pfizer Inc.

23. Order: *ceftazidime 200 mg IM q6h*

    Reconstitute with ________ mL diluent for a concentration of ________ mg/mL.

    Give: ________ mL

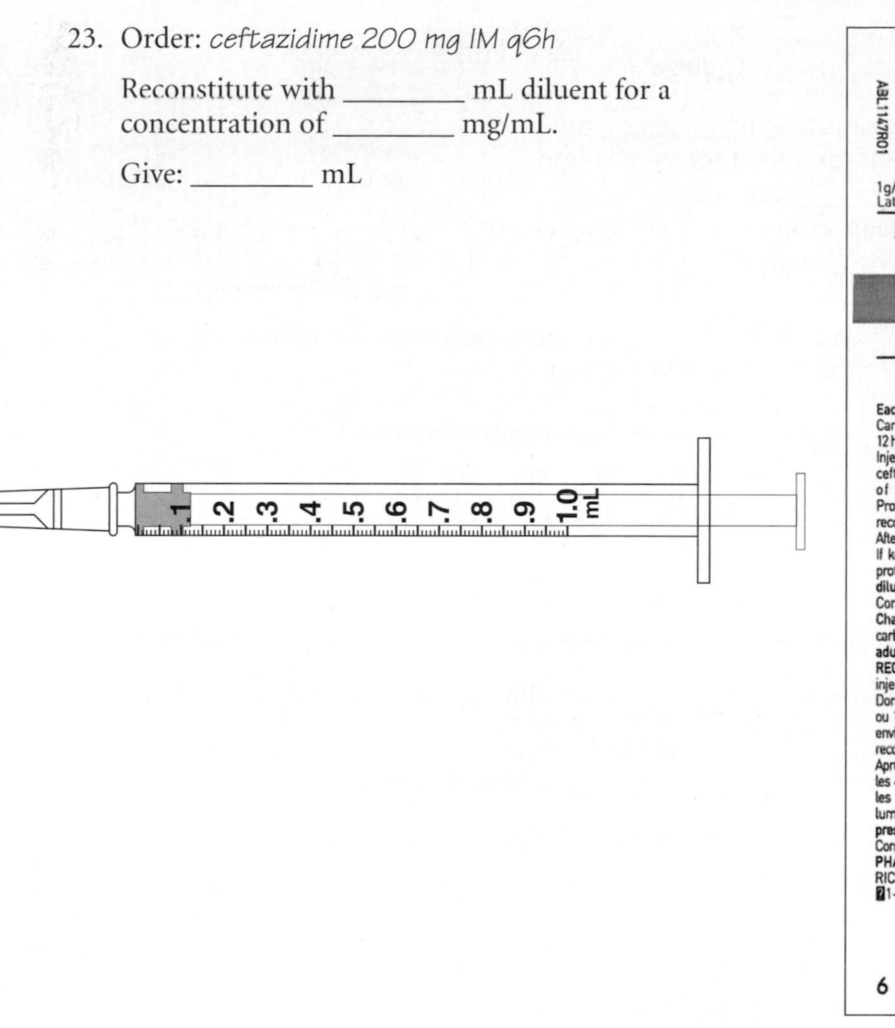

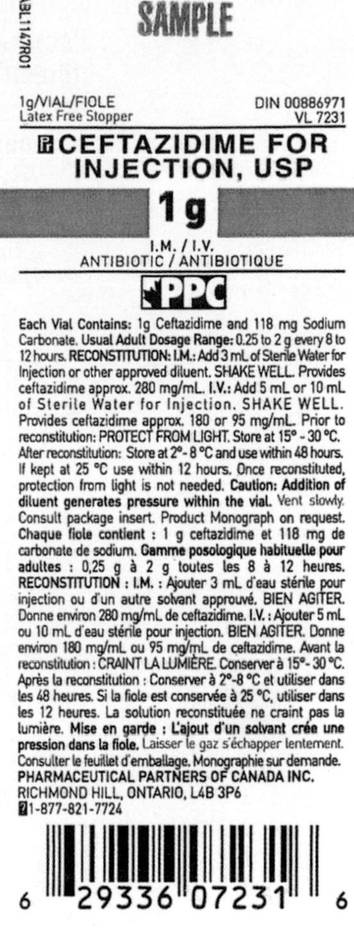

Pharmaceutical Partners of Canada Inc.

24. Order: *cefazolin sodium 750 mg IM q8h*

    Reconstitute with ________ mL diluent for a concentration of ________ mg/mL

    Give: ________ mL

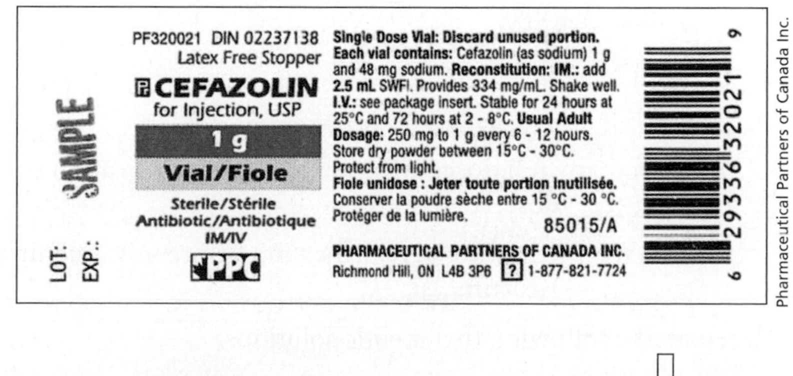

Pharmaceutical Partners of Canada Inc.

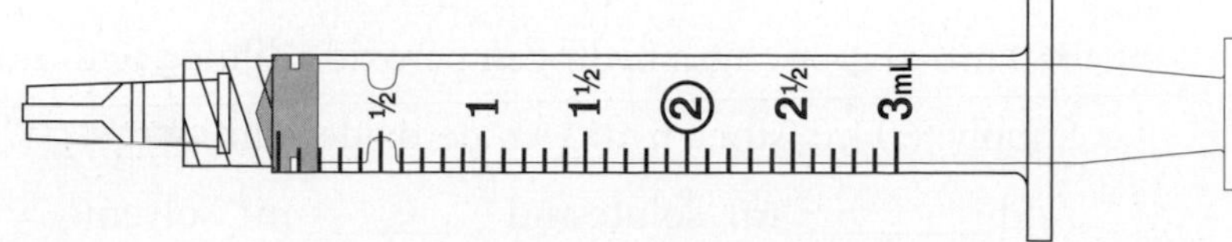

25. Order: *methylprednisolone sodium succinate 250 mg IV q6h*

Reconstitute with ________ mL diluent for a total solution volume of ________ mL with a concentration of ________ mg/mL.

Give: ________ mL

Sterile/Stérile DIN 02231895
METHYLPREDNISOLONE Sodium Succinate for Injection, USP
Succinate sodique de MÉTHYLPREDNISOLONE pour injection, USP
500 mg
methylprednisolone per vial / de méthylprednisolone par fiole
IM or IV Use / Usage IM ou IV
Novopharm Limited

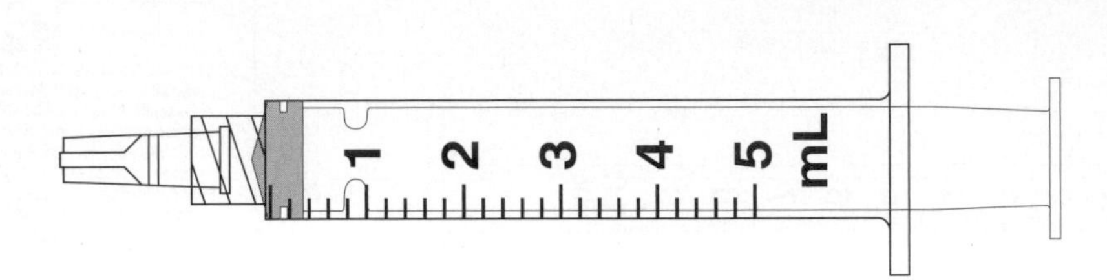

26. Order: *tobramycin sulfate 100 mg IV q8h*

Reconstitute with ________ mL diluent for a total solution volume of ________ mL with a concentration of ________ mg/mL.

Withdraw: ________ mL and further dilute before administration

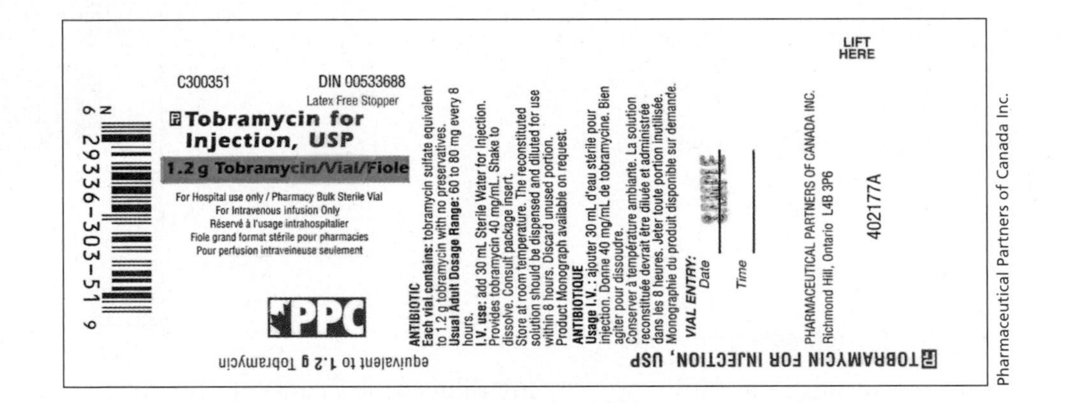

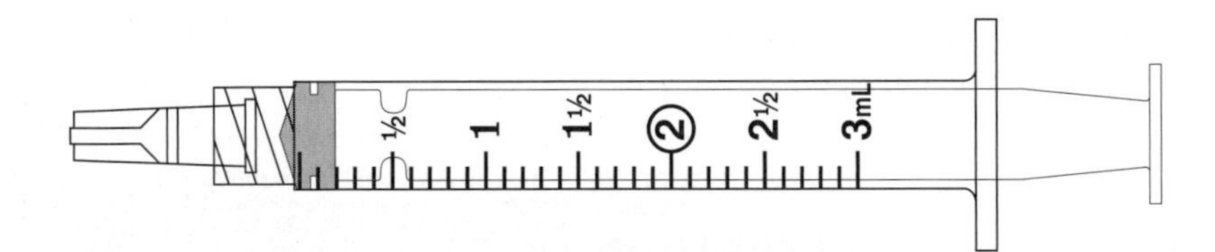

27. How many full doses are available of the medication supplied for question 26? ________ dose(s)

28. Will the medication supplied expire before it is used up for the order in question 26? ________ Explain: ________________________________

Prepare the following therapeutic solutions.

29. 360 mL of $\frac{1}{3}$-strength hydrogen peroxide diluted with normal saline

Supply: 60 mL stock hydrogen peroxide solution

Add ________ mL solute and ________ mL solvent

30. 240 mL $\frac{3}{4}$-strength Ensure

    Supply: 240-mL can of Ensure

    Add ________ mL Ensure and ________ mL water

Refer to the following order for questions 31 and 32.

Order: *Give $\frac{2}{3}$-strength Ensure 240 mL via NG tube q3h*

Supply: Ready-to-use Ensure 240-mL can and sterile water

31. How much Ensure and water are needed for a 24-hour supply for this patient? ________ mL Ensure and ___________mL water

32. How many cans of Ensure are needed to prepare this order for 1 day and how much would be discarded? ________ can(s) and discard ________ mL

Use the following information to answer questions 33 and 34.

You will prepare formula to feed nine infants in the nursery. Each infant has an order for *120 mL of $\frac{1}{2}$-strength Isomil formula q3h.* You have 240-mL cans of ready-to-use Isomil and sterile water.

33. How many cans of formula will you need to open to prepare the reconstituted formula for all nine infants for one feeding each? ________ can(s)

34. How many millilitres of sterile water will you add to the Isomil to reconstitute the formula for one feeding for all nine infants? ________ mL

Chapter 11: Pediatric and Adult Dosages Based on Body Weight

Calculate and assess the safety of the following dosages. Mark safe dosages on the syringe.

35. Order: *morphine sulfate 6 mg IV q4h prn severe pain* for a child who weighs 30.5 kg
    Recommended pediatric dosage: 100 to 200 mcg/kg q4h, up to a maximum of 15 mg/dose

    If the dosage ordered is safe, give ________ mL. If not safe, explain why not and describe what you should do. ___________

    ____

    ____

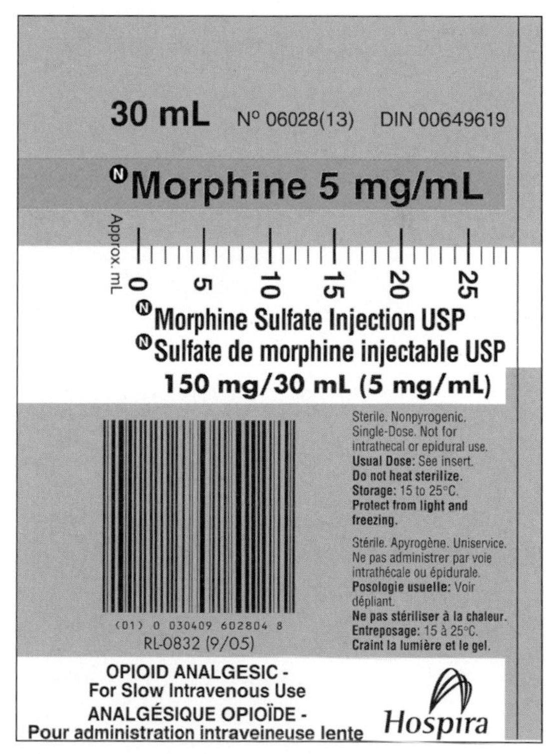

30 mL
Nº 06028(13) DIN 00649619
Morphine 5 mg/mL
Approx. mL
0 5 10 15 20 25
Morphine Sulfate Injection USP
Sulfate de morphine injectable USP
150 mg/30 mL (5 mg/mL)
Sterile. Nonpyrogenic. Single-Dose. Not for intrathecal or epidural use.
Usual Dose: See insert.
Do not heat sterilize.
Storage: 15 to 25°C.
Protect from light and freezing.
Stérile. Apyrogène. Uniservice. Ne pas administrer par voie intrathécale ou épidurale.
Posologie usuelle: Voir dépliant.
Ne pas stériliser à la chaleur.
Entreposage: 15 à 25°C.
Craint la lumière et le gel.
(01) 0 030409 602804 8
RL-0832 (9/05)
OPIOID ANALGESIC - For Slow Intravenous Use
ANALGÉSIQUE OPIOÏDE - Pour administration intraveineuse lente
Hospira

Courtesy of Pfizer Inc.

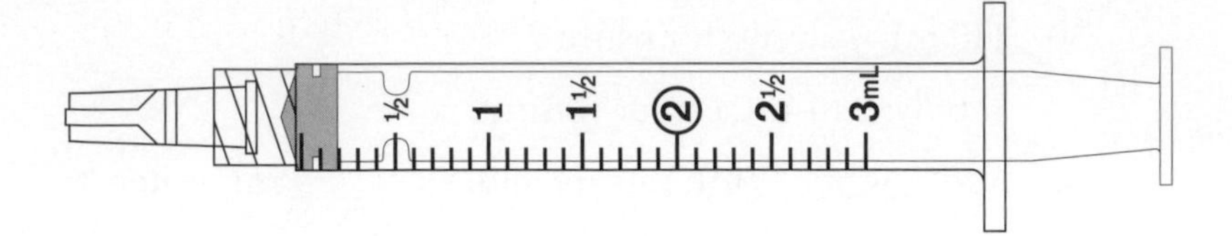

36. Order: *amoxicillin suspension 75 mg PO q8h* for a baby who weighs 6.8 kg.

Recommended dosage: See label.

If the dosage ordered is safe, reconstitute with ________ mL diluent for a total solution volume of ________ mL and a concentration of ________ mg/mL and give ___________ mL. If not safe, explain why not and describe what you should do. ____________________

____

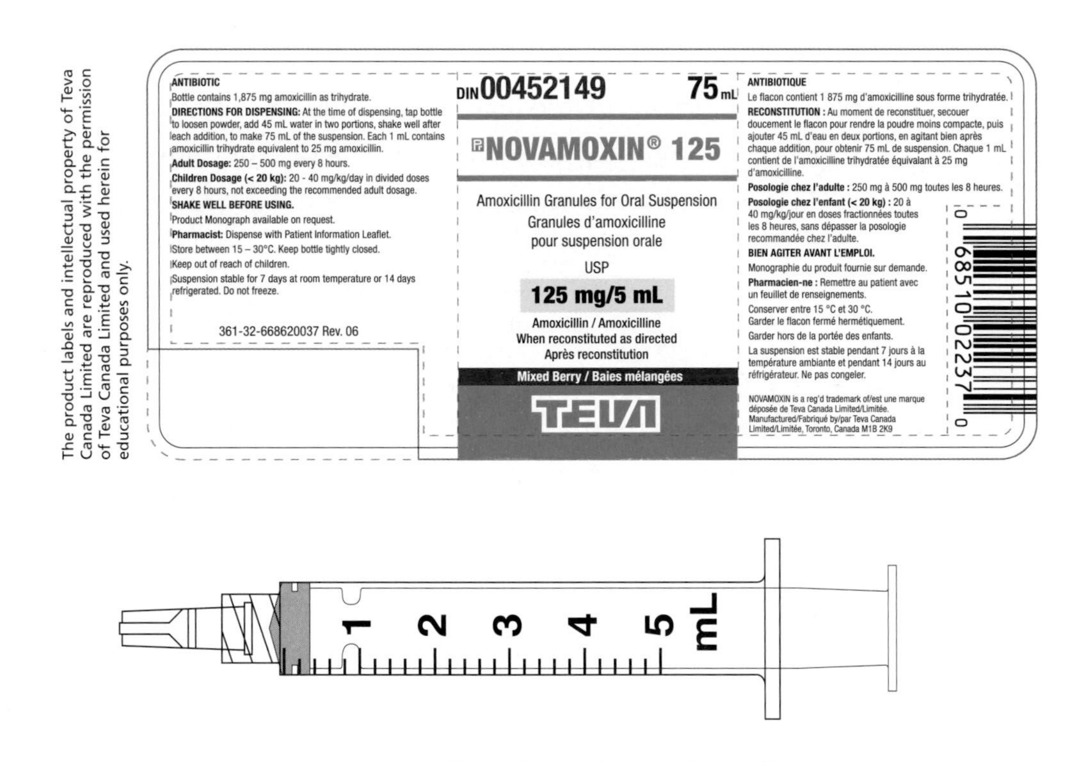

37. Order: *phenytoin sodium 200 mg IV* for a child who weighs 20 kg who is experiencing a generalized convulsive status epilepticus. Recommended pediatric IV dosage for short-term management of an acute seizure is 15 to 20 mg/kg. If the dosage ordered is safe and within effective range, give ________ mL. If not safe, explain why not and describe what you should do. ____

____

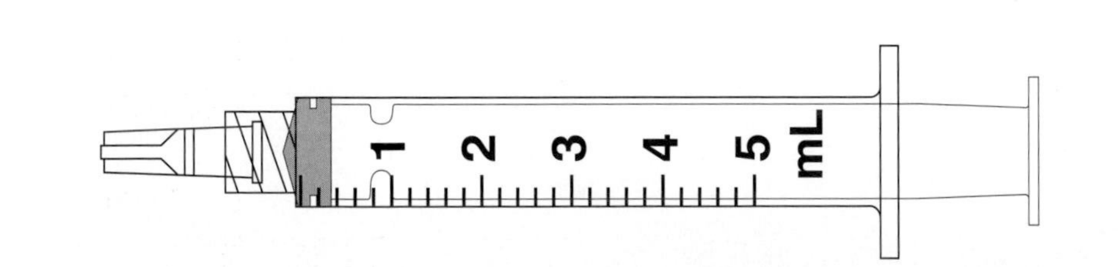

38. Order: *cefixime 60 mg PO daily* for a child with otitis media and who weighs 7.5 kg.

    Recommended dosage: See label.

    If the dosage ordered is safe, reconstitute with ________ mL diluent for a total solution volume of ________ mL and a concentration of ________ mg/mL. Give ________ mL. If not safe, explain why not and describe what you should do. ________________________

    ____

BIEN AGITER AVANT L'EMPLOI.
Le flacon contient de la céfixime sous forme de trihydrate correspondant à 1 g de céfixime anhydre.
POSOLOGIE – ADULTE : 400 mg, 1 fois par jour.
Si nécessaire, 200 mg, 2 fois par jour.
Infections urinaires : 400 mg, 1 fois par jour.
ENFANT : 8 mg/kg/jour, 1 fois par jour.
Si nécessaire, 4 mg/kg, 2 fois par jour.
Infections urinaires : 8 mg/kg/jour, 1 fois par jour.
RECONSTITUTION : Secouer légèrement le flacon plusieurs fois pour ameublir la poudre avant la reconstitution. Ajouter un volume total de 33 mL d'eau divisé en DEUX PORTIONS. Bien mélanger après chaque addition. Donne 20 mg/mL. La suspension peut être conservée pendant 14 jours à la température ambiante ou réfrigérée. **Jeter la portion non utilisée.**
Monographie du produit fournie sur demande ou disponible au www.sanofi.ca. Conserver la poudre à une température ambiante contrôlée se situant entre 15 et 30 °C.

(01)20065914106686

E50069005E

DIN 00868965
Suprax®
Cefixime for oral suspension, Mfr. Std. / Céfixime pour suspension orale, Norme-fabricant
100 mg / **5** mL*
Antibiotic / Antibiotique
50 mL
*when reconstituted / lorsque reconstitué
SANOFI

SHAKE WELL BEFORE USE.
The bottle contains cefixime as trihydrate, corresponding to 1 g cefixime anhydrous.
DOSAGE – ADULTS: 400 mg once daily. If necessary, 200 mg twice daily. **Urinary tract infections:** 400 mg once daily.
CHILDREN: 8 mg/kg/day once daily. If necessary, 4 mg/kg twice daily. **Urinary tract infections:** 8 mg/kg/day once daily.
RECONSTITUTION: Tap the bottle several times to loosen powder contents prior to reconstitution. Add a total volume of 33 mL of water split in TWO PORTIONS. Mix well after each addition. Provides 20 mg/mL. Suspension may be kept for 14 days at room temperature or under refrigeration. **Discard unused portion.** 1230421-E
Product Monograph available upon request or at www.sanofi.ca. Store powder at controlled room temperature between 15 and 30°C.
® Registered trade-mark of / Marque déposée de Astellas Pharma Inc., Osaka, Japan (Japon).
Mfd by / Fabr. par sanofi-aventis Canada Inc., Laval, Québec, Canada H7V 0A3
1 800 265-7927
Lot
Exp.

1 2 3 4 5 mL

39. Order: *tobramycin sulfate 30 mg IM q8h* for a child who weighs 7.3 kg. The recommended dosage of tobramycin for adults and children is 6–7.5 mg/kg/day in 3 divided doses, not to exceed 1.5 g/day.

    If the ordered dosage is safe, give ________ mL. If not safe, explain why not and describe what you should do. ________________________

    ____

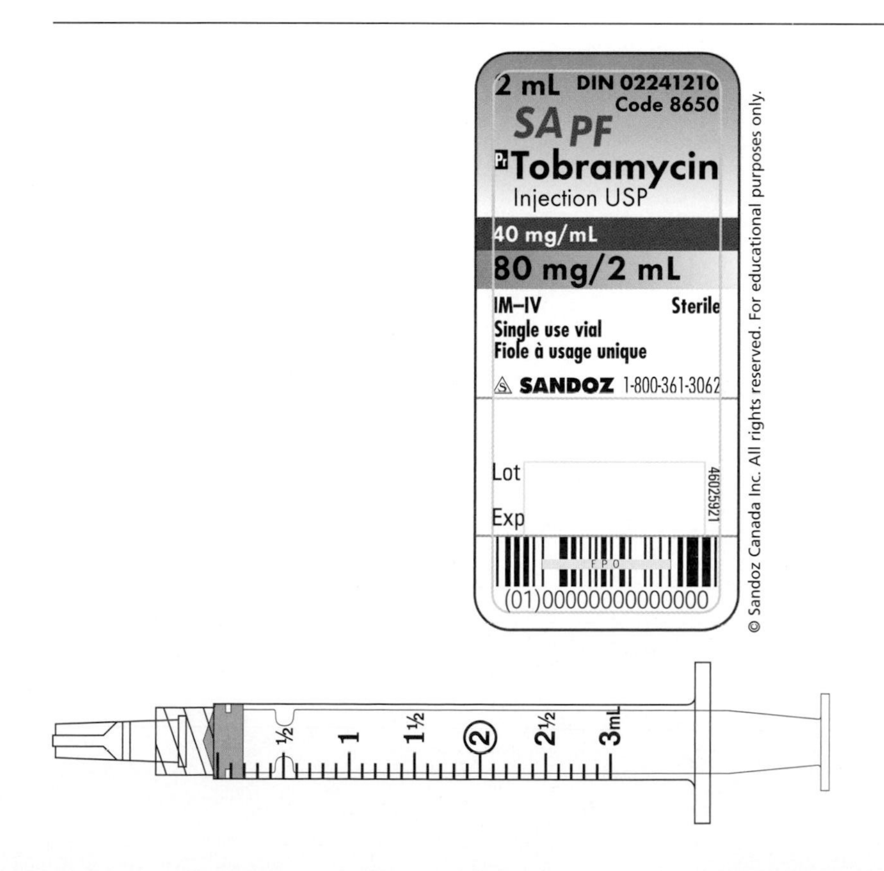

2 mL DIN 02241210
Code 8650
SA PF
Tobramycin
Injection USP
40 mg/mL
80 mg/2 mL
IM–IV
Sterile
Single use vial
Fiole à usage unique
SANDOZ 1-800-361-3062
Lot
Exp
46025921
FPO
(01)00000000000000
© Sandoz Canada Inc. All rights reserved. For educational purposes only.
½
1
1½
2
2½
3mL

40. Refer to the recommended dosage of tobramycin in question 39. What dosage range would you expect the single q8h dosage of tobramycin sulfate to be for an adult who weighs 125 kg?

    Minimum ________ mg/dose

    Maximum ________ mg/dose

After completing these problems, see the Answers section at the back of the book to check your answers. Give yourself 2 points for each correct answer.

Perfect score = 80 My score = ________

Mastery score = 74 or higher (37 or more correct)

Intravenous Solutions, Equipment, and Calculations

OBJECTIVES

1. Identify common intravenous (IV) solutions and equipment.
2. Calculate the amount of specific components in common IV fluids.
3. Define the following terms: *IV, peripheral line, central line, primary IV, secondary IV, saline lock, intravenous piggyback (IVPB),* and *direct IV.*
4. Calculate millilitres per hour, mL/h.
5. Recognize the calibration or drop factor in drops per mL (gtt/mL) from information on IV tubing packages.
6. Apply the formula method to calculate IV flow rate in gtt/min, as indicated on IV tubing packages.
7. Apply the shortcut method to calculate IV flow rate in gtt/min.
8. Calculate small-volume IVPBs.
9. Recalculate the IV flow rate when the IV is off-schedule.
10. Calculate the rate for direct IV medications.
11. Calculate the IV infusion time.
12. Calculate the IV infusion volume.

Intravenous (IV) refers to the administration of fluids, nutrients, and medications through a vein. IV fluids are ordered for a variety of reasons: to replace lost fluids, to maintain fluid and electrolyte balance, and to administer IV medications. *Replacement fluids* are often ordered to replace fluid losses resulting from hemorrhage, fluid shifts (ascites), capillary leaks (burns), vomiting, and diarrhea. *Maintenance fluids* sustain normal fluid and electrolyte balance. They may be used for the patient who is not yet depleted but is beginning to show symptoms of depletion. They may also be ordered for the patient who has fluid volume depletion has the potential to become volume depleted, such as the patient who is allowed nothing by mouth (NPO) prior to surgery.

IV fluids and drugs are administered by two methods: *continuous* and *intermittent* infusion. Continuous IV infusions replace or maintain fluid and electrolytes and are also used to administer drugs. Intermittent infusions, such as IVPB and direct IV, are used for IV administration of drugs and supplemental fluids. Intermittent peripheral infusion devices, also called saline or heparin locks, are used to maintain venous access without continuous fluid infusion.

IV therapy is an important and challenging nursing responsibility. The essential information and step-by-step calculations to help you gain a thorough understanding and mastery of this subject are presented in this chapter. To begin, we analyze IV solutions.

IV SOLUTIONS

IV solutions are ordered by a prescriber and are administered and monitored by the nurse. It is the responsibility of the nurse to ensure that the correct IV fluid is administered to the correct patient at the prescribed rate. IV fluids can be supplied in plastic solution bags (which is more common) or glass bottles, and the volume of the IV fluid container typically varies from 50 mL to 1000 mL. Some IV bags may contain more than 1000 mL. For example, solutions used for total parenteral nutrition usually contain 2000 mL or more in a single bag. The IV solution bag or bottle will be labelled with the exact components and amount of the IV solution. Prescribers frequently use abbreviations when communicating about the IV solution. Therefore, it is important to know the common IV solution components and the solution concentration strengths represented by such abbreviations.

Solution Components

Water, glucose (dextrose), saline (sodium chloride or NaCl), and selected electrolytes and salts are components of IV fluids. Dextrose and sodium chloride are the two most common solute components. Learn the following common IV component abbreviations.

REMEMBER

Common IV Component Abbreviations

Abbreviation	Solution Component
D	Dextrose
W	Water
S	Saline
NS	Normal saline (0.9% NaCl)
NaCl	Sodium chloride
RL	Ringer's Lactate
LR	Lactated Ringer's

Solution Strength

In the following examples, the abbreviation letters indicate the solution components, and the numbers indicate the solution strength or concentration of the components, for example, D_5W. The numbers may be written as subscripts in the patient care order.

Example 1:

Suppose an order specifies D_5W. This abbreviation means "dextrose 5% in water" and is supplied as 5% dextrose injection as shown in Figure 12-1. This means that the solution strength of the solute (dextrose) is 5%. The solvent is water. Recall from Chapter 7 that parenteral solutions expressed in a percent indicate X g per 100 mL. The IV bag label reads, "each 100 mL contains 5 g dextrose. . . ."

Example 2:

Suppose a nurse writes D_5LR in the progress notes. This abbreviation means "dextrose 5% in Lactated Ringer's" and is supplied as Lactated Ringer's and 5% dextrose injection as shown in Figure 12-2.

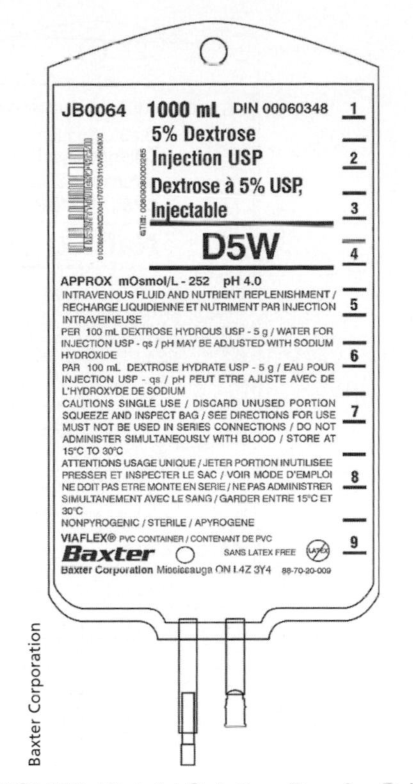
JB0064 1000 mL DIN 00060348
5% Dextrose
Injection USP
Dextrose à 5% USP,
Injectable
D5W
APPROX mOsmol/L - 252 pH 4.0
INTRAVENOUS FLUID AND NUTRIENT REPLENISHMENT / RECHARGE LIQUIDIENNE ET NUTRIMENT PAR INJECTION INTRAVEINEUSE
PER 100 mL DEXTROSE HYDROUS USP - 5 g / WATER FOR INJECTION USP - qs / pH MAY BE ADJUSTED WITH SODIUM HYDROXIDE
PAR 100 mL DEXTROSE HYDRATE USP - 5 g / EAU POUR INJECTION USP - qs / pH PEUT ETRE AJUSTE AVEC DE L'HYDROXYDE DE SODIUM
CAUTIONS SINGLE USE / DISCARD UNUSED PORTION SQUEEZE AND INSPECT BAG / SEE DIRECTIONS FOR USE MUST NOT BE USED IN SERIES CONNECTIONS / DO NOT ADMINISTER SIMULTANEOUSLY WITH BLOOD / STORE AT 15°C TO 30°C
ATTENTIONS USAGE UNIQUE / JETER PORTION INUTILISEE PRESSER ET INSPECTER LE SAC / VOIR MODE D'EMPLOI NE DOIT PAS ETRE MONTE EN SERIE / NE PAS ADMINISTRER SIMULTANEMENT AVEC LE SANG / GARDER ENTRE 15°C ET 30°C
NONPYROGENIC / STERILE / APYROGENE
VIAFLEX® PVC CONTAINER / CONTENANT DE PVC
Baxter
SANS LATEX FREE
Baxter Corporation Mississauga ON L4Z 3Y4 88-70-20-009
1
2
3
4
5
6
7
8
9
Baxter Corporation

FIGURE 12-1 IV Solution Bag for D_5W

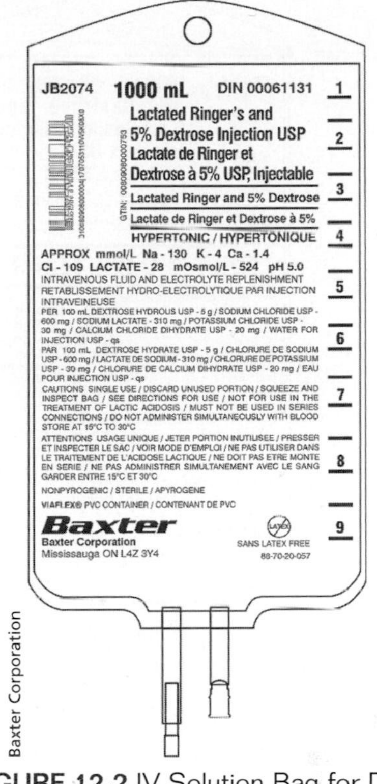
JB2074 1000 mL DIN 00061131
Lactated Ringer's and
5% Dextrose Injection USP
Lactate de Ringer et
Dextrose à 5% USP, Injectable
Lactated Ringer and 5% Dextrose
Lactate de Ringer et Dextrose à 5%
HYPERTONIC / HYPERTONIQUE
APPROX mmol/L Na - 130 K - 4 Ca - 1.4
Cl - 109 LACTATE - 28 mOsmol/L - 524 pH 5.0
INTRAVENOUS FLUID AND ELECTROLYTE REPLENISHMENT RETABLISSEMENT HYDRO-ELECTROLYTIQUE PAR INJECTION INTRAVEINEUSE
PER 100 mL DEXTROSE HYDROUS USP - 5 g / SODIUM CHLORIDE USP - 600 mg / SODIUM LACTATE - 310 mg / POTASSIUM CHLORIDE USP - 30 mg / CALCIUM CHLORIDE DIHYDRATE USP - 20 mg / WATER FOR INJECTION USP - qs
PAR 100 mL DEXTROSE HYDRATE USP - 5 g / CHLORURE DE SODIUM USP - 600 mg / LACTATE DE SODIUM - 310 mg / CHLORURE DE POTASSIUM USP - 30 mg / CHLORURE DE CALCIUM DIHYDRATE USP - 20 mg / EAU POUR INJECTION USP - qs
CAUTIONS SINGLE USE / DISCARD UNUSED PORTION / SQUEEZE AND INSPECT BAG / SEE DIRECTIONS FOR USE / NOT FOR USE IN THE TREATMENT OF LACTIC ACIDOSIS / MUST NOT BE USED IN SERIES CONNECTIONS / DO NOT ADMINISTER SIMULTANEOUSLY WITH BLOOD STORE AT 15°C TO 30°C
ATTENTIONS USAGE UNIQUE / JETER PORTION INUTILISEE / PRESSER ET INSPECTER LE SAC / VOIR MODE D'EMPLOI / NE PAS UTILISER DANS LE TRAITEMENT DE L'ACIDOSE LACTIQUE / NE DOIT PAS ETRE MONTE EN SERIE / NE PAS ADMINISTRER SIMULTANEMENT AVEC LE SANG GARDER ENTRE 15°C ET 30°C
NONPYROGENIC / STERILE / APYROGENE
VIAFLEX® PVC CONTAINER / CONTENANT DE PVC
Baxter
Baxter Corporation
Mississauga ON L4Z 3Y4
SANS LATEX FREE
88-70-20-057
1
2
3
4
5
6
7
8
9
Baxter Corporation

FIGURE 12-2 IV Solution Bag for D_5LR

Example 3:

A written order is for *D_5NS 1000 mL IV q8h.* This order means "administer 1000 mL 5% dextrose in normal saline intravenously every 8 hours" and is supplied as 5% dextrose and 0.9% sodium chloride as shown in Figure 12-3. *Normal saline* is the common term for 0.9% NaCl. Another name is *physiologic saline.* The concentration of sodium chloride in normal saline is 0.9 g (or 900 mg) per 100 mL of solution.

Another common saline IV concentration is 0.45% NaCl, as shown in Figure 12-4. Note that 0.45% NaCl is $\frac{1}{2}$ the strength of 0.9% NaCl. Thus, it is typically written as $\frac{1}{2}$ NS for $\frac{1}{2}$ normal saline. There are other saline solution strengths, including 0.3% NaCl (also abbreviated as $\frac{1}{3}$ NS) and 0.225% NaCl (also abbreviated as $\frac{1}{4}$ NS).

The goal of IV therapy, achieved through fluid infusion, is to maintain or regain fluid and electrolyte balance. When dextrose or saline (*solute*) is diluted in water for injection (*solvent*), the result is a *solution* that can be administered to maintain or approximate the normal blood plasma. Blood or serum concentration is described in terms of *tonicity* or *osmolarity* and is measured in milliOsmoles per litre, or mOsm/L. IV fluids are concentrated and classified as *isotonic* (the same tonicity or osmolarity as blood and other body serums), *hypotonic* (lower tonicity or osmolarity than blood and other body serums), or *hypertonic* (higher tonicity or osmolarity than blood and other body serums). Normal saline (0.9% NaCl, or physiologic saline) is an isotonic solution. The osmolarity of a manufactured solution is detailed on the printed label. Look for the mOsm/L in the fine print under the solution names in Figures 12-1 through 12-4.

In Figure 12-5, the three solution concentrations are compared according to normal serum osmolarity. Parenteral therapy is determined by unique patient needs, and these basic factors must be considered when ordering and infusing IV solutions.

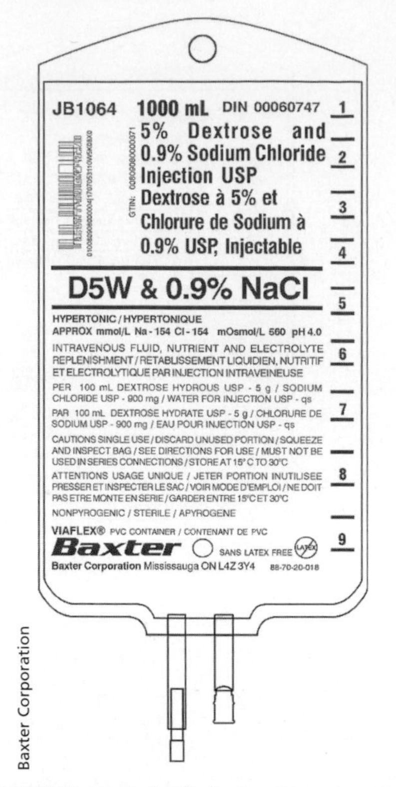

Baxter Corporation

FIGURE 12-3 IV Solution Bag for D_5NS

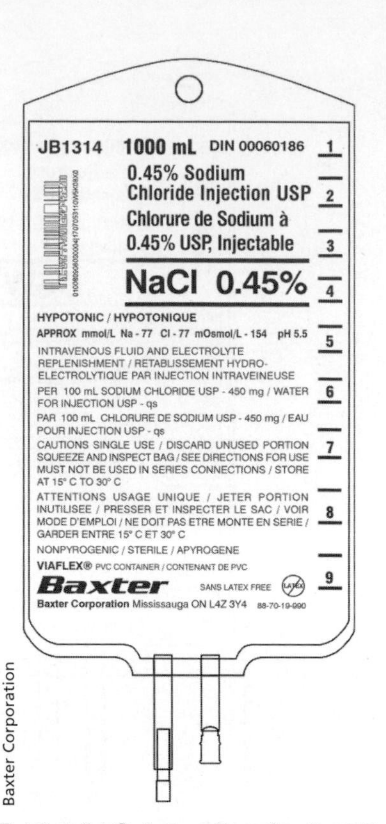

Baxter Corporation

FIGURE 12-4 IV Solution Bag for 0.45% NaCl

Normal Serum Osmolarity (Normal Average Tonicity—All Ages): 280–320 mOsm/L

Hypotonic (less than 250 mOsm/L) *Solvent exceeds solute—* used to dilute excess serum electrolytes, as in hyperglycemia	**Isotonic** (250–375 mOsm/L) *Solvent and solutes are* balanced—used to expand volume and maintain normal tonicity	**Hypertonic** (more than 375 mOsm/L) *Solutes exceed solvent—* used to correct electrolyte imbalances, as in loss from excess vomiting and diarrhea
Example of IV solution: *0.45% saline* (154 mOsm/L)	Examples of IV solution: *0.9% saline* (308 mOsm/L) *Lactated Ringer's* (273 mOsm/L) *5% dextrose in water** (252 mOsm/L)	Example of IV solution: *5% dextrose and 0.9% NaCl* (560 mOsm/L) *5% dextrose and Lactated Ringer's* (525 mOsm/L)

FIGURE 12-5 Comparison of IV Solution Concentrations by Osmolarity

*__Note:__ D_5W is initially isotonic; however, dextrose is rapidly metabolized by the body, such that no osmotically active particles remain, making it a hypotonic solution.

Solution Additives

Electrolytes may also be added to the basic IV fluid. Potassium chloride (KCl) is a common IV electrolyte and is measured in *milliequivalents* (mEq). The order is usually written to indicate the amount of milliequivalents *per litre* (1000 mL) to be added to the IV fluid. Potassium chloride is a high-alert medication, so standardized premixed IV solutions are available on units, and prescribing practices are standardized to meet available premixed solutions.

Example:

The order is for *D_5NS with 20 mEq KCl/L q8h*. This means that 20 milliequivalents potassium chloride per litre of 5% dextrose and 0.9% sodium chloride IV solution are to be administered every 8 hours.

QUICK REVIEW

- Pay close attention to IV abbreviations: *letters* indicate the solution components, and *numbers* indicate the concentration or solution strength.
- Dextrose and sodium chloride (NaCl) are common IV solutes.
- Normal saline is 0.9% sodium chloride: 0.9 g NaCl/100 mL solution.
- IV solution tonicity or osmolarity is measured in mOsm/L.
- D_5W and normal saline are common isotonic solutions.

REVIEW SET 12-1

For each of the IV solution bags labelled A through H,

a. Specify the *letter* of the solution bag corresponding to the fluid abbreviation.

b. List the *solute(s)* of each solution, and identify the *strength (g/mL)* of each solute.

c. Identify the *osmolarity (mOsm/L)* of each solution.

d. Identify the *tonicity (isotonic, hypotonic, or hypertonic)* of each solution.

	a. Letter of Matching Solution Bag	b. Solutes and Strength	c. Osmolarity (mOsm/L)	d. Tonicity
1. NS	______	______	______	______
2. D_5W	______	______	______	______
3. D_5NS	______	______	______	______
4. $D_5 \frac{1}{2}$NS	______	______	______	______
5. D_5 0.2% NS	______	______	______	______
6. D_5LR	______	______	______	______
7. NS with 20 mEq KCl/L	______	______	______	______
8. $\frac{1}{2}$NS	______	______	______	______

Check your work! Answers to all Review Sets are provided at the end of each chapter. Worked solutions for selected Review Sets are also available there.

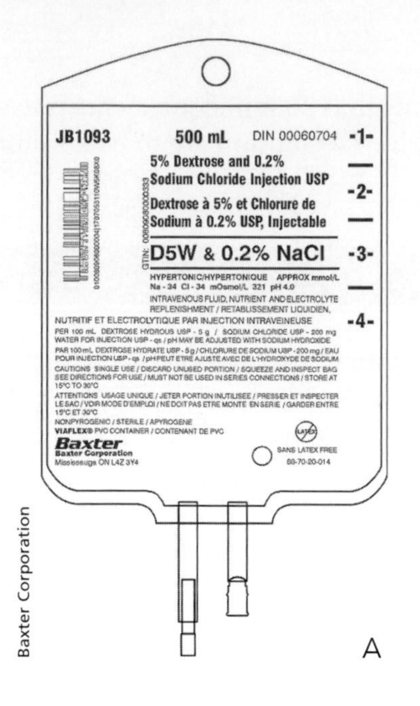

Baxter Corporation

A

JB1764 1000 mL DIN 00786209 1

(20 mmol/L) Potassium Chloride in 0.9% Sodium Chloride Injection USP 2

(20 mmol/L) Chlorure de Potassium dans du Chlorure de Sodium à 0.9% USP, Injectable 3 4

KCl 0.9% NaCl 20 mmol 5

6

HYPERTONIC/HYPERTONIQUE APPROX mOsmol/L - 348 / APPROX mmol/L Na - 154 K - 20 Cl - 174 pH 5.0

INTRAVENOUS FLUID AND ELECTROLYTE REPLENISHMENT RETABLISSEMENT HYDRO-ELECTROLYTIQUE PAR INJECTION INTRAVEINEUSE

7

PER 100 mL POTASSIUM CHLORIDE USP - 150 mg / SODIUM CHLORIDE USP - 900 mg / WATER FOR INJECTION USP - qs

CAUTIONS SINGLE USE / DISCARD UNUSED PORTION / SQUEEZE AND INSPECT BAG / SEE DIRECTIONS FOR USE / MUST NOT BE USED IN SERIES CONNECTIONS / STORE AT 15° C TO 30° C

PAR 100 mL CHLORURE DE POTASSIUM USP - 150 mg / CHLORURE DE SODIUM USP - 900 mg / EAU POUR INJECTION USP - qs

8

ATTENTIONS USAGE UNIQUE / JETER PORTION INUTILISEE / PRESSER ET INSPECTER LE SAC / VOIR MODE D'EMPLOI / NE DOIT PAS ETRE MONTE EN SERIE / GARDER ENTRE 15° C ET 30° C

NONPYROGENIC / STERILE / APYROGENE

VIAFLEX® PVC CONTAINER CONTENANT DE PVC

20 mmol

9

Baxter

SANS LATEX FREE

Baxter Corporation Mississauga ON L4Z 3Y4

88-70-19-961

Baxter Corporation

B

JB1324 1000 mL DIN 00060208 1

0.9% Sodium Chloride Injection USP 2

Chlorure de Sodium à 0.9% USP, Injectable 3

NaCl 0.9% 4

APPROX mmol/L Na - 154 Cl - 154 mOsmol/L - 308 pH 5.5

5

INTRAVENOUS FLUID AND ELECTROLYTE REPLENISHMENT / RETABLISSEMENT HYDRO-ELECTROLYTIQUE PAR INJECTION INTRAVEINEUSE

6

PER 100 mL SODIUM CHLORIDE USP - 900 mg / WATER FOR INJECTION USP - qs

PAR 100 mL CHLORURE DE SODIUM USP - 900 mg / EAU POUR INJECTION USP - qs

7

CAUTIONS SINGLE USE / DISCARD UNUSED PORTION SQUEEZE AND INSPECT BAG / SEE DIRECTIONS FOR USE MUST NOT BE USED IN SERIES CONNECTIONS / STORE AT 15° C TO 30° C

8

ATTENTIONS USAGE UNIQUE / JETER PORTION INUTILISEE / PRESSER ET INSPECTER LE SAC / VOIR MODE D'EMPLOI / NE DOIT PAS ETRE MONTE EN SERIE / GARDER ENTRE 15° C ET 30° C

NONPYROGENIC / STERILE / APYROGENE

VIAFLEX® PVC CONTAINER / CONTENANT DE PVC

9

Baxter

SANS LATEX FREE

Baxter Corporation Mississauga ON L4Z 3Y4 88-70-19-986

Baxter Corporation

C

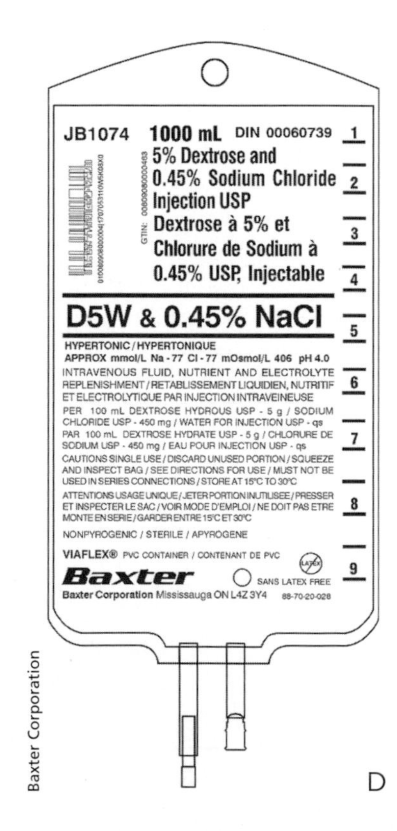

Baxter Corporation

D

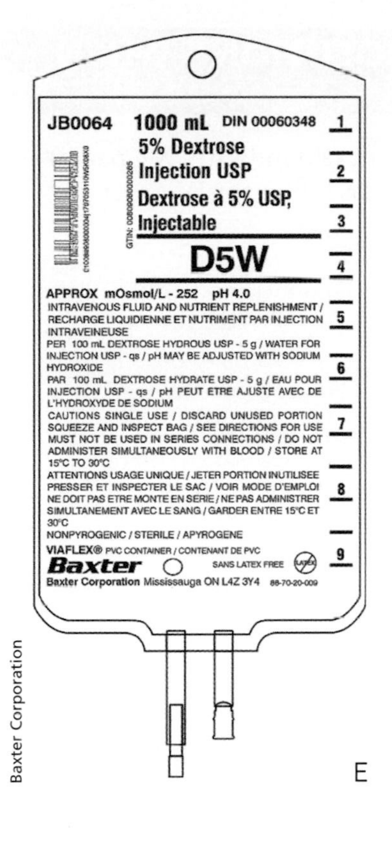

Baxter Corporation

E

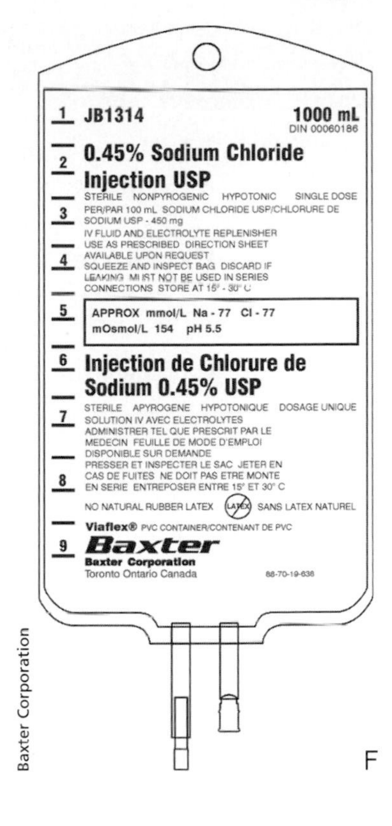

Baxter Corporation

F

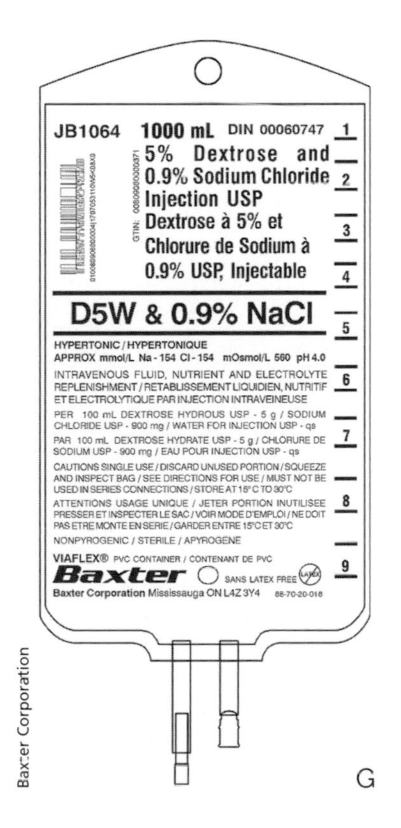

Baxter Corporation

G

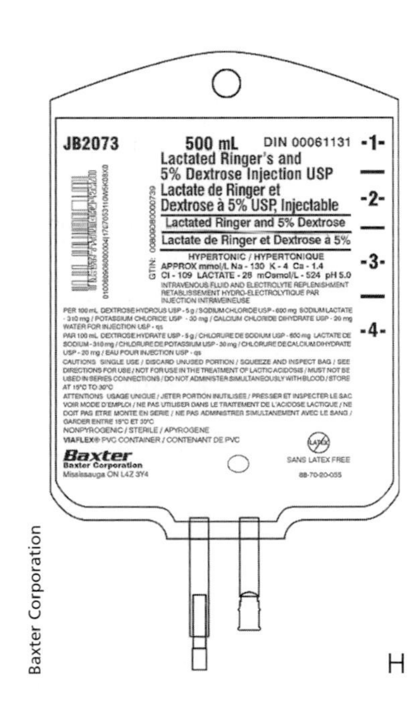

JB2073 500 mL DIN 00061131
Lactated Ringer's and
5% Dextrose Injection USP
Lactate de Ringer et
Dextrose à 5% USP, Injectable
Lactated Ringer and 5% Dextrose
Lactate de Ringer et Dextrose à 5%
HYPERTONIC / HYPERTONIQUE
APPROX mmol/L Na - 130 K - 4 Ca - 1.4
Cl - 109 LACTATE - 28 mOsmol/L - 524 pH 5.0
NONPYROGENIC / STERILE / APYROGENE
VIAFLEX® PVC CONTAINER / CONTENANT DE PVC
Baxter
Baxter Corporation
Mississauga ON L4Z 3Y4
SANS LATEX FREE
88-70-20-055
-1-
-2-
-3-
-4-

Baxter Corporation

H

CALCULATING COMPONENTS OF IV SOLUTIONS WHEN EXPRESSED AS A PERCENT

Recall that solution strength expressed as a percent (%) indicates X g per 100 mL. Understanding this concept allows you to calculate the total amount of solute per IV order.

Example 1a:

Order: *D_5W 1000 mL*

Calculate the amount of dextrose in 1000 mL D_5W.

This can be calculated using the ratio and proportion method.

% indicates g per 100 mL; for example, 5% dextrose is 5 g dextrose per 100 mL of solution.

$$\frac{5\text{ g}}{100\text{ mL}} \times \frac{X\text{ g}}{1000\text{ mL}}$$

$$100X = 5000$$

$$\frac{100X}{100} = \frac{5000}{100}$$

$$X = 50\text{ g}$$

1000 mL of D_5W contains 50 g of dextrose.

Example 1b:

The following alternative formula can also be used to determine the amount of solute:

$$\frac{\text{Concentration \%}}{100\text{ mL}} \times \text{Volume (mL)} = \text{Y (Dosage amount in g)}$$

The solutions percentage represents the number of grams of medication.

Using the above example:

$$\frac{5\%}{100\text{ mL}} \times 1000\text{ mL} = 50\text{ g}$$

Therefore, 1000 mL of D_5W contains 50 g of dextrose.

Example 2a:

Order: *$D_5 \frac{1}{4}$NS 500 mL*

Calculate the amount of dextrose and sodium chloride in 500 mL.

D_5 = dextrose 5% = 5 g dextrose per 100 mL

$$\frac{5\text{ g}}{100\text{ mL}} \times \frac{X\text{ g}}{500\text{ mL}}$$

$$100X = 2500$$

$$\frac{100X}{100} = \frac{2500}{100}$$

$$X = 25\text{ g}$$

500 mL of $D_5 \frac{1}{4}NS$ contains 25 g of dextrose.

$\frac{1}{4}NS = 0.225\%$ NaCl = 0.225 g NaCl per 100 mL

(NS, or normal saline, is 0.9% NaCl; therefore, $\frac{1}{4}$ NS is $\frac{1}{4} \times 0.9\% = 0.225\%$ NaCl.)

$$\frac{0.225 \text{ g}}{100 \text{ mL}} \;\; \frac{X \text{ g}}{500 \text{ mL}}$$

$$100X = 112.5$$

$$\frac{100X}{100} = \frac{112.5}{100}$$

$$X = 1.125 \text{ g}$$

500 mL $D_5 \frac{1}{4}$ NS contains 1.125 g of sodium chloride.

Example 2b:

Or, using the alternative formula, as shown in Example 1b:

Dextrose: $\frac{5\%}{100 \text{ mL}} \times 500 \text{ mL} = 25 \text{ g}$

Normal saline: $\frac{0.225\%}{100 \text{ mL}} \times 500 \text{ mL} = 1.125 \text{ g}$

Therefore, 500 mL of $D_5W \frac{1}{4}$ NS contains 25 g of dextrose and 1.125 g of sodium chloride.

This concept is important because it helps you understand that IV solutions provide much more than fluid. They also provide other components. Now you know what you are administering to your patient. For example, when the IV order prescribes *D_5W*, think, "I am hanging D_5W IV solution. Do I know what this fluid contains? Yes, it contains dextrose as the solute and water as the solvent in the concentration of 5 g of dextrose in every 100 mL of solution." Regular monitoring and careful understanding of IV infusions cannot be stressed enough.

QUICK REVIEW

- Solution strength expressed as a percent is the number of g of solute per 100 mL solution.

REVIEW SET 12-2

Calculate the amount of dextrose and/or sodium chloride in each of the following IV solutions.

1. 1000 mL of D_5NS

   dextrose ________ g

   sodium chloride ________ g

2. 500 mL of $D_5 \frac{1}{2}NS$

   dextrose ________ g

   sodium chloride ________ g

3. 250 mL of $D_{10}W$

   dextrose ________ g

4. 750 mL of NS

   sodium chloride ________ g

5. 500 mL of D_5 0.33% NaCl

   dextrose ________ g

   sodium chloride ________ g

6. 3 L of D_5NS

   dextrose ________ g

   sodium chloride ________ g

7. 0.5 L of $D_{10}\,\frac{1}{4}$NS
   dextrose ________ g
   sodium chloride ________ g
8. 300 mL of D_{12} 0.9% NaCl
   dextrose ________ g
   sodium chloride ________ g
9. 2 L of D_5 0.225% NaCl
   dextrose ________ g
   sodium chloride ________ g
10. 0.75 L of 0.45% NaCl
    sodium chloride ________ g

Check your work! Answers to all Review Sets are provided at the end of each chapter. Worked solutions for selected Review Sets are also available there.

IV SITES

IV fluids are administered through a *peripheral line,* such as a vein in the arm, leg, or sometimes a scalp vein for infants if other sites are inaccessible. Blood flowing through these veins can usually sufficiently dilute the components in IV fluids. Glucose and dextrose are usually concentrated between 5% and 10% for short-term IV therapy. Peripheral veins can accommodate a maximum glucose concentration of 12%. The rate of infusion in peripheral veins should not exceed 200 mL in 1 hour.

IV fluids that are transparent flow smoothly into relatively small peripheral veins. When blood transfusion or replacement is needed, a larger vein is preferred to ease blood flow. Whole blood or its components, especially packed cells, can be viscous and must be infused within a short period of time.

IV fluids may also be administered through a *central line,* in which a special catheter is inserted to access a large vein. The subclavian vein is a common site for central line placement. The internal jugular vein may also be used. A *peripherally inserted central catheter,* or *PICC line,* refers to the technique of using a peripheral vein to access a central vein. Access for a PICC line is usually through the cephalic vein, basilic vein, or brachial vein. The catheter is then advanced proximally toward the heart through increasingly larger veins until the tip of the catheter rests in the distal superior vena cava or cavoatrial junction. Larger veins can accommodate higher concentrations of glucose (up to 35%) and other nutrients, and at faster rates of IV fluids (more than 200 mL in 1 hour). They are often used when the patient is expected to need IV therapy for an extended period.

REMEMBER

The flow in central lines is determined not only by the diameter of the catheter but also by the length of the line. For example, a 16-gauge peripheral intravenous line will have a greater flow rate than a double or triple lumen central venous catheter.

QUICK REVIEW

Types of Intravenous Infusions

- Continuous Infusion: The administration of a prescribed volume of solution, with or without medication, over an ordered period of time and/or at a specified rate of infusion.
- Intermittent Infusion: The administration of a dose of medication or IV fluid at a prescribed rate, over a specified time, using an auxiliary IV unit (e.g., Buretrol®, Volutrol®, Soluset®, minibag, syringe on pump, or any small-volume unit).
- Direct: The administration of medications manually injected into a vein, an injection cap (e.g., a saline lock) on an existing central or peripheral IV site, or an injection port closest to the venipuncture site on an existing central or peripheral tubing set.

MONITORING IVs

The nurse is responsible for monitoring the patient regularly during an IV infusion.

CAUTION

Generally, the IV site and infusion should be checked at least every 30 minutes to 1 hour (or according to institution policy) for volume of remaining fluids and correct infusion rate.

PRIMARY AND SECONDARY IVs

Primary IV tubing packaging and set are shown in Figures 12-6 and 12-7. This IV set is used to set up a typical or *primary IV line*. Primary IV tubing includes a drip chamber, one or more injection ports, and a roller clamp. The tubing is long enough to be attached to the hub of the IV catheter positioned in the patient's vein. The drip chamber is squeezed until it is approximately half full of IV fluid, and IV fluid is run through the tubing prior to attaching it to the IV catheter to ensure that no air is in the tubing. The nurse can either regulate the rate manually using the roller clamp (see Figure 12-7(a)) or place the tubing in an electronic infusion pump (see Figures 12-11 through 12-13).

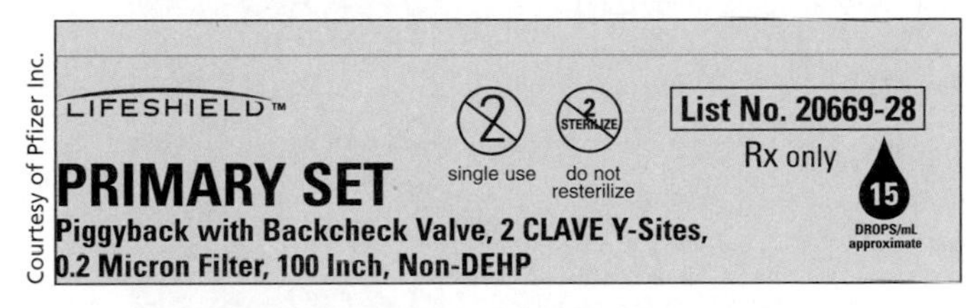

FIGURE 12-6 Primary IV Infusion Set

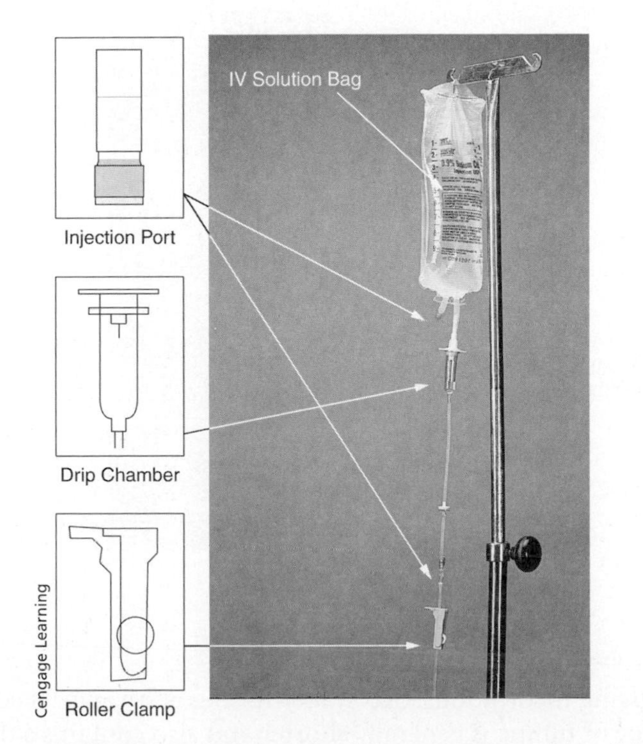

FIGURE 12-7(a) Standard Straight Gravity Flow IV System

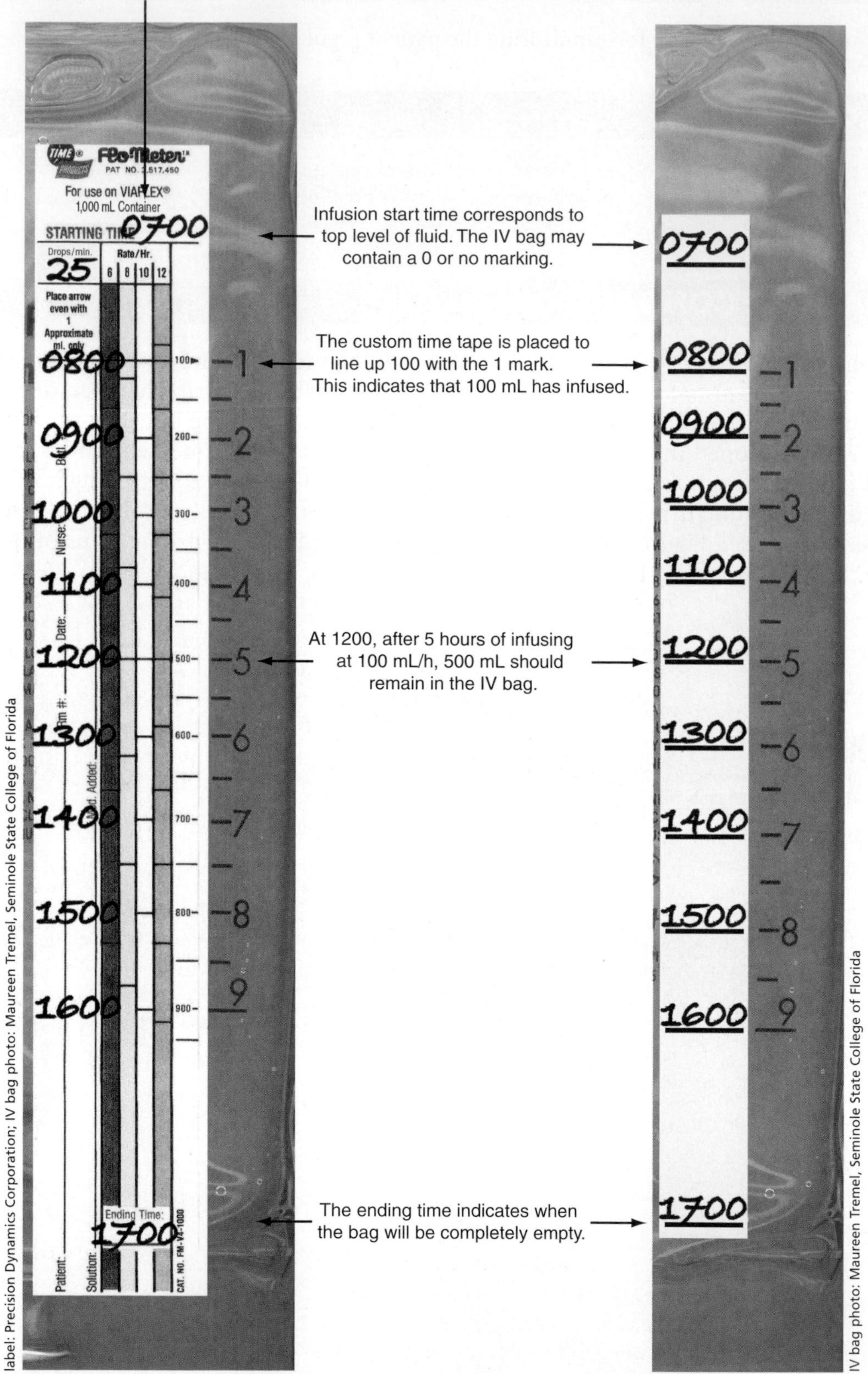

FIGURE 12-7(b) Infusion Label

Secondary IV tubing is used when giving medications. Secondary tubing is "piggybacked" into the primary line (see Figure 12-8). This type of tubing is generally shorter and also contains a drip chamber and roller clamp. This configuration provides access to the primary IV catheter without having to

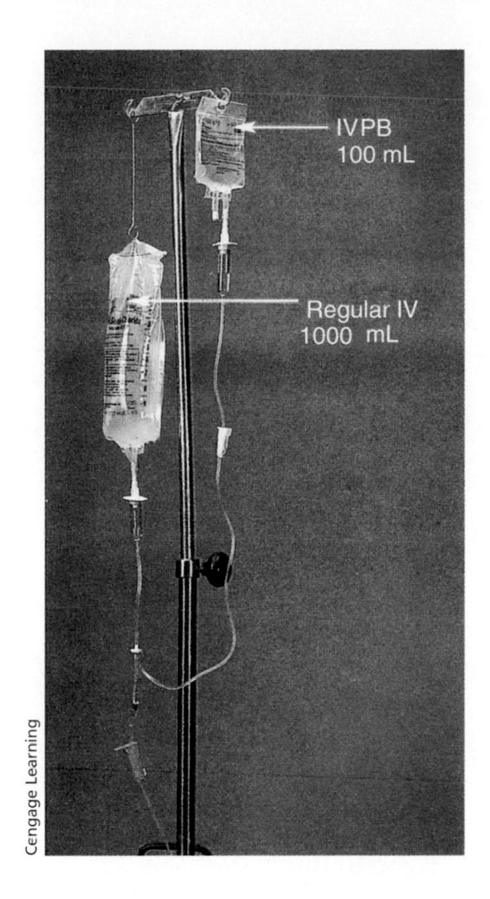

FIGURE 12-8 IV with Piggyback (IVPB)

start another IV. Notice that in this type of setup, the *secondary IV* set or *intravenous piggyback* (IVPB) is hung higher than the primary IV to allow the secondary set of medication to infuse first. When administering primary IV fluids, choose primary IV tubing; when hanging piggybacks, select secondary IV tubing. IVPBs are discussed further later in this chapter.

BLOOD ADMINISTRATION TUBING

When blood is administered, a Y-type blood set is commonly used (see Figure 12-9). The "Y" refers to the two spikes that are attached above the drip chamber. One spike is attached to the blood container, and the other spike is attached to normal saline. Normal saline is used to dilute packed cells and to flush the IV tubing at the beginning and at the end of the transfusion. Blood is usually infused manually by gravity, and the roller clamp on the line is used to adjust the rate. Some electronic pumps may also be used for infusion of blood. In such cases, the nurse programs the pump in mL/h, and the pump regulates the blood infusion.

IV FLOW RATE

The *flow rate* of an IV infusion is ordered by the prescriber. It is usually specified in mL/h and measured in mL/h or gtt/min. These calculations are described later in this chapter. It is the nurse's responsibility to regulate, monitor, and maintain the flow rate. Regulation of IV therapy is a critical skill in nursing. Because the fluids administered are infusing directly into the patient's circulatory system, careful monitoring is essential to ensure that the patient does not receive too much or too little IV fluid and medication. It is also important for the nurse to accurately set and maintain the flow rate to administer the prescribed volume of the IV solution within the specified time period. The nurse records the IV fluids administered and IV flow rates on the IV administration record (see Figure 12-10).

IV solutions are usually ordered for a certain volume to run for a period of time, such as *125 mL/h* or *1000 mL/8 h*. The nurse will use electronic or manual regulating equipment to monitor the flow rate. The calculations performed to set the flow rate depend on the equipment used to administer the IV solutions.

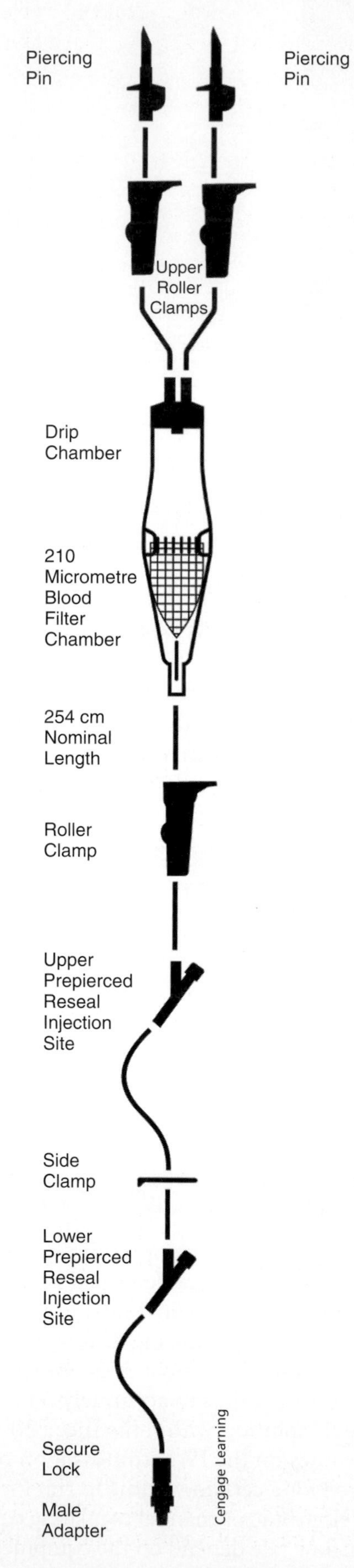
Piercing Pin
Piercing Pin
Upper Roller Clamps
Drip Chamber
210 Micrometre Blood Filter Chamber
254 cm Nominal Length
Roller Clamp
Upper Prepierced Reseal Injection Site
Side Clamp
Lower Prepierced Reseal Injection Site
Secure Lock
Male Adapter
Cengage Learning

FIGURE 12-9 Y-Type Blood Set

Nurses may label IV bags with a tape marking the infusion times (Figure 12-7(b)), which provides a quick visual check to see whether the IV is infusing on time as prescribed. These labels are attached to the IV bag and indicate the start and stop times of the infusion. They also provide an indication of how the IV should be progressing. Each hour, from the start time to the stop time, the nurse should mark the label at the level where the solution should be. For convenience, stock IV bags may be supplied with custom labels with premarked time intervals (see the left side of Figure 12-7(b)). The hourly intervals are marked for litre bags infusing over 6, 8, 10, and 12 hours. Nurses may also use plain tape and mark the hourly time intervals manually—the right side of Figure 12-7(b) shows an infusion tape adhered to a litre IV with a flow rate set at 25 gtt/min. The nurse intends to infuse the 1 L in 10 hours at 100 mL/h. Each hour is marked on the tape, beginning at 0700 when the IV started and ending at 1700 when the IV should be complete.

Page: 1 of 1 DATE: 11/10/xx through

Correct	I.V. Order	Rate	Time	Initial	Site / Infusion Port	Pump / Other	Tubing Change
✓	D_5 ½ NS	100 mL/h	0900	BS	LH / PIV	☐✓	✓
					/	☐	
					/	☐	
					/	☐	

CIRCULATORY ACCESS SITE

Time	Gauge	Length	Type	Site	# Attempts	Dressing Change	Site Condition	IV Lock	Initial	Time Catheter D/C	Intact	Site Condition	Reason Code	Initial
0800	22	1½″	I	LH	1	✓	0	☐	BS					
								☐						
								☐						
								☐						

Type:
I - Insyte
B - Butterfly
C - Cathlon
CVC - CVC
T - Tunnelled
IP - Implanted Port
PICC - PICC
A - Arterial Line
SG - Swan Ganz
DL - Dual Lumen Peripheral
UAC - UAC
UVC - UVC

Site:
L - Left
R - Right
H - Hand
FA - Forearm
UA - Upper Arm
SC - Subclavian
C - Chest
A - Antecubital
F - Femoral
J - Jugular
FT - Foot
S - Scalp
U - Umbilical
RA - Radial

Dressing Change:
T - Transparent
A - Air Occlusive
B - Bandaid
PR - Pressure Dressing

Reason Code:
1 - Infiltrate
2 - Physician Order
3 - Client Removed
4 - Clotted
5 - Phlebitis
6 - Site Rotation
7 - Leaking
8 - Positional
9 - Not Patent
10 - Family Refused
Other:
D - Dial-a-flow

Infusion Port:
PIV - Peripheral IV
CVC - CVC
SG - Swan Ganz
D - Distal
M - Middle
P - Proximal
R - Red
BL - Blue
V - Venous
S - Sideport
AN - Access Needle
A - Arterial

Site Condition:
0
1+
2+
3+
4+
5+

Tubing Change:
P - Primary
S - Secondary
E - Extension
T - 3 Way Stopcock
H - Hemodynamic

ALLERGIES: NKA

Initial / Signature - Circulatory Access Site(s) checked hourly.
BS / B. Swart, RN

Reconciled by:

Smith, James 43y M
Dr. Jones Medical Service
Admitted 08-10-xx Rm 237-1
Adm. # 6634297

IV ADMINISTRATION RECORD

602-0203 (2-94)dlg)MPC#32258)

Cengage Learning

FIGURE 12-10 IV Administration Record

ELECTRONICALLY REGULATED IVs

Usually, IV solutions are regulated electronically by an infusion device, or an IV pump. IV infusion pumps can deliver IV infusion therapy continuously, intermittently, or on command (as in patient-controlled analgesia, for example). The use of an electronic IV pump is determined by the need to strictly

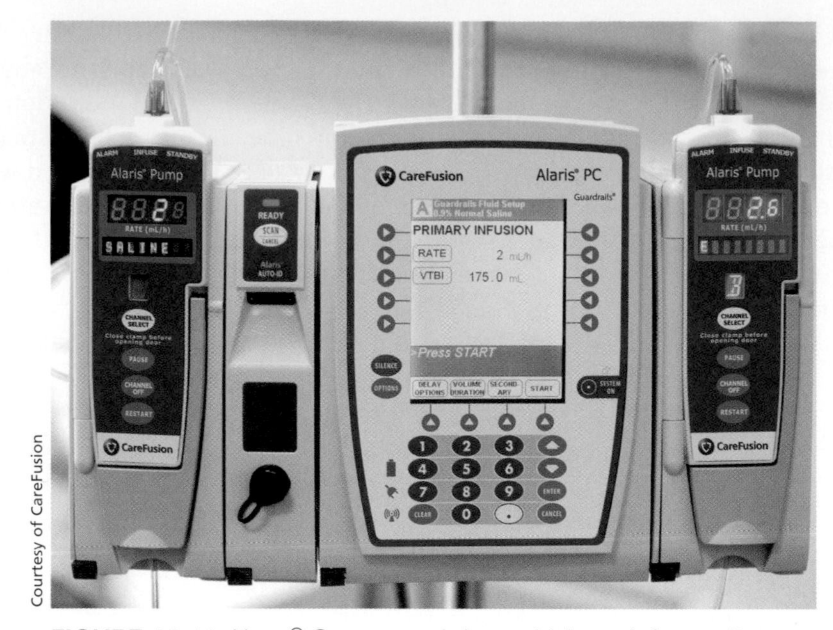

Courtesy of CareFusion

FIGURE 12-11 Alaris® System with Large Volume Infusion Pumps and Auto-ID Module for Medication Administration (Primary Infusion Pump and Two Secondary Pumps)

regulate the IV. Manufacturers supply special volumetric tubing that must be used with their infusion pumps. This special tubing ensures accurate, consistent IV infusions. Each device can be set for a specific flow rate and will set off an alarm when this rate is interrupted. Electronic units today are powered by direct current (from a wall outlet) as well as an internal rechargeable battery. The battery takes over when the unit is unplugged, to allow for portability and patient ambulation.

Infusion pumps represent significant threats to patient safety because various performance problems have resulted in overinfusion, underinfusion, and delays in therapy administration. The authors of the Canadian Adverse Events Study (2004) determined that events associated with drug or other fluid delivery were the second most common type of adverse event.

A key Patient Safety Goal from Accreditation Canada is to ensure the safe administration of parenteral medications. The related Required Organizational Practices (ROPs) require documentation and evidence for continuous effective training on all infusion pumps. An independent double-check by a second practitioner is recommended on initiation of infusion, change in infusion rate, and change of infusion bag for high-alert medications.

Infusion pumps do not rely on gravity but maintain the flow by displacing fluid at the prescribed rate. Resistance to flow within the system causes positive pressure in relation to the flow rate. The nurse or other user may preset a pressure alarm threshold. When the pressure sensed by the device reaches this threshold, the device stops pumping and sets off an alarm. The amount of change in pressure that results from infiltration or phlebitis may be insufficient to reach the alarm threshold. Therefore, users should not expect the device to stop infusing in the presence of these conditions. Infusion systems are becoming increasingly more sophisticated, designed with more safety features to reduce patient safety incidents and improve the dosing and rate of infusions. Accreditation Canada requires demonstration of infusion pump competency on an ongoing basis.

New pumps (e.g., "smart pumps") feature dose error reduction systems that include institution-defined drug lists, with standard drug concentrations and dose limits that are programmed into the pumps in an effort to improve the safety of IV medication administration.

A *syringe pump* or module is a type of electronic infusion pump (see Figures 12(a) and (b)), which is used to infuse fluids or medications directly from a syringe. It is most often used in the neonatal and pediatric areas, when small volumes of medication are delivered at low rates. It is also used in anaesthesia, hospice, labour and delivery, and critical care when the drug cannot be mixed with other solutions or medications or to reduce the volume of diluent delivered to the patient. Syringe pumps can deliver in up to 16 different modes, including millilitres per hour, volume/time, dose or body weight mode, mass modes such as units per hour, and other specialty modes.

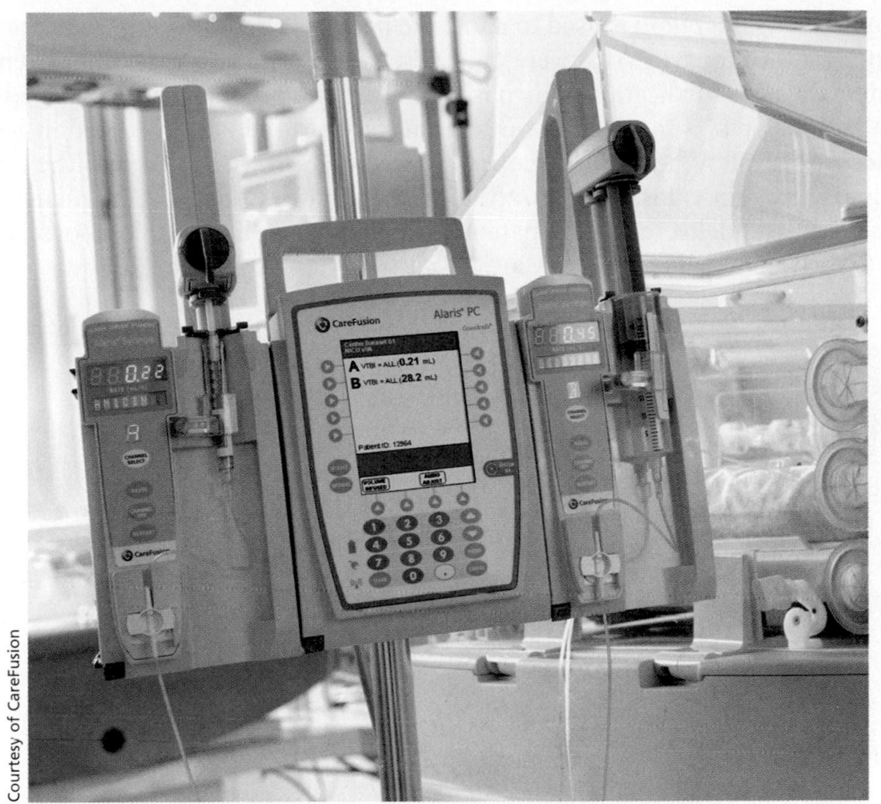

Courtesy of CareFusion

FIGURE 12-12(a) Alaris® System with Syringe Module Used in Neonatal Unit

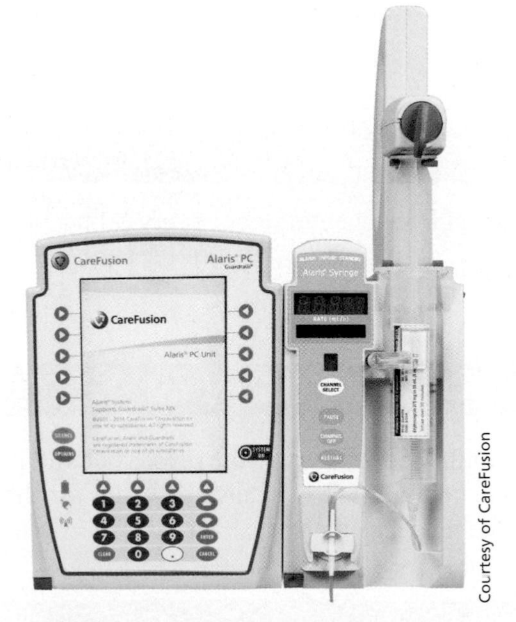

Courtesy of CareFusion

FIGURE 12-12(b) Syringe Monitor: Referred to as an Integrated Platform Designed for Infusions and Patient Monitoring

A *patient-controlled analgesia pump* is used to allow the patient to self-administer IV medication to control postoperative and other types of severe pain (see Figure 12-13 as part of a system module). The prescriber orders the pain medication, which is contained in a prefilled syringe locked securely in the IV pump. The patient presses the control button and receives the pain medication immediately. The dose, frequency, and a safety "lockout" time are ordered and programmed into the pump, which delivers an individual therapeutic dose. The pump stores information about the frequency and dosage of the drug requested by and delivered to the patient. The nurse can display this information to document and evaluate pain management effectiveness.

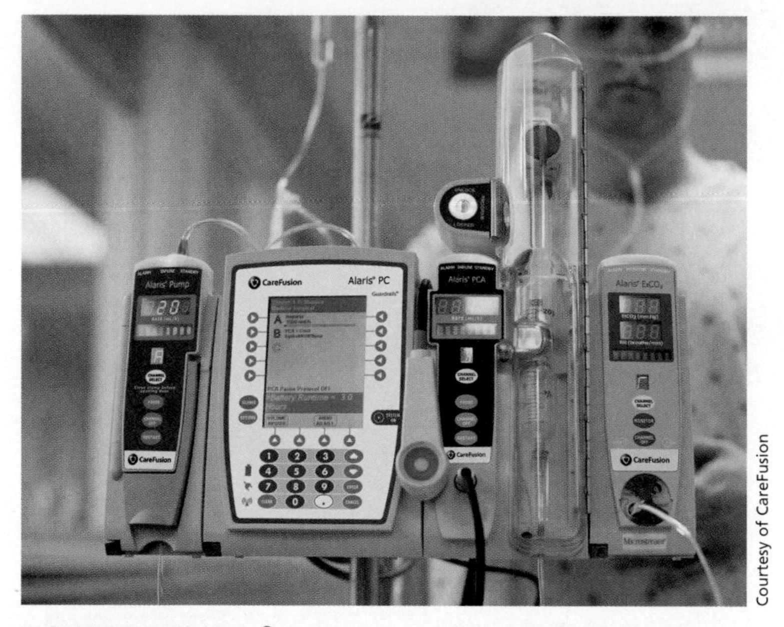

Courtesy of CareFusion

FIGURE 12-13 Alaris® System with PCA (Patient-Controlled Analgesia) Module, Pump Module for Use as Primary and Secondary Infusions, and Physiological Respiratory Monitoring Modules

CAUTION

All electronic infusion devices must be monitored frequently (at least every 30 minutes to 1 hour) to ensure proper and safe functioning. Check the policy in your facility.

CALCULATING FLOW RATES FOR INFUSION PUMPS IN mL/h

When an electronic infusion pump is used, the IV volume is ordered by the prescriber and programmed into the device by the nurse. These devices are regulated in mL/h. Usually, the order for the IV volume to be delivered is provided in mL/h. If not, the nurse must calculate it.

RULE

To regulate an IV volume by electronic infusion pump calibrated in millilitres per hour, calculate

$$\frac{\text{Total mL ordered}}{\text{Total h ordered}} = \text{mL/h (rounded to a whole number or tenths, depending on equipment)}$$

CAUTION

Some IV pumps are capable of delivering IV fluids in tenths of a mL. Check the equipment you have available before deciding to **round flow rates to whole mL/h**. For this text, it is assumed that the equipment available is programmable in whole mL unless directed otherwise.

Example:

Order: *D_5W 250 mL IV over the next 2 h by infusion pump*

Step 1 Think The pump is set by the rate of millilitres per hour. So, if 250 mL is to be infused in 2 hours, how much will be infused in 1 hour? 125 mL will be infused in 1 hour; the pump should be set at 125 mL per hour.

Step 2 Calculate Use the formula:

$$\frac{\text{Total mL ordered}}{\text{Total h ordered}} = \text{mL/h}$$

$$\frac{\overset{125}{\cancel{250}}\text{ mL}}{\underset{1}{\cancel{2}}\text{ h}} = \frac{125\text{ mL}}{1\text{ h}}$$

Therefore, set the pump at 125 mL per hour (125 mL/h).

In most cases, it is easy to calculate mL/h by dividing total millilitres by total hours. However, an IV with medication added or an IVPB may be ordered to be administered in *less than 1 hour* by an electronic infusion device, but the pump must still be set in mL/h.

RULE

$$\frac{\textbf{Total mL ordered}}{\textbf{Total } \cancel{\textbf{min}} \textbf{ ordered}} \times 60\ \cancel{\text{min}}/\text{h} = \text{mL/h}$$ **(rounded to a whole number or tenths depending on equipment). Notice that min cancel out.**

Example:

Order: *ampicillin 500 mg IV in 50 mL $D_5\frac{1}{2}$NS in 30 min by infusion pump*

Step 1 Think The infusion pump is set at the rate of mL/h. If 50 mL is to be infused in 30 minutes, then 100 mL will be infused in 60 minutes because 100 mL is twice as much as 50 mL and 60 minutes is twice as much as 30 minutes. Set the rate of the pump at 100 mL/h to infuse 50 mL/30 minutes.

Step 2 Calculate $$\frac{\text{Total mL ordered}}{\text{Total min ordered}} \times 60\text{ min/h} = \text{mL/h}$$

$$\frac{50\text{ mL}}{\underset{1}{\cancel{30}}\ \cancel{\text{min}}} \times \frac{\overset{2}{\cancel{60}}\ \cancel{\text{min}}}{1\text{ h}} = 100\text{ mL/h}$$

CAUTION

Typical values of mL/h to expect in calculations are in the range of 50 to 200 mL/h. Use this guideline as part of checking for reasonable answers.

QUICK REVIEW

For electronic infusion regulation,

- $\frac{\text{Total mL ordered}}{\text{Total h ordered}} = \text{mL/h}$
- If the infusion time is less than 1 hour, then $\frac{\text{Total mL ordered}}{\text{Total min ordered}} \times 60 \text{ min/h} = \text{mL/h}$
- **Round mL/h to a whole number or tenths, depending on equipment.**

REVIEW SET 12-3

Calculate the flow rate at which you will program the electronic infusion pump for the following IV orders.

1. *D_5W 1 L IV to infuse in 10 h*

   Flow rate: ________ mL/h

2. *NS 1800 mL IV to infuse in 15 h*

   Flow rate: ________ mL/h

3. *D_5W 2000 mL IV in 24 h*

   Flow rate: ________ mL/h

4. *NS 100 mL IVPB in 30 min*

   Flow rate: ________ mL/h

5. *An antibiotic in 30 mL D_5W IV in 15 min*

   Flow rate: ________ mL/h

6. *NS 2.5 L IV in 20 h*

   Flow rate: ________ mL/h

7. *D_5LR 500 mL IV in 4 h*

   Flow rate: ________ mL/h

8. *0.45% 600 mL NaCl IV in 3 h*

   Flow rate: ________ mL/h

9. An *antibiotic in 150 mL D_5W IV in 2 h*

   Flow rate: ________ mL/h

10. *NS 3 L IV in 24 h*

    Flow rate: ________ mL/h

11. *LR 1.5 L Injection IV in 24 h*

    Flow rate: ________ mL/h

12. *$D_{10}W$ 540 mL IV in 10 h*

    Flow rate: ________ mL/h

13. *D_5W 750 mL IV in 5 h*

    Flow rate: ________ mL/h

14. *D_5NS 1.5 L IV in 12 h*

    Flow rate: ________ mL/h

15. *D_5 0.45% 680 mL NaCl IV in 9 h*

    Flow rate: ________ mL/h

Check your work! Answers to all Review Sets are provided at the end of each chapter. Worked solutions for selected Review Sets are also available there.

MANUALLY REGULATED IVs

As a backup to an IV pump or when an electronic infusion pump is not available, the nurse can use a standard, straight gravity-flow IV system to administer fluids, medications, and nutrients. In this case, the nurse must manually regulate the IV flow rate. To do this, the nurse must calculate the ordered IV rate based on a certain *number of drops per minute (gtt/min)*. This actually represents the ordered mL/h, as will be seen in the calculation.

The number of drops falling per minute into the IV drip chamber (Figures 12-14 and 12-15) is counted and regulated by opening or closing the roller clamp. Place your digital or analogue watch with a second hand at the level of the drip chamber and count the drops as they fall during a 1-minute period or fraction thereof (called the *watch count*). This manual, gravity-flow rate depends on the IV tubing calibration called the *drop factor.*

RULE

Drop factor = gtt/mL

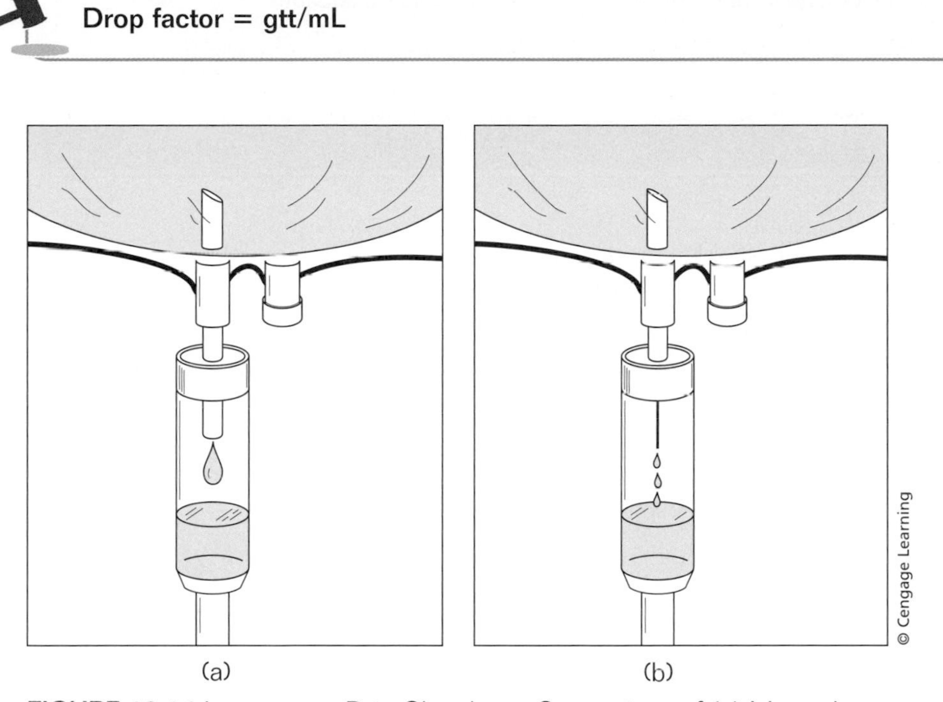

FIGURE 12-14 Intravenous Drip Chambers. Comparison of (a) Macrodrops and (b) Microdrops

The drop factor is the number of drops per millilitre (gtt/mL) a particular IV tubing set will deliver. It is determined by the size of the tubing or needle releasing the drops into the drip chamber (see Figure 12-14). The drip factor is written on the IV tubing package and varies according to the manufacturer of the IV equipment. The wider tubing delivers larger drops (macrodrops); therefore, there are fewer drops in 1 mL (Figure 12-14(a)). The standard macrodrop tubing is available in sizes that deliver a drop factor of 10 or 15 gtt/mL. The small needle delivers tiny drops; therefore, there are more drops in 1 mL (Figure 12-14(b)). All microdrop tubing delivers 60 gtt/mL. Hospitals typically stock one macrodrop tubing for routine adult IV administration and the microdrop tubing for situations requiring more exact measurement, or to manage a slow infusion rate.

Figure 12-14 compares macrodrop and microdrops. See Figure 12-15 for an illustration of the size and number of drops in 1 mL for each drop factor. Notice that the fewer the number of drops per millilitre, the larger the actual drop size.

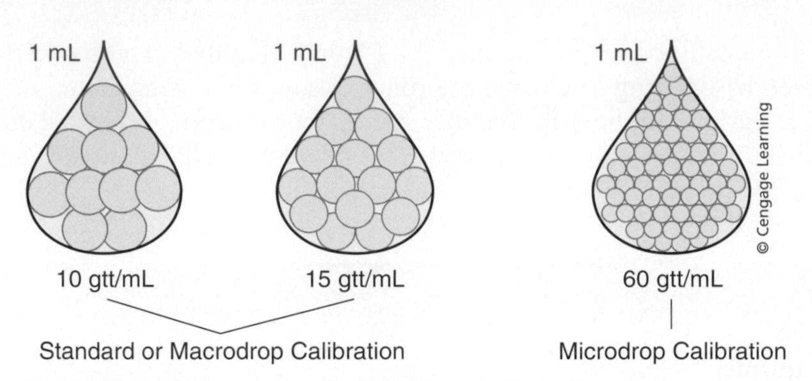

FIGURE 12-15 Comparison of Calibrated Drop Factors

QUICK REVIEW

- Drop factor = gtt/mL
- The drop factor is stated on the IV tubing package.
- Macrodrop factor: 10 or 15 gtt/mL
- Microdrop factor: 60 gtt/mL

REVIEW SET 12-4

Identify the drop factor calibration of the IV tubing shown.

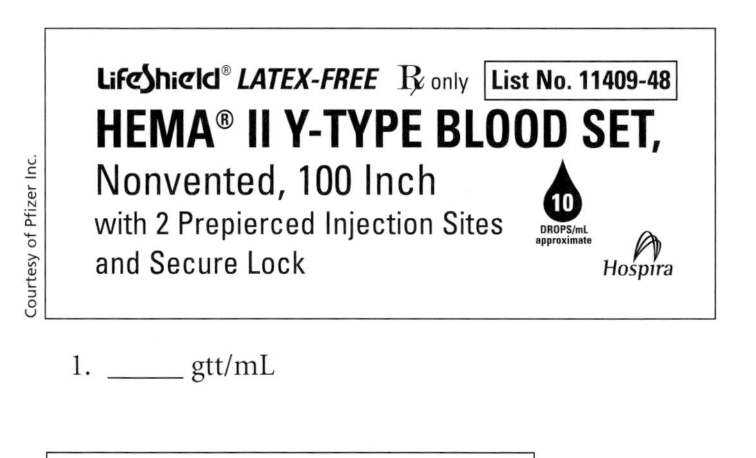

LifeShield® LATEX-FREE ℞ only List No. 11409-48
HEMA® II Y-TYPE BLOOD SET,
Nonvented, 100 Inch
with 2 Prepierced Injection Sites
and Secure Lock
10
DROPS/mL approximate
Hospira
Courtesy of Pfizer Inc.

1. _____ gtt/mL

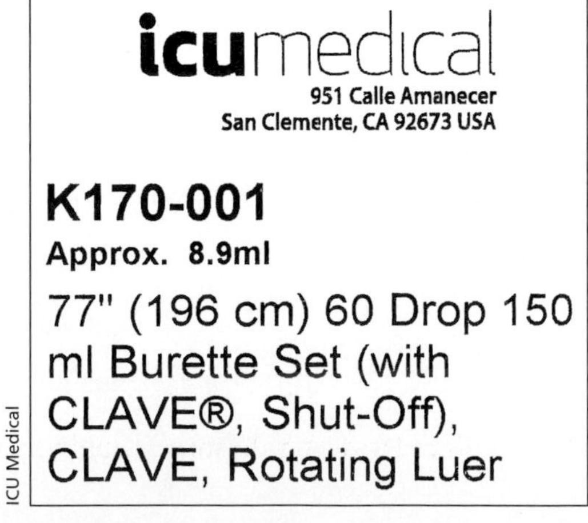

icumedical
951 Calle Amanecer
San Clemente, CA 92673 USA
K170-001
Approx. 8.9ml
77" (196 cm) 60 Drop 150 ml Burette Set (with CLAVE®, Shut-Off), CLAVE, Rotating Luer
ICU Medical

2. _____ gtt/mL

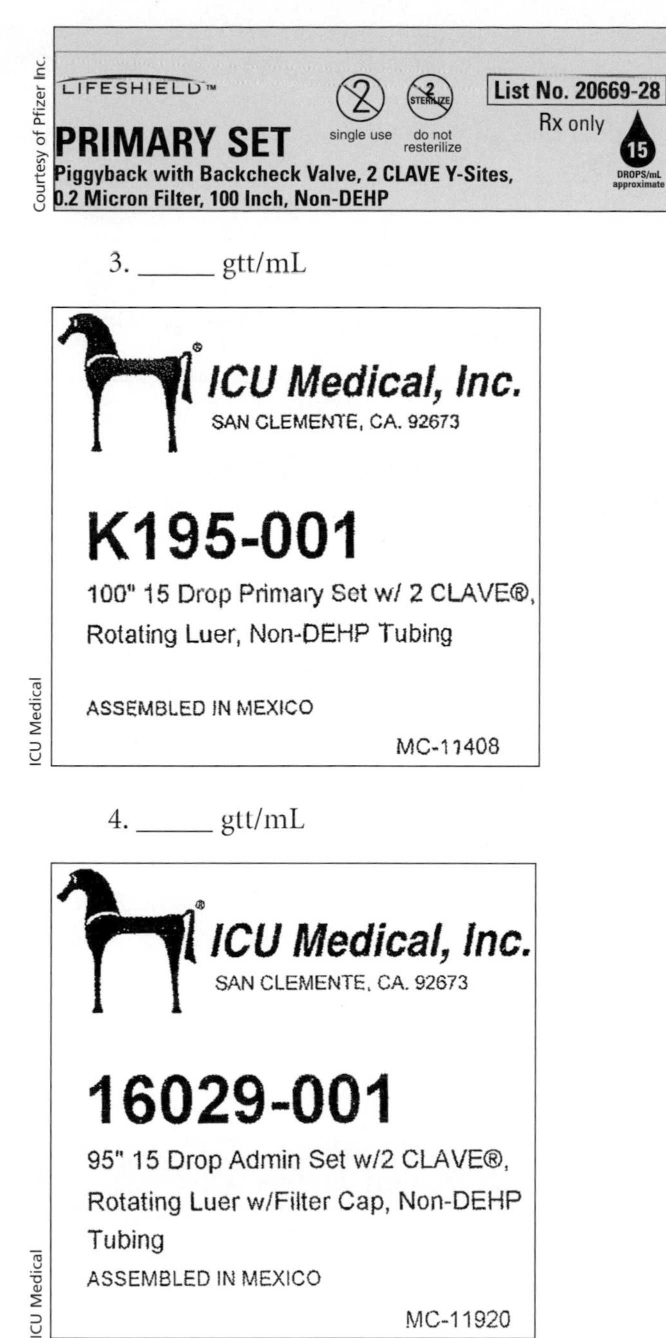

3. ______ gtt/mL

4. ______ gtt/mL

5. ______ gtt/mL

Check your work! Answers to all Review Sets are provided at the end of each chapter. Worked solutions for selected Review Sets are also available there.

CALCULATING FLOW RATES FOR MANUALLY REGULATED IVs IN gtt/min

In this section, you will learn two methods to calculate IV flow rate for manually regulated IVs: the formula method and the shortcut method.

The Formula Method

The formula method can be used to determine the flow rate in drops per minute (*gtt/min*).

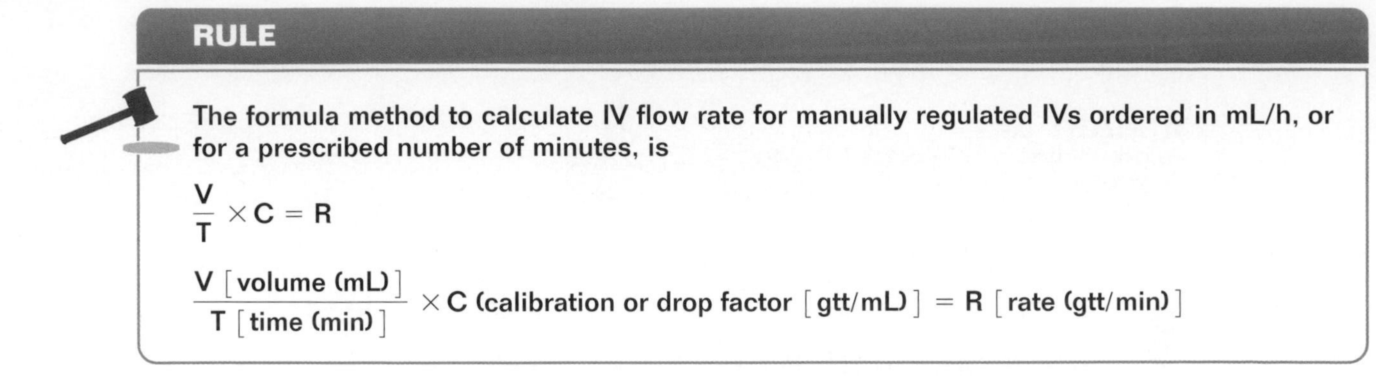

RULE

The formula method to calculate IV flow rate for manually regulated IVs ordered in mL/h, or for a prescribed number of minutes, is

$$\frac{V}{T} \times C = R$$

$$\frac{V\ [\text{volume (mL)}]}{T\ [\text{time (min)}]} \times C\ (\text{calibration or drop factor}\ [\text{gtt/mL}]) = R\ [\text{rate (gtt/min)}]$$

In this formula,

V = *volume* per hour to be infused designated in mL; ordered by the prescriber (primary infusion) or recommended by the pharmacist, drug reference guide, or drug insert (e.g., for an IVPB medication)

T = *time required to infuse V*; converted to minutes; ordered by the prescriber (primary infusion) or recommended by the pharmacist, drug reference guide, or drug insert (e.g., for an IVPB medication)

C = *calibration* of tubing (drop factor) in gtt/mL; noted on package

R = *rate* of flow in gtt/min. Think: The unknown is the "watch count."

The rate of IV fluid and IV medications is expressed as a specific volume to be infused in a certain time period. Most IV fluid orders are written as X mL/h, which means X mL in 60 minutes. However, some IV medications are administered in less than 1 hour (e.g., over 30 minutes).

MATH TIP

When using the formula method to calculate IV flow rates, carry calculations to one decimal place. Round gtt/min to the nearest whole number because you can watch-count only whole drops.

ALERT

Always round drops per minute (gtt/min) to the nearest whole number.

Some examples of how to calculate the flow rate or "watch count" in gtt/min follow.

Example 1:

Order: *D_5W IV at 125 mL/h.* The infusion set is calibrated for a drop factor of 10 gtt/mL. Calculate the IV flow rate in gtt/min. Notice that the mL cancel out, leaving *gtt/min.*

$$\frac{V}{T} \times C = \frac{125\text{ mL}}{60\text{ min}} \times 10\text{ gtt/mL} = \frac{125\ \cancel{\text{mL}}}{\underset{6}{\cancel{60}}\text{ min}} \times \frac{\overset{1}{\cancel{10}}\text{ gtt}}{1\ \cancel{\text{mL}}} = \frac{125\text{ gtt}}{6\text{ min}} = 20.8\text{ gtt/min} = 21\text{ gtt/min}$$

Use your watch to count the drops, and adjust the roller clamp to deliver 21 gtt/min.

Example 2:

Order: *Lactated Ringer's IV at 150 mL/h.* The drop factor is 15 gtt/mL.

$$\frac{V}{T} \times C = \frac{150\ \cancel{\text{mL}}}{\underset{4}{\cancel{60}}\text{ min}} \times \overset{1}{\cancel{15}}\text{ gtt/}\cancel{\text{mL}} = \frac{150\text{ gtt}}{4\text{ min}} = 37.5\text{ gtt/min} = 38\text{ gtt/min}$$

Example 3:

Order: *ampicillin 500 mg IV in 100 mL of NS, infuse over 20 min*

The drop factor is 10 gtt/mL. Notice that the time is less than 1 hour. Also notice that the 500 mg is not included in the calculation because it is the dose of ampicillin dissolved in the IV fluid. Only *the total volume of 100 mL* is needed to complete the calculation.

$$\frac{V}{T} \times C = \frac{100\ \cancel{mL}}{20\ min} \times 10\ gtt/\cancel{mL} = \frac{1000\ gtt}{20\ min} = 50\ gtt/min$$

MATH TIP

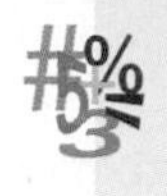

When the IV drop factor is 60 gtt/mL (microdrip sets), the flow rate in gtt/min is the same as the volume ordered in mL/h.

Example 4:

Order: *D_5W NS IV at 50 mL/h.* The drop factor is 60 gtt/mL. Notice that the order, 50 mL/h, is *the same as the flow rate* of 50 gtt/min when the drop factor is 60 gtt/mL.

$$\frac{V}{T} \times C = \frac{50\ \cancel{mL}}{\cancel{60}\ min} \times \cancel{60}\ gtt/\cancel{mL} = 50\ gtt/min$$

Sometimes, the prescriber will order a total IV volume to be infused over a total number of hours. In such cases, first calculate the mL/h (rounded to tenths), then calculate gtt/min (rounded to a whole number).

RULE

The formula method to calculate IV flow rate for manually regulated IVs ordered in total volume and total hours is

Step 1 $\frac{\text{Total mL}}{\text{Total hours}} = \text{mL/h}$

Step 2 $\frac{V}{T} \times C = R$

Example:

Order: *NS IV 3000 mL/24 h.* The drop factor is 15 gtt/min.

Step 1 $\frac{\text{Total mL}}{\text{Total h}} = \frac{3000\ mL}{24\ h} = 125\ mL/h$

Step 2 $\frac{V}{T} \times C = R$:

$$\frac{125\ mL}{60\ min} \times 15\ gtt/mL = \frac{125\ \cancel{mL}}{\underset{4}{\cancel{60}}\ min} \times \frac{\overset{1}{\cancel{15}}\ gtt}{1\ \cancel{mL}} = \frac{125\ gtt}{4\ min} = 31.3\ gtt/min = 31\ gtt/min$$

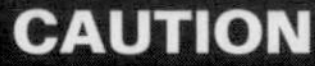

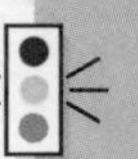

Typical values of gtt/min to expect in calculations are in the range of 20 to 100 gtt/min. Use this guideline as part of checking for reasonable answers.

QUICK REVIEW

- The formula method to calculate the flow rate, or watch count, in gtt/min for manually regulated IV rates ordered in mL/h or mL/min is

$$\frac{\text{Volume (mL)}}{\text{Time (min)}} \times \text{Calibration or drop factor (gtt/mL)} = \text{Rate (gtt/min)}$$

- When total volume and total hours are ordered, first calculate mL/h.
- When the drop factor calibration is 60 (microdrop sets), then the flow rate in gtt/min is the same as the ordered volume in mL/h.
- Round gtt/min to a whole number. Only whole drops can be counted.

REVIEW SET 12-5

1. State the rule for the formula method to calculate IV flow rate in gtt/min when mL/h is known. ____________________

Calculate the flow rate or watch count in gtt/min.

2. Order: *D_5W 3 000 mL IV at 125 mL/h*

   Drop factor: 10 gtt/mL

   ________ gtt/min

3. Order: *LR 250 mL IV at 50 mL/h*

   Drop factor: 60 gtt/mL

   ________ gtt/min

4. Order: *NS 100 mL bolus IV to infuse in 60 min*

   Drop factor: 10 gtt/mL

   ________ gtt/min

5. Order: *$D_5 \frac{1}{2}$ NS IV with 20 mEq KCl per litre to run at 25 mL/h*

   Drop factor: 60 gtt/mL

   ________ gtt/min

6. Order: *Two 500-mL units of whole blood IV to be infused in 4 h*

   Drop factor: 10 gtt/mL

   ________ gtt/min

7. Order: *D5 $\frac{1}{4}$ NS 1 L to infuse in 6 h*

   Drop factor: 15 gtt/mL

   ________ gtt/min

8. Order: *D_5NS IV at 150 mL/h*

   Drop factor: 10 gtt/mL

   ________ gtt/min

9. Order: *NS 150 mL bolus IV to infuse in 45 min*

   Drop factor: 15 gtt/mL

   ________ gtt/min

10. Order: *D_5W antibiotic solution 80 mL IV to infuse in 60 min*

    Drop factor: 60 gtt/mL

    ________ gtt/min

11. Order: *packed red blood cells 480 mL IV to infuse in 4 h*

    Drop factor: 10 gtt/mL

    ________ gtt/min

12. Order: *D_5W IV at 120 mL/h*

    Drop factor: 15 gtt/mL

    ________ gtt/min

13. Order: *D_5 0.33% NaCl IV at 50 mL/h*

    Drop factor: 10 gtt/mL

    ________ gtt/min

14. Order: *2500 mL LR IV at 165 mL/h*

    Drop factor: 10 gtt/mL

    ________ gtt/min

15. Order: *3500 mL D_5LR IV to run at 160 mL/h*

    Drop factor: 15 gtt/mL

    ________ gtt/min

Check your work! Answers to all Review Sets are provided at the end of each chapter. Worked solutions for selected Review Sets are also available there.

The Shortcut Method

By converting the volume and time in the formula method to mL/h (or mL/60 min), you can use a shortcut to calculate flow rate. This shortcut is derived from the drop factor (C), which cancels out each time and reduces the 60 minutes (T). You are left with the *drop factor constant.* Look at these examples.

Example 1:

Administer *normal saline 1000 mLIV at 125 mL/h* with a microdrop infusion set calibrated for *60 gtt/mL*. Use the formula $\frac{V}{T} \times C = R$.

$$\frac{V}{T} \times C = \frac{125\ \cancel{mL}}{\overset{}{\cancel{60}}\underset{1}{}\ min} \times \overset{1}{\cancel{60}}\ gtt/\cancel{mL} = \frac{125\ gtt}{\textcircled{1}\ min} = 125\ gtt/min$$

The drop factor constant for an infusion set with 60 gtt/mL is 1. Therefore, to administer 125 mL/h, set the flow rate at 125 gtt/min. Recall that when the drop factor is 60, then gtt/min = mL/h.

Example 2:

Administer *125 mL/h IV* with a *10 gtt/mL* infusion set.

$$\frac{V}{T} \times C = \frac{125\ \cancel{mL}}{\underset{6}{\cancel{60}}\ min} \times \overset{1}{\cancel{10}}\ gtt/\cancel{mL} = \frac{125\ gtt}{\textcircled{6}\ min} = 20.8\ gtt/min = 21\ gtt/min$$

Drop factor constant = 6

Each drop factor constant is obtained by dividing 60 by the drop factor calibration from the infusion set.

REMEMBER

Drop Factor	Drop Factor Constant
10 gtt/mL	$\frac{60}{10} = 6$
15 gtt/mL	$\frac{60}{15} = 4$
60 gtt/mL	$\frac{60}{60} = 1$

Most hospitals consistently use infusion equipment manufactured by one company. Each manufacturer typically supplies one macrodrop and one microdrop system. Once you become familiar with the supplier used where you work, the shortcut method will be practical, quick, and simple to use.

RULE

The shortcut method to calculate IV flow rate is

$$\frac{\text{mL/h}}{\text{Drop factor constant}} = \text{gtt/min}$$

Review the following three examples that use the shortcut method.

Example 1:

Order: *D_5W IV at 125 mL/h.* The infusion set is calibrated for a drop factor of 10 gtt/mL. Drop factor constant: 6

$$\frac{\text{mL/h}}{\text{Drop factor constant}} = \text{gtt/min}$$

$$\frac{125\text{ mL/h}}{6} = 20.8\text{ gtt/min} = 21\text{ gtt/min}$$

Example 2:

Order: *LR IV at 150 mL/h.* The drop factor is 15 gtt/mL. Drop factor constant: 4

$$\frac{\text{mL/h}}{\text{Drop factor constant}} = \text{gtt/min}$$

$$\frac{150\text{ mL/h}}{4} = 37.5\text{ gtt/min} = 38\text{ gtt/min}$$

Example 3:

Order: *D_5W NS IV at 50 mL/h.* The drop factor is 60 gtt/mL. Drop factor constant: 1

$$\frac{\text{mL/h}}{\text{Drop factor constant}} = \text{gtt/min}$$

$$\frac{50\text{ mL/h}}{1} = 50\text{ gtt/min}$$

Remember, when the drop factor is 60 (microdrop), set the flow rate at the same gtt/min as the mL/h.

CAUTION

For the shortcut method to work, the rate needs to be written in mL/h. The shortcut method will not work if the time is less than 1 hour or is calculated in minutes, such as 30 or 90 minutes.

QUICK REVIEW

- The drop factor constant is 60 divided by the drop factor.

Drop Factor	Drop Factor Constant
10 gtt/mL	6
15 gtt/mL	4
60 gtt/mL	1 → Set the flow rate at the same gtt/min as the mL/h.

- $\frac{\text{mL/h}}{\text{Drop factor constant}} = \text{gtt/min}$

REVIEW SET 12-6

1. The drop factor constant is derived by dividing ________ by the drop factor calibration.

Determine the drop factor constant for each of the following infusion sets.

2. 60 gtt/mL ________
3. 15 gtt/mL ________
4. 10 gtt/mL ________
5. State the rule for the shortcut method to calculate the IV flow rate in gtt/min. ________

____

Calculate the IV flow rate in gtt/min using the shortcut method.

6. Order: *D_5W 1000 mL IV to infuse at 200 mL/h*

   Drop factor: 15 gtt/mL

   Flow rate: ________ gtt/min

7. Order: *D_5W 750 mL IV to infuse at 125 mL/h*

   Drop factor: 15 gtt/mL

   Flow rate: ________ gtt/min

8. Order: *D_5W 0.45% Saline 500 mL IV to infuse at 165 mL/h*

   Drop factor: 10 gtt/mL

   Flow rate: ________ gtt/min

9. Order: *NS 2 L IV to infuse at 60 mL/h with microdrop infusion set of 60 gtt/mL*

   Flow rate: ________ gtt/min

10. Order: *D_5W 400 mL IV to infuse at 50 mL/h*

    Drop factor: 10 gtt/mL

    Flow rate: ________ gtt/min

11. Order: *NS 3 L IV to infuse at 125 mL/h*

    Drop factor: 15 gtt/mL

    Flow rate: ________ gtt/min

12. Order: *D_5LR 500 mL IV to infuse in 6 h*

    Drop factor: 10 gtt/mL

    Flow rate: ________ gtt/min

13. Order: *0.45% NaCl 0.5 L IV to infuse in 20 h*

    Drop factor: 60 gtt/mL

    Flow rate: ________ gtt/min

14. Order: *D_5 0.33% NaCl 650 mL IV to infuse in 10 h*

    Drop factor: 10 gtt/mL

    Flow rate: ________ gtt/min

15. Order: *$\frac{2}{3}$; $\frac{1}{3}$ 250 mL IV to infuse in 5 h*

    Drop factor: 60 gtt/mL

    Flow rate: ________ gtt/min

Check your work! Answers to all Review Sets are provided at the end of each chapter. Worked solutions for selected Review Sets are also available there.

CHECK POINT

To program electronic IV infusion devices, you learned to calculate mL/h. To watch-count manually regulated IVs, you learned to calculate gtt/min, including a shortcut method. Further, you now know how to calculate the supply dosage of certain IV solutes. These important topics warrant additional reinforcement and review.

QUICK REVIEW

- When regulating IV flow rate for an electronic infusion device, calculate mL/h.
- When calculating IV flow rate to regulate an IV manually, calculate mL/h, find the drop factor, and calculate gtt/min by using the

Formula method: $\frac{V}{T} \times C = R$

or Shortcut method: $\frac{\text{mL/h}}{\text{Drop factor constant}} = \text{gtt/min}$

REVIEW SET 12-7

Calculate the IV flow rate for these manually regulated IV administrations.

1. Order: *0.45% NaCl 3000 mL IV for 24 h*

   Drop factor: 15 gtt/mL

   Flow rate: ________ mL/h

   Flow rate: ________ gtt/min

2. Order: *D_5W 200 mL IV to run at 100 mL/h*

   Drop factor: 60 gtt/mL

   Flow rate: ________ gtt/min

3. Order: *$D_5 \frac{1}{3}$ NS 800 mL IV for 8 h*

   Drop factor: 10 gtt/mL

   Flow rate: ________ mL/h

   Flow rate: ________ gtt/min

4. Order: *NS IV 1000 mL at 50 mL/h*

   Drop factor: 60 gtt/mL

   Flow rate: ________ gtt/min

5. Order: *D_5W 1500 mL IV for 12 h*

   Drop factor: 15 gtt/mL

   Flow rate: ________ mL/h

   Flow rate: ________ gtt/min

6. Order: *theophylline 0.5 g IV in 250 mL D_5W to run over 2 h*

   Drop factor: 60 gtt/mL

   Flow rate: ________ mL/h

   Flow rate: ________ gtt/min

7. Order: *D_5 0.45% NaCl 2500 mL IV at 105 mL/h*

   Drop factor: 10 gtt/mL

   Flow rate: ________ gtt/min

8. Order: *D_5 0.45% NaCl 500 mL IV at 100 mL/h*

   Drop factor: 10 gtt/mL

   Flow rate: ________ gtt/min

9. Order: *NS 1200 mL IV at 150 mL/h*

   Drop factor: 10 gtt/mL

   Flow rate: ________ gtt/min

10. Order: *D_5 0.45% NaCl 1000 mL to infuse over 8 h*

    Drop factor: On electronic infusion pump

    Flow rate: ________ mL/h

Calculate the IV flow rate for these electronically regulated IV administrations.

11. Order: *D_5NS 2000 mL to infuse over 24 h*

    Flow rate: ________ mL/h

12. Order: *LR 500 mL to infuse over 4 h*

    Flow rate: ________ mL/h

13. Order: *100 mL IV antibiotic to infuse in 30 min*

    Flow rate: ________ mL/h

14. Order: *50 mL IV antibiotic to infuse in 20 min*

    Flow rate: ________ mL/h

15. Order: *150 mL IV antibiotic to infuse in 45 min*

    Flow rate: ________ mL/h

What is the total dosage of the solute(s) the patient will receive for each of the following orders?

16. *3000 mL $\frac{1}{2}$ NS IV* NaCl: ________ g
17. *200 mL D_{10} NS IV* D: ________ g NaCl: ________ g
18. *2500 mL NS IV* NaCl: ________ g
19. *650 mL D_5 0.33% NaCl IV* D: ________ g NaCl: ________ g
20. *1000 mL D_5 $\frac{1}{4}$ NS IV* D: ________ g NaCl: ________ g

Check your work! Answers to all Review Sets are provided at the end of each chapter. Worked solutions for selected Review Sets are also available there.

ADJUSTING IV FLOW RATE

IV fluids, particularly those with medications added (called *additives*), are viewed as solutions requiring specific dosages (rates of infusion, in this case). It is the responsibility of the nurse to maintain this rate of flow through careful calculations and close observation at regular intervals. Various circumstances, such as gravity, condition, and movement of the patient, can alter the set flow rate of an IV, causing the IV to run ahead of or behind schedule.

CAUTION

It is not up to the discretion of the nurse to arbitrarily speed up or slow down the flow rate to catch up the IV. This practice can result in serious conditions of overhydration, underhydration, and electrolyte imbalance. Avoid off-schedule IV flow rates by regularly monitoring IVs at least every 30 minutes to 1 hour. Check the institution policy.

During regular monitoring of the IV, if you find that the rate is not progressing as scheduled or is significantly ahead of or behind schedule, the prescriber may need to be notified as warranted by the patient's condition, hospital policy, and good clinical judgment. Some hospital policies allow the flow rate per minute to be adjusted a certain percentage of variation. A rule of thumb is that the flow rate per minute may be adjusted by **up to 25% more or less** than the original rate, depending on the condition of the patient. In such cases, assess the patient. If the patient is stable, recalculate the flow rate to administer the total millilitres remaining over the number of hours remaining of the original order.

RATIONALE FOR PRACTICE

- **Check the institution policy regarding correcting off-schedule IV rates and the percentage of variation allowed. This variation generally should not exceed 25%.**
- **If adjustment is permitted, use the following steps to recalculate the mL/h and gtt/min for the time remaining and the percentage of variation:**

Step 1 $\frac{\text{Remaining volume}}{\text{Remaining hours}} = \text{Recalculated mL/h}$

Step 2 $\frac{V}{T} \times C = \text{gtt/min}$

Step 3 $\frac{\text{Adjusted gtt/min} - \text{Ordered gtt/min}}{\text{Ordered gtt/min}} = \%\ \text{variation}$

The *% variation* will be positive (+) if the administration is slow and the rate needs to be increased, and negative (−) if the administration is too fast and the rate needs to be decreased.

Example 1:

The order is for *D_5W 1000 mL IV at 125 mL/h for 8 h.* The drop factor is 10 gtt/mL, and the IV is correctly set at 21 gtt/min. You would expect that after 4 hours, one-half of the total, or 500 mL, of the solution would be infused ($125\ \text{mL}/\cancel{\text{h}} \times 4\ \cancel{\text{h}} = 500\ \text{mL}$). However, during regular IV monitoring at the fourth hour after starting the IV, you find 600 mL remaining. The rate of flow is *behind schedule*, and the hospital allows a 25% IV flow variation after careful patient assessment and if the patient's condition is stable. The patient is stable, so you decide to calculate a new flow rate for the remaining 600 mL to complete the IV fluid order in the remaining 4 hours.

Step 1 $\frac{\text{Remaining volume}}{\text{Remaining hours}} = \text{Recalculated mL/h}$

$$\frac{600\ \text{mL}}{4\ \text{h}} = 150\ \text{mL/h}$$

Step 2 $\frac{V}{T} \times C = \frac{150\ \cancel{\text{mL}}}{\underset{6}{\cancel{60}}\ \text{min}} \times \overset{1}{\cancel{10}}\ \text{gtt}/\cancel{\text{mL}} = \frac{150\ \text{gtt}}{6\ \text{min}} = 25\ \text{gtt/min (adjusted flow rate)}$

You could also use the shortcut method.

$$\frac{\text{mL/h}}{\text{Drop factor constant}} = \text{gtt/min}$$

$$\frac{150\ \text{mL/h}}{6} = 25\ \text{gtt/min}$$

Step 3 $\frac{\text{Adjusted gtt/min} - \text{Ordered gtt/min}}{\text{Ordered gtt/min}} = \%\ \text{of variation}$

$\frac{25 - 21}{21} = \frac{4}{21} = 0.19 = 19\%$; within the acceptable 25% of variation depending on the institution policy and the patient's condition

Compare 25 gtt/min (in Example 1) with the starting flow rate of 21 gtt/min. You can see now that adjusting the total remaining volume over the total remaining hours slightly changes the flow rate per minute. Most patients can tolerate this small amount of increase per minute over several hours.

However, trying to catch up the lost 100 mL in 1 hour can be dangerous. To infuse an extra 100 mL in 1 hour, with a drop factor of 10 gtt/mL, you would need to speed up the IV to a much faster rate. Calculate what that rate would be.

$$\frac{V}{T} \times C = \frac{100 \not{mL}}{\not{60}_{6} \text{ min}} \times \not{10}^{1} \text{ gtt}/\not{mL} = \frac{100 \text{ gtt}}{6 \text{ min}} = 16.7 \text{ gtt/min} = 17 \text{ gtt/min more than the original rate}$$

To catch up the IV over the next hour, the flow rate would need to be 17 drops per minute faster than the original 21 drops per minute rate. The infusion would need to be set at 17 + 21 = 38 gtt/min for 1 hour and then slowed to the original rate. Such an increase would be $\frac{38 - 21}{21} = \frac{17}{21} = 81\%$ greater than the ordered rate. Changing the flow rate could present a serious problem. **Do not do it! If permitted by institution policy, the flow rate for the remainder of the order must be recalculated when the IV is off-schedule, and should never exceed a 25% adjustment.**

Example 2:

The order is for *LR 500 mL to run over 10 h at 50 mL/h.* The drop factor is 60 gtt/mL and the IV is correctly infusing at 50 gtt/min. It has been $2\frac{1}{2}$ hours, since the IV was started, but there has been no regular IV monitoring. You find 300 mL remaining. Almost one-half of the total volume has already infused in about one-quarter the time. This IV infusion is *ahead of schedule.* You would calculate a new flow rate of 300 mL to complete the IV fluid order in the remaining $7\frac{1}{2}$ hours. The patient would require close assessment for fluid overload.

Step 1 $\frac{\text{Remaining volume}}{\text{Remaining hours}} = \text{Recalculated mL/h}$

$\frac{300 \text{ mL}}{7.5 \text{ h}} = 40 \text{ mL/h}$

Step 2 $\frac{V}{T} \times C = \frac{40 \not{mL}}{\not{60}_{1} \text{ min}} \times \not{60}^{1} \text{ gtt/mL} = 40 \text{ gtt/min (adjusted flow rate)}$

Or, you know when the drop factor is 60, then mL/h = gtt/min.

Step 3 $\frac{\text{Adjusted gtt/min} - \text{Ordered gtt/min}}{\text{Ordered gtt/min}} = \% \text{ of variation}$

$\frac{40 - 50}{50} = \frac{-10}{50} = -0.2 = -20\%$ within the acceptable 25% of variation

Remember, the negative percent of variation (−20%) indicates that the adjusted flow rate will be decreased.

A safe rule is that the recalculated flow rate should not vary from the original rate by more than 25%. If the recalculated rate does vary from the original by more than 25%, contact your supervisor or the prescriber for further instructions. The original order may need to be revised. Regular monitoring helps prevent or minimize this problem.

Patients who require close monitoring for IV fluids will most likely have their IV regulated by an electronic infusion device. Because of the nature of the patient's condition, speeding up or slowing down these IVs, if off-schedule, is not recommended. If an IV regulated by an electronic infusion pump is off-schedule or inaccurate, suspect that the infusion pump may need recalibration. Consult with your supervisor, as appropriate.

QUICK REVIEW

- Regular IV monitoring and patient assessment at least every 30 minutes to 1 hour is important to maintain the prescribed IV flow rate.
- Do not arbitrarily speed up or slow down IV flow rates that are off-schedule.
- Check institution policy regarding adjustment of off-schedule IV flow rates and the percentage of variation allowed. If permitted, a rule of thumb is a maximum 25% variation for patients in stable condition.
- To recalculate off-schedule IV flow rate, use the remaining time and the remaining IV fluid volume:

Step 1 $\frac{\text{Remaining volume}}{\text{Remaining hours}} = \text{Recalculated mL/h}$

Step 2 $\frac{V}{T} \times C = \text{gtt/min}$

Step 3 $\frac{\text{Adjusted gtt/min} - \text{Ordered gtt/min}}{\text{Ordered gtt/min}} = \text{\% variation}$

- Contact the prescriber for a new IV fluid order if the recalculated IV flow rate variation exceeds the allowed variation or if the patient's condition is unstable.
- Carefully monitor patients receiving IV fluids every 30 minutes to 1 hour.
  - Check remaining IV fluids.
  - Check IV flow rate.
  - Observe IV site for complications.
  - Plan ahead for mechanical failures.
  - Place time labels on IV bags.

REVIEW SET 12-8

Calculate the flow rate in drops per minute. Institution policy permits recalculation of IVs when off-schedule, with a maximum variation in rate of 25% for stable patients. Calculate the percentage of variation.

1. Order: *Lactated Ringer's 1500 mL IV for 12 h at 125 mL/h*

   Drop factor: 10 gtt/mL

   Original flow rate: ________ gtt/min

   After 6 hours, there are 850 mL remaining; describe the appropriate nursing action now.

   Time remaining: ________ h

   Recalculated flow rate: ________ mL/h

   Recalculated flow rate: ________ gtt/min

   Variation: ________ %

   Action: ____

2. Order: *Lactated Ringer's 1000 mL IV for 6 h at 167 mL/h*

   Drop factor: 15 gtt/mL

   Original flow rate: ________ gtt/min

After 4 hours, there are 360 mL remaining; describe the appropriate nursing action now.

Time remaining: ________ h

Recalculated flow rate: ________ mL/h

Recalculated flow rate: ________ gtt/min

Variation: ________ %

Action: ____

3. Order: *D_5W 1000 mL IV for 8 h at 125 mL/h*

   Drop factor: 10 gtt/mL

   Original flow rate: ________ gtt/min

   After 4 hours, there are 800 mL remaining; describe the appropriate nursing action now.

   Time remaining: ________ h

   Recalculated flow rate: ________ mL/h

   Recalculated flow rate: ________ gtt/min

   Variation: ________ %

   Action: ____

4. Order: *NS 2000 mL IV for 12 h at 167 mL/h*

   Drop factor: 10 gtt/mL

   Original flow rate: ________ gtt/min

   After 8 hours, there are 750 mL remaining; describe the appropriate nursing action now.

   Time remaining: ________ h

   Recalculated flow rate: ________ mL/h

   Recalculated flow rate: ________ gtt/min

   Variation: ________ %

   Action: ____

5. Order: *NS 1000 mL IV for 8 h at 125 mL/h*

   Drop factor: 10 gtt/mL

   Original flow rate: ________ gtt/min

   After 4 hours, there are 750 mL remaining; describe the appropriate nursing action now.

   Time remaining: ________ h

   Recalculated flow rate: ________ mL/h

   Recalculated flow rate: ________ gtt/min

   Variation: ________ %

   Action: ____

6. Order: *NS 2000 mL IV for 16 h at 125 mL/h*

   Drop factor: 15 gtt/mL

   Original flow rate: ________ gtt/min

   After 6 hours, 650 mL of fluid have infused; describe the appropriate nursing action now.

Solution remaining: ________ mL Time remaining: ________ h

Recalculated flow rate: ________ mL/h

Recalculated flow rate: ________ gtt/min

Variation: ________ %

Action: ____

7. Order: *NS 900 mL IV for 6 h at 150 mL/h*

   Drop factor: 10 gtt/mL

   Original flow rate: ________ gtt/min

   After 3 hours, there are 700 mL remaining; describe the appropriate nursing action now.

   Time remaining: ________ h

   Recalculated flow rate: ________ mL/h

   Recalculated flow rate: ________ gtt/min

   Variation: ________ %

   Action: ____

8. Order: *D_5NS 500 mL IV for 5 h at 100 mL/h*

   Drop factor: 10 gtt/mL

   Original flow rate: ________ gtt/min

   After 2 hours, there are 250 mL remaining; describe the appropriate nursing action now.

   Time remaining: ________ h

   Recalculated flow rate: ________ mL/h

   Recalculated flow rate: ________ gtt/min

   Variation: ________ %

   Action: ____

9. Order: *NS 1 L IV for 20 h at 50 mL/h*

   Drop factor: 15 gtt/mL

   Original flow rate: ________ gtt/min

   After 10 hours, there are 600 mL remaining; describe the appropriate nursing action now.

   Time remaining: ________ h

   Recalculated flow rate: ________ mL/h

   Recalculated flow rate: ________ gtt/min

   Variation: ________ %

   Action: ____

10. Order: *D_5W 1000 mL IV for 10 h at 100 mL/h*

    Drop factor: 60 gtt/mL

    Original flow rate: ________ gtt/min

    After 5 hours, there are 500 mL remaining; describe the appropriate nursing action now.

    Time remaining: ________ h

Recalculated flow rate: ________ mL/h

Recalculated flow rate: ________ gtt/min

Variation: ________ %

Action: ____

Check your work! Answers to all Review Sets are provided at the end of each chapter. Worked solutions for selected Review Sets are also available there.

INTERMITTENT IV INFUSIONS

Sometimes the patient requires supplemental fluid therapy and/or IV medications but does not need continuous replacement or maintenance IV fluids. Several intermittent IV infusion systems are available to administer direct IV drugs. These include IVPB, IV locks for direct IV drugs, the ADD-Vantage system, and volumetric control sets (such as a Buretrol). Volumetric control sets are discussed in Chapter 13.

IV Piggybacks

A medication may be ordered to be dissolved in a small amount of IV fluid (usually 50 to 100 mL) and run piggyback to the regular IV fluids (Figure 12-8). The IVPB (or secondary IV) requires a secondary IV set.

The IVPB medication may come premixed by the manufacturer or pharmacy, or the nurse may need to prepare it. Whichever the case, it is always the responsibility of the nurse to accurately and safely administer the medication. The infusion time may be less than 60 minutes, so it is important to carefully read the order and recommended infusion time.

Sometimes, the patient care order for the IVPB medication will not include an infusion time or rate. When this is the case, it is understood that the nurse will follow the manufacturer's guidelines for infusion rates, keeping in mind the amount of fluid accompanying the medication and any standing orders that limit fluid amounts or rates. Appropriate infusion times are readily available in many drug reference books. Reference books are usually available in most nursing units; if not, you can consult a hospital pharmacist.

Example 1:

Order: *cephazolin 0.5 g in 100 mL D_5W IVPB to run over 30 min*

Drop factor: 10 gtt/mL

What is the flow rate in gtt/min?

$$\frac{V}{T} \times C = \frac{100 \text{ \cancel{mL}}}{\overset{}{\underset{3}{\cancel{30}}} \text{ min}} \times \overset{1}{\cancel{10}} \text{ gtt/}\cancel{\text{mL}} = \frac{100 \text{ gtt}}{3 \text{ min}} = 33.3 \text{ gtt/min} = 33 \text{ gtt/min}$$

Example 2:

An infusion pump is used to administer the same order as in Example 1. Calculate the flow rate, and remember to program the device in *mL/h*.

Step 1 Think If 100 mL will be administered in 30 minutes, or 1/2 hour, then 200 mL will be administered in 60 minutes.

Step 2 Calculate $\frac{\text{Total mL ordered}}{\text{Total min ordered}} \times 60 \text{ min/h} = \text{mL/h}$

$$\frac{100 \text{ mL}}{\cancel{30}_{1} \cancel{\text{min}}} \times \overset{2}{\cancel{60}} \cancel{\text{min}}/\text{h} = 200 \text{ mL/h}$$

Set the electronic IVPB regulator to 200 mL/h. The actual volume of 100 mL will be infused in 30 minutes.

Saline and Heparin IV Locks for Direct IV Drugs

IV locks can be attached to the hub of the peripheral IV catheter that is positioned in the vein. The lock may be referred to as a *saline lock*, meaning that saline is used to flush or maintain the IV catheter patency, or a *heparin lock* if heparin sodium is used to maintain the IV catheter patency. Sometimes a more general term, such as *intermittent peripheral infusion device*, may be used. Concentrated amounts of medications and a smaller amount of fluid can be administered via the direct IV route (often referred to as push or bolus). A syringe is attached to the lock, and the medication is pushed in. As well, a quantity of IV fluid can be run over a specified period of time through an IV setup that is attached to the lock. The use of the IV lock also allows for intermittent medication and fluid administration. The lock is commonly used in emergencies when a fast-acting medication requires immediate administration. Because evidence is lacking to support flushing catheters with heparin sodium, many institutions are now recommending the use of 0.9% sodium chloride injection as a flush (Bellini, 2012; Kumar, Vandermeer, Bassler, & Mansoor, 2013; Mitchell, Anderson, Williams, & Umsheid, 2009). The use of saline eliminates the risks associated with heparin sodium use. Saline locks are also being used for outpatient and home care medication therapy. Refer to the policy at your hospital or healthcare agency regarding the frequency, volume, and concentration of saline or heparin sodium to be used to maintain the IV lock.

CAUTION

Heparin sodium is a high-alert drug and is available in many dosage strengths. A heparin lock flush solution is available in concentrations of 10 units/mL or 100 units/mL. Much higher concentrations of heparin sodium are given intravenously or subcutaneously, so carefully check the concentration. Refer to the institution policy for the frequency, volume, and concentration of heparin sodium to be used to maintain a heparin lock.

Dosage calculations for direct IV injections are the same as calculations for intramuscular injections. The direct IV route of administration is often preferred when immediate onset of action is desired for persons with small or wasted muscle mass, poor circulation, or for drugs that have limited absorption from body tissues. The IV route of administration is preferred over the intramuscular route when IV access is available because repeated intramuscular injections can be painful. Use of the direct IV route is limited to healthcare providers who have this skill within their scope of practice.

An acceptable rate (per minute or per incremental amount of time) for direct IV drug administration is generally determined by institution guidelines, although many drug references have recommended rates of administration. Most timed direct IV administration recommendations are for one to five minutes or more. For smooth manual administration of direct IV drugs, calculate the incremental volume to administer over 15-second intervals. The administration should be timed with either a digital watch or clock or an analogue watch or clock that has a sweep–second hand. Once administration is complete, a new flush syringe is attached. Inject the normal saline flush at the same rate as the medication for first 1 mL to clear any residual medication from the port's dead space.

CAUTION

The purpose of administering drugs intravenously is to start a rapid systemic response to the medication. Use caution when using this method as there is no time to correct errors. Never infuse direct IV drugs more rapidly than recommended by institution policy or pharmacology literature. Some drugs require further dilution after reconstitution for direct IV administration. Carefully read package inserts and reputable drug resources for minimum dilution and minimum time for IV administration.

Example 1:

Order: *lorazepam 3 mg direct IV 20 min preoperatively*

Supply: lorazepam 4 mg/mL with drug literature guidelines: "IV infusion not to exceed 2 mg/min"

How much lorazepam should you prepare?

Step 1 Convert No conversion is necessary.

Step 2 Think You want to give less than 1 mL.

Step 3 Calculate $\frac{D}{H} \times Q = \frac{3 \cancel{mg}}{4 \cancel{mg}} \times 1 \text{ mL} = 0.75 \text{ mL}$

What is a safe infusion time?

RULE

To calculate the amount of time required to administer an ordered dosage according to the recommended dosage rate, use a modification of the dosage calculation formula:

$$\frac{\text{D (dosage desired)}}{\text{H (recommended supply rate)}} \times \text{T (time recommended)} = \text{X (infusion time)}$$

$$\frac{D}{H} \times T = \frac{3 \cancel{mg}}{2 \cancel{mg}} \times 1 \text{ min} = \frac{3}{2} \text{ min} = 1.5 \text{ min}$$

Administer 0.75 mL over 1.5 min

How much should you infuse every 15 seconds?

Convert: 1 min = 60 sec; 1.5 $\cancel{min}$ × 60 sec/$\cancel{min}$ = 90 sec

$$\frac{0.75 \text{ mL}}{90 \text{ sec}} \times \frac{X \text{ mL}}{15 \text{ sec}}$$

$90X = 11.25$

$$\frac{90X}{90} = \frac{11.25}{90}$$

$X = 0.125 \text{ mL}$

0.13 mL of lorazepam 4 mg/mL will be infused by direct IV every 15 seconds to deliver 3 mg of lorazepam at the recommended rate of 2 mg/min.

This is a small amount. Use a 1-mL syringe to prepare 0.75 mL and slowly administer 0.13 mL every 15 seconds.

Example 2:

Order: *cefazolin 1500 mg direct IV q8h*

Supply: cefazolin 1 g powder with directions, "For direct IV administration, reconstitute each 1 g in 10 mL sterile water and give slowly over 3 to 5 minutes."

How much cefazolin should you prepare?

Step 1 **Convert** 1 g = 1.000. = 1000 mg

Step 2 **Think** If 1 g (or 1000 mg) requires 10 mL for dilution, then two 1-g vials will be required. Therefore, to administer 1500 mg, you will prepare more than 10 mL and less than 20 mL.

Step 3 **Calculate** $\frac{D}{H} \times Q = \frac{\overset{3}{\cancel{1500}}\ \cancel{mg}}{\underset{1}{\cancel{2000}}\ \cancel{mg}} \times \overset{5}{\cancel{20}}\ mL = 15\ mL$

What is a safe infusion time?

This amount is larger than the lorazepam dosage from Example 1, so you should use the longer infusion time recommendation (1 g/5 min). Remember, *T* is the amount of time to infuse the dosage available.

$$\frac{D}{H} \times T = \frac{\overset{3}{\cancel{1500}}\ \cancel{mg}}{\underset{2}{\cancel{1000}}\ \cancel{mg}} \times 5\ min = \frac{15}{2}\ min = 7.5\ min$$

Administer 15 mL over 7.5 min.

How much should you infuse every 15 seconds?

Convert: 1 min = 60 sec

7.5 min = 7.5 min × 60 sec/min = 450 sec

$$\frac{15\ mL}{450\ sec} \times \frac{X\ mL}{15\ sec}$$

450X = 225

$$\frac{450X}{450} = \frac{225}{450}$$

X = 0.5 mL

0.5 mL of cefazolin 2 g per 20 mL will be infused by direct IV every 15 seconds to deliver 1500 mg of cefazolin at the rate of 1 g per 5 min.

Use a 20-mL syringe to withdraw 15 mL and slowly infuse 0.5 mL every 15 seconds.

The ADD-Vantage System

Another type of IV medication setup commonly used in hospitals is the ADD-Vantage system by Abbott Laboratories (Figure 12-16). This system uses a specially designed IV bag with a medication vial port. The medication vial comes with the ordered dosage and medication prepared in powder form. The medication vial is attached to the special IV bag, and together they become the IVPB container. The powder is dissolved by the IV fluid and used within a specified time. This system maintains asepsis and eliminates the extra time and equipment (syringe and diluent vials) associated with reconstitution of powdered medications. Several drug manufacturers market many common IV antibiotics that use products similar to the ADD-Vantage system.

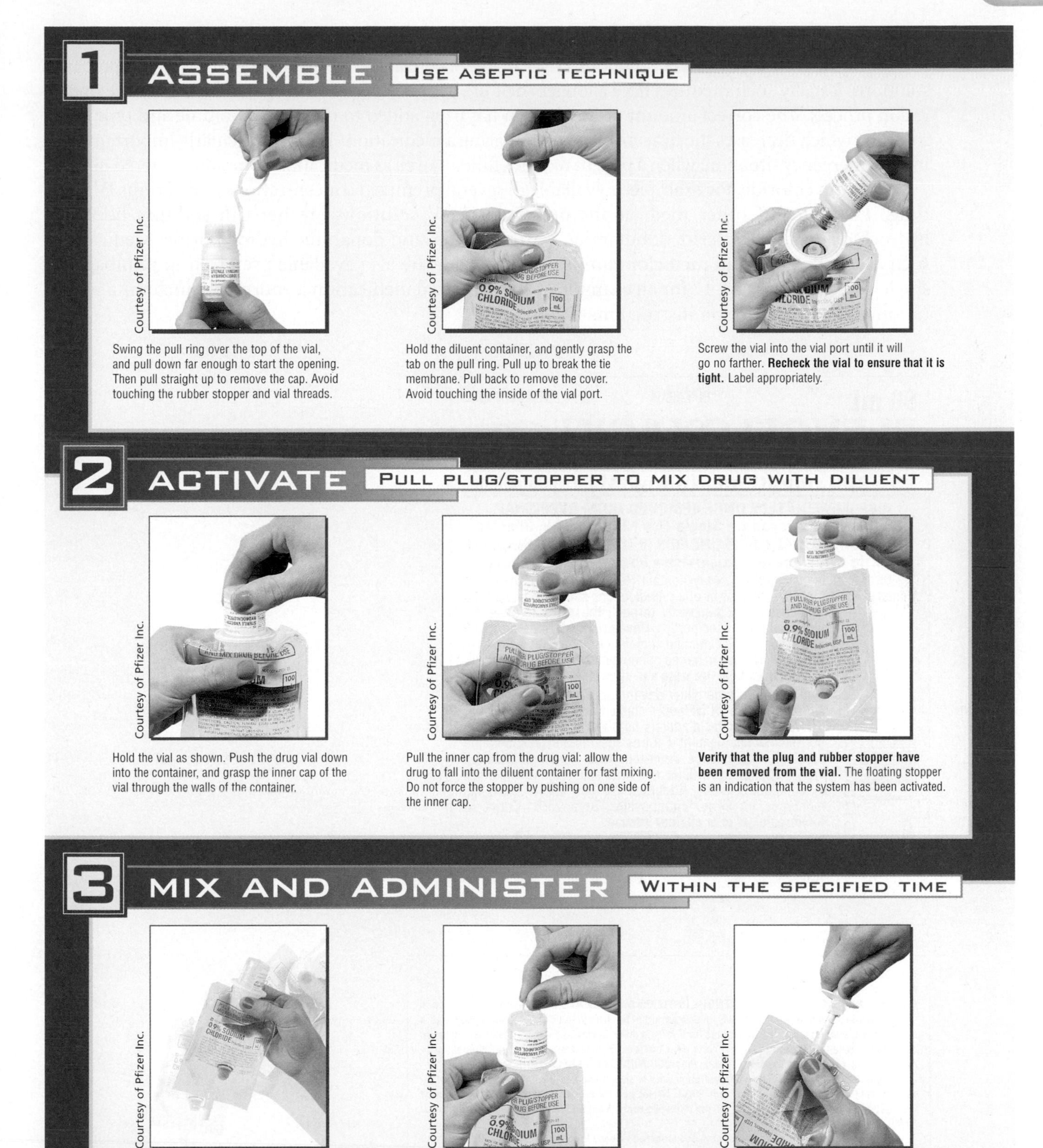

1 ASSEMBLE
USE ASEPTIC TECHNIQUE
Courtesy of Pfizer Inc.
Swing the pull ring over the top of the vial, and pull down far enough to start the opening. Then pull straight up to remove the cap. Avoid touching the rubber stopper and vial threads.
Courtesy of Pfizer Inc.
Hold the diluent container, and gently grasp the tab on the pull ring. Pull up to break the tie membrane. Pull back to remove the cover. Avoid touching the inside of the vial port.
Courtesy of Pfizer Inc.
Screw the vial into the vial port until it will go no farther. Recheck the vial to ensure that it is tight. Label appropriately.
2 ACTIVATE
PULL PLUG/STOPPER TO MIX DRUG WITH DILUENT
Courtesy of Pfizer Inc.
Hold the vial as shown. Push the drug vial down into the container, and grasp the inner cap of the vial through the walls of the container.
Courtesy of Pfizer Inc.
Pull the inner cap from the drug vial: allow the drug to fall into the diluent container for fast mixing. Do not force the stopper by pushing on one side of the inner cap.
Courtesy of Pfizer Inc.
Verify that the plug and rubber stopper have been removed from the vial. The floating stopper is an indication that the system has been activated.
3 MIX AND ADMINISTER
WITHIN THE SPECIFIED TIME
Courtesy of Pfizer Inc.
Mix container contents thoroughly to ensure complete dissolution. Look through the bottom of the vial to verify complete mixing. Check for leaks by squeezing the container firmly. If leaks are found, discard the unit.
Courtesy of Pfizer Inc.
Pull up the hanger on the vial.
Courtesy of Pfizer Inc.
Remove the white administration port cover, and spike (pierce) the container with the piercing pin. Administer within the specified time.

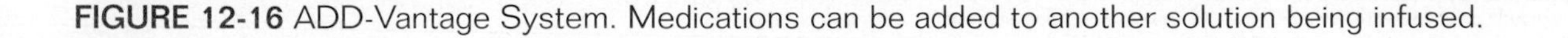
FIGURE 12-16 ADD-Vantage System. Medications can be added to another solution being infused.

Premixed Intravenous Solutions

A large number of premixed IV solutions are available. There are some advantages to using preprepared solutions. Usually such mixtures have a longer shelf life because they have been sterilized after the preparation process. The correct amount of medication has been added to the correct volume and type of IV solution, which decreases the time involved in preparing a medication. This is particularly important during an emergency situation, when a patient requires fluids as well as medication to be administered quickly.

Potassium chloride, for example, is available in several premixed concentrations and various IV solutions. Examples of other medications premixed in IV solutions are heparin sodium, lidocaine hydrochloride, nitroglycerin, dobutamine hydrochloride, and dopamine hydrochloride. Medications such as levofloxacin and metoclopramide hydrochloride are also available premixed in minibags for single use. See Figure 12-17 for an example of the premixed medication levofloxacin, including preparation and administration instructions.

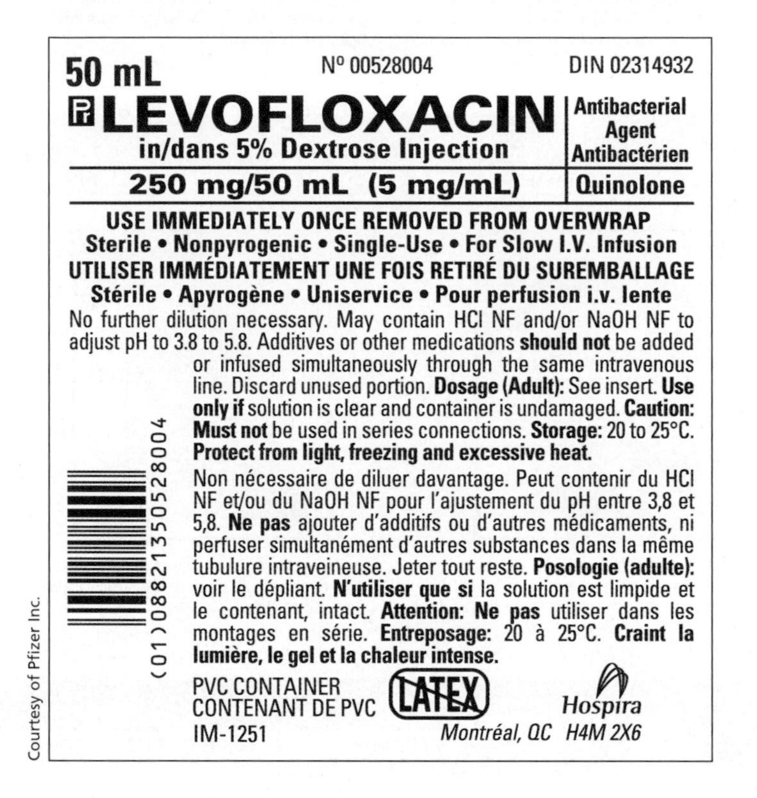

Courtesy of Pfizer Inc.

Administration
Injection
CAUTION: RAPID OR BOLUS INTRAVENOUS INFUSION MUST BE AVOIDED. Levofloxacin injection should be infused intravenously, slowly, over a period of not less than 60 minutes for a 250 mg or a 500 mg dose, and not less than 90 minutes for a 750 mg dose. Levofloxacin in 5% Dextrose Injection should only be administered by intravenous infusion. It is not for intramuscular, intrathecal, intraperitoneal, or subcutaneous administration (see **WARNINGS AND PRECAUTIONS**).

Levofloxacin in 5% Dextrose Injection premix in single-use flexible containers does not require further dilution. Consequently, each 50 mL, 100 mL and 150 mL of PREMIXED solution contains the equivalent of 250 mg, 500 mg and 750 mg of levofloxacin (5 mg/mL) respectively, in 5% Dextrose (D_5W).

This parenteral drug product should be inspected visually for clarity, discolouration, particulate matter, precipitate, and leakage prior to administration. Samples containing visible particles should be discarded.

Since the premix flexible containers are for single use only, any unused portion should be discarded.

Since only limited data are available on the compatibility of levofloxacin intravenous injection with other intravenous substances, **additives or other medications should not be added to Levofloxacin in 5% Dextrose Injection or infused simultaneously through the same intravenous line**. If the same intravenous line is used for sequential infusion of several different drugs, the line should be flushed before and after infusion of Levofloxacin in 5% Dextrose Injection with an infusion solution compatible with Levofloxacin in 5% Dextrose Injection and with any other drug(s) administered via this common line.

Courtesy of Pfizer Inc.

FIGURE 12-17 Premixed Medication Solution

QUICK REVIEW

- Intermittent IV infusions usually require more or less than 60 minutes of infusion time.
- Calculate the IVPB flow rate in gtt/min: $\frac{V}{T} \times C = R$.
- Calculate the IVPB flow rate in mL/h for an electronic infusion device:

$$\frac{\text{Total mL ordered}}{\text{Total min ordered}} \times 60 \text{ min/h} = \text{mL/h}$$

- Use the Three-Step Approach to dosage calculation to calculate the amount to give for direct IV medications: convert, think, calculate X.
- Use $\frac{D}{H} \times T = X$ to calculate safe direct IV time in minutes and seconds as recommended by a reputable drug reference. T is the amount of time to infuse the dosage available.

REVIEW SET 12-9

Calculate the IVPB or direct IV flow rate.

1. Order: *cefazolin 1 g in 100 mL D_5W IVPB to be administered by electronic infusion pump to infuse in 45 min*

   Flow rate: ________ mL/h

2. Order: *cefazolin 1 g in 100 mL D_5W IVPB to be infused over 45 min*

   Drop factor: 60 gtt/mL

   Flow rate: ________ gtt/min

3. Order: *cefazolin 500 mg IVPB diluted in 50 mL D_5W to infuse in 15 min by an electronic infusion pump*

   Flow rate: ________ mL/h

4. Order: *cefazolin 2 g IVPB diluted in 50 mL D_5W to infuse in 15 min*

   Drop factor: 15 gtt/mL

   Flow rate: ________ gtt/min

5. Order: *50 mL IVPB antibiotic solution to infuse in 30 min*

   Drop factor: 60 gtt/mL

   Flow rate: ________ gtt/min

6. Order: *piperacillin/tazobactam 3 g in 100 mL D_5W IVPB to be infused over 40 min*

   Drop factor: 10 gtt/mL

   Flow rate: ________ gtt/min

7. Order: *cefazolin 1.5 g in 50 mL D_5W IVPB to be infused over 15 min*

   Drop factor: 15 gtt/mL

   Flow rate: ________ gtt/min

8. Order: *meropenem 1 g in 100 mL D_5W IVPB to be infused over 30 min*

   Use electronic infusion pump.

   Flow rate: ________ mL/h

9. Order: *cefazolin 750 mg in 50 mL NS IVPB to be infused over 20 min*

   Use electronic infusion pump.

   Flow rate: ________ mL/h

10. Order: *oxacillin sodium 900 mg in 125 mL D_5W IVPB to be infused over 45 min*

    Use electronic infusion pump.

    Flow rate: ________ mL/h

11. Order: *cefazolin 0.5 g in 100 mL D_5W IVPB to be infused over 15 min*

    Drop factor: 10 gtt/mL

    Flow rate: ________ gtt/min

12. Order: *cefazolin 500 mg in 50 mL NS IVPB to be infused over 20 min*

    Drop factor: 10 gtt/mL

    Flow rate: ________ gtt/min

13. Order: *meropenem 1 g in 100 mL D_5W IVPB to be infused over 50 min*

    Use infusion pump.

    Flow rate: ________ mL/h

14. Order: *ampicillin 900 mg in 125 mL D_5W IVPB to be infused over 20 min*

    Drop factor: 10 gtt/mL

    Flow rate: ________ gtt/min

15. Order: *piperacillin/tazobactam 1.3 g in 100 mL D_5W IVPB to be infused over 30 min*

    Drop factor: 60 gtt/mL

    Flow rate: ________ gtt/min

16. Order: *furosemide 120 mg direct IV stat*

    Supply: furosemide 10 mg/mL with drug insert, which states, "IV injection not to exceed 40 mg/min"

    Give: ________ mL/ ________ min or ________ mL/15 sec

17. Order: *phenytoin sodium 150 mg direct IV stat*

    Supply: phenytoin sodium 250 mg/5 mL with drug insert, with these instructions: "IV infusion not to exceed 50 mg/min."

    Give: ________ mL/ ________ min or ________ mL/15 sec

18. Order: *morphine sulfate 6 mg direct IV q3h prn, pain*

    Supply: morphine sulfate 10 mg/mL with drug reference recommendation: "IV infusion not to exceed 2.5 mg/min."

    Give: ________ mL/ ________ min and ________ sec or ________ mL/15 sec

19. Order: *ranitidine hydrochloride 300 mg direct IV stat*

    Supply: ranitidine hydrochloride 300 mg/2 mL

    Package insert instructions: "For direct IV injection, dilute 300 mg in 0.9% NaCl to a total volume of 20 mL. Inject over at least 2 minutes."

    Prepare ________ mL ranitidine.

    Dilute with ________ mL 0.9% NaCl for a total of 20 mL of solution.

    Administer ________ mL/min or ________ mL/15 sec.

20. Order: *midazolam 1.5 mg direct IV stat*

    Supply: midazolam 1 mg/mL

    Instructions: "Slowly titrate to the desired effect using no more than 2.5 mg initially given over 2-min period."

    Prepare ________ mL midazolam.

    Give ________ mL/min or ________ mL/15 sec.

Check your work! Answers to all Review Sets are provided at the end of each chapter. Worked solutions for selected Review Sets are also available there.

CALCULATING IV INFUSION TIME AND VOLUME

IV solutions are usually ordered to be administered at a prescribed number of millilitres per hour, such as *Lactated Ringer's 1000 mL IV to run at 125 mL per hour.* You may need to calculate the total infusion time so that you can anticipate when to add a new bag or when to discontinue the IV.

RULE

To calculate IV infusion time,

- $\frac{\textbf{Total volume}}{\textbf{L/h}} = \textbf{Total hours}$

Example 1:

LR 1000 mL IV to run at 125 mL/h. How long will this IV last?

$$\frac{\overset{8}{\cancel{1000}}\ \cancel{mL}}{\underset{1}{\cancel{125}}\ \cancel{mL}/h} = 8\ h$$

MATH TIP

When calculating IV infusion time, use fractions for hours that are not whole numbers. They are more exact than decimals, which often need to be rounded. For calculations involving time, rounded decimals are more difficult to use.

Example 2:

D_5W 1000 mL IV to infuse at 60 mL/h to begin at 0600. At what time will this IV be complete?

$$\frac{1000\ \cancel{mL}}{60\ \cancel{mL}/h} = 16.67\ h = 16\frac{2}{3}\ h$$

$$\frac{2}{3}\ h = \frac{2}{3}\ h \times 60\ min/h = 40\ min;\ \text{Total time: 16 h and 40 min}$$

The IV will be complete at 0600 + 1640 = 2240.

If the IV is regulated in mL/h, you can also calculate the total volume that will infuse over a specific time.

RULE

To calculate IV volume,
Total hours × mL/h = Total volume

Example:

Your patient's IV is running on an infusion pump set at the rate of 100 mL/h. How much will be infused during the next 8 hours?

$8\ \cancel{h} \times 100\ mL/\cancel{h} = 800\ mL$

QUICK REVIEW

- The formula to calculate IV infusion time, when mL is known, is

  $$\frac{\text{Total volume}}{\text{mL/h}} = \text{Total hours}$$

- The formula to calculate total infusion volume, when mL/h is known, is
  Total hours × mL/h = Total mL

REVIEW SET 12-10

Calculate the infusion time and rate (as requested) for the following IV orders.

1. Order: *D_5W 500 mL at 90 mL/h*

   Drop factor: 10 gtt/mL

   Time: ________ h and ________ min

2. Order: *Lactated Ringer's 1000 mL at 100 mL/h*

   Drop factor: 10 gtt/mL

   Time: ________ h and ________ min

3. Order: *D_5 Lactated Ringer's 800 mL at 125 mL/h*

   Drop factor: 15 gtt/mL

   Time: ________ h and ________ min

Calculate the infusion time and completion time for the following IVs.

4. At 1600, the nurse started D_5W 1200 mL at 100 mL/h. The infusion set used is calibrated for a drop factor of 15 gtt/mL.

   Infusion time: ________ h and ________ min

   Completion time: ________

5. At 1530, the nurse starts D_5W 2000 mL to run at 125 mL/h.

   Infusion time: ________ h and ________ min

   Completion time: ________

Calculate the total volume (mL) to be infused per 24 hours.

6. An IV of D_5 Lactated Ringer's is infusing on an electronic infusion pump at 125 mL/h.

   Total volume: ________ mL/24 h

Calculate the total volume and completion time (if requested) for the following IV orders.

7. Order: *0.9% sodium chloride IV infusing at 65 mL/h for 4 h*

   Volume: ________ mL

8. Order: *D_5W IV infusing at 150 mL/h for 2 h*

   Volume: ________ mL

9. Order: *D_5LR IV at 75 mL/h for 8 h*

   Volume: ________ mL

10. Order: *0.45% NaCl IV at 90 mL/h for 4 h*

    Drop factor: 10 gtt/mL

    Volume: ________ mL

Check your work! Answers to all Review Sets are provided at the end of each chapter. Worked solutions for selected Review Sets are also available there.

APPLICATION OF CLINICAL REASONING

It is important to know the equipment you are using. An example in which the nurse was unfamiliar with the IVPB setup follows.

Potential Patient Safety Incident

Failing to follow the manufacturer's directions when using a new IVPB system.

Possible Scenario

Suppose the order is *ceftriaxone sodium 1 g IV q12h* for an older adult patient who has streptococcus pneumonia. The medication was sent to the unit by pharmacy using the ADD-Vantage system. Ceftriaxone sodium 1 g was supplied in a powder form and attached to a 50-mL IV bag of D_5W. The directions for preparing the medication were attached to the label. The nurse, who was unfamiliar with the new ADD-Vantage system, hung the IV medication, calculated the drip rate, and infused the 50 mL of fluid. The nurse cared for the patient for 3 days. During walking rounds on the third day, the incoming nurse noticed that the ceftriaxone sodium powder remained in the vial and was never diluted in the IV bag. The nurse realized that the vial stopper inside the IV bag was not open. Therefore, the medication powder had not been mixed in the IV fluid during this shift for the past 3 days.

Potential Outcome

The omission by the nurse resulted in the patient missing 3 doses of the ordered IV antibiotic. The delay in administering the medication could have serious consequences for the patient, such as worsening pneumonia, and septicemia, and potential death, especially in an older adult. The patient received one-half of the daily dose ordered by the prescriber for 3 days. The prescriber would be notified of the incident and would likely order additional diagnostic studies, such as chest X-ray, blood cultures, and an additional one-time dose of ceftriaxone sodium.

Prevention

This incident could easily have been avoided had the nurse read the directions for preparing the medication or consulted with another nurse who was familiar with the system.

Application of Critical Reasoning Additional application problems are provided at the end of the chapter. Answers are provided at the end of the book.

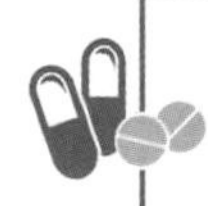

UNDERSTANDING NCLEX QUESTIONS

Here's an example of a standard question used in textbooks:

Rafael has been ordered heparin sodium 1500 units/h by IV infusion. The IV contains 25 000 units of heparin sodium in 250 mL of D_5W. The IV infusion pump would be set at:

a. 15 mL/h
b. 16 mL/h
c. 17 mL/h
d. 20 mL/h

Here's how the question would look in an NCLEX examination:

The patient is to receive heparin sodium 1500 units/h by IV infusion. The IV contains 25 000 units of heparin sodium in 250 mL of D_5W. At what rate would the nurse set the IV infusion pump?

a. 15 mL/h
b. 16 mL/h
c. 17 mL/h
d. 20 mL/h

Answer: a

25 000 units : 250 mL = 1500 units : x mL
Note: Remember, a pump setting is always in mL per hour.

PRACTICE PROBLEMS—CHAPTER 12

Calculate the flow rate in drops per minute or millilitres per hour as requested. For these situations, hospital policy permits recalculating IVs when off-schedule with a maximum variation in rate of 25%.

1. Order: *ampicillin 500 mg dissolved in 100 mL D_5W IV to run for 1 h*

   Drop factor: 10 gtt/mL

   Flow rate: ________ gtt/min

2. Order: *D_5W 1000 mL IV per 24h*

   Drop factor: 60 gtt/mL

   Flow rate: ________ gtt/min

3. Order: *D_5LR 1500 mL IV to run for 12 h*

   Drop factor: 10 gtt/mL

   Flow rate: ________ gtt/min

4. Order: *D_5RL 200 mL IV for 24 h*

   Drop factor: 60 gtt/mL

   Flow rate: ________ gtt/min

5. Order: *$D_{10}W$ 1 L IV to run from 1000 to 1800 h*

   Drop factor: On electronic infusion pump

   Flow rate: ________ mL/h

6. See question 5. At 1100, 800 mL remains. Describe the appropriate nursing action now.

   ____

   ____

7. Order: *NS 1000 mL followed by D_5W 2000 mL IV to run for 24 h*

   Drop factor: 15 gtt/mL

   Flow rate: ________ gtt/min

8. Order: *NS 2.5 L IV to infuse at 125 mL/h*

   Drop factor: 10 gtt/mL

   Flow rate: ________ gtt/min

9. Order: *D_5W 1000 mL IV for 6 h*

   Drop factor: 15 gtt/mL

   After 2 hours, 800 mL remains. Describe the appropriate nursing action now. ________________

   ____

Questions 10 through 20 refer to the following situation: The IV tubing package in the accompanying figure is the IV system available in the hospital for manually regulated, straight gravity-flow IV administration with macrodrop. At 1515, the doctor ordered *D_5W 500 mL IV q4h*, and the nurse started the IV at 1530.

LIFESHIELD™
PRIMARY SET
single use
do not resterilize
List No. 20669-28
Rx only
15
DROPS/mL approximate
Piggyback with Backcheck Valve, 2 CLAVE Y-Sites, 0.2 Micron Filter, 100 Inch, Non-DEHP

Courtesy of Pfizer Inc.

10. How much IV fluid will the patient receive in 24 hours? ________ mL
11. Who is the manufacturer of the IV infusion set tubing? ________
12. What is the drop factor calibration for the IV infusion set tubing? ________
13. What is the drop factor constant for the IV infusion set tubing? ________
14. Using the shortcut (drop factor constant) method, calculate the flow rate of the IV as ordered. Show your work.

    Shortcut method calculation: ________________

    Flow rate: ________ gtt/min
15. Using the formula method, calculate the flow rate of the IV as ordered. Show your work.

    Formula method calculation: ________________

    Flow rate: ________ gtt/min
16. At what time should the nurse anticipate the first IV bag of 500 mL D_5W to be completely infused? ________
17. How much IV fluid should be infused by 1730? ________ mL
18. At 1730, the nurse notices that the IV has 210 mL remaining. After assessing the patient and confirming that her condition is stable, what should the nurse do? ________________

    ____
19. After consulting the prescriber, the nurse decides to use an electronic infusion pump to better regulate the flow rate. The prescriber orders the pump to infuse 500 mL every 4 hours. The nurse should set the pump for ________ mL/h.
20. The next day, the prescriber adds the order *ampicillin 250 mg in 50 mL D_5W IVPB to infuse in 30 min QID*. The patient is still on the IV pump. To infuse the ampicillin via the IVPB, the nurse should set the pump for ________ mL/h.
21. List the components and concentration strengths of the fluid $D_{2.5}\frac{1}{2}$ NS.

    ____
22. Calculate the amount of dextrose and sodium chloride in D_5NS 500 mL.

    dextrose ________ g

    NaCl ________ g

23. Define a central line. ____

____

24. Define a primary line. ____

____

25. Describe the purpose of a saline lock. ____

____

26. A safe direct IV infusion rate of protamine sulfate is 5 mg/min. What is a safe infusion time to administer 50 mg? ________ min

    Protamine sulfate is available in a supply dosage of 10 mg/mL. To administer 50 mg by direct IV, prepare ________ mL and slowly inject into the IV at the rate of ________ mL/min or ________ mL/15 sec.

27. Describe the purpose of a patient-controlled analgesia pump. ____

____

28. Identify three advantages of a syringe pump. ____

____

29. How often should an IV site be monitored? ____

____

30. Describe the purpose of the Y-set IV system. ____

____

For each IV order in questions 31 through 42, use the drop factor to calculate the flow rate in gtt/min.

Order: *D_5W 1 L IV to infuse in 12 h*

31. Drop factor 10 gtt/mL   Flow rate: ________ gtt/min
32. Drop factor 15 gtt/mL   Flow rate: ________ gtt/min
33. Drop factor 60 gtt/mL   Flow rate: ________ gtt/min

Order: *D_5NS 2 L IV to infuse in 20 h*

34. Drop factor 10 gtt/mL   Flow rate: ________ gtt/min
35. Drop factor 15 gtt/mL   Flow rate: ________ gtt/min
36. Drop factor 60 gtt/mL   Flow rate: ________ gtt/min

Order: *0.45% NaCl 1000 mL IV at 200 mL/h*

37. Drop factor 10 gtt/mL   Flow rate: ________ gtt/min
38. Drop factor 15 gtt/mL   Flow rate: ________ gtt/min
39. Drop factor 60 gtt/mL   Flow rate: ________ gtt/min

Order: *D_5 0.9% NaCl 540 mL IV at 45 mL/h*

40. Drop factor 10 gtt/mL   Flow rate: ________ gtt/min
41. Drop factor 15 gtt/mL   Flow rate: ________ gtt/min
42. Drop factor 60 gtt/mL   Flow rate: ________ gtt/min

43. The nurse makes rounds before his lunch break and finds that a patient has 60 mL of IV fluid remaining of an intermittent IV ordered at 125 mL/h on an IV pump and with a saline lock. What volume will be infused during the 30 minutes that he will be at lunch? ________ mL. What should he alert the relief nurse to watch for while he is off the unit? ________________________

44. The nurse's shift is 0700–1500. She makes rounds at 0730 and finds 400 mL remaining on an IV of D_5 0.45% NaCl that is regulated on an electronic infusion pump at the ordered rate of 75 mL/h. The order specifies a continuous infusion. At what time should she anticipate hanging the next IV bag? ________

45. The patient is receiving 250 mL of D_5W infusing at 15 gtt/min. The available IV tubing is 10 gtt/mL. Calculate the infusion time.

46. The patient is receiving 250 mL of D_5NS to run over 6 h. The available tubing is 15 gtt/mL. Calculate the gtt/min for infusion over 6 h.

47. A patient is to receive 800 mL of Ringer's Lactate to infuse at 75 mL/h.

    a) How many hours will the IV run?

    b) Select the most appropriate IV tubing. Available is macrodrip tubing at 10 gtt/mL and microdrop tubing at 60 gtt/mL.

    c) Calculate the drops per minute for the selected tubing.

48. A patient has the following IV order: NS to run at 30 mL/h. The supply cupboard has 250-mL, 500-mL, and 1000-mL bags of NS, as well as macrodrip (10 gtt/mL) and microdrip IV tubing. There is no infusion pump available.

    a) Calculate the infusion rate using both macrodrip and microdrip tubing.

    b) Which bag size and which type of IV tubing should the nurse utilize to complete this order? Provide rationale. ________________

49. A patient has the following IV order: NS to run at 125 mL/h. The supply cupboard has 250-mL, 500-mL, and 1000-mL bags of NS, as well as macrodrip (10 gtt/mL) and microdrip IV tubing. There is no infusion pump available.

    a) Calculate the infusion rate using both macrodrip and microdrip tubing.

    b) Which bag size and which type of IV tubing should the nurse utilize to complete this order? Provide rationale. ________________

Check your work! Answers to all problems are provided at the end of the book, in the Answers section. Worked solutions for some Practice Problems are also provided there.

APPLICATION OF CLINICAL REASONING

12-1 Describe the clinical reasoning you would implement to prevent this patient safety incident.

Possible Scenario

Suppose the prescriber ordered *D_5LR at 125 mL/h* for an older adult patient just returning from the operating room following abdominal surgery. The nurse gathered the IV solution and IV tubing, which had a drop factor of 10 gtt/mL. The nurse did not check the package for the drop factor and assumed it was 60 gtt/mL. The manual rate was calculated this way:

$$\frac{125\ \cancel{mL}}{\cancel{60}\ min} \times \cancel{60}\ gtt/\cancel{mL} = 125\ gtt/min$$

The nurse infused the D_5LR at 125 gtt/min for 8 hours. While reporting to the incoming nurse, the patient called for the nurse, reporting shortness of breath. On further assessment, the nurse heard crackles in the patient's lungs and noticed that the patient's third 1000-mL bottle of D_5LR this shift was nearly empty. At this point, the nurse realized the IV rate was in error. The nurse was accustomed to using the 60-gtt/mL IV setup and therefore calculated the drip rate using the 60 gtt/mL (microdrop) drop factor. However, the tubing used delivered a 10-gtt/mL (macrodrop) drop factor. The nurse never looked at the drop factor on the IV set package and assumed it was a 60 gtt/mL setup.

Potential Outcome

The patient developed signs of fluid overload and could have developed heart failure due to the excessive IV rate. The prescriber would have been notified and would have probably ordered furosemide (a diuretic) to help eliminate the excess fluid. The patient would possibly have been transferred to the ICU for closer monitoring.

Prevention

___

___

Check your work! Answers to all Application for Clinical Reasoning problems are provided at the end of the book, in the Answers section.

ANSWERS TO REVIEW SETS

Review Set 12-1

1) C; sodium chloride 0.9%, 0.9 g/100 mL; 308 mOsm/L; isotonic

2) E; dextrose 5%, 5 g/100 mL; 252 mOsm/L; isotonic (**Note:** Although isotonic in the bag, D_5W acts like a hypotonic solution once it enters the bloodstream because its low concentration of dextrose is quickly metabolized by the cells of the lining of the vein and the circulating cells in the bloodstream.)

3) G; dextrose 5%, 5 g/100 mL; sodium chloride 0.9%, 0.9 g/100 mL; 560 mOsm/L; hypertonic

4) D; dextrose 5%, 5 g/100 mL, sodium chloride 0.45%, 0.45 g/100 mL; 406 mOsm/L; hypertonic

5) A; dextrose 5%, 5 g/100 mL, sodium chloride 0.2%, 0.2 g/100 mL; 321 mOsm/L; hypertonic

6) H; dextrose 5%, 5 g/100 mL; sodium lactate 0.31 g/100 mL, NaCl 0.6 g/100 mL; KCl 0.03 g/100 mL; CaCl 0.02 g/100 mL; 525 mOsm/L; hypertonic

7) B; sodium chloride 0.9%; 0.9 g/100 mL; potassium chloride 20 mEq per litre (0.149 g/100 mL); 348 mOsm/L; hypertonic

8) F; sodium chloride 0.45%, 0.45 g/100 mL; 154 mOsm/L; hypotonic

Review Set 12-2

1) 50; 9 **2)** 25; 2.25 **3)** 25 **4)** 6.75 **5)** 25; 1.65 **6)** 150; 27 **7)** 50; 1.125 **8)** 36; 2.7 **9)** 100; 4.5 **10)** 3.375

Review Set 12-3

1) 100 **2)** 120 **3)** 83 **4)** 200 **5)** 120 **6)** 125 **7)** 125 **8)** 200 **9)** 75 **10)** 125 **11)** 63 **12)** 54 **13)** 150 **14)** 125 **15)** 76

Review Set 12-4

1) 10 **2)** 60 **3)** 15 **4)** 15 **5)** 15

Review Set 12-5

1) $\frac{V}{T} \times C = R$ **2)** 21 **3)** 50 **4)** 17 **5)** 25 **6)** 42 **7)** 42 **8)** 25 **9)** 50 **10)** 80 **11)** 20 **12)** 30 **13)** 8 **14)** 28 **15)** 40

Review Set 12-6

1) 60 **2)** 1 **3)** 4 **4)** 6 **5)** $\frac{\text{mL/h}}{\text{Drop factor constant}} = \text{gtt/min}$ **6)** 50 **7)** 31 **8)** 28 **9)** 60 **10)** 8 **11)** 31 **12)** 14 **13)** 25 **14)** 11 **15)** 50

Review Set 12-7

1) 125; 31 **2)** 100 **3)** 100; 17 **4)** 50 **5)** 125; 31 **6)** 125; 125 **7)** 18 **8)** 17 **9)** 25 **10)** 125 **11)** 83 **12)** 125 **13)** 200 **14)** 150 **15)** 200 **16)** 13.5 **17)** 20; 1.8 **18)** 22.5 **19)** 32.5; 2.145 **20)** 50; 2.25

Review Set 12-8

1) 21; 6; 142; 24; 14%; reset to 24 gtt/min (14% increase is acceptable).

2) 42; 2; 180; 45; 7%; reset to 45 gtt/min (7% increase is acceptable).

3) 21; 4; 200; 33; 57%; recalculated rate 33 gtt/min (57% increase is unacceptable). Consult the prescriber.

4) 28; 4; 188; 31; 11%; reset to 31 gtt/min (11% increase is acceptable).

5) 21; 4; 188; 31; 48% (48% increase is unacceptable). Consult the prescriber.

6) 31; 1350; 10; 135; 34; 10%; reset to 34 gtt/min (10% increase is acceptable).

7) 25; 3; 233; 39; 56% (56% increase is unacceptable). Consult the prescriber.

8) 17; 3; 83; 14; −18%; (−18% variation is acceptable). IV is ahead of schedule. Slow rate to 14 gtt/min, and observe patient's condition.

9) 13; 10; 60; 15; 15%; reset to 15 gtt/min (15% increase is acceptable).

10) 100; 5; 100; 100; 0%; IV is on time, so no adjustment is needed.

Review Set 12-9

1) 133 **2)** 133 **3)** 200 **4)** 50 **5)** 100 **6)** 25 **7)** 50 **8)** 200 **9)** 150 **10)** 167 **11)** 67 **12)** 25 **13)** 120 **14)** 63 **15)** 200 **16)** 12; 3; 1 **17)** 3; 3; 0.25 **18)** 0.6; 2; 24; 0.06 **19)** 2; 18; 10; 2.5 **20)** 1.5; 1.25; 0.3

Review Set 12-10

1) 5 h and 33 min **2)** 10 h and 0 min **3)** 6 h and 24 min **4)** 12 h; 0400 **5)** 16 h; 0730 **6)** 3000 **7)** 260 **8)** 300 **9)** 600 **10)** 360

SELECTED SOLUTIONS TO REVIEW SETS

Review Set 12-2

1) D_5 NS = 5 g dextrose per 100 mL and 0.9 g NaCl per 100 mL

Dextrose:

$$\frac{5 \text{ g}}{100 \text{ mL}} \times \frac{X \text{ g}}{1000 \text{ mL}}$$

$$100X = 5000$$

$$\frac{100X}{100} = \frac{5000}{100}$$

$$X = 50 \text{ g}$$

NaCl:

$$\frac{0.9 \text{ g}}{100 \text{ mL}} \times \frac{X \text{ g}}{1000 \text{ mL}}$$

$$100X = 900$$

$$\frac{100X}{100} = \frac{900}{100}$$

$$X = 9 \text{ g (NaCl)}$$

7) $D_{10}\frac{1}{4}NS$ = 10 g dextrose per 100 mL and 0.225 g NaCl per 100 mL

Dextrose:

$$\frac{10 \text{ g}}{100 \text{ mL}} \times \frac{X \text{ g}}{500 \text{ mL}}$$

$$100X = 5000$$

$$\frac{100X}{100} = \frac{5000}{100}$$

$$X = 50 \text{ g}$$

NaCl:

$$\frac{0.225 \text{ g}}{100 \text{ mL}} \times \frac{X \text{ g}}{500 \text{ mL}}$$

$$100X = 112.5$$

$$\frac{100X}{100} = \frac{112.5}{100}$$

$$X = 1.125 \text{ g (NaCl)}$$

Review Set 12-3

1) 1 L = 1000 mL

$$\frac{\text{Total mL}}{\text{Total h}} = \frac{1000 \text{ mL}}{10 \text{ h}} = 100 \text{ mL/h}$$

3) $$\frac{\text{Total mL}}{\text{Total h}} = \frac{2000 \text{ mL}}{24 \text{ h}} = 83.3 \text{ mL/h} = 83 \text{ mL/h}$$

4) $$\frac{100 \text{ mL}}{\cancel{30}_{1} \text{ min}} \times \frac{\cancel{60}^{2} \text{ min}}{\text{h}} = 200 \text{ mL/h}$$

5) $$\frac{30 \text{ mL}}{\cancel{15}_{1} \text{ min}} \times \frac{\cancel{60}^{4} \text{ min}}{\text{h}} = 120 \text{ mL/h}$$

6) 2.5 L = 2.5 × 1000 = 2500 mL

$$\frac{\text{Total mL}}{\text{Total h}} = \frac{2500 \text{ mL}}{20 \text{ h}} = 125 \text{ mL/h}$$

Review Set 12-5

1) $$\frac{V}{T} \times C = R \text{ or } \frac{\text{Volume}}{\text{Time in min}} \times \text{Drop factor} = \text{Rate}$$

Volume in mL divided by *time* in minutes, multiplied by the *drop factor calibration* in drops per millilitre, equals the flow *rate* in drops per minute.

2) $$\frac{V}{T} \times C = \frac{125 \cancel{\text{mL}}}{\cancel{60}_{6} \text{ min}} \times \cancel{10}^{1} \text{ gtt}/\cancel{\text{mL}}$$

$$= \frac{125 \text{ gtt}}{6 \text{ min}} = 20.8 \text{ gtt/min} = 21 \text{ gtt/min}$$

3) $$\frac{V}{T} \times C = \frac{50 \cancel{\text{mL}}}{\cancel{60}_{1} \text{ min}} \times \cancel{60}^{1} \text{ gtt}/\cancel{\text{mL}} = 50 \text{ gtt/min}$$

Recall that when the drop factor is 60 mL/60 minutes, mL/60 minutes = gtt/min.

4) $$\frac{V}{T} \times C = \frac{100 \cancel{\text{mL}}}{\cancel{60}_{6} \text{ min}} \times \cancel{10}^{1} \text{ gtt}/\cancel{\text{mL}}$$

$$= \frac{100 \text{ gtt}}{6 \text{ min}} = 16.6 \text{ gtt/min} = 17 \text{ gtt/min}$$

6) Two 500 mL units of blood = 1000 mL total volume

$$\text{mL/60 minutes} = \frac{1000 \text{ mL}}{4 \text{ h}} = 250 \text{ mL/60 minutes}$$

$$\frac{V}{T} \times C = \frac{250 \cancel{\text{mL}}}{\cancel{60}_{6} \text{ min}} \times \cancel{10}^{1} \text{ gtt}/\cancel{\text{mL}}$$

$$= \frac{250 \text{ gtt}}{3 \text{ min}} = 41.6 \text{ gtt/min} = 42 \text{ gtt/min}$$

7) $$\frac{\text{Total mL}}{\text{Total h}} = \frac{1000 \text{ mL}}{6 \text{ h}} = 166.7 \text{ mL/60 minutes}$$

= 167 mL/60 minutes

$$\frac{V}{T} \times C = \frac{167 \cancel{\text{mL}}}{\cancel{60}_{4} \text{ min}} \times \cancel{15}^{1} \text{ gtt}/\cancel{\text{mL}}$$

$$= \frac{167 \text{ gtt}}{4 \text{ min}} = 41.75 \text{ gtt/min} = 42 \text{ gtt/min}$$

9) $$\frac{150 \cancel{\text{mL}}}{\cancel{45}_{3} \text{ min}} \times \cancel{15}^{1} \text{ gtt}/\cancel{\text{mL}} = \frac{\cancel{150}^{50} \text{ gtt}}{\cancel{3}_{1} \text{ min}} = 50 \text{ gtt/min}$$

Review Set 12-6

3) $$\frac{60}{15} = 4$$

6) $$\frac{\text{mL/h}}{\text{drop factor constant}} = \text{gtt/min: } \frac{200 \text{ mL/h}}{4}$$

= 50 gtt/min

7) $$\frac{\text{mL/h}}{\text{drop factor constant}} = \text{gtt/min: } \frac{125 \text{ mL/h}}{4}$$

= 31.2 gtt/min = 31 gtt/min

8) $$\frac{\text{mL/h}}{\text{drop factor constant}} = \text{gtt/min: } \frac{165 \text{ mL/h}}{6}$$

= 27.5 gtt/min = 28 gtt/min

9) $\frac{\text{mL/h}}{\text{drop factor constant}} = \text{gtt/min: } \frac{60 \text{ mL/h}}{1}$

$= 60 \text{ gtt/min}$

(Set the flow rate at the same number of gtt/min as the number of mL/h when the drop factor is 60 gtt/mL because the drop factor constant is 1.)

13) $0.5 \text{ L} = 500 \text{ mL}; \frac{500 \text{ mL}}{20 \text{ h}} = 25 \text{ mL/h}$; since drop factor is 60 gtt/mL, then mL/h = gtt/min; so rate is 25 gtt/min.

14) $650 \text{ mL in } 10 \text{ h} = \frac{650 \text{ mL}}{10 \text{ h}} = 65 \text{ mL/h}$

$\frac{\text{mL/h}}{\text{drop factor constant}} = \text{gtt/min: } \frac{65 \text{ mL/h}}{6}$

$= 10.8 \text{ gtt/min} = 11 \text{ gtt/min}$

Review Set 12-7

1) $\frac{\text{Total mL}}{\text{Total h}} = \frac{3000 \text{ mL}}{24 \text{ h}} = 125 \text{ mL/h}$

$\frac{V}{T} \times C = \frac{125 \cancel{\text{mL}}}{\cancelto{4}{60} \text{ min}} \times \cancelto{1}{15} \text{ gtt}/\cancel{\text{mL}} = \frac{125 \text{ gtt}}{4 \text{ min}}$

$= 31.3 \text{ gtt/min} = 31 \text{ gtt/min}$

7) $\frac{\text{mL/h}}{\text{drop factor constant}} = \text{gtt/min: } \frac{105 \text{ mL/h}}{6}$

$= 18 \text{ gtt/min}$

8) $\frac{\text{mL/h}}{\text{drop factor constant}} = \text{gtt/min: } \frac{100 \text{ mL/h}}{6}$

$= 16.6 \text{ gtt/min} = 17 \text{ gtt/min}$

10) $\frac{\text{Total mL}}{\text{Total h}} = \frac{1000 \text{ mL}}{8 \text{ h}} = 125 \text{ mL/h}$

13) $\frac{100 \text{ mL}}{\cancelto{1}{30 \text{ min}}} \times \frac{\cancelto{2}{60 \text{ min}}}{\text{h}} = 200 \text{ mL/h}$

15) $\frac{150 \text{ mL}}{\cancelto{3}{45 \text{ min}}} \times \frac{\cancelto{4}{60 \text{ min}}}{\text{h}} = 200 \text{ mL/h}$

16) $\frac{1}{2} \text{ NS} = 0.45\% \text{ NaCl} = 0.45 \text{ g NaCl per } 100 \text{ mL}$

$\frac{0.45 \text{ g}}{100 \text{ mL}} \times \frac{X \text{ g}}{3000 \text{ mL}}$

$100X = 1350$

$\frac{100X}{100} = \frac{1350}{100}$

$X = 13.5 \text{ g (NaCl)}$

17) $D_{10}NS = 10\% \text{ dextrose} = 10 \text{ g dextrose per } 100 \text{ mL and } 0.9\% \text{ NaCl} = 0.9 \text{ g NaCl per } 100 \text{ mL}$

Dextrose:

$\frac{10 \text{ g}}{100 \text{ mL}} \times \frac{X \text{ g}}{200 \text{ mL}}$

$100X = 2000$

$\frac{100X}{100} = \frac{2000}{100}$

$X = 20 \text{ g (dextrose)}$

$NS = 0.9\% \text{ NaCl} = 0.9 \text{ g NaCl per } 100 \text{ mL}$

NaCl:

$\frac{0.9 \text{ g}}{100 \text{ mL}} \times \frac{X \text{ g}}{200 \text{ mL}}$

$100X = 180$

$\frac{100X}{100} = \frac{180}{100}$

$X = 1.8 \text{ g (NaCl)}$

Review Set 12-8

1) $\frac{V}{T} \times C = \frac{125 \cancel{\text{mL}}}{\cancelto{6}{60} \text{ min}} \times \cancelto{1}{10} \text{ gtt}/\cancel{\text{mL}} = \frac{125 \text{ gtt}}{6 \text{ min}} = 20.8 \text{ gtt/min} = 21 \text{ gtt/min (ordered rate)}$

$12 \text{ h} - 6 \text{ h} = 6 \text{ h}$

$\frac{\text{Remaining volume}}{\text{Remaining hours}} = \text{Recalculated mL/h; } \frac{850 \text{ mL}}{6 \text{ h}} = 141.6 \text{ mL/h} = 142 \text{ mL/h}$

$\frac{V}{T} \times C = \frac{142 \cancel{\text{mL}}}{\cancelto{6}{60} \text{ min}} \times \cancelto{1}{10} \text{ gtt}/\cancel{\text{mL}} = \frac{142 \text{ gtt}}{6 \text{ min}} = 23.5 \text{ gtt/min} = 24 \text{ gtt/min (adjusted rate)}$

$\frac{\text{Adjusted gtt/min} - \text{Ordered gtt/min}}{\text{Ordered gtt/min}} = \text{\% of variation; } \frac{24 - 21}{21} = \frac{3}{21} = 0.14 = 14\%$ (within the acceptable % of variation); reset rate to 47 gtt/min

3) $\frac{V}{T} \times C = \frac{125\ \cancel{mL}}{\underset{6}{\cancel{60}}\ min} \times \overset{1}{\cancel{10}}\ gtt/\cancel{mL} = = \frac{125\ gtt}{6\ min} = 20.8\ gtt/min = 21\ gtt/min$ (ordered rate)

$8\ h - 4\ h = 4\ h$

$\frac{800\ mL}{4\ h} = 200\ mL/h; \frac{V}{T} \times C = \frac{200\ \cancel{mL}}{\underset{6}{\cancel{60}}\ min} \times \overset{1}{\cancel{10}}\ gtt/\cancel{mL} = = \frac{200\ gtt}{6\ min} = 33.3 = 33\ gtt/min$ (adjusted rate)

$\frac{\text{Adjusted gtt/min} - \text{Ordered gtt/min}}{\text{Ordered gtt/min}} = \%$ of variation; $\frac{33 - 21}{21} = \frac{12}{21} = 0.3 = 57\%$ faster; unacceptable % of variation—call prescriber for a revised order

6) $\frac{V}{T} \times C = \frac{125\ \cancel{mL}}{\underset{4}{\cancel{60}}\ min} \times \overset{1}{\cancel{15}}\ gtt/\cancel{mL} = = \frac{125\ gtt}{4\ min} = 31.3\ gtt/min = 31\ gtt/min$ (ordered rate)

$2000\ mL - 650\ mL = 1350\ mL$ remaining; $16\ h - 6\ h = 10\ h$

$\frac{1350\ mL}{10\ h} = 135\ mL/h; \frac{V}{T} \times C = \frac{135\ \cancel{mL}}{\underset{4}{\cancel{60}}\ min} \times \overset{1}{\cancel{15}}\ gtt/\cancel{mL} = \frac{135\ gtt}{4\ min} = 33.7\ gtt/min = 34\ gtt/min$

$\frac{\text{Adjusted gtt/min} - \text{Ordered gtt/min}}{\text{Ordered gtt/min}} = \%$ of variation; $\frac{34 - 31}{31} = \frac{3}{31} = 0.096 = 0.10 = 10\%$ (within acceptable % of variation); reset rate to 34 gtt/min

8) $\frac{V}{T} \times C = \frac{100\ \cancel{mL}}{\underset{6}{\cancel{60}}\ min} \times \overset{1}{\cancel{10}}\ gtt/\cancel{mL} = \frac{100\ gtt}{6\ min} = 16.7\ gtt/min = 17\ gtt/min$ (ordered rate)

$5\ h - 2\ h = 3\ h$

$\frac{250\ mL}{3\ h} = 83.3\ mL/h = 83\ mL/h; \frac{V}{T} \times C = \frac{83\ \cancel{mL}}{\underset{6}{\cancel{60}}\ min} \times \overset{1}{\cancel{10}}\ gtt/\cancel{mL} = \frac{83\ gtt}{6\ min} = 13.7\ gtt/min$

$= 14\ gtt/min$ (adjusted rate)

$\frac{\text{Adjusted gtt/min} - \text{Ordered gtt/min}}{\text{Ordered gtt/min}} = \%$ of variation; $\frac{14 - 17}{17} = \frac{-3}{17} = -0.176 = -18\%$

(Remember, the minus sign indicates the IV is ahead of schedule and rate must be decreased.) Within the acceptable % of variation. Slow IV to 14 gtt/min, and closely monitor patient.

Review Set 12-9

1) $\frac{\text{Total mL ordered}}{\text{Total min ordered}} \times 60\ min/h = mL/h$

$\frac{100\ mL}{\underset{3}{\cancel{45}}\ \cancel{min}} \times \overset{4}{\cancel{60}}\ \cancel{min}/h = \frac{400}{3}\ mL/h$

$= 133\ mL/h = 133\ mL/h$

2) $\frac{V}{T} \times C = \frac{100\ \cancel{mL}}{\underset{3}{\cancel{45}}\ min} \times \overset{4}{\cancel{60}}\ gtt/\cancel{mL} = \frac{400\ gtt}{3\ min}$

$= 133.3\ gtt/min = 133\ gtt/min$

3) $\frac{\text{Total mL ordered}}{\text{Total min ordered}} \times 60\ min/h = mL/h$

$\frac{50\ mL}{\underset{1}{\cancel{15}}\ \cancel{min}} \times \overset{4}{\cancel{60}}\ \cancel{min}/h = 200\ mL/h$

4) $\frac{V}{T} \times C = \frac{50\ \cancel{mL}}{\underset{1}{\cancel{15}}\ min} \times \overset{1}{\cancel{15}}\ gtt/\cancel{mL} = 50\ gtt/min$

11) $\frac{V}{T} \times C = \frac{100\ \cancel{mL}}{\underset{3}{\cancel{15}}\ min} \times \overset{2}{\cancel{10}}\ gtt/\cancel{mL} = \frac{200\ gtt}{3\ min}$

$= 66.6\ gtt/min = 67\ gtt/min$

16) $\frac{D}{H} \times Q = \frac{12\cancel{0}\ \cancel{mg}}{1\cancel{0}\ \cancel{mg}} \times 1\ mL = 12\ mL$

$\frac{D}{H} \times Q = \frac{\overset{3}{\cancel{120}}\ mg}{\underset{1}{\cancel{40}}\ mg} \times 1\ min = 3\ min$

Administer 12 mL over at least 3 min.

$1\ min = 60\ sec$

$3\ min = 3 \times 60 = 180\ sec$

$\frac{12\ mL}{180\ sec} = \frac{X\ mL}{15\ sec}$

$180X = 180$

$\frac{180X}{180} = \frac{180}{180}$

$X = 1\ mL$ per 15 sec

17) $\frac{D}{H} \times Q = \frac{150 \text{ mg}}{250 \text{ mg}} \times 5 \text{ mL} = \frac{150}{50} \text{ mL} = 3 \text{ mL}$

$\frac{D}{H} \times Q = \frac{150 \text{ mg}}{50 \text{ mg}} \times 1 \text{ min} = 3 \text{ min}$

Administer 3 mL over 3 min.

1 min = 60 sec

3 min = 3 × 60 = 180 sec

$\frac{3 \text{ mL}}{180 \text{ sec}} \times \frac{X \text{ mL}}{15 \text{ sec}}$

180X = 45

$\frac{180X}{180} = \frac{45}{180}$

X = 0.25 mL (per 15 sec)

18) $\frac{D}{H} \times Q = \frac{6 \text{ mg}}{10 \text{ mg}} \times 1 \text{ mL} = \frac{6}{10} \text{ mL} = 0.6 \text{ mL}$

$\frac{D}{H} \times Q = \frac{6 \text{ mg}}{2.5 \text{ mg}} \times 1 \text{ min} = 2.4 \text{ min}$

1 min = 60 sec

2 min = 2 × 60 = 120 sec; 0.4 min = 0.4 × 60 = 24 sec

120 sec + 24 sec = 144 sec

$\frac{0.6 \text{ mL}}{144 \text{ sec}} \times \frac{X \text{ mL}}{15 \text{ sec}}$

144X = 9

$\frac{144X}{144} = \frac{9}{144}$

X = 0.06 mL (per 15 sec)

Review Set 12-10

1) Infusion time $= \frac{\text{Total volume}}{\text{mL/h}} = \frac{500 \text{ mL}}{90 \text{ mL/h}}$

= 5.55 hours

0.55 h × 60 min/h = 33 minutes

Therefore, the infusion time is 5 hours and 33 minutes.

2) Infusion time $= \frac{\text{Total volume}}{\text{mL/h}} = \frac{1000 \text{ mL}}{100 \text{ mL/h}}$

= 10 hours

4) Infusion time $= \frac{\text{Total volume}}{\text{mL/h}} = \frac{1200 \text{ mL}}{100 \text{ mL/h}}$

= 12 hours

1600 + 1200 = 2800 = 2400 + 400; therefore, the completion time is 0400.

5) Time: $\frac{\text{Total vol}}{\text{mL/h}} = \text{Total h}$

$\frac{2000 \text{ mL}}{125 \text{ mL/h}} = 16 \text{ h}$

1530 + 1600 = 3130 − 2400 = 0730

6) Total hours × mL/h = Total volume

24 h × 125 mL/h = 3000 mL

7) 65 mL/h × 4 h = 260 mL

10) 90 mL/h × 4 h = 360 mL

CHAPTER

13

Body Surface Area and Advanced Pediatric Calculations

OBJECTIVES

1. Determine the body surface area (BSA) using a calculation formula or a nomogram scale.
2. Calculate the safe amount of drug to be administered when ordered according to the BSA.
3. Calculate intermittent intravenous (IV) medications administered with IV infusion control sets.
4. Calculate the amount to mix proportionate IV additive medications into small-volume IV solutions.
5. Calculate the minimal and maximal dilution in which an IV medication can be safely prepared and delivered.
6. Calculate pediatric IV maintenance fluids.

The focus of this chapter is on more advanced calculations frequently used by pediatric nurses. The concepts in this chapter will help you understand the unique drug and fluid management required by a growing child. These concepts are also applied to adults in special situations. This chapter begins by looking at the BSA method of calculating a dosage, followed by a discussion on checking the accuracy and safety of a particular drug order.

BODY SURFACE AREA METHOD

Two methods are used to calculate the safe dosage of a drug for a child: the weight in kilograms method and the BSA method. Because a child's BSA is thought to parallel organ growth, maturation, and metabolic rate, it is considered a safer way to measure dosage calculations. The BSA method is also used for accurate dosage calculations in some adult patients (e.g., those undergoing open heart surgery or radiation and patients with severe burns or kidney disease). Regardless of age, chemotherapy drugs and an increasing number of other highly potent drug classifications are being prescribed based on BSA.

BSA is a mathematical estimate based on a formula that uses the patient's *height* and *weight*. BSA is expressed in metres squared (**m^2**). BSA is also determined by using a chart, called a *nomogram*, that estimates the BSA. Because drug dosages recommended by BSA measurement are potent, and because the formula calculation is the most accurate, we will begin with the formula. In most situations, the prescriber or pharmacist will calculate the BSA for drugs ordered by this method. However, the nurse who administers the drug is responsible for verifying safe dosage, which may require calculating the BSA.

The BSA Formula

The BSA formula, based on the metric measurement of height in centimetres and weight in kilograms, is easy to calculate using the square root function on a calculator. Many institutions have BSA calculators on their intranets. BSA calculators are also readily available on the Internet.

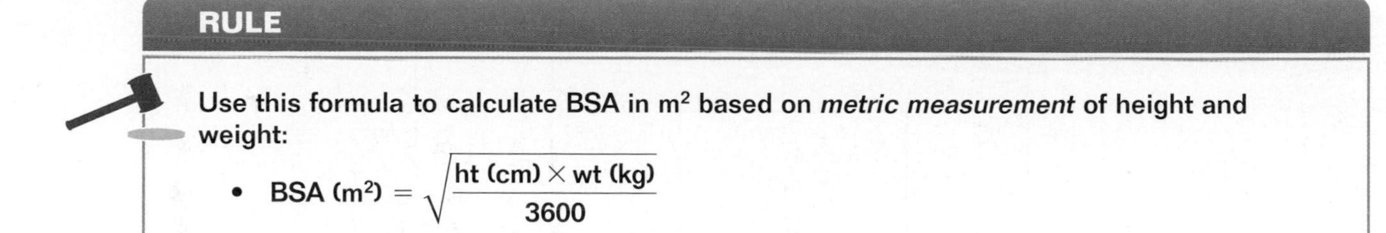

RULE

Use this formula to calculate BSA in m² based on *metric measurement* of height and weight:

- **BSA (m²)** $= \sqrt{\dfrac{\text{ht (cm)} \times \text{wt (kg)}}{3600}}$

Now apply the metric formula in the following examples.

Example 1:

Use the metric formula to calculate the BSA of an infant whose length is 50 cm and weight is 6.8 kg.

$$\text{BSA (m}^2\text{)} = \sqrt{\frac{\text{ht (cm)} \times \text{wt (kg)}}{3600}} = \sqrt{\frac{50 \times 6.8}{3600}} = \sqrt{\frac{340}{3600}} = \sqrt{0.094} = 0.307 \text{ m}^2 = 0.31 \text{ m}^2$$

MATH TIP

To perform BSA calculations using the metric formula on most calculators, follow this sequence: multiply height in cm by weight in kg, divide by 3600, press =, then press $\sqrt{\ }$ to arrive at m². Round m² to hundredths (two decimal places). For Example 1 above, enter $50 \times 6.8 \div 3600 = 0.094$, and press $\sqrt{\ }$ to arrive at 0.307, rounded to 0.31 m².

There is another formula that uses household measurements of inches and pounds. That formula is shown here, but the metric formula is preferred.

$$\text{BSA (m}^2\text{)} = \sqrt{\frac{\text{ht (in)} \times \text{wt (lb)}}{3131}} = \sqrt{\frac{20 \times 15}{3131}} = \sqrt{\frac{300}{3131}} = \sqrt{0.095} = 0.309 \text{ m}^2 = 0.31 \text{ m}^2$$

Example 2:

Calculate the BSA of a child whose height is 105 cm and weight is 31.8 kg.

$$\text{BSA (m}^2\text{)} = \sqrt{\frac{\text{ht (cm)} \times \text{wt (kg)}}{3600}} = \sqrt{\frac{105 \times 31.8}{3600}} = \sqrt{\frac{3339}{3600}} = \sqrt{0.927} = 0.963 \text{ m}^2 = 0.96 \text{ m}^2$$

Example 3:

Calculate the BSA of an adult whose height is 173 cm and weight is 88.8 kg.

$$\text{BSA (m}^2\text{)} = \sqrt{\frac{\text{ht (cm)} \times \text{wt (kg)}}{3600}} = \sqrt{\frac{173 \times 88.8}{3600}} = \sqrt{\frac{15\,362.4}{3600}} = \sqrt{4.267} = 2.065 \text{ m}^2 = 2.07 \text{ m}^2$$

The BSA Nomogram

Some practitioners use a chart called a *nomogram* that *estimates* the BSA using the patient's height and weight. Look at Figure 13-1: Locate the height on the left side of the nomogram and the weight on the right side. Draw a line connecting the two points—the point where the lines meet is the BSA in square metres. The nomogram in Figure 13-1 is the most well known BSA chart, the West Nomogram. It is used for both children and adults for heights up to 240 cm and weights up to 80 kg.

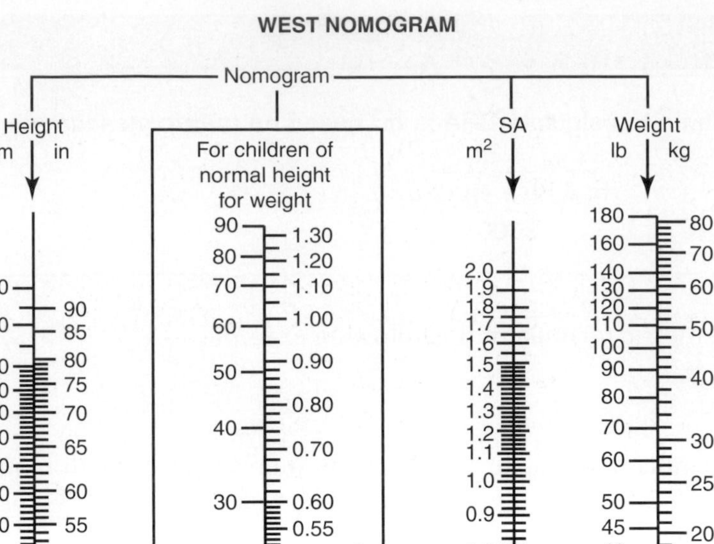
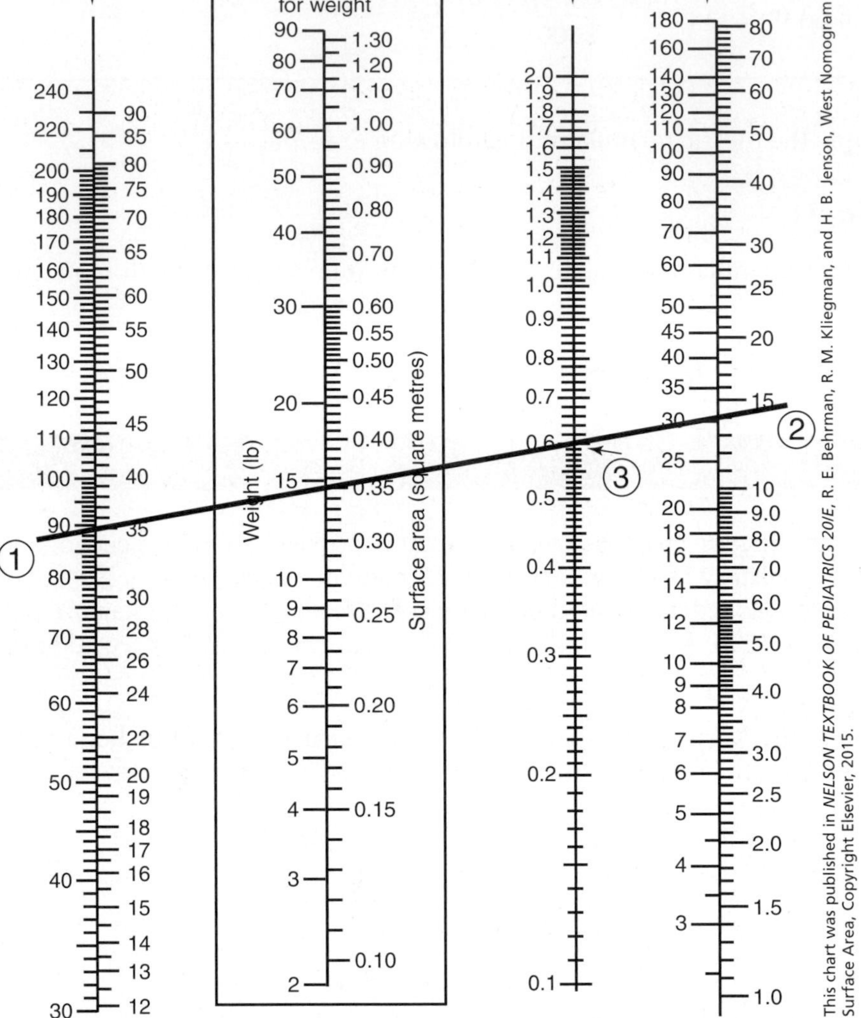

FIGURE 13-1 Using the West Nomogram, body surface area (BSA) is determined by drawing a straight line from the patient's height (1) in the far left column to her weight (2) in the far right column. Intersection of the line with the surface area (SA) column (3) is the estimated BSA (m^2). For infants and children of normal height and weight, BSA may be estimated from weight alone by referring to the data within the black rectangle.

CAUTION

The increments of measurement and the spaces on a BSA nomogram are not consistent. Be sure you correctly read the numbers and the calibration values between them.

For a child of normal height for weight, the BSA can be determined on the West Nomogram using the weight alone. Notice the column within the black rectangle to the centre left in Figure 13-1. Normal height and weight standards can be found on pediatric growth and development charts.

CAUTION

To use the normal height and weight column on the West Nomogram, you must be familiar with normal height and weight standards for children. If you are unsure, use both height and weight to estimate BSA. Do not guess.

QUICK REVIEW

- BSA is used to calculate select dosages across the life span, most often for children.
- BSA is calculated using the patient's height and weight and expressed in metres squared (m^2).
- The following metric formula is the preferred method of calculating BSA:

  $$\text{BSA} (m^2) = \sqrt{\frac{\text{ht (cm)} \times \text{wt (kg)}}{3600}}$$

- Nomograms can be used to estimate BSA by correlating height and weight measures to m^2.

REVIEW SET 13-1

Use the formula method to determine the BSA. Round to two decimal places.

1. An adult is 190 cm tall and weighs 105 kg. ________ m^2
2. A child is 94 cm tall and weighs 18 kg. ________ m^2
3. A teenager is 153 cm tall and weighs 46 kg. ________ m^2
4. An adult is 175 cm tall and weighs 85 kg. ________ m^2
5. An adult is 62 inches tall and weighs 140 lb. ________ m^2
6. A teenager is 160 cm tall and weighs 64 kg. ________ m^2
7. A child is 65 cm tall and weighs 15 kg. ________ m^2
8. A child is 92 cm tall and weighs 24 kg. ________ m^2

Find the BSA on the West Nomogram (Figure 13-1) for a child of normal height and weight.

9. 4 lb ________ m^2
10. 42 lb ________ m^2
11. 17 lb ________ m^2

Find the BSA on the West Nomogram (Figure 13-1) for children with the following height and weight.

12. 41 inches and 32 lb ________ m^2
13. 140 cm and 30 kg ________ m^2
14. 80 cm and 11 kg ________ m^2
15. 106 cm and 25 kg ________ m^2

Check your work! Answers to all Review Sets are provided at the end of each chapter. Worked solutions for selected Review Sets are also available there.

BSA Dosage Calculations

Once the BSA is obtained, the drug dosage can be verified by consulting a reputable drug resource for the recommended dosage. Package inserts, the hospital formulary, and other dosage handbooks contain pediatric and adult dosages. Remember to carefully read the reference to verify whether the drug dosage is calculated in *m^2 per dose* or *m^2 per day.*

Use the following rule to calculate dosage based on body mass measurement in m^2. Notice that the calculation is similar to that used for determining dosage based on body weight (e.g., mg/kg) learned previously.

RULE

To verify safe pediatric dosage based on BSA,

1. **Determine the BSA in m^2;**
2. **Calculate the safe dosage based on BSA:**

   $mg/m^2 \times m^2$

3. **Compare the ordered dosage to the recommended dosage, and decide whether the dosage is safe; and**
4. **If the dosage is safe, calculate the amount to give and administer the dose. If the dosage seems unsafe, consult the prescriber before administering the drug.**

Note: Recommended dosage may specify mg/m^2, mcg/m^2, g/m^2, $units/m^2$, $microunits/m^2$, or mEq/m^2.

Example 1:

A child is 126 cm tall and weighs 23 kg. Drug order: *vincristine 1.8 mg IV at 1000.* Is this dosage safe for this child? The recommended dosage as noted on the package insert is 2 mg/m^2. Supply: See the label in Figure 13-2.

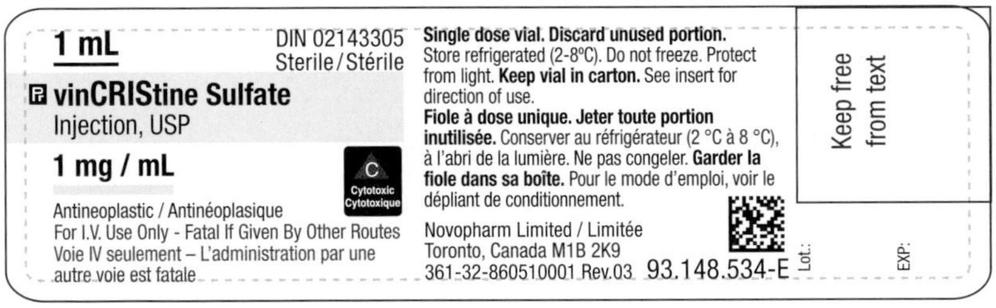

FIGURE 13-2 Vincristine Label

1. **Determine the BSA.**

$$\text{BSA } (m^2) = \sqrt{\frac{\text{ht (cm)} \times \text{wt (kg)}}{3600}} = \sqrt{\frac{126 \times 23}{3600}} = \sqrt{\frac{2898}{3600}} = \sqrt{0.805} = 0.897 \text{ m}^2 = 0.9 \text{ m}^2$$

   The child's BSA is 0.9 m^2.

2. **Calculate the recommended dosage.** $mg/m^2 \times m^2$; $2\ mg/\cancel{m^2} \times 0.9\ \cancel{m^2} = 1.8\ mg$
3. **Decide whether the dosage is safe.** The dosage ordered is 1.8 mg, and 1.8 mg is the amount recommended by the BSA. The dosage is safe. How much should you give?
4. **Calculate one dose.**

Step 1 Convert No conversion is necessary.

Step 2 Think You want to give more than 1 mL and less than 2 mL.

Step 3 Calculate $\frac{D}{H} \times Q = \frac{1.8 \cancel{mg}}{\cancel{1} \cancel{mg}} \times \cancel{1} mL = 1.8 mL$

Example 2:

A 2-year-old child with herpes simplex is 35 inches tall and weighs 30 lb. The drug order is *acyclovir 100 mg IV BID*. Is this order safe? The recommendation from the drug reference is 250 mg/m^2 q8h for children younger than 12 years and older than 6 months. Acyclovir is supplied as a 500-mg injection with directions to reconstitute with 10 mL sterile water for injection for a concentration of 50 mg/mL.

1. **Determine the BSA.** According to the West Nomogram, the child's BSA is 0.6 m^2.
2. **Calculate the recommended dosage.** mg/m^2 × m^2; $250 \text{ mg}/\cancel{m^2} \times 0.6 \cancel{m^2} = 150 \text{ mg}$
3. **Decide whether the dosage is safe.** The dosage of 100 mg BID is not safe—the single dosage is too low. Further, the drug should be administered 3 times per day or q8h, not BID or 2 times per day.
4. **Confer with the prescriber.**

Example 3:

It is also possible to determine the pediatric drug dosage when the child's BSA is known (or calculated) and the adult dose is based on the average adult BSA (1.7 m^2).

$$\frac{\text{Child's known BSA}}{1.7 \text{ m}^2 \text{ (usual adult BSA)}} \times \text{Usual adult dose} = \text{child's dose}$$

The child's BSA is 0.36 m^2 and the normal adult dose is 250 mg.

$$\frac{0.36 \cancel{m^2}}{1.7 \cancel{m^2}} \times 250 \text{ mg} = \frac{90}{1.7} = 52.94 = 53 \text{ mg}$$

Recommended dosage: The drug is available as 100 mg in 5 mL.

Calculate the dosage:

$$\frac{D}{H} \times Q = \frac{53 \text{ mg}}{100 \text{ mg}} \times 5 \text{ mL} = \frac{53}{20} = 2.65 \text{ mL} = 2.7 \text{ mL}$$

QUICK REVIEW

- Safe dosage based on BSA: mg/m^2 × m^2, compared to recommended dosage.

REVIEW SET 13-2

1. What is the dosage of one dose of interferon alpha-2b required for a child with a BSA of 0.82 m^2 if the recommended dosage is 2 000 000 units/m^2? ________ units
2. What is the total daily dosage range of mitomycin required for a child with a BSA of 0.59 m^2 if the recommended dosage range is 10 to 20 mg/m^2/day? ________ mg/day to ________ mg/day
3. What is the dosage of a drug required for an adult with a BSA of 1.47 m^2 if the recommended dosage is 500 mg/m^2? ________ mg

4. What is the daily dosage of cyclophosphamide required for an adult with a BSA of 2.64 m^2 if the recommended dosage is 600 mg/m^2 for one dose on day 1? ________ mg/day
5. What is the dosage of acyclovir required for a child with a BSA of 1 m^2 if the recommended dosage is 250 mg/m^2? ________ mg
6. A child is 30 inches tall and weighs 25 pounds.

   Order: *acyclovir 122.5 mg IV q8h*

   Supply: acyclovir 500 mg with directions to reconstitute with 10 mL sterile water for injection for a final concentration of 50 mg/mL

   Recommended dosage from drug insert: 250 mg/m^2

   BSA = ________ m^2

   Recommended dosage for this child: ________ mg

   Is the ordered dosage safe? ________

   If safe, give ________ mL.

   If not safe, what should the nurse do? ________________
7. A child is 114 cm tall and weighs 25 kg.

   Order: *methotrexate 2.9 mg IV daily*

   Supply: methotrexate 2.5 mg/mL

   Recommended dosage from drug insert: 3.3 mg/m^2

   BSA = ________ m^2

   Recommended dosage for this child: ________ mg

   Is the ordered dosage safe? ________

   If safe, give ________ mL.

   If not safe, what should the nurse do? ________________
8. Order: *diphenhydramine 22 mg IV q8h*. A child has a BSA of 0.44 m^2. Recommended safe dosage of diphenhydramine is 150 mg/m^2/day in divided dosages every 8 hours.

   Recommended daily dosage for this child: ________ mg/day

   Recommended single dosage for this child: ________ mg/dose

   Is the ordered dosage safe? ________

   If not safe, what should the nurse do? ________________
9. Order: *quinidine 198 mg PO; daily for 5 days*. A child has a BSA of 0.22 m^2. Recommended safe dosage of quinidine is 900 mg/m^2/day given in 5 daily doses.

   Recommended dosage for this child: ________ mg/dose

   Is the dosage ordered safe? ________

   If not safe, what should the nurse do? ________

   How much quinidine would this child receive over 5 days of therapy? ________ mg
10. Order: *deferoxamine mesylate IV per protocol*. A child has a BSA of 1.02 m^2.

    Protocol: 600 mg/m^2 initially followed by 300 mg/m^2 at 4-hour intervals for 2 doses; then give 300 mg/m^2 q12h for 2 days. Calculate the total dosage received.

    Initial dosage: ________ mg

Two q4h dosages: ________ mg

Two days of q12h dosages: ________ mg

Total dosage child would receive: ________ mg

11. Order: *fludarabine 10 mg/m² bolus over 15 minutes followed by a continuous IV infusion of 30.5 mg/m²/day*. A child has a BSA of 0.81 m^2. The bolus dosage is ________ mg, and the continuous 24-hour IV infusion will contain ________ mg of fludarabine.

12. Order: *drug X 83.75 mg IV q12h* for a child with a BSA of 0.67 m^2. The recommended dosage range is 100 to 250 mg/m^2/day in 2 divided doses.

    Recommended daily dosage range for this child: ________ mg/day to ________ mg/day

    Recommended single dosage range for this child: ________ mg/dose to ________ mg/dose

    Is the ordered dosage safe? ________

    If not, what should the nurse do? ________________________________

13. Order: *daunorubicin 9.6 mg IV on day 1 and day 8 of cycle*

    Protocol: 25 to 45 mg/m^2 on days 1 and 8 of cycle. A child has a BSA of 0.32 m^2.

    Recommended dosage range for this child: ________ mg/dose to ________ mg/dose

    Is the ordered dosage safe? ________

    If not safe, what should the nurse do? ________________________________

Answer questions 14 and 15 based on the following information.

The recommended dosage of pegaspargase is 2500 units/m^2/dose IV daily $\times$ 14 days for adults and children with a BSA more than 0.6 m^2.

Supply: pegaspargase 750 units/mL with directions to dilute in 100 mL D_5W and give over 2 hours. The nurse will administer the drug through an infusion pump.

14. Order: *Give pegaspargase 2050 units IV today at 1600.* The child is 100 cm tall and weighs 24 kg. The child's BSA is ________ m^2.

    The recommended dosage for this child is ________ units. Is the ordered dosage of pegaspargase safe? ________

    If yes, add ________ mL of pegaspargase for a total IV fluid volume of ________ mL. Set the IV infusion pump at ________ mL/h.

    If the order is not safe, what should the nurse do? ________

15. Order: *pegaspargase 4050 units IV stat* for an adult patient who is 162 cm tall and weighs 58.2 kg. The patient's BSA is ________ m^2. The recommended dosage of pegaspargase for this adult is ________ units.

    Is the ordered dosage of pegaspargase safe? ________

    If safe, the nurse should add ________ mL of pegaspargase for a total IV fluid volume of ________ mL. Set the infusion pump at ________ mL/h.

    If the order is not safe, what should the nurse do? ________________________________

Check your work! Answers to all Review Sets are provided at the end of each chapter. Worked solutions for selected Review Sets are also available there.

SYRINGE PUMPS

Syringe pumps (sometimes called syringe pump modules, depending on the manufacturer) continuously and accurately deliver a controlled volume of fluids or drugs including bolus infusions (Figure 13.3(a) and Figure 13.3(b)). Some units provide million unit dosing and nanogram precision for administration to adults, children, and infants. Syringe sizes are flexible and can vary from 1 to 60 mL, with the unit automatically detecting the size. These pumps also have other features, including automatic alerts such as pressure-sensing discs that monitor when a dosing limit, bolus limit, concentration limit, or weight limit has been exceeded. Specified syringes and volume sets are used for syringe pumps.

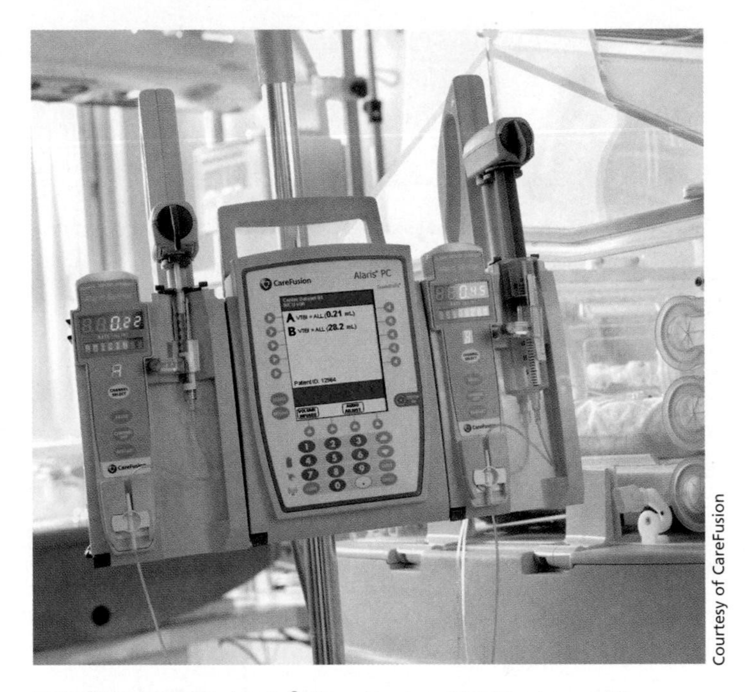

Courtesy of CareFusion

FIGURE 13.3(a) Alaris® CareFusion PC System with Large-Volume Infusion Pumps and Auto-ID Module for Medication Administration (Primary Infusion Pump and Two Secondary Pumps)

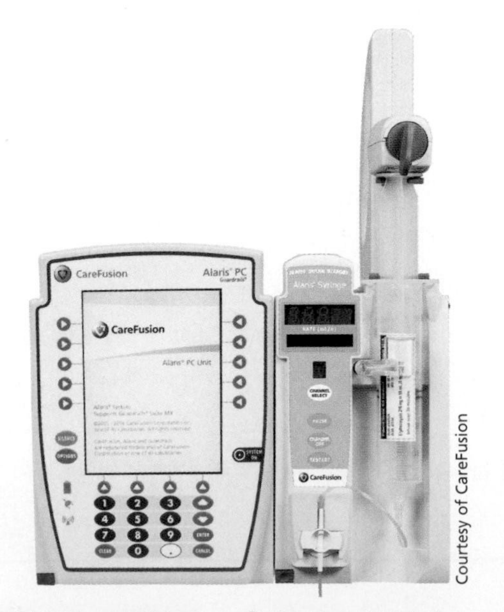

Courtesy of CareFusion

FIGURE 13.3(b) Alaris® Syringe Module

PEDIATRIC VOLUMETRIC CONTROL SETS

Volumetric control sets, or volumetric cylinders, are being used less often to administer hourly fluids and intermittent IV medications to children (Figure 13-4). Indeed, the majority of pediatric hospitals in Canada no longer routinely use in-line volumetric cylinders for pediatric IV infusions. However, as they may still be used in some institutions, they are discussed here. The fluid chamber holds 100 to 150 mL of fluid to be infused over a specified time period as ordered, usually in 60 minutes or less. The medication is added to the IV fluid in the chamber for a prescribed dilution volume.

The volume of fluid in the chamber is filled by the nurse every one to two hours or as needed. Only small, prescribed quantities of fluid are added, and the clamp above the chamber is fully closed. The IV bag acts only as a reservoir to hold future fluid infusions. The patient is protected from receiving more volume than intended, which is especially important for children, who can tolerate only a narrow range of fluid volume. This process differs from standard IV infusions that run directly from the IV bag through the drip chamber and IV tubing into the patient's vein.

Volumetric control sets may also be used to administer intermittent IV medications to adults who have fluid restrictions, as a result of heart disease or kidney disease. An electronic pump may be used to regulate the flow rate. When used, an electronic device will sound an alarm when the chamber empties.

With the expanded use of IV pumps, volumetric control devices (such as the Buretrol) are now less common in practice. However, as a safety device for controlling the volume of fluid administered to children and patients of any age who are critically ill, they are still available. Nurses should be familiar with how to use them and how to calculate the IV flow rate when using them.

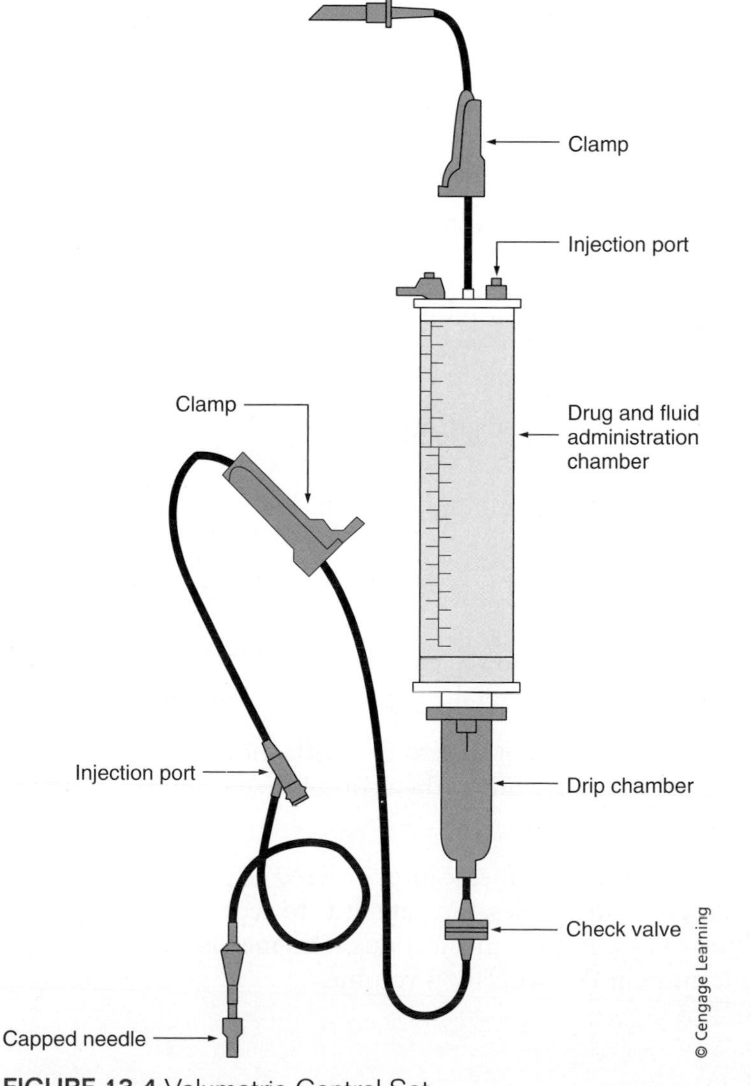

FIGURE 13-4 Volumetric Control Set

Intermittent IV Medication Infusion with a Volumetric Control Set

Children receiving IV medications may have a saline lock in place of a continuous IV infusion. The nurse will inject the medication into the volumetric control set chamber, add an appropriate volume of IV fluid to dilute the drug, and attach the IV tubing to the child's IV lock to infuse over a specified period of time. Once the chamber empties, some medication still remains in the drip chamber, IV tubing, and the IV lock above the child's vein. After the chamber has emptied and the medication has infused, a flush of IV fluid is given to ensure that all the medication has cleared the tubing. There is no standard amount of fluid used to flush peripheral and central IV lines. Because tubing varies by manufacturer, the flush can vary from 15 mL to as much as 50 mL, according to the overall length of the tubing and extra extensions added. Verify the institution policy on the correct volume to flush peripheral and central IV lines in children. For the purpose of sample calculations, this text uses a 15-mL volume to flush a peripheral IV line, unless specified otherwise.

To calculate the IV flow rate for the volumetric control set, consider the total fluid volume of the medication, the IV fluid used for dilution, and the volume of IV flush fluid. Volumetric control sets are microdrip sets with a drop factor of 60 gtt/mL.

Example:

Order: *cefotaxime sodium 250 mg IV q6h in 50 mL $D_5 \frac{1}{4}$ NS to infuse in 30 min followed by a 15-mL flush*. The child has a saline lock.

Supply: See label.

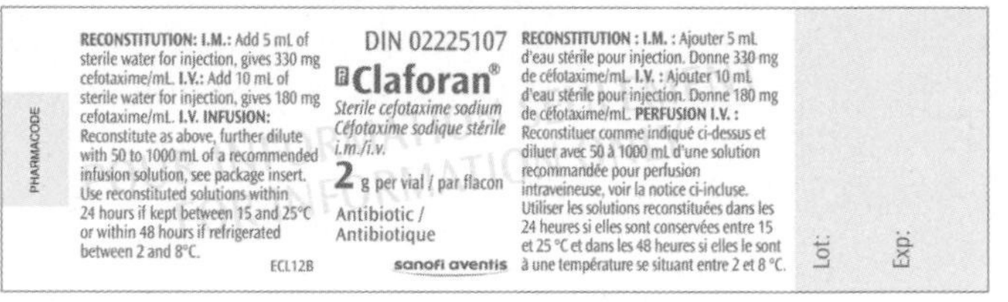

Instructions from the package insert for IV are to add 10 mL diluent for a total volume of 11 mL with a concentration of 180 mg/mL.

Step 1 Calculate the total volume of the intermittent IV medication and the IV flush.
50 mL + 15 mL = 65 mL

Step 2 Calculate the flow rate of the IV medication and the IV flush. Remember: The drop factor is 60 gtt/mL.

$$\frac{V}{T} \times C = \frac{65 \text{ mL}}{\cancel{30}_{1} \text{ min}} \times \cancel{60}^{2} \text{ gtt}/\cancel{\text{mL}} = 130 \text{ gtt/min}$$

Step 3 Calculate the volume of the medication to be administered.

$$\frac{D}{H} \times Q = \frac{250 \cancel{\text{mg}}}{180 \cancel{\text{mg}}} \times 1 \text{ mL} = 1.39 \text{ mL} = 1.4 \text{ mL}$$

Step 4 Add 1.4 mL cefotaxime sodium 2 g to the chamber and fill with IV fluid to a volume of 50 mL. This provides the prescribed total volume of 50 mL in the chamber.

Step 5 Set the flow rate of the 50 mL of intermittent IV medication to 130 gtt/min. Follow with the 15-mL flush, also set to 130 gtt/min. When complete, detach the IV tubing and follow saline lock policy.

The patient may also have an intermittent medication ordered as part of a continuous infusion at a prescribed IV volume per hour. In such cases, the patient is to receive the same fluid volume each hour, regardless of the addition of intermittent medications. This means that the total prescribed fluid volume must include the intermittent IV medication volume.

Example:

Order: *D_5NS IV at 30 mL/h for continuous infusion and methylprednisolone sodium succinate 30 mg IV q8h over 30 min*

Supply: See the label in Figure 13-5.

An electronic infusion pump is in use with the volumetric control set.

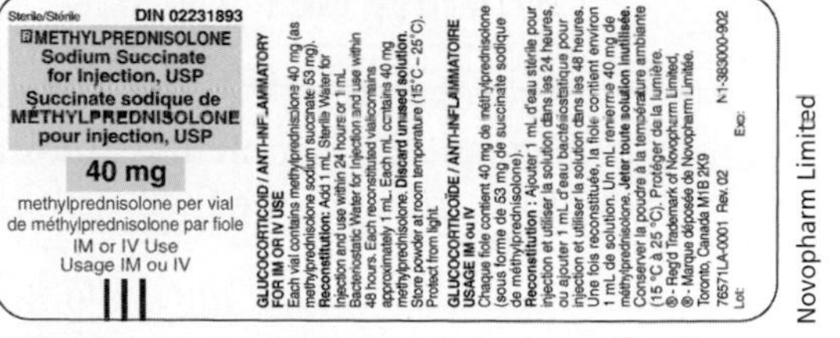

FIGURE 13-5 Methylprednisolone Sodium Succinate Label

Step 1 Calculate the dilution volume required to administer the methylprednisolone sodium succinate at the prescribed continuous flow rate of 30 mL/h.

Think If 30 mL infuses in 1 hour, then $\frac{1}{2}$ of 30, or 15 mL, will infuse in $\frac{1}{2}$ hour or 30 minutes.

Calculate Use ratio and proportion to verify your estimate.

$$\frac{30 \text{ mL}}{60 \text{ min}} \times \frac{X \text{ mL}}{30 \text{ min}}$$

$$60X = 900$$

$$\frac{60X}{60} = \frac{900}{60}$$

$$X = 15 \text{ mL}$$

Therefore, the IV fluid dilution volume required to administer 30 mg of methylprednisolone sodium succinate in 30 minutes is 15 mL to maintain the prescribed, continuous infusion rate of 30 mL/h.

Step 2 Determine the volume of methyprednisolone sodium succinate and IV fluid to add to the volumetric control chamber.

$$\frac{D}{H} \times Q = \frac{\overset{3}{\cancel{30 \text{ mg}}}}{\underset{4}{\cancel{40 \text{ mg}}}} \times 1 \text{ mL} = \frac{3}{4} \text{ mL} = 0.75 \text{ mL}$$

Add 0.75 mL methyprednisolone sodium succinate, and fill the chamber with D_5NS to the total volume of 15 mL.

Step 3 Set the infusion pump to 30 mL/h to deliver 15 mL of intermittent IV methylprednisolone sodium succinate solution in 30 minutes. Resume the regular IV, which will also flush out the tubing. The continuous flow rate will remain at 30 mL/h.

QUICK REVIEW

- Volumetric control sets have a drop factor of 60 gtt/mL.
- The total volume of the medication, IV dilution fluid, and the IV flush fluid must be considered to calculate flow rates when using volumetric control sets.
- Use ratio and proportion to calculate flow rates for intermittent medications when a continuous IV rate in mL/h is prescribed.

REVIEW SET 13-3

Calculate the IV flow rate to administer the following IV medications using a volumetric control set, and determine the amount of IV fluid and medication to be added to the chamber. The ordered time includes the flush volume.

1. Order: *amikacin 125 mg IV q8h in 50 mL $D_5 \frac{1}{3}$ NS over 45 min. Flush with 15 mL.*

   Supply: amikacin 250 mg/mL

   Flow rate: ________ gtt/min

   Add ________ mL medication and add IV fluid to make a total of ________ mL in the chamber.

2. Order: *cefuroxime sodium 500 mg IV q6h in 50 mL $D_5 \frac{1}{4}$ NS over 30 min. Flush with 15 mL.*

   Supply: cefuroxime sodium 750 mg vial. Reconstitute with 8.0 mL for injection to yield 90-mg/mL solution.

   Flow rate: ________ gtt/min

   Add ________ mL medication and add IV fluid to make a total of ________ mL in the chamber.

3. Order: *ampicillin 150 mg IV BID in 25 mL 0.9% NaCl over 20 min. Flush with 15 mL.*

   Supply: ampicillin 250 mg/3 mL

   Flow rate: ________ gtt/min

   Add ________ mL medication and add IV fluid to make a total of ________ mL in the chamber.

4. Order: *cefazolin sodium 0.6 g IV q12h in 50 mL D_5NS over 60 min on an infusion pump. Flush with 30 mL.*

   Supply: cefazolin sodium 1 g/10 mL

   Flow rate: ________ mL/h

   Add ________ mL medication and add IV fluid to make a total of ________ mL in the chamber.

5. Order: *clindamycin phosphate 150 mg IV q8h in 32 mL D_5NS over 60 min on an infusion pump. Flush with 28 mL.*

   Supply: clindamycin phosphate 150 mg/mL

   Flow rate: ________ mL/h

   Add ________ mL medication and add IV fluid to make a total of ________ mL in the chamber.

   Total IV volume after three doses are given is ________ mL.

6. Order: *0.9% NaCl at 50 mL/h for continuous infusion with cefazolin sodium 250 mg IV q8h to be infused over 30 min by volumetric control set.*

   Supply: cefazolin 125 mg/mL

   Add ________ mL medication and add IV fluid to make a total of ________ mL in the chamber.

7. Order: *D_5W at 30 mL/h for continuous infusion with dexamethasone sodium phosphate 2 mg BID to be infused over 20 min by volumetric control set*

   Supply: dexamethasone sodium phosphate 4 mg/mL

   Add ________ mL medication and add IV fluid to make a total of ________ mL in the chamber.

8. Order: *D_5 0.225% NaCl IV at 85 mL/h with erythromycin 600 mg IV q6h to be infused over 40 min by volumetric control set*

   Supply: erythromycin 50 mg/mL

   Add ________ mL medication and add IV fluid to make a total of ________ mL in the chamber.

9. Order: *D_5 0.33% NaCl IV at 66 mL/h with ceftazidime 720 mg IV q8h to be infused over 40 min by volumetric control set*

   Supply: ceftazidime 1 g/10 mL

   Add ________ mL medication and add IV fluid to make a total of ________ mL in the chamber.

10. Order: *D_5 0.45% NaCl IV at 90 mL/h with cefotetan disodium 1 g IV q6h to be infused over 30 min by volumetric control set*

    Supply: cefotetan disodium 1 g/vial. Add 10 mL to provide 10.5 mL of volume.

    Add ________ mL medication and add IV fluid to make a total of ________ mL in the chamber.

Check your work! Answers to all Review Sets are provided at the end of each chapter. Worked solutions for selected Review Sets are also available there.

MINIMAL DILUTIONS FOR IV MEDICATIONS

Intravenous medications in infants and young children (and adults on limited fluids) are often ordered to be given in the smallest volume or maximal safe concentration to prevent fluid overload. Consult a pediatric reference, hospital formulary, or drug insert to assist you in problem solving. These types of medications are usually given with an electronic infusion pump.

Many pediatric IV medications allow a dilution range or a minimum and maximum allowable concentration. A solution of lower concentration may be given if the patient can tolerate the added volume (called minimal safe concentration, maximal dilution, or largest volume). A solution of higher concentration (called maximal safe concentration, minimal dilution, or smallest volume) must not exceed the recommended dilution instructions. Recall that the greater the volume of diluent or solvent, the less concentrated the resulting solution. Likewise, less volume of diluent or solvent results in a more concentrated solution.

CAUTION

An excessively high concentration of an IV drug can cause vein irritation and potentially life-threatening toxic effects. Dilution calculations are critical skills.

Examine how to follow the drug reference recommendations for a minimal IV drug dilution, when a minimal and maximal range is given for an IV drug dilution.

RULE

Ratio for recommended drug dilution equals ratio for desired drug dilution.

Example 1:

The prescriber orders *vancomycin 40 mg IV q12h* for an infant who weighs 4000 g. What is the minimal amount of IV fluid in which the vancomycin can be safely diluted? The package insert indicates that a "concentration of no more than 10 mg/mL is recommended." This is the *recommended maximal safe concentration.*

$$\frac{10 \text{ mg}}{1 \text{ mL}} \times \frac{40 \text{ mg}}{X \text{ mL}}$$

$$10X = 40$$

$$\frac{10X}{10} = \frac{40}{10}$$

$$X = 4 \text{ mL}$$

This is the minimal amount of IV fluid.

Example 2:

The prescriber orders *cefotaxime sodium 1.2 g IV q8h* for a child who weighs 36 kg. The recommended safe administration of cefotaxime sodium for intermittent IV administration is a final concentration of 20 to 60 mg/mL to infuse over 15 to 30 minutes. What is the minimal amount of IV fluid to safely dilute this dosage? (Remember, this represents the **maximal safe concentration.**)

Step 1 Convert $1.2 \text{ g} = 1.2 \cancel{\text{g}} \times 1000 \text{ mg}/\cancel{\text{g}} = 1200 \text{ mg}$

Step 2 Think 1200 is more than 10 times 60; in fact, it is 20 times 60. So you need at least 20 mL to dilute the drug.

Step 3 Calculate

$$\frac{60 \text{ mg}}{1 \text{ mL}} \times \frac{1200 \text{ mg}}{X \text{ mL}}$$

$$60X = 1200$$

$$\frac{60X}{60} = \frac{1200}{60}$$

$$X = 20 \text{ mL}$$

This is the minimal dilution for maximal safe concentration.

What is the maximal amount of IV fluid recommended to safely dilute this drug to the minimal safe concentration?

Step 1 Convert 1.2 g = 1.2 g × 1000 mg/g = 1200 mg

Step 2 Think 1200 is more than 50 times 20; in fact, it is 60 times 20. So you can use up to 60 mL to dilute the drug.

Step 3 Calculate

$$\frac{20 \text{ mg}}{1 \text{ mL}} \times \frac{1200 \text{ mg}}{X \text{ mL}}$$

$$20X = 1200$$

$$\frac{20X}{20} = \frac{1200}{20}$$

$$X = 60 \text{ mL}$$

This is the maximal dilution for minimal safe concentration.

CALCULATION OF DAILY VOLUME FOR MAINTENANCE FLUIDS

Another common pediatric IV calculation is to calculate daily rates for 24-hour maintenance IV fluids.

RULE

Use this calculation to determine the daily rate of pediatric maintenance IV fluids:

- **100 mL/kg/day for the first 10 kg of body weight;**
- **50 mL/kg/day for the next 10 kg of body weight; and**
- **20 mL/kg/day for each kilogram above 20 kg of body weight.**

This formula uses the child's weight in kilograms to estimate the 24-hour total fluid need, including oral intake. It does not include replacement for losses, such as due to diarrhea, vomiting, and fever. This accounts only for fluid needed to maintain normal cellular metabolism and fluid turnover.

Pediatric IV solutions that run over 24 hours usually include a combination of glucose, saline, and potassium chloride and are *hypertonic* solutions (see Figure 12-5). Dextrose (glucose) for energy is usually concentrated between 5% and 12% for peripheral infusions. Sodium chloride is usually concentrated between 0.225% and 0.9% ($\frac{1}{4}$ NS up to 0.9% NS). Further, 20 mEq per litre of potassium chloride (20 mEq KCl/L) is usually added to continuous pediatric infusions. Any dextrose and saline combination without potassium should be used only as an intermittent or short-term IV fluid in children. Be wary of isotonic solutions such as 5% dextrose in water and 0.9% sodium chloride. They do not contribute enough electrolytes and can quickly lead to water intoxication.

CAUTION

A red flag should be raised if either plain 5% dextrose in water or 0.9% sodium chloride (normal saline) is running continuously on an infant or child. Consult the prescriber immediately!

Examine the daily rate of maintenance fluids and the hourly flow rate for the children in the following examples. For these examples, assume that the IV pump is programmable in whole numbers and tenths of a millilitre.

Example 1:

A child weighs 6 kg. Calculate the hourly flow rate.

$100 \text{ mL/}\cancel{\text{kg}}\text{/day} \times 6 \cancel{\text{kg}} = 600 \text{ mL/day}$ or per 24 hours

$$\frac{600 \text{ mL}}{24 \text{ h}} = 25 \text{ mL/h}$$

Example 2:

A child weighs 12 kg. Calculate the hourly flow rate.

$100 \text{ mL/}\cancel{\text{kg}}\text{/day} \times 10 \cancel{\text{kg}} = 1000 \text{ mL/day}$ (for first 10 kg)

$50 \text{ mL/}\cancel{\text{kg}}\text{/day} \times 2 \cancel{\text{kg}} = 100 \text{ mL/day}$ (for the remaining 2 kg)

Total: $1000 \text{ mL/day} + 100 \text{ mL/day} = 1100 \text{ mL/day}$ or per 24 hours

$$\frac{1100 \text{ mL}}{24 \text{ h}} = 45.8 \text{ mL/h} = 46 \text{ mL/h}$$

Example 3:

A child weighs 24 kg. Calculate the hourly flow rate.

$100 \text{ mL/}\cancel{\text{kg}}\text{/day} \times 10 \cancel{\text{kg}} = 1000 \text{ mL/day}$ (for first 10 kg)

$50 \text{ mL/}\cancel{\text{kg}}\text{/day} \times 10 \cancel{\text{kg}} = 500 \text{ mL/day}$ (for next 10 kg)

$20 \text{ mL/}\cancel{\text{kg}}\text{/day} \times 4 \cancel{\text{kg}} = 80 \text{ mL/day}$ (for the remaining 4 kg)

Total: $1000 \text{ mL/day} + 500 \text{ mL/day} + 80 \text{ mL/day} = 1580 \text{ mL/day}$ or per 24 hours

$$\frac{1580 \text{ mL}}{24 \text{ h}} = 65.8 \text{ mL/h} = 66 \text{ mL/h}$$

QUICK REVIEW

- Minimal and maximal dilution volumes for some IV drugs are recommended to prevent fluid overload and to minimize vein irritation and toxic effects.
- The ratio for recommended dilution equals the ratio for desired drug dilution.
- When mixing IV drug solutions,
  - the *smaller* the added volume, the *stronger* or *higher* the resulting *concentration* (minimal dilution); and
  - the *larger* the added volume, the *weaker (more dilute)* or *lower* the resulting *concentration* (maximal dilution).
- Daily volume of pediatric maintenance IV fluids based on body weight is
  - 100 mL/kg/day for first 10 kg;
  - 50 mL/kg/day for next 10 kg; and
  - 20 mL/kg/day for each kilogram above 20.

REVIEW SET 13-4

1. If a child is receiving *chloramphenicol 400 mg IV q6h* and the maximum concentration is 100 mg/mL, what is the minimum volume of fluid in which the medication can be safely diluted? ________ mL
2. If a child is receiving *gentamicin sulfate 25 mg IV q8h* and the minimal concentration is 1 mg/mL, what is the maximum volume of fluid in which the medication can be safely diluted? ________ mL
3. Calculate the total volume and hourly IV flow rate for a 25-kg child receiving maintenance IV fluids. Infuse ________ mL at ________ mL/h
4. Calculate the total volume and hourly IV flow rate for a 13-kg child receiving maintenance IV fluids. Infuse ________ mL at ________ mL/h
5. Calculate the total volume and hourly IV flow rate for a 77-lb child receiving maintenance fluids. Infuse ________ mL at ________ mL/h
6. Calculate the total volume and hourly IV flow rate for a 3500-g infant receiving maintenance fluids. Infuse ________ mL at ________ mL/h
7. A child is receiving 350 mg IV of a medication, and the minimal and maximal dilution range is 30 to 100 mg/mL. What is the minimum volume (maximal concentration) and the maximum volume (minimal concentration) for safe dilution?
   ________ mL (minimum volume); ________ mL (maximum volume)
8. A child is receiving 52 mg IV of a medication, and the minimal and maximal dilution range is 0.8 to 20 mg/mL. What is the minimum volume and the maximum volume of fluid for safe dilution? ________ mL (minimum volume); ________ mL (maximum volume)
9. A child is receiving 175 mg IV of a medication, and the minimal and maximal dilution range is 5 to 75 mg/mL. What is the minimum volume and the maximum volume of fluid for safe dilution?
   ________ mL (minimum volume); ________ mL (maximum volume)
10. The nurse is making rounds and notices that a 2-year-old child who weighs 14 kg has 1000 mL of normal saline infusing at the rate of 50 mL/h. The nurse decides to question this order. What is the rationale for this decision? ________________________________

    ____

Check your work! Answers to all Review Sets are provided at the end of each chapter. Worked solutions for selected Review Sets are also available there.

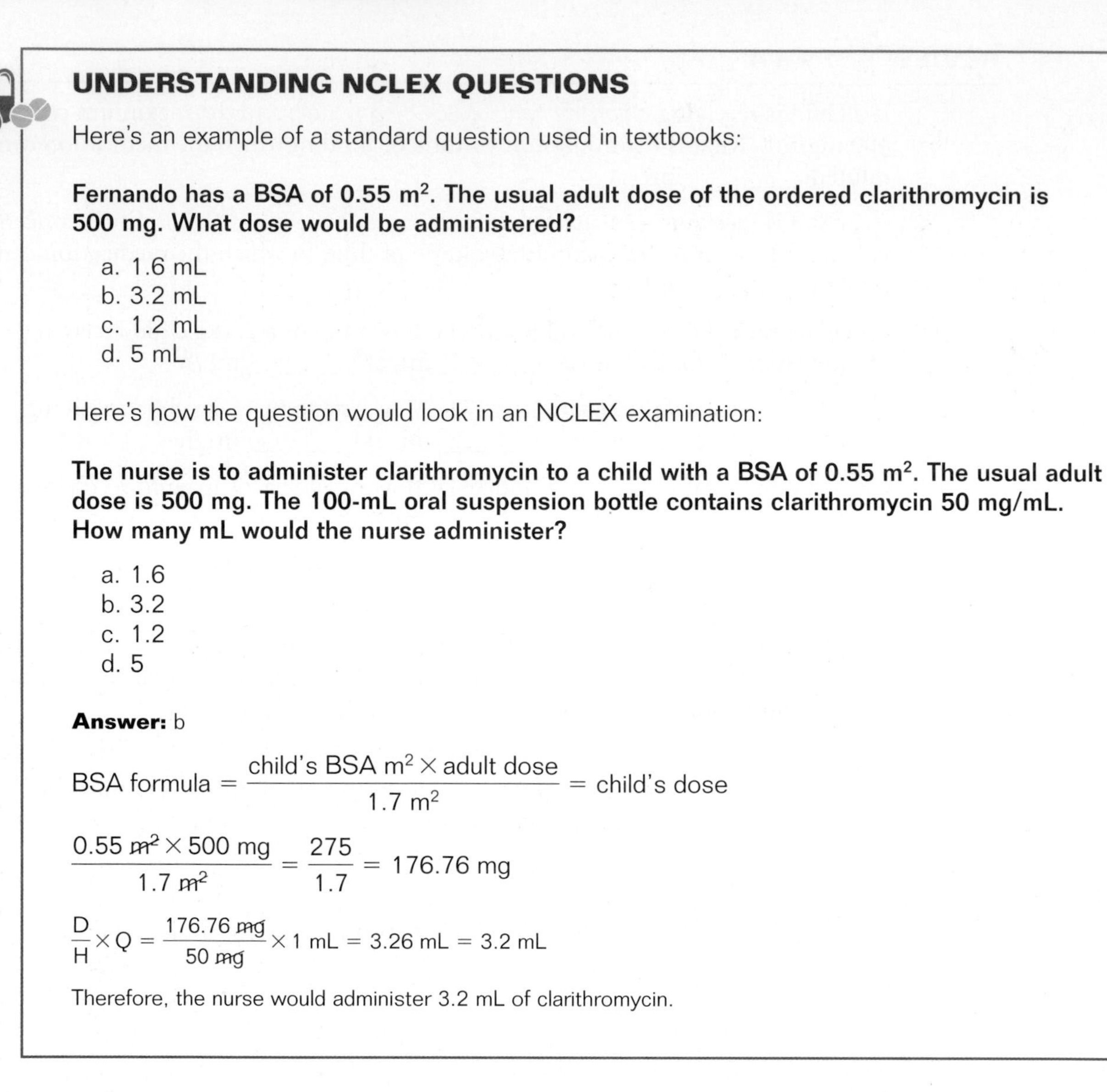

UNDERSTANDING NCLEX QUESTIONS

Here's an example of a standard question used in textbooks:

Fernando has a BSA of 0.55 m^2. The usual adult dose of the ordered clarithromycin is 500 mg. What dose would be administered?

a. 1.6 mL
b. 3.2 mL
c. 1.2 mL
d. 5 mL

Here's how the question would look in an NCLEX examination:

The nurse is to administer clarithromycin to a child with a BSA of 0.55 m^2. The usual adult dose is 500 mg. The 100-mL oral suspension bottle contains clarithromycin 50 mg/mL. How many mL would the nurse administer?

a. 1.6
b. 3.2
c. 1.2
d. 5

Answer: b

$$\text{BSA formula} = \frac{\text{child's BSA m}^2 \times \text{adult dose}}{1.7 \text{ m}^2} = \text{child's dose}$$

$$\frac{0.55 \cancel{\text{m}^2} \times 500 \text{ mg}}{1.7 \cancel{\text{m}^2}} = \frac{275}{1.7} = 176.76 \text{ mg}$$

$$\frac{D}{H} \times Q = \frac{176.76 \cancel{\text{mg}}}{50 \cancel{\text{mg}}} \times 1 \text{ mL} = 3.26 \text{ mL} = 3.2 \text{ mL}$$

Therefore, the nurse would administer 3.2 mL of clarithromycin.

PRACTICE PROBLEMS—CHAPTER 13

Calculate the volume for one safe dosage. Refer to the BSA formula or the West Nomogram in Figure 13-6 on the next page to answer questions 1 through 10.

1. Order: *vincristine 2 mg direct IV stat* for a child who weighs 85 pounds and is 50 inches tall

   Recommended dosage of vincristine for children: 1.5 to 2 mg/m^2 1 time/week; inject slowly over a period of 1 minute.

   Supply: vincristine 1 mg/mL

   BSA (per formula) of this child: ________ m^2

   Recommended dosage range for this child: ________ mg to ________ mg

   Is the ordered dosage safe? ________

   If safe, give ________ mL/min or ________ mL/15 seconds

   If not, what should the nurse do? ________________________________

2. Use the BSA nomogram to determine the BSA; then calculate the safe oral dosage and amount to give of mercaptopurine for a child of normal proportions who weighs 11.4 kg.

   Recommended dosage: 80 mg/m²/day once daily PO

   Supply: mercaptopurine 50 mg/mL

   BSA: ________ m²

   Safe dosage: ________ mg

   Give: ________ mL

Metric:

$$\text{BSA (m}^2\text{)} = \sqrt{\frac{\text{ht (cm)} \times \text{wt (kg)}}{3600}}$$

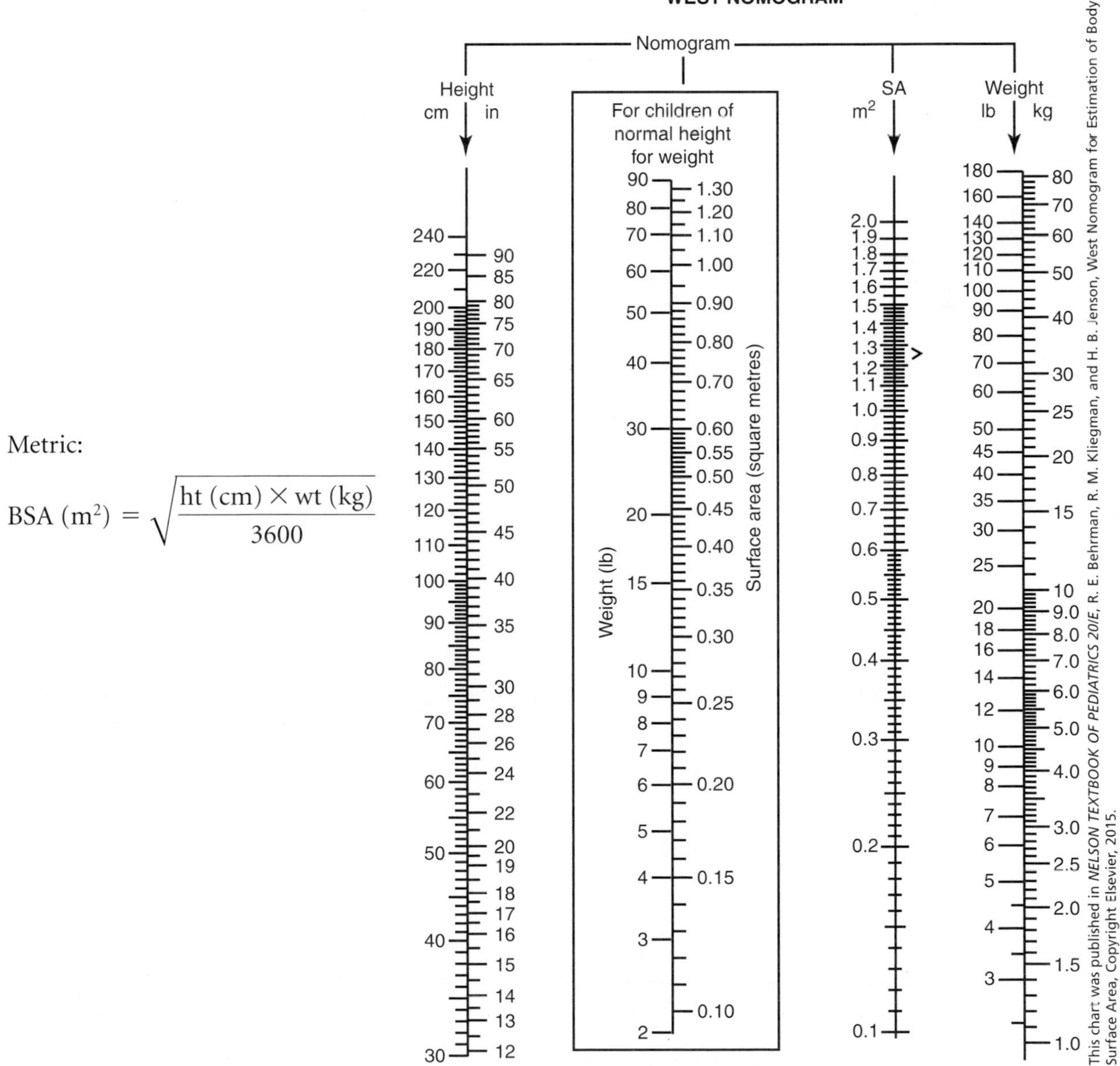

FIGURE 13-6 West Nomogram for Estimation of Body Surface Area

3. Use the BSA nomogram to determine the BSA; then calculate the safe IV dosage of sargramostim for a 1-year-old child who is 63.5 cm tall and weighs 9.1 kg. **Note:** Sargramostim is available in Canada only through the Special Access Programme.

   Recommended dosage: 250 mcg/m^2/day once daily IV

   BSA: ________ m^2

   Safe dosage: ________ mcg

4. Sargramostim is available in a solution strength of 500 mcg/10 mL. Calculate one dose for the child in question 3.

   Give: ________ mL

5. Use the BSA nomogram to determine the BSA for a child who is 88.9 cm tall and weighs 18 kg.

   BSA: ________ m^2

6. Use the BSA nomogram to determine the BSA; then calculate the safe IM dosage of pegaspargase for a child who is 107 cm tall and weighs 20.5 kg. The recommended IM dosage is 2500 units/m^2/dose. **Note:** Pegaspargase is available in Canada only through the Special Access Programme.

   BSA: ________ m^2

   Safe dosage: ________ units

7. Pegaspargase is reconstituted to 750 units per 1 mL. Calculate one dose for the child in question 6.

   Give: ________ mL

8. Should the pegaspargase in question 7 be given in one injection? ________

9. A child is 140 cm tall and weighs 43.5 kg. The recommended IV dosage of doxorubicin is 20 mg/m^2. Use the BSA formula to determine the BSA; then calculate the safe IV dosage of doxorubicin for this child.

   BSA: ________ m^2

   Safe dosage: ________ mg

10. Calculate the dose amount of doxorubicin for the child in question 9.

    Supply: doxorubicin 2 mg/mL

    Give: ________ mL

For questions 11 through 16, use the BSA formulas to calculate the BSA values.

11. Height: 60 cm Weight: 6 kg BSA: ________ m^2
12. Height: 68 in Weight: 170 lb BSA: ________ m^2
13. Height: 164 cm Weight: 58 kg BSA: ________ m^2
14. Height: 100 cm Weight: 17 kg BSA: ________ m^2
15. Height: 160 cm Weight: 63 kg BSA: ________ m^2
16. Height: 85 cm Weight: 11.5 kg BSA: ________ m^2
17. What is the safe dosage of one dose of interferon alpha-2b required for a child with a BSA of 0.28 m^2 if the recommended dosage is 2 000 000 units/m^2? ________ units
18. What is the safe dosage of a drug required for an adult with a BSA of 2.17 m^2 if the recommended dosage is 500 mg/m^2? ________ mg or ________ g

19. What is the total daily dosage range of mitomycin required for a child with a BSA of 0.19 m^2 if the recommended dosage range is 10 to 20 $mg/m^2/day$? ________ to ________ mg/day

20. What is the total safe daily dosage of cyclophosphamide required for an adult with a BSA of 1.34 m^2 if the recommended dosage is 6 $mg/m^2/day$? ________ mg/day

21. After 5 full days of therapy receiving the recommended dosage, the patient in question 20 will have received a total of ________ mg of cyclophosphamide.

For questions 22 through 29, the IV pump measures whole millilitres.

22. Order: *cefazolin 0.42 g IV q12h in 30 mL D_5NS over 30 min by volumetric control set on an infusion pump. Flush with 15 mL.*

    Supply: cefazolin 500 mg/5 mL

    Total IV fluid volume: ________ mL

    Flow rate: ________ mL/h

    Add ________ mL cefazolin and fill chamber to ________ mL with D_5NS.

23. After 7 days of IV therapy, the patient referred to in question 22 will have received a total of ________ mL of cefazolin.

24. Order: *clindamycin 285 mg IV q8h in 45 mL D_5NS over 60 min by volumetric control set on an infusion pump. Flush with 15 mL.*

    Supply: clindamycin 75 mg/0.5 mL

    Total IV fluid volume: ________ mL

    Flow rate: ________ mL/h

    Add ________ mL clindamycin and fill the chamber to ________ mL with D_5NS.

25. When the patient in question 24 has received 4 days therapy of clindamycin, he will have received a total IV medication volume of ________ mL.

26. Order: *D_5 0.33% NaCl IV at 65 mL/h with ampicillin 500 mg IV q6h to be infused over 20 min*

    You will use a volumetric control set and flush with 15 mL.

    Supply: ampicillin 250 mg/mL

    Add ________ mL of ampicillin and fill chamber to ________ mL with D_5 0.33% NaCl.

27. When the patient in question 26 has received 5 days of treatment with ampicillin, he will have received a total IV medication volume of ________ mL.

28. Order: *D_5 0.45% NaCl IV at 66 mL/h with ceftazidime 620 mg IV q8h to be infused over 40 min*

    You will use a volumetric control set and flush with 15 mL.

    Supply: ceftazidime 0.5 g/5 mL

    Add ________ mL ceftazidime and fill chamber to ________ mL with D_5 0.45% NaCl.

29. When the patient in question 28 has received 5 days of treatment with ceftazidime, she will have received a total IV medication volume of ____________mL.

For questions 30 through 33, calculate the daily volume of pediatric maintenance IV fluids.

30. Calculate the total volume and hourly IV flow rate for a 21-kg child receiving maintenance fluids.

    Infuse ________ mL at ________ mL/h.

31. Calculate the total volume and hourly IV flow rate for a 78-lb child receiving maintenance fluids.

    Infuse ________ mL at ________ mL/h.

32. Calculate the total volume and hourly IV flow rate for a 15-kg child receiving maintenance fluids.

    Infuse ________ mL at ________ mL/h.

33. Calculate the total volume and hourly IV flow rate for a 2-kg infant receiving maintenance fluids.

    Infuse ________ mL at ________ mL/h.

For questions 34 through 44, verify the safety of the pediatric dosages ordered. If the dosage is safe, calculate one dose and the IV volume to infuse one dose.

Order for a child weighing 15 kg:

D_5 0.45% NaCl IV at 53 mL/h with ampicillin 275 mg IV q4h infused over 40 min by volumetric control set

Recommended dosage: ampicillin 100 to 125 mg/kg/day in 6 divided doses

Supply: ampicillin 1 g/10 mL

34. Safe daily dosage range for this child: ________ mg/day to ________ mg/day

    Safe single dosage range for this child: ________ mg/dose to ________ mg/dose

    Is the ordered dosage safe? ________. If safe, give ________ mL/dose.

    If not safe, describe the appropriate action. ________________________________

35. IV fluid volume to be infused in 40 min: ________ mL

    Add ________ mL ampicillin and fill chamber to ________ mL with D_5 0.45% NaCl.

Order for a child who weighs 12.3 kg:

D_5 0.33% NaCl IV at 46 mL/h. The child is to receive vancomycin 100 mg IV q6h to be infused over 60 min in 100 mL D_5W by volumetric control set in 100 mL D_5W

Recommended dosage: vancomycin 10 mg/kg/dose given q6h

Supply: vancomycin 50 mg/ mL

36. Safe single dosage for this child: ________ mg/dose

    Is the ordered dosage safe? ________. If safe, give ________ mL/dose.

    If not safe, describe the appropriate action. ________________________________

37. IV fluid volume to be infused in 60 min: ________ mL

    Add ________ mL vancomycin and fill chamber to ________ mL with D_5W. Infuse over 60 min at a rate of 100 mL/h. Once the medication has been infused, readjust the IV to the ordered rate.

Order for a child who weighs 22 kg:

D_5 0.225% NaCl IV at 50 mL/h with tranexamic acid 165 mg IV q8h to be infused over 30 min by volumetric control set

Recommended dosage: tranexamic acid 15 to 22.5 mg/kg/day in 3 divided doses q8h

Supply: tranexamic acid 100 mg/mL

38. Safe daily dosage range for this child: ________ mg/day to ________ mg/day

    Safe single dosage range for this child: ________ mg/dose to ________ mg/dose

    Is the ordered dosage safe? ________. If safe, give ________ mL/dose.

    If not safe, describe the appropriate action. ________________________________

39. IV fluid volume to be infused in 30 min: ________ mL

    Add ________ mL tranexamic acid and fill chamber to ________ mL with D_5 0.225% NaCl.

Order for a child who weighs 9 kg:

D_5 0.33% NaCl IV at 38 mL/h with ticarcillin disodium/clavulanate potassium 800 mg IV q4h to be infused over 40 min by volumetric control set

Recommended dosage: 200 to 300 mg/kg/day based on ticarcillin disodium content in 6 divided doses every 4 hours

Supply: ticarcillin disodium 200 mg/mL (when the vial is reconstituted with sterile water)

40. Safe daily dosage range for this child: ________ mg/day to ________ mg/day

    Safe single dosage range for this child: ________ mg/dose to ________ mg/dose

    Is the ordered dosage safe? ________. If safe, give ________ mL/dose.

    If not safe, describe the appropriate action. ________________________________

41. IV fluid volume to be infused in 40 min: _____ mL

    Add ________ mL ticarcillin disodium and fill chamber to ________ mL with D_5 0.33% NaCl.

Order for a child who weighs 25 kg:

D_5NS IV at 60 mL/h with penicillin G sodium 525 000 units q4h to be infused over 20 min by volumetric control set

Recommended dosage: penicillin G sodium 100 000 to 250 000 units/kg/day in 6 divided doses q4h

Supply: penicillin G sodium 200 000 units/mL

42. Safe daily dosage for this child: ________ units/day to ________ units/day

    Safe single dosage for this child: ________ units/dose to ________ units/dose

43. Is the ordered dosage safe? ________. If safe, give ________ mL/dose.

    If not safe, describe the appropriate action. ________________________________

44. IV fluid volume to be infused in 20 min: ________ mL

    Add ________ mL penicillin G sodium and fill chamber to ________ mL with D_5 NS.

Check your work! Answers to all problems are provided at the end of the book, in the Answers section. Worked solutions for some Practice Problems are also provided there.

ANSWERS TO REVIEW SETS

Review Set 13-1

1) 2.35 **2)** 0.69 **3)** 1.4 **4)** 2.03 **5)** 1.66 **6)** 1.69 **7)** 0.52 **8)** 0.78 **9)** 0.15 **10)** 0.78 **11)** 0.39 **12)** 0.64 **13)** 1.08 **14)** 0.5 **15)** 0.88

Review Set 13-2

1) 1 640 000 **2)** 5.9; 11.8 **3)** 735 **4)** 1584 **5)** 250 **6)** 0.49; 122.5; yes; 2.5 **7)** 0.89; 2.9; Yes; 1.2 **8)** 66; 22; Yes; **9)**198; Yes; 990 **10)** 612; 612; 1224; 2448 **11)** 8.1; 24.7 **12)** 67–167.5; 33.5–83.8; Yes **13)** 8–14.4; Yes **14)** 0.82; 2050; Yes; 2.7; 102.7; 51 **15)** 1.62; 4050; Yes; 5.4; 105.4; 53

Review Set 13-3

1) 87; 0.5; 50 **2)** 130; 5.6; 50 **3)** 120; 1.8; 25 **4)** 80; 6; 50 **5)** 60; 1; 32; 96 **6)** 2; 25 **7)** 0.5; 10 **8)** 12; 57 **9)** 7.2; 44 **10)** 10.5; 45

Review Set 13-4

1) 4 **2)** 25 **3)** 1600; 67 **4)** 1150; 48 **5)** 1800; 75 **6)** 350; 15 **7)** 3.5 or 4; 11.6 or 12 **8)** 2.6 or 3; 65 **9)** 2.3 or 3; 35 **10)** This order should be questioned because normal saline is an isotonic solution and appears to be a continuous infusion for this child. This solution does not contribute enough electrolytes for the child, and water intoxication may result. A 1000-mL bag would last 20 h (too long to hang one bag; it is better to use a 250-mL or 500-mL bag for children).

SELECTED SOLUTIONS TO REVIEW SETS

Review Set 13-1

1) Metric: $\text{BSA (m}^2) = \sqrt{\frac{\text{ht (cm)} \times \text{wt (kg)}}{3600}} = \sqrt{\frac{190 \times 105}{3600}} = \sqrt{\frac{19\,950}{3600}} = \sqrt{5.542} = 2.354 \text{ m}^2 = 2.35 \text{ m}^2$

Review Set 13-2

1) $2\,000\,000 \text{ units}/\cancel{\text{m}^2} \times 0.82 \cancel{\text{m}^2} = 1\,640\,000 \text{ units}$

2) $10 \text{ mg}/\cancel{\text{m}^2}/\text{day} \times 0.59 \cancel{\text{m}^2} = 5.9 \text{ mg/day}$

(minimum safe dosage)

$20 \text{ mg}/\cancel{\text{m}^2}/\text{day} \times 0.59 \cancel{\text{m}^2} = 11.8 \text{ mg/day}$

(maximum safe dosage)

3) $500 \text{ mg}/\cancel{\text{m}^2} \times 1.47 \cancel{\text{m}^2} = 735 \text{ mg}$

4) $600 \text{ mg}/\cancel{\text{m}^2}/\text{dose} \times 2.64 \cancel{\text{m}^2} = 1584 \text{ mg/day}$

8) $150 \text{ mg}/\cancel{\text{m}^2}/\text{day} \times 0.44 \cancel{\text{m}^2} = 66 \text{ mg/day;}$

$66 \text{ mg/day} \div 3 \text{ doses/day} = 22 \text{ mg/dose}$

The ordered dose of 22 mg is exactly the recommended dose so the order is safe.

10) $600 \text{ mg}/\cancel{\text{m}^2} \times 1.02 \cancel{\text{m}^2} = 612 \text{ mg, initially}$

$300 \text{ mg}/\cancel{\text{m}^2} \times 1.02 \cancel{\text{m}^2} = 306 \text{ mg; for 2 doses:}$

$306 \text{ mg} \times 2 = 612 \text{ mg}$

q12h is 2 doses/day and

$2 \text{ doses}/\cancel{\text{day}} \times 2 \cancel{\text{days}} = 4 \text{ doses}$

$306 \text{ mg} \times 4 = 1224 \text{ mg}$

$612 \text{ mg} + 612 \text{ mg} + 1224 \text{ mg} = 2448 \text{ mg (total)}$

12) $100 \text{ mg}/\cancel{\text{m}^2}/\text{day} \times 0.67 \cancel{\text{m}^2} = 67 \text{ mg/day}$

$250 \text{ mg}/\cancel{\text{m}^2}/\text{day} \times 0.67 \cancel{\text{m}^2} = 167.5 \text{ mg/day}$

$67 \text{ mg/day} \div 2 \text{ doses/day} = 33.5 \text{ mg}$

$167.5 \text{ mg/day} \div 2 \text{ doses/day} = 83.75 \text{ mg}$

Ordered dose of 83.75 mg is between the minimum dose of 33.5 mg and the maximum dose of 83.8 mg, and is safe.

13) $25 \text{ mg}/\cancel{\text{m}^2} \times 0.32 \cancel{\text{m}^2} = 8 \text{ mg}$

$45 \text{ mg}/\cancel{\text{m}^2} \times 0.32 \cancel{\text{m}^2} = 14.4 \text{ mg}$

Ordered dose of 9.6 mg is between the minimum dose of 8 mg and the maximum dose of 14.4 mg, and is safe.

Review Set 13-3

1) Total volume: 50 mL + 15 mL = 65 mL

$\frac{V}{T} \times C = \frac{65 \cancel{\text{mL}}}{\cancel{45}_{3} \text{ min}} \times \cancel{60}^{4} \text{ gtt}/\cancel{\text{mL}} =$

$\frac{260 \text{ gtt}}{3 \text{ min}} = 86.6 \text{ gtt/min} = 87 \text{ gtt/min}$

$\frac{D}{H} \times Q = \frac{\cancel{125 \text{ mg}}}{\cancel{250 \text{ mg}}} \times 1 \text{ mL} = 0.5 \text{ mL (medication)}$

9.5

Add 0.5 mL amikacin to the chamber and fill with IV fluid to a volume of 50 mL. Follow with the 15-mL flush also set at 87 gtt/min.

4) Total volume: 50 mL + 30 mL = 80 mL

80 mL/60 min = 80 mL/h

$\frac{D}{H} \times Q = \frac{0.6\ \cancel{g}}{1\ \cancel{g}} \times 10\ mL = 6\ mL\ (medication)$

Add 6 mL cefazolin sodium to the chamber and fill with IV fluid to a volume of 50 mL. Follow with the 30 mL flush.

6) $\frac{50\ mL}{60\ min} \times \frac{X\ mL}{30\ min}$

$60X = 1500$

$\frac{60X}{60} = \frac{1500}{60}$

$X = 25\ mL\ (total\ volume)$

$\frac{D}{H} \times Q = \frac{\overset{2}{\cancel{250}}\ mg}{\underset{1}{\cancel{125}}\ mg} \times 1\ mL = 2\ mL\ (medication)$

Add 2 mL cefazolin sodium to the chamber and fill with IV fluid to a volume of 25 mL.

8) $\frac{85\ mL}{60\ min} \times \frac{X\ mL}{40\ min}$

$60X = 3400$

$\frac{60X}{60} = \frac{3400}{60}$

$X = 56.6\ mL = 57\ mL\ (total\ volume)$

$\frac{D}{H} \times Q = \frac{\overset{12}{\cancel{600}}\ \cancel{mg}}{\underset{1}{\cancel{50}}\ \cancel{mg}} \times 1\ mL = 12\ mL\ (medication)$

Add 12 mL erythromycin to the chamber and fill with IV fluid to a volume of 57 mL.

9) $\frac{66\ mL}{60\ min} = \frac{X\ mL}{40\ min}$

$60X = 2640$

$\frac{60X}{60} = \frac{2640}{60}$

$X = 44\ mL\ (total\ volume)$

$\frac{D}{H} \times Q = \frac{720\ \cancel{mg}}{\underset{100}{\cancel{1000}}\ \cancel{mg}} \times \overset{1}{\cancel{10}}\ mL$

Add 7.2 mL ceftazidime to the chamber and fill with IV fluid to a volume of 44 mL.

Review Set 13-4

1) $\frac{100\ mg}{1\ mL} \times \frac{400\ mg}{X\ mL}$

$100X = 400$

$\frac{100X}{100} = \frac{400}{100}$

$X = 4\ mL$

3) 100 mL/~~kg~~/day × 10 ~~kg~~ = 1000 mL/day for first 10

50 mL/~~kg~~/day × 10 ~~kg~~ = 500 mL/day for next 10

20 mL/~~kg~~/day × 5 ~~kg~~ = 100 mL/day for remaining

1600 mL/day or per 24 h

$\frac{1600\ mL}{24\ h} = 66.7\ mL/h = 67\ mL/h$

4) 100 mL/~~kg~~/day × 10 ~~kg~~ = 1000 mL/day for first 10 kg

150 mL/day × 3 ~~kg~~ = 150 mL/day for next 10 kg

1150 mL/day or per 24 h

$\frac{1150\ mL}{24\ h} = 47.9\ mL/h = 48\ mL/h$

5) $77\ lb = \frac{77}{2.2} = 35\ kg$

100 mL/~~kg~~/day × 10 ~~kg~~ = 1000 mL/day for first 10

50 mL/kg/day × 10 kg = 500 mL/day for next 10

20 mL/kg/day × 15 kg = 300 mL/day for remaining

1800 mL/day or per 24 h

$\frac{1800\ mL}{24\ h} = 75\ mL/h$

7) $\frac{100\ mg}{1\ mL} \times \frac{350\ mg}{X\ mL}$

$100X = 350$

$\frac{100X}{100} = \frac{350}{100}$

$X = 3.5\ or\ 4\ mL\ (min.\ dilution\ volume)$

$\frac{30\ mg}{1\ mL} \times \frac{350\ mg}{X\ mL}$

$30X = 350$

$\frac{30X}{30} = \frac{350}{30}$

$X = 11.6\ or\ 12\ mL\ (max.\ dilution\ volume)$

CHAPTER

14

Advanced Adult Intravenous Calculations

OBJECTIVES

1. Initiate and manage continuous infusions of high-alert medications using a protocol to calculate a bolus dosage and volume, calculate a continuous infusion dosage (units/h) and rate (mL/h), monitor and make necessary adjustments to continuous intravenous therapy, and observe patients for serious adverse reactions and administer the appropriate antidote as needed.
2. Calculate the flow rate and assess safe dosages for critical care IV medications administered over a specified time period.
3. Calculate the flow rate for primary IV and IV piggyback (IVPB) solutions for patients with restricted fluid intake requirements.

Nurses are responsible for the administration of many high-alert medications in both critical care areas and general nursing units. These specialized potent life-sustaining medications are required for optimal management of patients who are critically ill and may have life-threatening conditions. Such medications require tight control of dosing, as minute changes in the infusion rate can alter the therapeutic effect. Knowing the therapeutic dosage for the desired effect is just as important as knowing the correct calculations for the drug. For example, dopamine hydrochloride at doses of 3 to 5 mcg/kg/minute provides a gentle dilation of the renal arteries, increasing urine output with no effect on blood pressure (BP). At higher doses (up to 20 mcg/kg/minute), dopamine hydrochloride is used for BP support. It is crucial to be knowledgeable about the medication, the effect it is expected to deliver, and the maximum recommended safe infusion dosage. The focus of this chapter is advanced adult IV calculations with special requirements that can be applied to patients across the life span.

CALCULATING IV DOSAGES AND FLOW RATES USING CLINICAL PROTOCOLS

Clinical protocols are preapproved orders that provide a precise sequence of activities to be adhered to in the management of specific clinical conditions for patients with specific clinical problems. These orders are common in practice settings where patients' needs require immediate attention. Based on these protocols, the nurse makes a clinical judgment regarding the rate and amount of drug the patient receives. Clinical protocols provide the nurse with legal protection to intervene appropriately and administer medication without contacting the prescriber each time the patient's condition changes. Heparin sodium and insulin, two high-alert medications, are examples of medications given intravenously that are ordered using standard protocols. Specific protocols will vary slightly between prescribers and institutions; however, two typical protocols (Figures 14-1 and 14-5) are provided in this chapter as samples for study purposes.

Because patients vary in weight, the intravenous heparin sodium dosage is individualized based on the patient's weight. The heparin sodium protocol orders shown in Figure 14-1 are based on patient weight rounded to the nearest 10 kg (line 1). Some institutions use the patient's exact weight in kilograms. It is important to know the protocol for your institution. When the patient's response to heparin sodium therapy changes, as measured by the activated partial thromboplastin time (aPTT) blood clotting value (measured in seconds), the heparin sodium dosage is adjusted as indicated in lines 11 to 15 of Figure 14-1.

Insulin dosage must be closely matched with insulin needs. For patients who are hospitalized, the dosage must be monitored and adjusted to meet special conditions such as infection, surgery, pregnancy, and drug-to-drug interactions. Nurses follow standard protocols to ensure that insulin dosage is coordinated with insulin requirements through rigorous blood glucose monitoring and insulin replacement therapy. The insulin protocol orders in Figure 14-5 provide instructions to use specific dosage grids for three levels of therapy based on potential resistance to insulin. If the patient does not have diabetes, the insulin infusion is started on the lowest level, that is, level 1. Patients who have diabetes begin insulin replacement on level 2 and may need to move to the level 3 insulin dosage grid if the therapy is ineffective.

For both the heparin sodium and insulin protocols, as well as other protocols for critical medications, the administration process is the same and includes three sequential actions: (1) bolus, (2) continuous infusion, and (3) rebolus and adjust the infusion rate.

RULE

To administer critical intravenous medications according to protocol, follow three sequential actions:

Action 1 **Bolus:** Determine the need for a bolus dose (a large dose to rapidly achieve a therapeutic effect) according to the patient condition specified in the protocol. Select the right supplied drug, calculate, and administer the right amount by direct IV bolus or direct IV infusion.

Action 2 **Continuous infusion:** Acquire the right concentration of the continuous solution from the pharmacy (or mix the IVPB bag by selecting the right supplied drug), calculate the amount required to provide the ordered dosage, and calculate and set the flow rate as determined by protocol.

Action 3 **Rebolus and/or adjust the infusion rate:** Based on patient monitoring, determine whether an additional bolus is needed or whether the continuous infusion rate needs to be increased, decreased, or discontinued.

CAUTION

Remember that high-alert drugs require independent double verification (of the order, test results, calculations, and drug preparation) by two clinicians who are alone and apart from each other, and who later compare results.

First, all three actions beginning with the heparin sodium protocol will be applied, followed by the same process with the insulin protocol.

IV Heparin Sodium Protocol

Heparin sodium protocols may vary slightly between institutions. For problems in this text, a sample Standard Weight-Based Heparin Sodium Protocol is used (Figure 14-1), but always use the protocol that has been adopted by the specific institution where you practise.

Action 1: Bolus

A bolus dosage is a large dose of a medication given to rapidly achieve the needed therapeutic concentration in the bloodstream. Notice that the heparin sodium protocol defines the bolus dosage that should be given based on the patient's weight and the results of the patient's blood tests. First consider the initial bolus dosage ordered.

Example 1:

The patient, who weighs 110 lb, has orders to start on Standard Weight-Based Heparin Sodium Protocol. The result of the baseline aPTT is 29 sec. Refer to Figure 14-1, lines 1, 2, and 10 as you work through this example.

Order: *bolus with 80 units/kg* (line 10, Figure 14-1)

Supply: vials of heparin sodium in various concentrations (Figure 14-2)

SAMPLE STANDARD WEIGHT-BASED HEPARIN SODIUM PROTOCOL	
For all patients on heparin sodium drips:	
1. Weight in KILOGRAMS. Required for order to be processed: ________ kg (round to nearest 10 kg).	
2. Heparin sodium 25 000 units in 250 mL of NS; boluses to be given as 1000 units/mL.	
3. aPTT q6h or 6 hours after rate change; daily after two consecutive therapeutic aPTTs.	
4. CBC initially and repeat every ________ day(s).	
5. Obtain aPTT and PT/INR on day 1 prior to initiation of therapy.	
6. Guaiac stool initially, then every ________ day(s) until heparin sodium discontinued. Notify if positive.	
7. Neuro checks every ________ hours while on heparin sodium. Notify prescriber of any changes.	
8. Discontinue aPTT and CBC once heparin sodium drip is discontinued unless otherwise ordered.	
9. Notify physician of any bleeding problems.	
10. Bolus with 80 units/kg. Start drip at 18 units/kg/h.	
11. If aPTT is less than 35 sec	Rebolus with 80 units/kg and increase rate by 4 units/kg/h.
12. If aPTT is 36 to 44 sec	Rebolus with 40 units/kg and increase rate by 2 units/kg/h.
13. If aPTT is 45 to 75 sec	Continue current rate.
14. If aPTT is 76 to 90 sec	Decrease rate by 2 units/kg/h.
15. If aPTT is greater than 90 sec	Hold heparin sodium for 1 hour and decrease rate by 3 units/kg/h.
ONLY USE 1000 unit/mL HEPARIN SODIUM FOR BOLUSES	

WEIGHT	**INITIAL BOLUS** (VOL.)	**INITIAL INFUSION** (rate)
40 kg	3 200 units (3.2 mL)	700 units/h (7 mL/h)
50 kg	4 000 units (4 mL)	900 units/h (9 mL/h)
60 kg	4 800 units (4.8 mL)	1 100 units/h (11 mL/h)
70 kg	5 600 units (5.6 mL)	1 300 units/h (13 mL/h)
80 kg	6 400 units (6.4 mL)	1 400 units/h (14 mL/h)
90 kg	7 200 units (7.2 mL)	1 600 units/h (16 mL/h)
100 kg	8 000 units (8 mL)	1 800 units/h (18 mL/h)
110 kg	8 800 units (8.8 mL)	2 000 units/h (20 mL/h)
120 kg	9 600 units (9.6 mL)	2 200 units/h (22 mL/h)
130 kg	10 400 units (10.4 mL)	2 300 units/h (23 mL/h)
140 kg	11 200 units (11.2 mL)	2 500 units/h (25 mL/h)
150 kg	12 000 units (12 mL)	2 700 units/h (27 mL/h)

FIGURE 14-1 Sample Heparin Sodium Therapy Protocol

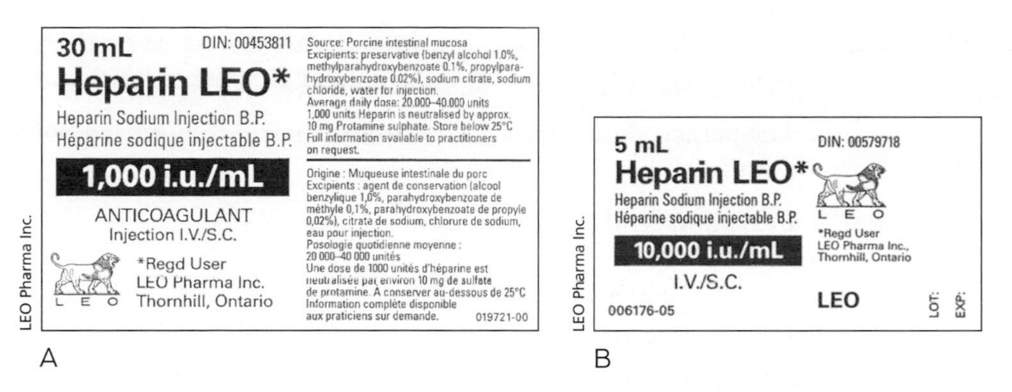

FIGURE 14-2(a) Heparin Sodium 1000 units/mL; (b) Heparin Sodium 10 000 units/mL

RULE

To calculate the heparin sodium bolus,

1. **Calculate the dosage (units) of the heparin sodium bolus based on patient's weight (kg): units/kg × kg = units.**
2. **Calculate the volume (mL) of the bolus to prepare using the dosage calculation formula:**

$$\frac{D}{H} \times Q = X.$$

Note: **This rule also applies to other bolus drugs ordered in units/kg, milliunits/kg, mg/kg, mcg/kg, g/kg, or mEq/kg.**

Now prepare the initial IV bolus, using the Three-Step Approach to dosage calculations that has been used throughout the book.

Step 1 Convert No conversion is necessary for the medications, but the patient's weight needs to be converted to kilograms to calculate the correct bolus dosage by weight.

Approximate equivalent: 1 kg = 2.2 lb; conversion factor is 2.2 lb/kg

$110 \text{ lb} \div 2.2 \text{ lb/kg} = 110 \cancel{\text{lb}} \times 1 \text{ kg}/2.2 \cancel{\text{lb}} = 50 \text{ kg}$

Step 2 Think The patient is ordered to receive an initial bolus of 80 units/kg. According to the grid provided the initial bolus dosage for a patient weighing 50 kg is 4000 units or 4 mL. But because heparin sodium is supplied in various concentrations, it is important to know which concentration; not just any 4-mL vial of heparin sodium is appropriate. The protocol specifically requires the use of the 1000 units/mL concentration of heparin sodium (line 2). The grid provides only the initial bolus, so the nurse will need to calculate any additional boluses needed throughout the therapy. Calculate the bolus now to verify the grid, and then use this same calculation process for additional boluses. Carefully compare the two supplied concentrations. Select one vial labelled 1000 units/mL, and check the label again to be certain it is the desired concentration.

Step 3 Calculate the dosage (units) of the heparin sodium bolus based on the patient's weight (kg): units/kg × kg = 80 units/~~kg~~ × 50 ~~kg~~ = 4000 units

The patient should receive 4000 units heparin sodium as a bolus (verifies grid).

Calculate the volume (mL) of the bolus to prepare.

$$\frac{D}{H} \times Q = \frac{\overset{4}{\cancel{4000}\ \cancel{\text{units}}}}{\underset{1}{\cancel{1000}\ \cancel{\text{units}}}} \times 1\text{ mL} = 4\text{ mL (verifies grid)}$$

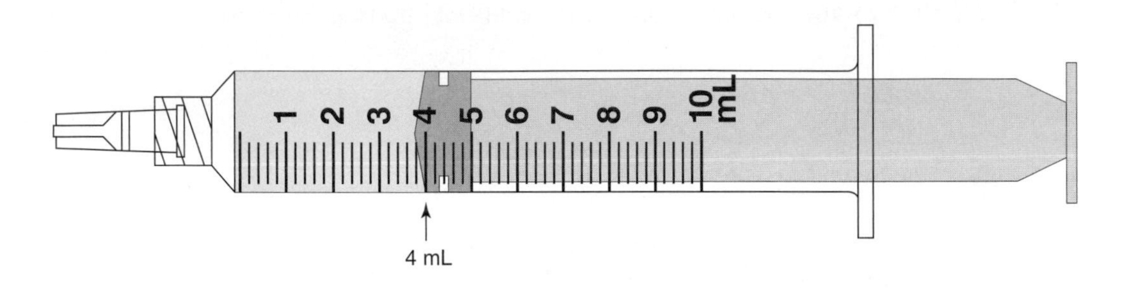

Measure 4 mL of heparin sodium from the 1000 units/mL supply in a 10 mL syringe. Because 6 mL remain in the vial, label the vial with the date and time opened, and store it safely for its next use. Give the order, vial, and syringe to another nurse for independent verification and documentation.

Action 2: Continuous Infusion

A continuous infusion is a controlled method of drug administration in which the rate and quality of drug administration can be precisely adjusted over time. Often, IV solutions with heparin sodium, insulin, or other added high-alert drugs come premixed from the hospital pharmacy. There may be times when nurses will need to mix the IV solution for the continuous infusion. Now continue with the patient in Example 1 by following the protocol to prepare the IV heparin sodium solution and calculate the initial infusion rate.

Example 2:

In addition to receiving the bolus dose, the patient from Example 1 will need to have the continuous infusion started according to protocol.

Order: *heparin sodium 25 000 units in 250 mL NS* (line 2, Figure 14-1)

Supply: vials of heparin sodium in various concentrations (Figure 14-2)

Now prepare the IV solution using the Three-Step Approach to dosage calculations.

Step 1 Convert Remember, 110 lb = 50 kg. The order and the supplied dosages are in the same unit. No conversion is necessary.

Step 2 Think The 10 000 units/mL supply dosage is the vial that will provide 25 000 units. If there are 10 000 units in 1 mL, there are 50 000 units in 5 mL. This order for 25 000 units is half the total volume in the vial, or 2.5 mL. Select one vial labelled 10 000 units/mL, and check the label again to ensure it is the desired concentration.

Step 3 Calculate

$$\frac{D}{H} \times Q = \frac{\overset{25}{\cancel{25\,000}\ \cancel{\text{units}}}}{\underset{10}{\cancel{10\,000}\ \cancel{\text{units}}}} \times 1\text{ mL} = \frac{25}{10}\text{ mL} = 2.5\text{ mL (verifies estimate)}$$

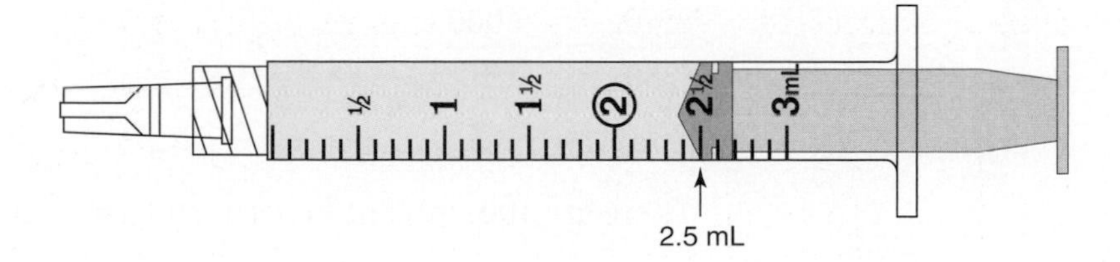

Measure 2.5 mL of heparin sodium from the 10 000 units/mL supply in a 3-mL syringe. Give the order, vial, and syringe to another nurse for independent verification and documentation. Add to the 250-mL IVPB bag of 0.9% sodium chloride through the injection port. There will be 2.5 mL of this highly concentrated, high-alert drug remaining in the vial. Either discard the vial immediately or label it with the date and time opened, and store the vial safely. Prepare a label with the patient's name, drug name and concentration, dosage and amount added, date and time prepared, and your signature, and place the label on the IVPB bag.

Order: *start drip at 18 units/kg/h* (line 10, Figure 14-1)

Supply: heparin sodium 25 000 units in 250 mL

RULE

To calculate the continuous flow rate of the IV heparin sodium solution in mL/h,

1. **Calculate the dosage (units/h) of the initial continuous infusion based on patient's weight (kg):**

   units/kg/h × kg = units/h

2. **Calculate the continuous infusion rate (mL/h) using a version of the dosage calculation formula:**

   $$\frac{\text{D (units/h desired)}}{\text{H (units available)}} \times \text{Q (mL available)} = \text{R (mL/h rate)}$$

Note: **This rule applies to drugs ordered in units/kg/h, milliunits/kg/h, mg/kg/h, mcg/kg/h, g/kg/h, or mEq/kg/h.**

Now calculate the initial infusion rate using the Three-Step Approach to dosage calculations.

Step 1 Convert The order and the supplied dosages are the same unit. No conversion is necessary. Remember, the patient's weight: 110 lb = 50 kg.

Step 2 Think According to the grid provided, the initial continuous infusion rate for a patient weighing 50 kg is 900 units/h (9 mL/h). Remember that the grid provides only the initial infusion rate, so the nurse will need to calculate any necessary infusion rate increases or decreases throughout the therapy. Calculate the infusion rate now to verify the grid, then use this same calculation process for any needed adjustments in the rate. The solution prepared is 25 000 units per 250 mL. You need 900 units for the dose; 900 units is less than $\frac{1}{2}$ but more than $\frac{1}{3}$ of 25 000 units. So you will need less than 125 mL but more than 80 mL. You can think about this in a different way by using ratio and proportion to determine how many units are in 1 mL. If there are 25 000 units per 250 mL, how many units are there in 1 mL? Set up the ratio-proportion like this:

$$\frac{25\,000 \text{ units}}{250 \text{ mL}} \times \frac{\text{X units}}{1 \text{ mL}}$$

$$250\text{X} = 25\,000$$

$$\frac{250X}{250} = \frac{25\,000}{250}$$

$X = 100$ units

There are 100 units of heparin sodium per 1 mL.

Now you know that with the concentration of heparin sodium solution used for this protocol, each mL infused will contain 100 units of heparin sodium. So if you want to administer 900 units of heparin sodium, you want 9 times 1 mL, or 9 mL.

Step 3 Calculate the dosage (units/h) of the continuous infusion increase based on the patient's weight (kg):

units/kg/h × kg = 18 units/~~kg~~/h × 50 ~~kg~~ = 900 units/h (verifies grid)

Calculate the new hourly infusion rate (mL/h) using a version of the dosage calculation formula:

$$\frac{D\text{ (units/h)}}{H\text{ (units)}} \times Q\text{ (mL)} = R\text{ (mL/h)};\ \frac{900\ \cancel{\text{units}}/\text{h}}{\underset{100}{\cancel{25\,000}}\ \cancel{\text{units}}} \times \overset{1}{\cancel{250}}\text{ mL} = \frac{9\cancel{00}}{1\cancel{00}}\text{ mL/h}$$

$= 9$ mL/h

or

$$\frac{D\text{ (units/h)}}{H\text{ (units)}} \times Q\text{ (mL)} = R\text{ (mL/h)};\ \frac{\overset{9}{\cancel{900}}\ \cancel{\text{units}}/\text{h}}{\underset{1}{\cancel{100}}\ \cancel{\text{units}}} \times 1\text{ mL} = 9\text{ mL/h}$$

(verifies grid and estimate)

Knowing the units per mL simplifies the calculation. In fact, for many protocols, the concentrations for the solutions are specifically chosen to help make the calculations easier, thereby reducing the risk of patient safety incident. The rate on the chart included with the protocol is verified by the calculations. Remember that, while the chart is convenient to refer to when setting up the initial infusion, it is not to be used for any needed adjustment to the infusion rate throughout the therapy. This high-alert medication will be infused using an electronic IV infusion pump. For this example, assume that the infusion pump available is designed to infuse at the mL/h rate using whole numbers only. It is important to verify the calibration of the IV pump in your clinical setting. Some IV pumps are programmable in tenths of a millilitre. Set the rate on the pump for the initial infusion at 9 mL/h. Ask another nurse for independent verification of the initial infusion rate.

Action 3: Rebolus and/or Adjust the Infusion Rate

The anticoagulant heparin sodium is used to prevent formation of thrombi (intravenous blood clots) by suppressing clotting factors, such as thrombin. The most significant complication of treatment is life-threatening hemorrhage. The goal of heparin sodium therapy is to reduce the body's ability to clot to a level that is low enough to prevent thrombosis but not so low that it causes spontaneous bleeding. Response to heparin sodium therapy is highly variable from one patient to another. The aPTT is a blood test that measures the time it takes blood to clot. The aPTT is used during anticoagulation therapy to determine the right dosage of the drug. It is the nurse's responsibility to monitor the patient for bleeding and adjust the dosage of heparin sodium based on periodic measurements of aPTT and the heparin sodium protocol. To ensure consistent monitoring from shift to shift, the nurse must document the time and dose of the bolus and any changes in the infusion rate. Figure 14-3 is an example of a handwritten heparin sodium protocol worksheet that could be used for this patient.

STANDARD WEIGHT-BASED HEPARIN PROTOCOL WORKSHEET

Round patient's total body weight to nearest 10 kg: _______ kg.

DO NOT change the weight based on daily measurements.

FOUND ON THE ORDER FORM

Initial Bolus (80 units/kg): _______ units _______ mL

Initial Infusion Rate (18 units/kg/h): _______ units/h _______ mL/h

Make adjustments to the heparin drip rate as directed by the order form.

ALL DOSES ARE ROUNDED TO THE NEAREST 100 UNITS.

Date	Time	aPTT	Bolus	Rate Change		New Rate	RN 1	RN 2
				units/h	mL/h			

If aPTT is	Then
Less than 35 sec:	Rebolus with 80 units/kg and increase rate by 4 units/kg/h.
36 to 44 sec:	Rebolus with 40 units/kg and increase rate by 2 units/kg/h.
45 to 75 sec:	Continue current rate.
76 to 90 sec:	Decrease rate by 2 units/kg/h.
Greater than 90 sec:	Hold heparin sodium for 1 hour and decrease rate by 3 units/kg/h.

Signatures ______________________________ Initials

____

____

____

____

____

Fresenius Kabi USA

FIGURE 14-3 Sample Heparin Sodium Protocol Worksheet

Example 3:

After 6 hours of heparin sodium infusion, the patient on the heparin sodium protocol has an aPTT test (line 3, Figure 14-1). One hour later, the result is reported to be 43 seconds. The clotting time measured has lengthened from 26 seconds to 43 seconds but has not reached the target time. According to the protocol, the nurse will rebolus with 40 units/kg and increase the amount of IV heparin by 2 units/kg/h (line 12, Figure 14-1) and then recheck the aPTT in 6 hours. The same calculation skills learned in the previous examples are used for both the initial bolus and to set the initial infusion rate.

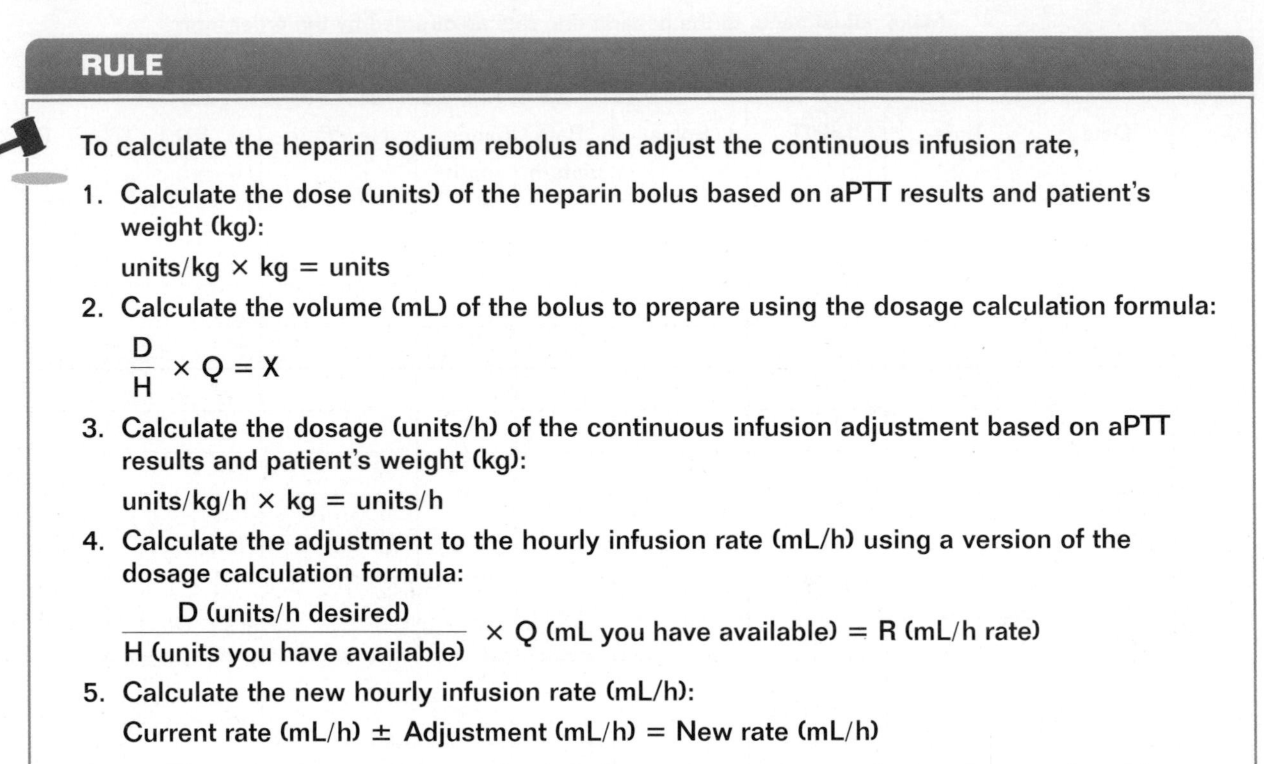

RULE

To calculate the heparin sodium rebolus and adjust the continuous infusion rate,

1. **Calculate the dose (units) of the heparin bolus based on aPTT results and patient's weight (kg):**

   units/kg × kg = units

2. **Calculate the volume (mL) of the bolus to prepare using the dosage calculation formula:**

   $$\frac{D}{H} \times Q = X$$

3. **Calculate the dosage (units/h) of the continuous infusion adjustment based on aPTT results and patient's weight (kg):**

   units/kg/h × kg = units/h

4. **Calculate the adjustment to the hourly infusion rate (mL/h) using a version of the dosage calculation formula:**

   $$\frac{\text{D (units/h desired)}}{\text{H (units you have available)}} \times \text{Q (mL you have available)} = \text{R (mL/h rate)}$$

5. **Calculate the new hourly infusion rate (mL/h):**

   Current rate (mL/h) ± Adjustment (mL/h) = New rate (mL/h)

Note: This rule also applies to other rebolus and continuous infusion drugs ordered in units/kg/h, milliunits/kg/h, mg/kg/h, mcg/kg/h, g/h, or mEq/kg/h.

Order: *rebolus with 40 units/kg and increase rate by 2 units/kg/h* (line 12, Figure 14-1)

Supply: vial of heparin sodium 1000 units/mL with 6 mL remaining; IVPB of heparin sodium 25 000 units in 250 mL

Calculate the adjusted infusion rate using the Three-Step Approach to dosage calculations.

Step 1 Convert You already know the patient's weight (50 kg) and that no unit conversion is necessary.

Step 2 Think The patient now needs to receive a bolus of 40 units/kg. You cannot use the grid provided because it lists the dosage for the initial bolus of 80 units/kg. You will need to calculate the dose, so think: if the patient now needs half the initial bolus order, the dose should be half the bolus dose, which was 4 mL. The bolus should now be 2 mL. In addition, the continuous infusion is set at a rate of 18 units/kg/h, or 9 mL per hour. The rate will need to be increased by 2 units/kg/h, which should provide an hourly rate of slightly more than 9 mL.

Step 3 Calculate the dosage (units) of the heparin sodium rebolus based on patient's weight (kg):

units/kg × kg; 40 units/~~kg~~ × 50 ~~kg~~ = 2000 units

The patient should receive 2000 units heparin sodium as a rebolus.

Calculate the volume (mL) of the rebolus to prepare. Remember that you will use the 1000 units/mL supply to measure the amount of heparin sodium for the rebolus.

$$\frac{D}{H} \times Q = \frac{\overset{2}{\cancel{2000}}\ \cancel{\text{units}}}{\underset{1}{\cancel{1000}}\ \cancel{\text{units}}} \times 1\text{ mL} = 2\text{ mL (verifies estimate)}$$

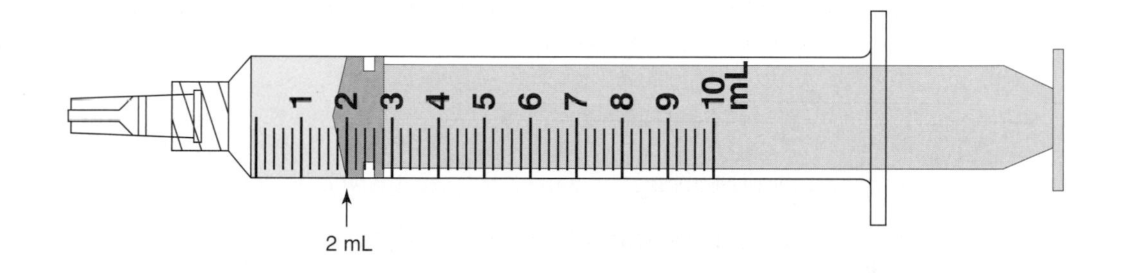

Measure 2 mL of heparin sodium from the 1000 units/mL supply in a 10-mL syringe. You may use the vial with 6 mL remaining from the initial bolus if it was safely labelled and stored. There will now be 4 mL remaining, which may be stored safely for the next use. Give the order, vial, and syringe to another nurse for independent verification and documentation.

Calculate the dosage (units/h) of the continuous infusion increase based on patient's weight (kg):

units/kg/h × kg = 2 units/~~kg~~/h × 50 ~~kg~~ = 100 units/h

The infusion rate should be increased by 100 units per hour.

Calculate the adjustment to the hourly infusion rate (mL/h):

$$\frac{D\text{ (units/h)}}{H\text{ (units)}} \times Q\text{ (mL)} = R\text{ (mL/h)}; \frac{\cancel{100}\ \cancel{\text{units}}/\text{h}}{\cancel{100}\ \cancel{\text{units}}} \times 1\text{ mL} = 1\text{ mL/h}$$

Calculate the new hourly infusion rate (mL/h):

9 mL/h + 1 mL/h = 10 mL/h (verifies estimate)

Increase the rate on the pump to 10 mL/h. Ask another nurse for independent verification of the infusion rate adjustment.

You have now worked through the three sequential actions needed to safely initiate, monitor, and maintain continuous intravenous infusions of high-alert medications. The principles learned with the heparin sodium examples may be applied to calculations of boluses and continuous infusions for other critical medications.

Heparin Sodium Overdose

Intravenous infusions of high-alert medications require vigilance to ensure that the patient receives the correct dosage and that serious harmful incidents are recognized and treated promptly. In addition to safely preparing the medication according to protocol, the nurse must be prepared to administer an antidote in case of life-threatening harmful incidents. Harmful incidents may be the result of expected risks due to individual patient variation, but may also occur due to a calculation error or an intravenous pump malfunction. Protamine sulfate is the antidote to severe heparin sodium overdose. Now consider a situation when protamine sulfate might be indicated.

Example 4:

The patient on the heparin sodium protocol has been receiving intravenous heparin sodium according to protocol for 21 hours. After periodic adjustments, the infusion rate is currently set for 12 mL/h, which is equal to 12 000 units/h. The most recent aPTT result was 94 seconds, which according to protocol required the infusion to be stopped for 1 hour and then decreased by 3 units/kg/h (line 15, Figure 14-1). While waiting to resume the heparin sodium infusion, the patient's blood pressure dropped, the pulse increased, and the urine became dark. Recognizing these signs of possible hemorrhage, the nurse contacts the prescriber, who orders *protamine sulfate 12 mg slow by direct IV*. The recommended infusion rate is no faster than 20 mg per minute. Calculate this emergency dose using the Three-Step Approach to dosage calculations.

Order: *protamine sulfate 12 mg slow direct IV*

Supply: See Figure 14-4

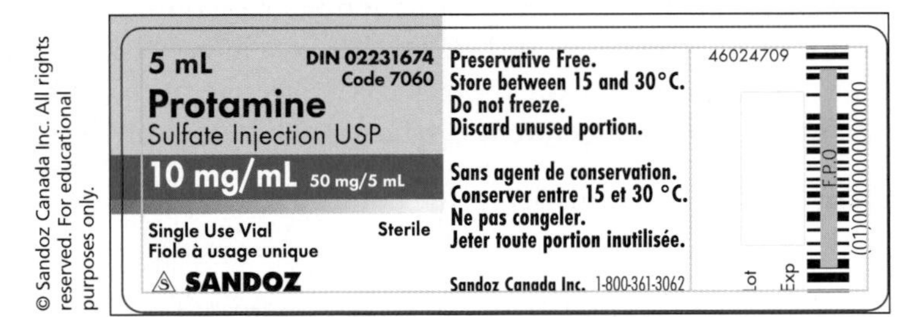

FIGURE 14-4 Protamine Sulfate 50 mg (10 mg/mL)

Step 1 Convert The order and the supplied dosages are the same unit. No conversion is necessary.

Step 2 Think There are 50 mg in the entire 5-mL vial, but the concentration is also stated as 10 mg/mL. Since 12 mg is slightly larger than 10 mg, you will need slightly more than 1 mL. The rate should be no faster than 20 mg per minute. Since 12 mg is slightly larger than $\frac{1}{2}$ of 20 mg, the dose should be injected in slightly more than $\frac{1}{2}$ minute.

Step 3 Calculate

$$\frac{D}{H} \times Q = \frac{\overset{6}{\cancel{12}}\ \cancel{\text{mg}}}{\underset{5}{\cancel{10}}\ \cancel{\text{mg}}} \times 1\text{ mL} = \frac{6}{5}\text{ mL} = 1.2\text{ mL (verifies estimate)}$$

Draw up 1.2 mL in a 3-mL syringe and inject as by direct IV.

Recall from Chapter 12 that $\frac{D}{H} \times T$ can be used to calculate the time required to administer a direct IV medication.

Rate: 20 mg/min or 20 mg per 60 seconds

$$\frac{D}{H} \times T = \frac{12 \text{ mg}}{20 \text{ mg}} \times 60 \text{ sec} = \frac{36}{1} \text{ sec} = 36 \text{ sec (verifies estimate)}$$

Infuse 1.2 mL of protamine sulfate over at least 36 seconds.

Use ratio and proportion to calculate how much to administer each 15 seconds, to slowly titrate the infusion.

$$\frac{1.2 \text{ mL}}{36 \text{ sec}} \times \frac{X \text{ mL}}{15 \text{ sec}}$$

$$36X = 18 \text{ sec}$$

$$\frac{36X}{36} = \frac{18}{36}$$

$$X = 0.5 \text{ mL (every 15 seconds)}$$

IV Insulin Protocol

It has been shown that for patients who are critically ill and have diabetes, tight management of blood glucose levels can reduce morbidity and mortality. There is an increased use of intravenous insulin protocols in critical care units and also in some medical surgical units to maintain tight control of hyperglycemia. While there is no universal protocol for intravenous insulin infusions, most are similar in approach. In this text, the sample critical care intravenous insulin protocol in Figure 14-5 will be used to calculate insulin dosage, but in your clinical practice, use the protocol that has been adopted by your institution. According to the sample protocol, the target level for blood glucose control is 4 to 6 mmol/L, although 4 to 7 mmol/L may also be correct.

As with the heparin sodium protocol, use the same three sequential actions: (1) bolus, (2) continuous infusion, and (3) rebolus and/or adjust the infusion rate.

Example 1:

Individual patients' have different insulin needs that are regulated based on the measurement of blood glucose. The sample insulin protocol provides three levels of insulin dosage, depending on the expected individual response to insulin therapy. Rapid- or short-acting insulin may be used for intravenous infusions. The sample protocol uses regular insulin. Choose Humulin R regular insulin, as shown in Figure 14-6.

For this example, we will provide insulin coverage for a patient who has insulin-dependent type 2 diabetes who is recovering in the intensive care unit from extensive surgery. According to protocol (line 3, Figure 14-5), the sample level 2 grid for titration of insulin will be used for this patient. (For simplicity, the level 1 and level 3 grids have been omitted.) The blood glucose measurement of this patient is 12.5 mmol/L, as tested upon admission to the intensive care unit.

	Sample Critical Care Intravenous Insulin Protocol Orders
TARGET	**BLOOD GLUCOSE LEVEL 4 to 6 mmol/L**
Insulin Solution	1. 100 units short-acting insulin in 100 mL of 0.9% NaCl, to be titrated based on grid for levels 1, 2, or 3.
Initial Infusion	2. Start patients who do not have diabetes at level 1. Advance to level 2 if TARGET range not reached after 2 hours on level 1. 3. Start patients who have diabetes at level 2. Advance to level 3 if TARGET range not reached after 2 hours on level 2. 4. Do not initiate insulin infusion unless blood glucose greater than 6 mmol/L.
Monitoring	5. Check blood glucose prior to start of insulin infusion. 6. Check blood glucose every hour thereafter. 7. When glucose is 4.4 to 6 mmol/L for 3 hours, check glucose every 2 hours. 8. Resume monitoring every hour if blood glucose greater than 6.7 mmol/L for 2 hours.
Blood Glucose Less than 4.4 mmol/L	9. If patient has blood glucose less than 4.4 mmol/L: a. Refer to regular insulin infusion rate column in grid tables for management instructions. b. If necessary to reinitiate insulin infusion, start one level below previous level. c. Call prescriber for symptomatic hypoglycemia or blood glucose less than 2.8 mmol/L, even if treated.

Sample Grid for Titration of Intravenous Insulin—Level 2

LEVEL 2: DO NOT INITIATE insulin drip unless blood glucose is greater than 6 mmol/L.

Blood Glucose (mmol/L)	Regular Insulin Bolus	Regular Insulin Infusion Rate
Less than 3.9	Give $\frac{1}{2}$ amp of 50% dextrose	HOLD insulin infusion × 60 minutes and check blood glucose every 15 minutes until equal to or greater than 4.4.
3.9 to 4.3	0	HOLD insulin infusion × 60 minutes and check blood glucose every 15 minutes until equal to or greater than 4.4.
4.4 to 6	0	2 units/h
6.1 to 6.9	0	3 units/h
7 to 8.2	0	4 units/h
8.3 to 9.1	0	5 units/h
9.2 to 9.9	0	6 units/h
10 to 11.5	0	8 units/h
11.6 to 13.2	10 units direct IV	12 units/h
13.3 to 14.9	10 units direct IV	16 units/h
15 to 16.5	10 units direct IV	20 units/h
16.6 to 19.4	10 units direct IV	25 units/h
greater than 19.4	Notify prescriber	

FIGURE 14-5 Sample Intravenous Insulin Therapy Protocol

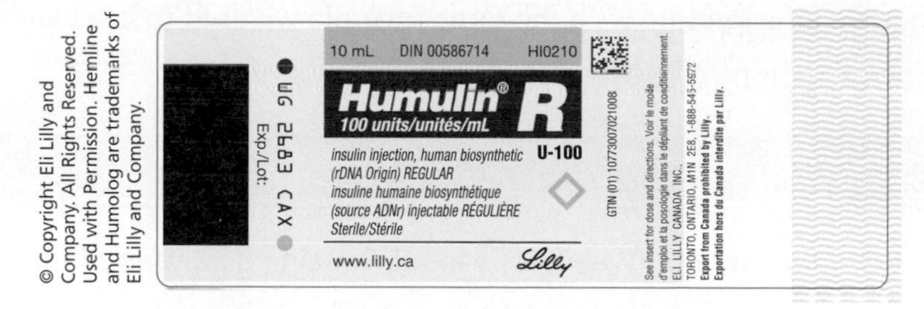

FIGURE 14-6 Humulin R Regular U-100 Insulin

Action 1 **Bolus:** Unlike the heparin sodium protocol, the initial insulin bolus dose is not based on patient weight, but glucose level alone. A bolus dose is not always required. In this instance, the patient's blood glucose level of 12.5 mmol/L falls between 11.6 and 13.2 mmol/L, which requires a bolus of 10 units regular insulin. Draw up 10 units in a 30-unit lo-dose insulin syringe.

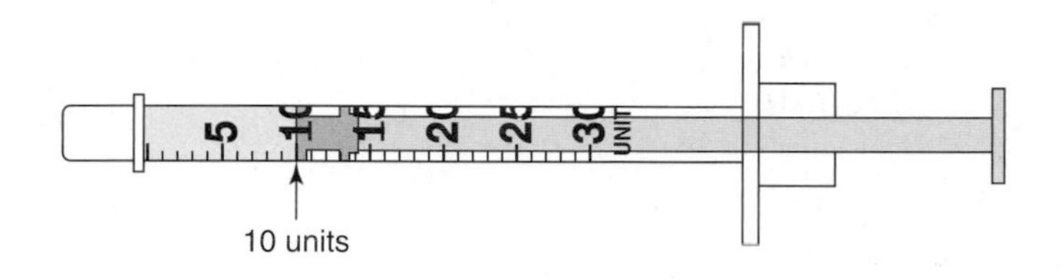

Give the order, glucose measurement, insulin vial, and syringe to another nurse for independent verification and documentation.

Action 2 **Continuous Infusion:** Often, insulin and other high-alert drugs come premixed from the hospital pharmacy. But nurses will sometimes need to mix the IV solution for the continuous infusion. Now continue with the patient example by following the protocol to prepare the IV insulin solution (line 1, Figure 14-5) and then by calculating the initial infusion rate for the blood glucose level of this patient (12.5 mmol/L, which is in the range on the level 2 grid of 11.6 to 13.2 mmol/L).

Order: *100 units Humulin R short-acting insulin in 100 mL of 0.9% NaCl*

Draw up 100 units of Humulin R short-acting insulin in a standard insulin syringe.

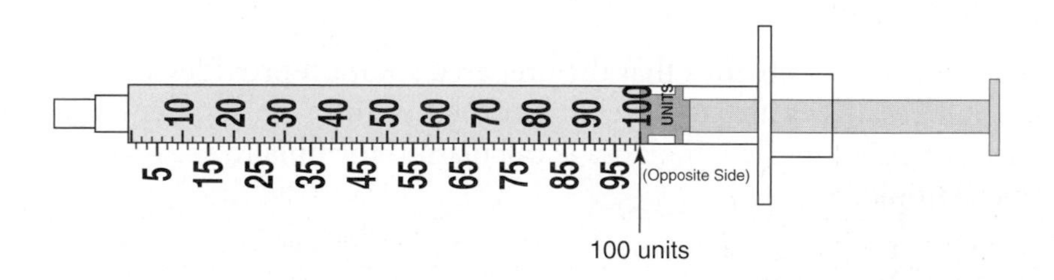

Give the order, glucose measurement, insulin vial, and syringe to another nurse for independent verification and documentation. Inject the 100 units into the 100-mL IVPB bag of 0.9% normal saline. Prepare a label with the patient's name, drug name and concentration, dosage and amount added, date and time prepared, and your signature. Secure the label on the IVPB bag.

Order: Now calculate the hourly infusion rate with the same formula we used to calculate the heparin infusion.

RULE

To calculate the continuous flow rate of IV solutions in mL/h using a version of the dosage calculation formula,

$$\frac{\text{D (units/h desired)}}{\text{H (units available)}} \times \text{Q (mL available)} = \text{R (mL/h rate)}$$

Note: This rule also applies to other continuous infusion drugs ordered in units/h, milliunits/h, mg/h, mcg/h, g/h, or mEq/h.

The patient's blood glucose level of 12.5 mmol/L falls between 11.6 and 14.2 mmol/L, which requires an infusion rate of 12 units/h.

$$\frac{\text{D (units/h)}}{\text{H (units)}} \times \text{Q (mL)} = \text{R (mL/h)}$$

$$\frac{12 \cancel{\text{units}}/\text{h}}{\cancel{100} \cancel{\text{units}}} \times \cancel{100} \text{ mL} = 12 \text{ mL/h}$$

Remember that you can think of this calculation in a different way by using ratio and proportion to determine how many units are in 1 mL. If there are 100 units per 100 mL, how many units are in 1 mL? Use ratio and proportion to calculate the amount.

$$\frac{100 \text{ units}}{100 \text{ mL}} \rightleftarrows \frac{\text{X units}}{1 \text{ mL}}$$

$$100\text{X} = 100$$

$$\frac{100}{100} = \frac{100\text{X}}{100}$$

$$\text{X} = 1 \text{ unit}$$

There is 1 unit of insulin in 1 mL.

After setting up the equation, it is obvious that the prepared solution provides 1 unit of insulin in each 1 mL of solution. It is safe practice to develop intravenous infusion protocols that require the simplest possible math calculations. Use the dosage calculation formula to see how using this calculation is so much simpler.

$$\frac{\text{D (units/h)}}{\text{H (units)}} \times \text{Q (mL)} = \text{R (mL/h)}$$

$$\frac{12 \cancel{\text{units}}/\text{h}}{1 \cancel{\text{unit}}} \times 1 \text{ mL} = 12 \text{ mL/h}$$

For this problem, assume that the infusion pump available is designed to infuse at a mL/h rate using whole numbers only. Set the rate on the pump for the initial infusion at 12 mL/h. Ask another nurse for independent verification of the initial infusion rate.

Action 3 **Rebolus and/or Adjust Infusion Rate:** The insulin protocol requires hourly blood glucose monitoring until the glucose level is 4.4 to 6 mmol/L for 3 hours (lines 6 and 7, Figure 14-5). For the patient in this example, one hour after the infusion is started, the blood glucose measurement is 11.4 mmol/L. What should the nurse do?

Rebolus: Is a bolus necessary now? 11.4 mmol/L falls between 10 and 11.5 mmol/L. According to the grid, no bolus is needed at this time.

Adjust Infusion Rate: According to the grid, for a glucose measurement of 11.4 mmol/L, the rate should be set for 8 units per hour. Now that you know there is 1 unit/mL, you will give 8 times as much, or 8 mL/h. While this calculation seems obvious, use the dosage calculation formula to verify this estimate.

$$\frac{\text{D (units/h)}}{\text{H (units)}} \times \text{Q (mL)} = \text{R (mL/h)}; \quad \frac{8\ \cancel{\text{units}}/\text{h}}{1\ \cancel{\text{units}}} \times 1\ \text{mL} = 8\ \text{mL/h}$$

Reduce the rate on the infusion pump from 12 mL/h to 8 mL/h. Ask another nurse for independent verification of the change in infusion rate. Remember: To ensure consistent monitoring from shift to shift, the nurse must document the time and dose of the bolus and infusion rate changes on a standard worksheet.

INSULIN OVERDOSE

Hypoglycemia (blood glucose below 2.8 mmol/L) occurs when insulin levels exceed insulin needs. This imbalance may result from an overdose of insulin during intravenous infusion due to expected risks because of individual patient variation, but may also occur because of a calculation error or an intravenous pump malfunction. Rapid treatment of hypoglycemia is required to prevent irreversible brain damage or even death. For this reason, protocols for insulin and other high-alert drugs frequently include standard orders for severe adverse reactions. The sample protocol for intravenous insulin infusion provides an order for 50% dextrose in the case of hypoglycemia. It is supplied for emergency use in a prefilled ampule of 25 g per 50 mL.

Example 2:

After periodic adjustments in the insulin infusion rate, the patient in Example 1 was acting confused during glucose monitoring, which was 3.6 mmol/L. According to the protocol, the nurse should give $\frac{1}{2}$ amp (ampule) of 50% dextrose, hold the insulin infusion for 60 minutes, and check blood glucose every 15 minutes until it is greater than or equal to 4.4 mmol/L.

Order: *Give $\frac{1}{2}$ amp of 50% dextrose*

Supply: 50 mL ampule of 50% dextrose

$$\text{Calculate: } \frac{1}{2} \times 50\ \text{mL} = \frac{\overset{25}{\cancel{50}}}{\underset{1}{\cancel{2}}}\ \text{mL} = 25\ \text{mL}$$

To administer $\frac{1}{2}$ amp of 50% dextrose, you will need to give 25 mL by direct IV. Discard 25 mL, leaving 25 mL in the ampule, and then administer the entire amount remaining through an infusion port near the IV insertion site. It is not safe to insert the ampule with the entire amount into the port and then try to administer only 25 mL. It is difficult to administer by direct IV a 50% dextrose solution, and you could administer forcefully and inject more than the ordered amount.

According to protocol, increase glucose monitoring to every 15 minutes until the blood glucose is greater than 4.4 mmol/L. The prescriber must be notified for symptomatic hypoglycemia or blood glucose that is less than 2.8 mmol/L, even if treated (line 9c, Figure 14-5). The patient showed the hypoglycemic symptom of confusion. Notify the prescriber.

QUICK REVIEW

- Many hospitals use standard protocols to initiate and maintain continuous infusion therapy for high-alert medications such as heparin sodium and insulin.
- Protocols may be based on weight in kilograms, and dose adjustments are made based on blood tests or other patient data such as physical assessment findings.
- To calculate mL/h when units/h and units/mL are known, use $\frac{D}{H} \times Q = R$.
- Document boluses and changes to infusion rate on the flowsheet for consistent monitoring and maintenance of infusions.
- Be prepared to administer an antidote if severe adverse reactions occur.

REVIEW SET 14-1

Calculate the flow rate. The infusion pumps are calibrated to deliver whole mL.

1. Order: *0.9% NS 1000 mL IV with heparin sodium 25 000 units to infuse at 1000 units/h*

   Flow rate: ________ mL/h

2. Order: *D_5W 500 mL IV with heparin sodium 40 000 units to infuse at 1100 units/h*

   Flow rate: ________ mL/h

3. Order: *0.9% NS 500 mL IV with heparin sodium 25 000 units to infuse at 500 units/h*

   Flow rate: ________ mL/h

4. Order: *D_5W 500 mL IV with heparin sodium 40 000 units to infuse at 1500 units/h*

   Flow rate: ________ mL/h

5. Order: *D_5W 1 L IV with heparin sodium 25 000 units to infuse at 1200 units/h.* On rounds, you assess the patient and observe that the infusion pump is set at 120 mL/h.

   At what rate should the pump be set? ________ mL/h

   What should the nurse's action be? ________________________________

6. Order: *D_5W 500 mL IV with heparin sodium 25 000 units to infuse at 800 units/h*

   Flow rate: ________ mL/h

Questions 7 through 10 refer to a patient who weighs 165 lb and has IV heparin sodium ordered according to the following Weight-Based Heparin Sodium Protocol. With this variation of the heparin sodium protocol, you will not round the patient's weight; instead, you will use the patient's actual weight. The infusion pumps are calibrated to deliver whole mL.

Weight-Based Heparin Sodium Protocol:

Heparin sodium IV infusion: Heparin sodium 25 000 units in 250 mL of 0.9% NS

IV boluses: Use heparin sodium 1000 units/mL.

Calculate the patient's weight in kg. Weight: ________ kg

Bolus with heparin sodium 80 units/kg. Then initiate heparin sodium drip at 18 units/kg/h. Obtain aPTT every 6 hours, and adjust dosage and rate as follows:

If aPTT is less than 35 seconds: Rebolus with 80 units/kg and increase rate by 4 units/kg/h.

If aPTT is 36 to 44 seconds: Rebolus with 40 units/kg and increase rate by 2 units/kg/h.

If aPTT is 45 to 75 seconds: Continue current rate.

If aPTT is 76 to 90 seconds: Decrease rate by 2 units/kg/h.

If aPTT is greater than 90 seconds: Hold heparin sodium for 1 hour and then decrease rate by 3 units/kg/h.

7. Convert the patient's weight to kg: ________ kg

   Calculate the initial heparin sodium bolus dosage: ________ units

   Calculate the bolus dose: ________ mL

   Calculate the initial heparin sodium infusion rate: ________ units/h, or ________ mL/h

8. At 0900, the patient's aPTT is 33 seconds. According to the protocol, what should the nurse do?

   Rebolus with ________ units, or ________ mL.

   Increase infusion rate by ________ units/h, or ________ mL/h, for a new rate of ________ mL/h.

9. At 1500, the patient's aPTT is 40 seconds. According to the protocol, what should the nurse do?

   Rebolus with ________ units or ________ mL.

   Increase infusion rate by ________ units/h, or ________ mL/h, for a new rate of ________ mL/h.

10. At 2100, the patient's aPTT is 60 seconds. According to the protocol what should the nurse do? ________________________________

Questions 11 through 15 refer to a patient who is seriously ill and in the critical care unit who requires insulin for management of type 2 diabetes. Use the following grid for titration of intravenous insulin. An IV pump is used, and it is calibrated to deliver whole millilitres.

Sample Grid for Titration of Intravenous Insulin—Level 2		
LEVEL 2: DO NOT INITIATE insulin drip unless blood glucose is greater than 6 mmol/L.		
Blood Glucose (mmol/L)	**Regular Insulin Bolus**	**Regular Insulin Infusion Rate**
Less than 3.9	Give $\frac{1}{2}$ amp of 50% dextrose	HOLD insulin infusion × 60 minutes and check blood glucose every 15 minutes until equal to or greater than 4.4.
3.9 to 4.3	0	HOLD insulin infusion × 60 minutes and check blood glucose every 15 minutes until equal to or greater than 4.4.
4.4 to 6	0	2 units/h
6.1 to 6.9	0	3 units/h
7 to 8.2	0	4 units/h
8.3 to 9.1	0	5 units/h
9.2 to 9.9	0	6 units/h
10 to 11.5	0	8 units/h
11.6 to 13.2	10 units direct IV	12 units/h
13.3 to 14.9	10 units direct IV	16 units/h
15 to 16.5	10 units direct IV	20 units/h
16.6 to 19.4	10 units direct IV	25 units/h
greater than 19.4	Notify prescriber	

11. The blood glucose level at the start of the infusion is 17.8 mmol/L. Is a bolus dose of insulin required? ________ If so, what is the required bolus dosage? ________ units
12. The insulin solution prepared for the continuous infusion is 100 units regular insulin 100-unit in 100 mL of 0.9% NaCl. What should be the rate at the start of the infusion? ________ mL/h
13. One hour later, the blood glucose level is 11 mmol/L. Is a bolus dose of insulin required? ________ If so, what is the required dosage? ________ units
14. What should be the new rate for the continuous infusion? ________ mL/h
15. After monitoring and adjustment to insulin doses over 4 hours, the blood glucose level is 4 mmol/L. What should the nurse do? ________________________________

Check your work! Answers to all Review Sets are provided at the end of each chapter. Worked solutions for selected Review Sets are also available there.

CRITICAL CARE IV CALCULATIONS: CALCULATING THE FLOW RATE OF AN IV MEDICATION TO BE GIVEN OVER A SPECIFIED TIME PERIOD

Medications are frequently ordered for patients in critical care situations as a prescribed amount to be administered in a specified time period, such as *X mg per minute.* Such medications are usually administered by electronic infusion devices programmed in mL/h. Unless stated otherwise, for calculations you can assume that the IV pump is calibrated to deliver whole millilitres. Careful monitoring of patients receiving life-threatening therapies is a critical nursing skill.

IV Medications Ordered per Minute

RULE

To determine the flow rate (mL/h) for IV medications ordered per minute (such as mg/min).

Step 1 Calculate the dosage in mL/min:

$$\frac{D}{H} \times Q = R \text{ (mL/min)}$$

Step 2 Calculate the flow rate in mL/h of the volume to administer per minute:

$$\text{mL/min} \times 60 \text{ min/h} = \text{mL/h}$$

Note: The order may specify mg/min, mcg/min, g/min, units/min, milliunits/min, or mEq/min.

In the formula $\frac{D}{H} \times Q = R \text{ (mL/min)}$,

D = dosage *desired:* mg/min

H = dosage you *have* available: mg

Q = *quantity* of solution you have available: mL

R = flow *rate:* mL/min

Example 1:

Order: *lidocaine hydrochloride 2 g IV in 500 mL D_5W at 2 mg/min via infusion pump.* You must prepare and hang 500 mL of D_5W IV solution that has 2 g of lidocaine hydrochloride added to it. Then, you must regulate the flow rate so the patient receives 2 mg of the lidocaine hydrochloride every minute. Determine the flow rate for the IV pump calibrated to deliver tenths of an mL/h.

Step 1 Calculate mL/min (change mg/min to mL/min)

Convert g to mg: $2 \text{ g} = 2 \cancel{\text{g}} \times 1000 \text{ mg}/\cancel{\text{g}} = 2000\text{mg}$

$$\frac{D}{H} \times Q = \frac{2 \cancel{\text{mg}}/\text{min}}{2000 \cancel{\text{mg}}} \times 500 \text{ mL} = R \text{ (mL/min)}$$

$$\frac{2 \cancel{\text{mg}}/\text{min}}{\underset{4}{\cancel{2000}} \cancel{\text{mg}}} \times \frac{\overset{1}{\cancel{500}} \text{ mL}}{1} = \frac{\overset{1}{\cancel{2}}}{\underset{2}{\cancel{4}}} \text{ mL/min} = \frac{1}{2} \text{ mL/min} = 0.5 \text{ mL/min}$$

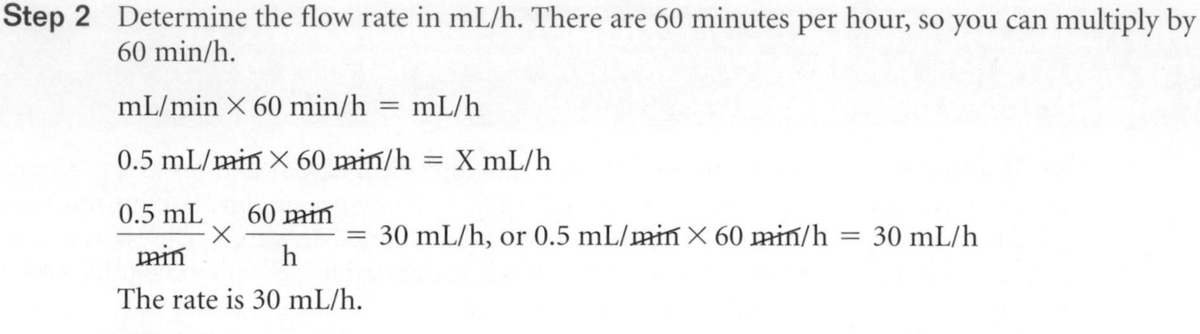

Step 2 Determine the flow rate in mL/h. There are 60 minutes per hour, so you can multiply by 60 min/h.

$\text{mL/min} \times 60 \text{ min/h} = \text{mL/h}$

$0.5 \text{ mL/}\cancel{\text{min}} \times 60 \text{ }\cancel{\text{min}}\text{/h} = X \text{ mL/h}$

$\frac{0.5 \text{ mL}}{\cancel{\text{min}}} \times \frac{60 \text{ }\cancel{\text{min}}}{\text{h}} = 30 \text{ mL/h, or } 0.5 \text{ mL/}\cancel{\text{min}} \times 60 \text{ }\cancel{\text{min}}\text{/h} = 30 \text{ mL/h}$

The rate is 30 mL/h.

Regulate the flow rate to 30 mL/h to deliver 2 mg/min of lidocaine that is prepared at the concentration of 2 g per 500 mL of D_5W IV solution.

Example 2:

Order: *nitroglycerin 125 mg IV in 500 mL D_5W to infuse at 42 mcg/min.*

Calculate the flow rate in mL/h to program the infusion pump calibrated to deliver tenths of a mL/h.

Step 1 Calculate mL/min (change mcg/min to mL/min)

First, convert mg to mcg: 1 mg = 1000 mcg; 125 mg = 125.000. = 125 000 mcg

Then, calculate mL/min:

$$\frac{D}{H} \times Q = \frac{42 \text{ }\cancel{\text{mcg}}\text{/min}}{\underset{250}{\cancel{125000}} \text{ }\cancel{\text{mcg}}} \times \overset{1}{\cancel{500}} \text{ mL} = \frac{42}{250} \text{ mL/min} = 0.168 \text{ mL/min} = 0.17 \text{ mL/min}$$

Step 2 Determine the flow rate in mL/h (change mL/min to mL/h).

$\text{mL/min} \times 60 \text{ min/h} = \text{mL/h}$

$0.17 \text{ mL/}\cancel{\text{min}} \times 60 \text{ }\cancel{\text{min}}\text{/h} = 10.2 \text{ mL/h}$

The rate is 10.2 mL/h, not 10 mL/h, because the IV pump is calibrated in tenths.

Regulate the flow rate to 10.2 mL/h to deliver 42 mcg/min of nitroglycerin, which is prepared at the concentration of 125 mg per 500 mL of D_5W IV solution.

IV Medication Ordered per Kilogram per Minute

The prescriber may also order the amount of medication in an IV solution that a patient should receive in a specified time period per kilogram of body weight. An electronic infusion device is usually used to administer these orders.

RULE

To determine the flow rate (mL/h) for IV medications ordered per minute (such as mg/kg/min).

Step 1 Convert to like units, such as mg to mcg or lb to kg;

Step 2 Calculate desired dosage per minute: mg/kg/min × kg = mg/min.;

Step 3 Calculate the dosage flow rate in mL/min: $\frac{D}{H} \times Q = R$ (mL/min);

Step 4 Calculate the flow rate in mL/h of the volume to administer per minute: mL/min × 60 min/h = mL/h

Note: The order may specify mg/min, mcg/min, g/min, units/min, milliunits/min, or mEq/min; or it may specify mg/h, mcg/h, g/h, units/h, milliunits/h, or mEq/h.

Example:

Order: *250 mL of IV solution with 225 mg of a medication to infuse at 3 mcg/kg/min via infusion pump* for a person who weighs 110 lb.

Determine the flow rate for the IV pump calibrated in whole mL/h.

Step 1 **Convert** mg to mcg: 1 mg = 1000 mcg; 225 mg = 225.000. = 225 000 mcg

Convert lb to kg: 1 kg = 2.2 lb; 110 lb ÷ 2.2 lb/kg = 110 ~~lb~~ × 1 kg/2.2 ~~lb~~ = 50 kg

Step 2 **Calculate** desired mcg/min.

3 mcg/~~kg~~/min × 50 ~~kg~~ = 150 mcg/min

Step 3 **Calculate** mL/min.

$$\frac{D}{H} \times Q = \frac{150 \text{ mcg/min}}{225000 \text{ mcg}} \times 250 \text{ mL} = \frac{150}{900} \text{ mL/min} = 0.166 \text{ mL/min} = 0.17 \text{ mL/min}$$

Step 4 **Calculate** mL/h.

mL/min × 60 min/h = 0.17 mL/~~min~~ × 60 ~~min~~/h = 10.2 mL/h = 10 mL/h

The rate is 10 mL/h. Remember, the IV pump is calibrated in whole mL/h.

For a person who weighs 110 lb, or 50 kg, regulate the IV flow rate to 10 mL/h to deliver 150 mcg/min (3 mcg/kg/min) of the drug, which is prepared at the concentration of 225 mg per 250 mL of IV solution.

Titrating IV Drugs

Sometimes, IV medications may be prescribed to be administered at an initial dosage over a specified time period and then continued at a different dosage and time period. These situations are common in obstetrics and critical care. Medications such as magnesium sulfate, dobutamine hydrochloride, dopamine hydrochloride, isoproterenol hydrochloride, and oxytocin are ordered to be *titrated,* or *regulated,* to obtain measurable physiologic responses. Dosages will be adjusted until the desired effect is achieved. In some cases, a loading or bolus dose is infused and monitored closely. Most IV medications that require titration usually start at the lowest dosage and are increased or decreased as needed. An upper titration limit is usually set and is not exceeded unless the desired response is not obtained. A new drug order is then required.

Let us examine some of these situations.

RULE

To calculate flow rate (mL/h) for IV medications ordered over a specific time period (such as mg/min),

Step 1 Calculate mg/mL;

Step 2 Calculate mL/h.

Note: The order may specify mg/min, mcg/min, g/min, units/min, milliunits/min, or mEq/min; or it may specify mg/h, mcg/h, g/h, units/h, milliunits/h, or mEq/h.

Example 1:

Order: *RL 1000 mL IV with magnesium sulfate 20 g. Start with bolus of 4 g for 30 min, then maintain a continuous infusion at 2 g/h*

1. What is the flow rate in whole mL/h for the bolus order?

Step 1 **Calculate** the bolus dosage in g/mL.

There are 20 g in 1000 mL. How many mL are necessary to infuse 4 g?

$$\frac{D}{H} \times Q = \frac{4\ \text{g}}{\cancel{20}_{1}\ \cancel{\text{g}}} \times \overset{50}{\cancel{1000}}\ \text{mL} = 200\ \text{mL}$$

Therefore, 200 mL contain 4 g, to be administered over 30 minutes.

Step 2 **Calculate** the bolus rate in mL/h.

What is the flow rate in mL/h to infuse 200 mL (which contain 4 g of magnesium sulfate)?

$$\frac{\text{Total mL}}{\text{Total min}} \times 60\ \text{min/h} = \frac{200\ \text{mL}}{\cancel{30}_{1}\ \cancel{\text{min}}} \times \frac{\overset{2}{\cancel{60}}\ \cancel{\text{min}}}{1\ \text{h}} = 400\ \text{mL/h}$$

The rate is 400 mL/h.

Set the infusion pump at 400 mL/h to deliver the bolus of 4 g per 30 minutes as ordered.

Now calculate the continuous IV rate in mL/h.

2. What is the flow rate in mL/h for the continuous infusion of magnesium sulfate of 2 g/h? You know from the bolus dosage calculation that 200 mL contain 4 g.

$$\frac{D}{H} \times Q = \frac{2\ \cancel{\text{g}}/\text{h}}{\cancel{4}_{1}\ \cancel{\text{g}}} \times \overset{50}{\cancel{200}}\ \text{mL} = 100\ \text{mL/h}$$

After the bolus has infused in the first 30 minutes, reset the infusion pump to 100 mL/h to deliver the continuous infusion of 2 g/h.

The next example uses oxytocin (a drug used to induce or augment labour) measured in units and milliunits.

Example 2:

A drug order is written to induce labour: *LR 1000 mL IV with oxytocin 20 units. Begin a continuous infusion IV at 1 milliunit/min, increase by 1 milliunit/min q15 min to a maximum of 20 milliunits/min*

1. What is the flow rate in whole mL/h to deliver 1 milliunit/min?

   In this example, the medication is measured in units.

Step 1 **Calculate** milliunits/mL.

Convert: 1 unit = 1000 milliunits; 20 units = 20 × 1000 milliunits = 20 000 milliunits

$$\frac{D}{H} \times Q = \frac{1\ \cancel{\text{milliunit}}}{\cancel{20\,000}_{20}\ \cancel{\text{milliunits}}} \times \overset{1}{\cancel{1000}}\ \text{mL} = \frac{1}{20}\ \text{mL} = 0.05\ \text{mL}$$

Therefore, 0.05 mL contains 1 milliunit of oxytocin, or there is 1 milliunit per 0.05 mL.

Step 2 **Calculate** mL/h.

What is the flow rate in mL/h to infuse 0.05 mL/min (which is 1 milliunit oxytocin/min)?

$$\frac{\text{Total mL}}{\text{Total min}} \times 60 \text{ min/h} = \frac{0.05 \text{ mL}}{1 \cancel{\text{min}}} \times \frac{60 \cancel{\text{min}}}{1 \text{ h}} = 3 \text{ mL/h}$$

Set the infusion pump at 3 mL/h to infuse oxytocin 1 milliunit/min as ordered.

2. What is the maximum flow rate in mL/h at which the oxytocin infusion can be set for the titration as ordered? Notice that the order allows a maximum of 20 milliunits/min. You know from the bolus dosage calculation that there is 1 milliunit per 0.05 mL.

$$\frac{D}{H} \times Q = \frac{20 \cancel{\text{milliunits}}/\text{min}}{1 \cancel{\text{milliunit}}} \times 0.05 \text{ mL} = 1 \text{ mL/min}$$

Now convert mL/min to mL/h so you can program the electronic infusion device.

$$\text{mL/min} \times 60 \text{ min/h} = 1 \text{ mL}/\cancel{\text{min}} \times 60 \cancel{\text{min}}/\text{h} = 60 \text{ mL/h}$$

The rate of 60 mL/h will deliver 20 milliunits/minute.

Verifying Safe IV Medication Dosage Recommended per Minute

It is also a critical nursing clinical judgment to ensure that patients are receiving safe dosages of medications. Therefore, you must also be able to convert critical care IVs with additive medications to *mg/h* or *mg/min* to check safe or normal dosage ranges.

RULE

To check safe dosage of IV medications ordered in mL/h,

Step 1 Calculate mg/h;

Step 2 Calculate mg/min;

Step 3 Compare recommended dosage and ordered dosage to decide whether the dosage is safe.

Note: The ordered and recommended dosages may specify mg/min, mcg/min, g/min, units/min, milliunits/min, or mEq/min.

Example:

According to the drug reference, the recommended dosage of lidocaine hydrochloride is 1 to 4 mg/min. The patient has an order for *D_5W 500 mL IV with lidocaine hydrochloride 1 g to infuse at 30 mL/h.* Is the lidocaine hydrochloride dosage within the safe range? **Note:** Lidocaine hydrochloride for continuous intravenous infusion is prepared by the manufacturer.

Step 1 **Calculate** mg/h

Convert: 1 g = 1000 mg

$$\frac{D}{H} \times Q = \frac{D \cancel{\text{mg}}/\text{h}}{\underset{2}{\cancel{1000}} \cancel{\text{mg}}} \times \overset{1}{\cancel{500}} \text{ mL} = 30 \text{ mL/h}$$

$$\frac{D}{2} = 30$$

$$\frac{D}{2} \times \frac{30}{1}$$

$$D = 60 \text{ mg/h}$$

You know the answer is in mg/h because D is measured in mg/h.

Step 2 **Calculate** mg/min.

Think: It is obvious that 60 mg/h is the same as 60 mg per 60 minute or 1 mg/min.

1 h = 60 min

$$\frac{\text{mg/h}}{\text{60 min/h}} = \text{mg/min}$$

$$\frac{\overset{1}{\cancel{60}}\ \text{mg/}\cancel{\text{h}}}{\underset{1}{\cancel{60}}\ \text{min/}\cancel{\text{h}}} = 1\ \text{mg/min}$$

The rate is 1 mg/min.

Step 3 Compare ordered and recommended dosages.

1 mg/min is within the safe range of 1 to 4 mg/min. The dosage is safe.

Likewise, IV medications ordered as mL/h and recommended in mg/kg/min require verification of their safety or normal dosage range.

RULE

To check safe dosage of IV medications recommended in mg/kg/min and ordered in mL/h.

Step 1 **Convert to like units, such as mg to mcg or lb to kg;**
Step 2 **Calculate recommended mg/min;**
Step 3 **Calculate ordered mg/h;**
Step 4 **Calculate ordered mg/min;**
Step 5 **Compare ordered and recommended dosages. Decide whether the dosage is safe.**

Note: The ordered and recommended dosages may specify mg/kg/min, mcg/kg/min, g/kg/min, units/kg/min, milliunits/kg/min, or mEq/kg/min.

Example:

The recommended dosage range of sodium nitroprusside for adults is 0.3 to 10 mcg/kg/min. The patient has an order for *D_5W 100 mL IV with sodium nitroprusside 420 mg to infuse at 1 mL/h.* The patient weighs 154 lb. Is the sodium nitroprusside dosage within the normal range?

Step 1 **Convert** lb to kg: 154 lb ÷ 2.2 lb/kg = 154 $\cancel{\text{lb}}$ × 1 kg/2.2 $\cancel{\text{lb}}$ = 70 kg

Convert mg to mcg: 420 mg = 420 mg × 1000 mcg/m = 420 000 mcg

Step 2 **Calculate** recommended mcg/min range.

Minimum: 0.3 mcg/$\cancel{\text{kg}}$/min × 70 $\cancel{\text{kg}}$ = 21 mcg/min

Minimum: 10 mcg/$\cancel{\text{kg}}$/min × 70 $\cancel{\text{kg}}$ = 700 mcg/min

Step 3 **Calculate** ordered mcg/h.

$$\frac{D}{H} \times Q = R$$

$$\frac{\text{D}\ \cancel{\text{mcg}}\text{/h}}{\underset{4200}{\cancel{420\,000}}\ \cancel{\text{mcg}}} \times \overset{1}{\cancel{100}}\ \text{mL} = 1\ \text{mL/h}$$

$$\frac{D}{4200} = 1$$

$$\frac{D}{4200} \times \frac{1}{1}$$

$D = 4200$ mcg/h

You know the answer is in mcg/h because D is measured in mcg/h.

Step 4 **Calculate** ordered mcg/min: 4200 mcg/h = 4200 mcg per 60 min

$$\frac{4200 \text{ mcg}}{60 \text{ min}} = 70 \text{ mcg/min}$$

Step 5 Compare the ordered and recommended dosages. Decide whether the dosage is safe. Because 70 mcg/min is within the allowable range of 21 to 700 mcg/min, the ordered dosage is safe.

QUICK REVIEW

- For IV medications ordered in mg/min,
  Step 1 Calculate mL/min;
  Step 2 Calculate mL/h.
- To check safe dosages of IV medications recommended in mg/min and ordered in mL/h,
  Step 1 Calculate mg/h;
  Step 2 Calculate mg/min;
  Step 3 Compare recommended and ordered dosages. Decide whether the dosage is safe.
- To check safe dosages of IV medications recommended in mg/kg/min and ordered in mL/h,
  Step 1 Convert to like units, such as mg to mcg or lb to kg;
  Step 2 Calculate recommended mg/min;
  Step 3 Calculate ordered mg/h;
  Step 4 Calculate ordered mg/min;
  Step 5 Compare ordered and recommended dosages. Decide whether the dosage is safe.

REVIEW SET 14-2

For questions 1 through 5, calculate the flow rate for the medications to be administered by IV pump calibrated in tenths of a mL/h.

1. Order: *lidocaine hydrochloride 2 g IV per 1000 mL D_5W at 4 mg/min*

   Rate: ________ mL/min and ________ mL/h

2. Order: *procanamide hydrochloride 0.5 g IV per 250 mL D_5W at 2 mg/min*

   Rate: ________ mL/min and ________ mL/h

3. Order: *isoproterenol hydrochloride 2 mg IV per 500 mL D_5W at 6 mcg/min*

   Rate: ________ mL/min and ________ mL/h

4. Order: *medication X 450 mg IV per 500 mL NS at 4 mcg/kg/min*

   Weight: 198 lb

   Weight: ________ kg Give: ________ mcg/min

   Rate: ________ mL/min and ________ mL/h

5. Order: *dopamine hydrochloride 800 mg in 500 mL NS IV at 15 mcg/kg/min*

   Weight: 70 kg

   Give: ________ mcg/min

   Rate: ________ mL/min and ________ mL/h

   Refer to the following order for questions 6 through 8.

   Order: *D_5W 500 mL IV with dobutamine hydrochloride 500 mg to infuse at 15 mL/h.* The patient weighs 125 lb. Recommended range: 2.5 to 10 mcg/kg/min

6. What mcg/min range of dobutamine hydrochloride should this patient receive? ________ to ________ mcg/min

7. What mg/min range of dobutamine hydrochloride should this patient receive? ________ to ________ mg/min

8. Is the dobutamine hydrochloride as ordered within the safe range? ________

   Refer to the following order for questions 9 and 10.

   Order: *D_5W 500 mL IV with procainamide 2 g to infuse at 60 mL/h.* Normal range: 2 to 6 mg/min

9. How many mg/min of procainamide is the patient receiving? ________ mg/min

10. Is the dosage of procainamide within the normal range? ________

11. Order: *magnesium sulfate 20 g IV in LR 500 mL. Start with a bolus of 2 g to infuse over 30 min. Then maintain a continuous infusion at 1 g/h.* IV pump delivers whole mL/h.

    Rate: ________ mL/h for bolus

    ________ mL/h for continuous infusion

12. The following order is to induce labour. The IV pump delivers whole mL/h.

    oxytocin 15 units IV in 250 mL LR. Begin a continuous infusion at the rate of 1 milliunit/min.

    Rate: ________ mL/h

    Refer to the following order for questions 13 through 15.

    Order: *D_5W 1000 mL IV with norepinephrine bitartrate 4 mg to infuse at 60 mL/h*

    Normal dosage range: 2 to 4 mcg/min

13. How many mg/min of norepinephrine bitartrate is the patient receiving? ________ mg/min

14. How many mcg/min of norepinephrine bitartrate is the patient receiving? ________ mcg/min

15. Is the dosage of norepinephrine bitartrate within the normal range? ________

Check your work! Answers to all Review Sets are provided at the end of each chapter. Worked solutions for selected Review Sets are also available there.

LIMITING INFUSION VOLUMES

Calculating IV rates to include the IV piggyback (IVPB) volume may be necessary to limit the total volume of IV fluid a patient receives. To do this, the nurse must calculate the flow rate for both the regular IV and the piggyback IV. In such instances of restricted fluids, the piggyback IVs are to be included as part of the total prescribed IV volume and time.

RULE

Follow these six steps to calculate the flow rate of an IV, which includes IVPB:

Step 1 IVPB flow rate: $\frac{V}{T} \times C = R$

or use $\frac{mL/h}{\text{Drop factor constant}} = R$

Step 2 Total IVPB time: Time for 1 dose × number of doses in 24 h

Step 3 Total IVPB volume: Volume of 1 dose × number of doses in 24 h

Step 4 Total regular IV volume: Total volume − IVPB volume = Regular IV volume

Step 5 Total regular IV time: Total time − IVPB time = Regular IV time

Step 6 Regular IV flow rate: $\frac{V}{T} \times C = R$

or use $\frac{mL/h}{\text{Drop factor constant}} = R$

Example 1:

Order: *LR 3000 mL IV for 24 h with cefazolin 1 g IVPB per 100 mL D_5W q6h to run 1 hour. Limit total fluids to 3000 mL daily.*

The drop factor is 10 gtt/mL.

Note: The order intends that the patient receive a maximum of 3000 mL in 24 hours. Remember, when fluids are restricted, the piggybacks are to be *included* in the total 24-hour intake, not added to it.

Step 1 **Calculate** the flow rate of the IVPB.

$$\frac{V}{T} \times C = \frac{100 \text{ mL}}{\overset{}{\underset{6}{\cancel{60}}} \text{ min}} \times \overset{1}{\cancel{10}} \text{ gtt/mL} = \frac{100 \text{ gtt}}{6 \text{ min}} = 16.6 \text{ gtt/min} = 17 \text{ gtt/min}$$

or $\frac{mL/h}{\text{Drop factor constant}}$ = gtt/min (drop factor constant is 6)

$$\frac{100 \text{ mL/h}}{6} = 16.6 \text{ gtt/min} = 17 \text{ gtt/min}$$

Set the flow rate for the IVPB at 17 gtt/min to infuse 1 g cefazolin in 100 mL over 1 hour, or 60 min.

Step 2 **Calculate** the total time the IVPB will be administered.

q6h = 4 times per 24 h; 4 × 1 h = 4 h

Step 3 **Calculate** the total volume of the IVPB.

$100 \text{ mL} \times 4 = 400 \text{ mL}$ IVPB per 24 hours

Step 4 **Calculate** the volume of the regular IV fluids to be administered between IVPB doses. Total volume of regular IV minus total volume of IVPB: $3000 \text{ mL} - 400 \text{ mL} = 2600 \text{ mL}$

Step 5 **Calculate** the total regular IV fluid time or the time between IVPB doses. Total IV time minus total IVPB time: $24 \text{ h} - 4 \text{ h} = 20 \text{ h}$

Step 6 **Calculate** the flow rate of the regular IV.

$$\text{mL/h} = \frac{2600 \text{ mL}}{20 \text{ h}} = 130 \text{ mL/h}$$

$$\frac{V}{T} \times C = \frac{130 \not{\text{mL}}}{\underset{6}{\not{60}} \text{ min}} \times \overset{1}{\not{10}} \text{ gtt}/\not{\text{mL}} = \frac{130 \text{ gtt}}{6 \text{ min}} = 21.6 \text{ gtt/min} = 22 \text{ gtt/min}$$

or $\frac{\text{mL/h}}{\text{Drop factor constant}} = \text{gtt/min}$ (drop factor constant is 6)

$$\frac{130 \text{ mL/h}}{6} = 21.6 \text{ gtt/min} = 22 \text{ gtt/min}$$

Set the regular IV of LR at the flow rate of 22 gtt/min. Then after 5 hours, switch to the cefazolin IVPB at the flow rate of 17 gtt/min for 1 hour. Repeat this process 4 times in 24 hours.

Example 2:

Order: *NS 2000 mL IV for 24 h with 80 mg gentamicin sulfate in 80 mL IVPB q8h to run for 30 min. Limit fluid intake to 2000 mL daily.*

Drop factor: 15 gtt/mL

Calculate the flow rate for the regular IV and for the IVPB. IV pump is calibrated in whole mL/h.

Step 1 IVPB flow rate:

$$\frac{V}{T} \times C = \frac{80 \not{\text{mL}}}{\underset{2}{\not{30}} \text{ min}} \times \overset{1}{\not{15}} \text{ gtt}/\not{\text{mL}} = = \frac{80 \text{ gtt}}{2 \text{ min}} = 40 \text{ gtt/min}$$

Step 2 Total IVPB time: q8h = 3 times per 24 h; $3 \times 30 \text{ min} = 90 \text{ min}$

$$90 \text{ min} \div 60 \text{ min/h} = 90 \not{\text{min}} \times 1 \text{ h}/60 \not{\text{min}} = 1\frac{1}{2} \text{ h}$$

Step 3 Total IVPB volume: $80 \text{ mL} \times 3 = 240 \text{ mL}$

Step 4 Total regular IV volume: $2000 \text{ mL} - 240 \text{ mL} = 1760 \text{ mL}$

Step 5 Total regular IV time: $24 \text{ h} - 1\frac{1}{2} \text{ h} = 22\frac{1}{2} \text{ h} = 22.5 \text{ h}$

Step 6 Regular IV flow rate:

$$\text{mL/h} = \frac{1760 \text{ mL}}{22.5 \text{ h}} = 78.2 \text{ mL/h} = 78 \text{ mL/h}$$

$$\frac{V}{T} \times C = \frac{78 \cancel{\text{mL}}}{\underset{4}{\cancel{60}} \text{ min}} \times \overset{1}{\cancel{15}} \text{ gtt/}\cancel{\text{mL}} = \frac{78 \text{ gtt}}{4 \text{ min}} = 19.5 \text{ gtt/min} = 20 \text{ gtt/min}$$

$$\text{or } \frac{\text{mL/h}}{\text{Drop factor constant}} = \text{R (drop factor is 4)}$$

$$\frac{78 \text{ mL/h}}{4} = 19.5 \text{ gtt/min} = 20 \text{ gtt/min}$$

Set the regular IV of NS at the flow rate of 20 gtt/min. After $7\frac{1}{2}$ hours, switch to the gentamicin IVPB at the flow rate of 40 gtt/min for 30 minutes. Repeat this process 3 times in 24 hours.

Patients receiving a primary IV at a specific rate with an electronic infusion pump may require that the infusion rate be altered when a secondary (piggyback) medication is being administered. To do this, calculate the flow rate of the secondary medication in mL/h as you would the primary IV, and reset the infusion device.

Some infusion pumps allow you to set the flow rate for the secondary IV independent of the primary IV. Upon completion of the secondary infusion, the infusion device automatically returns to the original flow rate. If this is not the case, be sure to manually readjust the primary flow rate after the completion of the secondary set.

QUICK REVIEW

- To calculate the flow rate of a regular IV with an IVPB and restricted fluids, calculate the
  - **Step 1** IVPB flow rate;
  - **Step 2** Total IVPB time;
  - **Step 3** Total IVPB volume;
  - **Step 4** Total regular IV volume;
  - **Step 5** Total regular IV time;
  - **Step 6** Regular IV flow rate.

REVIEW SET 14-3

Calculate the flow rates for the following IV and IVPB orders. These patients are on limited fluid volume (restricted fluids). IV pumps are calibrated in whole mL.

1. Orders: *NS 3000 mL IV for 24 h*

   Limit total IV fluids to 3000 mL daily

   penicillin G potassium 1000 000 units IVPB q4h in 100 mL NS to run for 30 min

   Drop factor: 10 gtt/mL

   IVPB flow rate: ________ gtt/min

   IV flow rate: ________ gtt/min

2. Orders: *D_5W 1000 mL IV for 24 h*

   Limit total IV fluids to 1000 mL daily

   gentamicin sulfate 40 mg qid in 40 mL IVPB to run 1 h

   Drop factor: 60 gtt/mL

   IVPB flow rate: ________ gtt/min

   IV flow rate: ________ gtt/min

3. Orders: *LR 3000 mL IV for 24 h*

   Limit total IV fluids to 3000 mL daily

   ampicillin sodium 0.5 g q6h IVPB in 50 mL D_5W to run 30 min

   Drop factor: 15 gtt/mL

   IVPB flow rate: ________ gtt/min

   IV flow rate: ________ gtt/min

4. Orders: *$\frac{1}{2}$NS 2000 mL IV for 24 h*

   Limit total IV fluids to 2000 mL daily

   chloramphenicol sodium succinate 500 mg per 50 mL NS IVPB q6h to run 1 h

   Drop factor: 60 gtt/mL

   IVPB flow rate: ________ gtt/min

   IV flow rate: ________ gtt/min

5. Orders: *LR 1000 mL IV for 24 h*

   Limit total IV fluids to 1000 mL daily

   cefazolin sodium 250 mg IVPB per 50 mL D_5W q8h to run 1 h

   Drop factor: 60 gtt/mL

   IVPB flow rate: ________ gtt/min

   IV flow rate: ________ gtt/min

6. Orders: *D_5W 2400 mL IV for 24 h*

   Limit total IV fluids to 2400 mL daily

   cefazolin sodium 1 g IVPB q6h in 50 mL D_5W to run 30 min

   Drop factor: On electronic infusion pump

   IVPB flow rate: ________ mL/h

   IV flow rate: ________ mL/h

7. Orders: *NS 2000 mL IV for 24 h*

   Limit total IV fluids to 2000 mL daily

   gentamicin sulfate 100 mg IVPB q8h in 100 mL D_5W to run in over 30 min

   Drop factor: On electronic infusion pump

   IVPB flow rate: ________ mL/h

   IV flow rate: ________ mL/h

8. Orders: *D_5 0.45% NS 3000 mL IV to run 24 h*

   Limit total IV fluids to 3000 mL daily

   ranitidine hydrochloride 50 mg q6h in 50 mL D_5W to infuse 15 min

   Drop factor: On electronic infusion pump

   IVPB flow rate: ________ mL/h

   IV flow rate: ________ mL/h

9. Orders: *NS 1500 mL IV to run 24 h*

   Limit total IV fluids to 1500 mL daily

   cefazolin 500 mg IVPB per 50 mL D_5W q8h to run 1 h

   Drop factor: 20 gtt/mL

   IVPB flow rate: ________ gtt/min

   IV flow rate: ________ gtt/min

10. Orders: *NS 2700 mL IV for 24 h*

    Limit total IV fluids to 2700 mL per day

    gentamicin sulfate 60 mg in 60 mL D_5W IVPB q8h to run for 30 min

    Drop factor: On electronic infusion pump

    IV PB flow rate: ________ mL/h

    IV flow rate: ________ mL/h

Check your work! Answers to all Review Sets are provided at the end of each chapter. Worked solutions for selected Review Sets are also available there.

APPLICATION OF CLINICAL REASONING

Knowing the therapeutic dosage of a given medication requires sound clinical judgment. In this example, the order was unclear and the nurse did not verify the order with the appropriate person.

Potential Patient Safety Incident

Failing to clarify an order.

Possible Scenario

Suppose the prescriber ordered a heparin sodium infusion for a 100-kg patient with thrombophlebitis. The institution uses the Standard Weight-Based Heparin Sodium Protocol (Figure 14-1). The order was written this way:

heparin sodium 25 000 units in 250 mL NS IV at 18 000/h

The order was difficult to read, and the nurse asked a coworker to help her decipher it. They both agreed that it read 18 000 units per hour. The nurse calculated mL/h to be

$$\frac{18\,000 \text{ units/h}}{25\,000 \text{ units}} \times 250 \text{ mL} = 180 \text{ mL/h}$$

(continues)

(continued)

The nurse proceeded to start the heparin sodium drip at 180 mL/h. The patient's aPTT prior to initiation of the infusion was 37 seconds. Six hours into the infusion, an aPTT was drawn according to protocol. The nurse was shocked when the results returned and were 95 seconds, which is abnormally high. The nurse called the prescriber, who asked, "What is the rate of the heparin sodium drip?" The nurse replied, "I have the infusion set at 180 mL/h so that the patient receives the prescribed amount of 18 000 units per hour." The prescriber replied, "I ordered the drip at 1800 units per hour, not 18 000 units per hour."

Potential Outcome

The prescriber would likely have discontinued the heparin sodium and ordered protamine sulfate, the antidote for heparin overdosage. Another aPTT would also likely be obtained. The patient may have started to show signs of abnormal bleeding, such as hematuria epistaxis, and increased tendency to bruise.

Prevention

When the prescriber wrote the order for 1800 U/h, the *U* for "units" looked like a 0, and the nurse misinterpreted the order as 18 000 units. The nurse missed three opportunities to prevent the patient safety incident. The order as written is unclear, unsafe, and incomplete. Contacting the prescriber and requesting a clarification of the order is an appropriate action for several reasons. First, the writing is unclear and does not follow ISMP-Canada guidelines, which are automatic cautions to contact the prescriber for clarification. The prescriber should have spelled out *units* rather than use the *U* abbreviation. Guessing about the exact meaning of an order is dangerous, as this scenario demonstrates.

Second, the Standard Weight-Based Heparin Sodium Protocol recommends a safe heparin sodium infusion rate of 1800 units/h, or 18 mL/h (with a supply dosage of 25 000 units per 250 mL or 100 units/mL), for an individual weighing 100 kg. It is the responsibility of the individual administering a medication to be sure the Rights of medication administration are observed. The first three rights are that the *"right patient must receive the right drug in the right amount."* The order of 18 000 units as understood by the nurse was unsafe. The patient was overdosed by 10 times the recommended amount of heparin sodium.

Third, if the nurse clearly interpreted the order as 18 000, then no unit of measure was specified, which is a patient safety incident that requires contact with the prescriber for correction. An incomplete order must not be filled.

Application of Critical Reasoning Additional application problems are provided at the end of the chapter. Answers are provided at the end of the book.

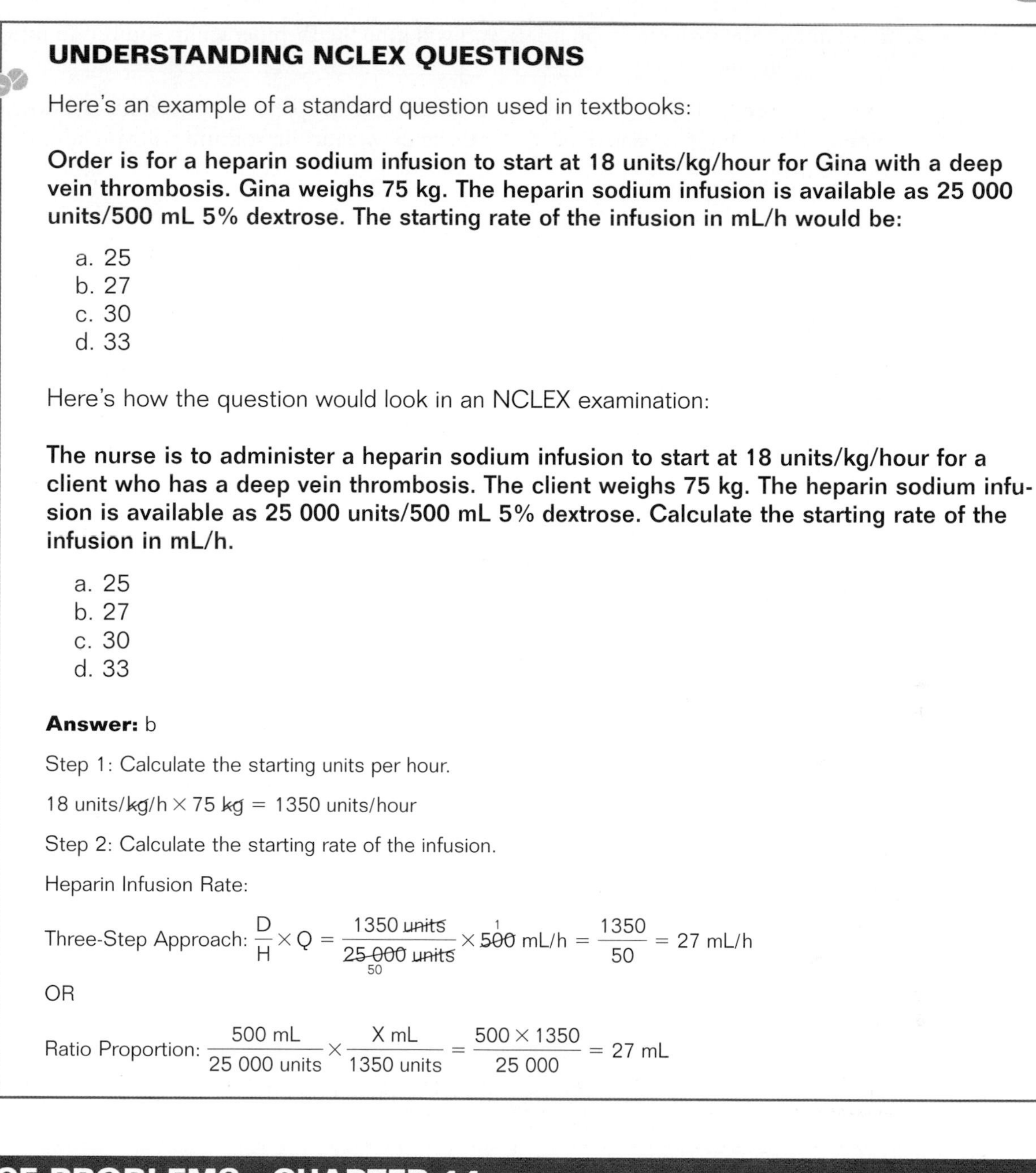

UNDERSTANDING NCLEX QUESTIONS

Here's an example of a standard question used in textbooks:

Order is for a heparin sodium infusion to start at 18 units/kg/hour for Gina with a deep vein thrombosis. Gina weighs 75 kg. The heparin sodium infusion is available as 25 000 units/500 mL 5% dextrose. The starting rate of the infusion in mL/h would be:

a. 25
b. 27
c. 30
d. 33

Here's how the question would look in an NCLEX examination:

The nurse is to administer a heparin sodium infusion to start at 18 units/kg/hour for a client who has a deep vein thrombosis. The client weighs 75 kg. The heparin sodium infusion is available as 25 000 units/500 mL 5% dextrose. Calculate the starting rate of the infusion in mL/h.

a. 25
b. 27
c. 30
d. 33

Answer: b

Step 1: Calculate the starting units per hour.

$18 \text{ units}/\cancel{\text{kg}}/\text{h} \times 75 \cancel{\text{kg}} = 1350 \text{ units/hour}$

Step 2: Calculate the starting rate of the infusion.

Heparin Infusion Rate:

Three-Step Approach: $\frac{D}{H} \times Q = \frac{1350 \cancel{\text{units}}}{\underset{50}{\cancel{25\,000}} \cancel{\text{units}}} \times \overset{1}{\cancel{500}} \text{ mL/h} = \frac{1350}{50} = 27 \text{ mL/h}$

OR

Ratio Proportion: $\frac{500 \text{ mL}}{25\,000 \text{ units}} \times \frac{X \text{ mL}}{1350 \text{ units}} = \frac{500 \times 1350}{25\,000} = 27 \text{ mL}$

PRACTICE PROBLEMS—CHAPTER 14

Unless stated otherwise, IV pumps are calibrated in whole mL/h.

Refer to the following patient information for questions 1 through 5. You are working on the day shift, 0700 to 1500. You observe that one of the patients assigned to you has an IV infusion with a volumetric control set (as shown in Figure 13-3). The patient's orders include

D_5W IV at 50 mL/h for continuous infusion piperacillin sodium 2 g IV q6h

Piperacillin sodium is available as a 2-g powder to be reconstituted with 10 mL of sterile water for injection (total volume = 11 mL), with instructions to add piperacillin sodium to volumetric control set, and infuse over 30 minutes. Answer questions 1 through 5.

1. What is the drop factor of the volumetric control set? ________ gtt/mL
2. What amount of piperacillin sodium will you add to the chamber? ________ mL
3. How much D_5W IV fluid will you add to the chamber with the piperacillin sodium? ________ mL

4. To maintain the flow rate at 50 mL/h, you will time the IV piperacillin sodium to infuse at ________ gtt/min.
5. The medication administration record indicates that the patient received his last dose of IV piperacillin sodium at 0600. How many doses of piperacillin sodium will you administer during your shift? ________
6. Order: *heparin sodium 25 000 units in 250 mL 0.9% NS to infuse at 1200 units/h*

   Drop factor: On electronic infusion pump

   Flow rate: ________ mL/h
7. Order: *thiamine 100 mg per L D_5W IV to infuse at 5 mg/h*

   Drop factor: On electronic infusion pump

   Flow rate: ________ mL/h
8. Order: *magnesium sulfate 4 g in 500 mL D_5W at 500 mg/h*

   Drop factor: On electronic infusion pump

   Flow rate: ________ mL/h
9. A patient is to receive *D_5W 500 mL with heparin sodium 20 000 units at 1400 units/h.*

   Set the infusion pump at ________ mL/h.
10. At the rate of 4 mL/min, how long will it take to administer 1.5 L of IV fluid? ________ h and ________ min
11. Order: *lidocaine hydrochloride 2 g in 500 mL D_5W IV to run at 4 mg/min*

    Drop factor: On electronic infusion pump calibrated in tenths of a mL/h

    Flow rate: ________ mL/h
12. Order: *lidocaine hydrochloride 1 g IV in 250 mL D_5W at 3 mg/min*

    Drop factor: On electronic infusion pump calibrated in tenths of a mL/h

    Flow rate: ________ mL/h
13. Order: *procainamide hydrochloride 1 g IV in 500 mL D_5W to infuse at 2 mg/min*

    Drop factor: On electronic infusion pump calibrated in tenths of a mL/h

    Flow rate: ________ mL/h
14. Order: *dobutamine hydrochloride 250 mg IV in 250 mL D_5W to infuse at 5 mcg/kg/min*

    Weight: 80 kg

    Drop factor: On electronic infusion pump calibrated in tenths of a mL/h

    Flow rate: ________ mL/h
15. A patient has an order for *D_5W 1 L IV with 2 g lidocaine hydrochloride added infusing at 75 mL/h.* The recommended continuous IV dosage of lidocaine is 1 to 4 mg/min. Is this dosage safe? ________
16. Orders: *Restricted fluids: 3000 mL D_5NS IV for 24 h*

    chloramphenicol sodium succinate 1 g IVPB in 100 mL NS q6h to run over 1 h

    Drop factor: 10 gtt/mL

    Flow rate: ________ gtt/min IVPB and ________ gtt/min primary IV

17. Order: *Restricted fluids: 3000 mL D_5W IV for 24 h*

    ampicillin sodium 500 mg in 50 mL D_5W IVPB qid for 30 min

    Drop factor: On electronic infusion pump

    Flow rate: ________ mL/h IVPB and ________ mL/h primary IV

18. Order: *50 mg nitroprusside sodium IV in 500 mL D_5W to infuse at 3 mcg/kg/min*

    Weight: 125 lb

    Drop factor: On electronic infusion pump calibrated in tenths of a mL/h

    Flow rate: ________ mL/h

19. Order: *KCl 40 mEq to each litre IV fluid*

    Situation: IV discontinued with 800 mL remaining

    How much KCl infused? ________

20. A patient's infusion rate is 125 mL/h. The rate is equivalent to ________ mL/min.

21. Order: *$\frac{2}{3}$ and $\frac{1}{3}$ solution (0.3% NaCl with 3.3% dextrose) 500 mL IV to run at 100 mL/h.*

    Calculate the infusion time. ________ h

22. Order: *KCl 40 mEq/L D_5W IV to infuse at 2 mEq/h*

    Rate: ________ mL/h

23. Order: *heparin sodium 50 000 units/L D_5W IV to infuse at 1250 units/h*

    Rate: ________ mL/h

24. If the minimal dilution for tobramycin is 5 mg/mL and you are giving 37 mg, what is the least amount of fluid in which you could safely dilute the dosage? ________ mL

25. Order: *oxytocin 10 units IV in 500 mL NS. Infuse 4 milliunits/min for 20 min, followed by 6 milliunits/min for 20 min. Use electronic infusion pump.*

    Rate: ________ mL/h for first 20 min

    Rate: ________ mL/h for next 20 min

26. Order: *magnesium sulfate 20 g IV in 500 mL of LR solution. Start with a bolus of 3 g to infuse over 30 min. Then maintain a continuous infusion at 2 g/h.*

    Use an electronic infusion pump.

    Rate: ________ mL/h for bolus

    Rate: ________ mL/h for continuous infusion

27. Order: *oxytocin 15 units IV in 500 mL of LR solution. Infuse at 1 milliunit/min.*

    Use an electronic infusion pump.

    Rate: ________ mL/h

28. Order: *heparin sodium drip 40 000 units/L D_5W IV to infuse at 1400 units/h*

    Drop factor: On infusion pump

    Flow rate: ________ mL/h

Refer to the following order for questions 29 and 30.

Order: *magnesium sulfate 4 g IV in 500 mL D_5W at 500 mg/h on an infusion pump*

29. What is the solution concentration? ________ mg/mL
30. What is the hourly flow rate? ________ mL/h

Calculate the drug concentrations of the following IV solutions as requested.

31. A solution containing 80 units of oxytocin in 1000 mL of D_5W: ________ milliunits/mL
32. A solution containing 200 mg of nitroglycerin in 500 mL of D_5W: ________ mg/mL
33. A solution containing 4 mg of isoproterenol hydrochloride in 1000 mL of D_5W: ________ mcg/mL
34. A solution containing 2 g of lidocaine hydrochloride in 500 mL of D_5W: ________ mg/mL

Refer to the following order for questions 35 through 37.

Order: *venuronium bromide IV 1 mg/kg/min* to control respirations for a patient who is ventilated

35. The patient weighs 220 pounds, which is equal to ________ kg.
36. The available venuronium bromide 20 mg is dissolved in 100 mL NS. This available solution concentration is ________ mg/mL, which is equivalent to ________ mcg/mL.
37. The IV is infusing at the rate of 1 mcg/kg/min on an infusion pump calibrated in tenths of a mL/h. The hourly rate is ________ mL/h.

Refer to these orders for questions 38 through 43.

Orders: *Restricted fluids: 3000 mL per 24 h. Primary IV of D_5LR running via infusion pump ampicillin sodium 3 g IVPB q6h in 100 mL of D_5W over 30 min*

gentamicin sulfate 170 mg IVPB q8h in 50 mL of D_5W to infuse in 1 h

38. Calculate the IVPB flow rates.

    ampicillin sodium: ________ mL/h; gentamicin sulfate: ________ mL/h
39. Calculate the total IVPB time. ________ h
40. Calculate the total IVPB volume. ________ mL
41. Calculate the total regular IV volume. ________ mL
42. Calculate the total regular IV time. ________ h
43. Calculate the regular IV flow rate. ________ mL/h
44. A patient who weighs 190 lb receives *dopamine 800 mg in 500 mL of D_5W IV at 4 mcg/kg/min.* As the patient's blood pressure drops, the nurse titrates the drip to *12 mcg/kg/min* as ordered.

    What is the initial flow rate for the IV pump calibrated in tenths of a mL/h? ________ mL/h

    After titration, what is the flow rate? ________ mL/h

Questions 45 through 49 refer to a patient who has left-leg deep vein thrombosis. He has orders for IV heparin sodium therapy. He weighs 225 lb. On admission, his aPTT is 25 seconds. You initiate therapy at 1130 on 5/10/xx. Follow the Standard Weight-Based Heparin Sodium Protocol in Figure 14-7, and record your answers on the Standard Weight-Based Heparin Sodium Protocol Worksheet in Figure 14-8.

Standard Weight-Based Heparin Sodium Protocol

For all patients on heparin drips:

1. Weight in kilograms (round to nearest 10 kg). Required for order to be processed: ________ kg
2. Heparin sodium 25 000 units in 250 mL of NS. Boluses to be given as 1000 units/mL.
3. aPTT q6h or 6 hours after rate change; daily after two consecutive therapeutic aPTTs.
4. CBC initially and repeat every ________ days(s).
5. Obtain aPTT and PT/INR on day 1 prior to initiation of therapy.
6. Guaiac stool initially, then every ________ day(s) until heparin sodium discontinued. Notify if positive.
7. Neuro checks every ________ hours while on heparin sodium. Notify physician of any changes.
8. Discontinue aPTT and CBC once heparin sodium drip is discontinued, unless otherwise ordered.
9. Notify physician of any bleeding problems.
10. Bolus with 80 units/kg. Start drip at 18 units/kg/h.
11. If aPTT is less than 35 sec: Rebolus with 80 units/kg and increase rate by 4 units/kg/h.
12. If aPTT is 36 to 44 sec: Rebolus with 40 units/kg and increase rate by 2 units/kg/h.
13. If aPTT is 45 to 75 sec: Continue current rate.
14. If aPTT is 76 to 90 sec: Decrease rate by 2 units/kg/h.
15. If aPTT is greater than 90 sec: Hold heparin sodium for 1 hour and decrease rate by 3 units/kg/h.

FIGURE 14-7 Standard Weight-Based Heparin Sodium Protocol

45. What is the patient's weight in kilograms? Calculate the weight as instructed in the protocol and record weight on the worksheet. ________ kg

    What does the protocol indicate for the standard bolus dosage of heparin sodium? ________ units/kg

46. Calculate the dosage of heparin sodium that should be administered for the bolus for this patient, and record your answer on the worksheet. ________ units

    What does the protocol indicate as the required solution concentration (supply dosage) of heparin sodium to use for the bolus? ________ units/mL

    Calculate the dose volume of heparin sodium that should be administered for the bolus for this patient, and record your answer on the worksheet. ________ mL

STANDARD WEIGHT-BASED HEPARIN PROTOCOL WORKSHEET

Round patient's total body weight to nearest 10 kg: ______ kg.

DO NOT change the weight based on daily measurements.

FOUND ON THE ORDER FORM

Initial Bolus (80 units/kg): ______ units ______ mL

Initial Infusion Rate (18 units/kg/h): ______ units/h ______ mL/h

Make adjustments to the heparin drip rate as directed by the order form.

ALL DOSES ARE ROUNDED TO THE NEAREST 100 UNITS.

Date	Time	aPTT	Bolus	Rate Change		New Rate	RN 1	RN 2
				units/h	mL/h			

If aPTT is	**Then**
Less than 35 sec:	Rebolus with 80 units/kg and increase rate by 4 units/kg/h.
36 to 44 sec:	Rebolus with 40 units/kg and increase rate by 2 units/kg/h.
45 to 75 sec:	Continue current rate.
76 to 90 sec:	Decrease rate by 2 units/kg/h.
Greater than 90 sec:	Hold heparin sodium for 1 hour and decrease rate by 3 units/kg/h.

Signatures ______________________________ Initials ______

____

____

____

____

____

Fresenius Kabi USA

FIGURE 14-8 Standard Weight-Based Heparin Sodium Protocol Worksheet

47. What does the protocol indicate for the initial infusion rate? ________ units/kg/h

    Calculate the dosage of heparin sodium this patient should receive each hour, and record your answer in the worksheet. ________ units/h

    What does the protocol indicate as the required solution concentration (supply dosage) of heparin sodium to use for the initial infusion? ________ units/mL

    Calculate the heparin sodium solution volume this patient should receive each hour to provide the correct infusion for his weight, and record your answer in the worksheet. ________ mL/h

48. According to the protocol, how often should the patient's aPTT be checked? q ________ h

    At 1730, the patient's aPTT is 37 seconds. Calculate the new heparin sodium bolus, and record your answer in the worksheet. Give ________ units/kg or ________ units measured as ________ mL.

    Calculate the change in heparin sodium infusion rate (increase or decrease), and record in worksheet. How much should you change the infusion rate? ________ by ________ units/kg/h or ________ units/h for a rate of ________ mL/h.

    Calculate the new infusion rate, and record in the worksheet. ________ mL/h

49. At 2330, the patient's aPTT is 77 seconds. What should the nurse do now?

    ____

    Calculate the new infusion rate, and record your answer in the worksheet. ________ mL/h

Check your work! Answers to all problems are provided at the end of the book, in the Answers section. Worked solutions for some practice problems are also provided there.

APPLICATION OF CLINICAL REASONING

14-1 Describe the clinical reasoning you would implement to prevent this patient safety incident.

Possible Scenario

Suppose the prescriber writes an order to induce labour as follows: *oxytocin 20 U IV added to 1 litre of LR beginning at 1 mU/min, then increase by 1 mU/min q15 min to a maximum of 20 mU/min until adequate labour is reached.* The labour and delivery unit stocks oxytocin ampules 10 units per mL in boxes of 50 ampules. The nurse preparing the IV solution misread the order as "20 mL of oxytocin added to 1 litre of Lactated Ringer's . . . " and pulled 20 ampules of oxytocin from the supply shelf. Another nurse, seeing this nurse drawing up medication from several ampules, asked what the nurse was preparing. When the nurse described the IV solution being prepared, he suddenly realized he had misinterpreted the order.

Potential Outcome

The amount of oxytocin that was being drawn up (20 mL) to be added to the IV solution would have been 10 units/mL $\times$ 20 mL = 200 units of oxytocin, 10 times the ordered amount of 20 units. Starting this oxytocin solution, even at the usual slow rate, would have delivered an excessively high amount of oxytocin that could have led to fatal consequences for both the fetus and mother who is in labour. What should the nurse have done to avoid this type of patient safety incident?

Prevention

____

____

Check your work! Answers to all Applications for Clinical Reasoning are provided at the end of the book, in the Answers section.

ANSWERS—REVIEW SETS

Review Set 14-1

1) 40 **2)** 14 **3)** 10 **4)** 19 **5)** 48; consult prescriber **6)** 16 **7)** 75; 6000; 6; 1350; 14 **8)** 6000; 6; 300; 3; 17 **9)** 3000; 3; 150; 2; 19 **10)** Continue current rate of 19 mL/h **11)** 10 **12)** 25 **13)** No **14)** 8 **15)** Hold insulin infusion for 60 minutes and check blood glucose every 15 minutes until greater than or equal to 4.4 mmol/L.

Review Set 14-2

1) 2; 120 **2)** 1; 60 **3)** 1.5; 90 **4)** 90; 360; 0.4; 24 **5)** 1 050; 0.66; 39.6 **6)** 142–568 **7)** 0.14–0.57 **8)** Yes **9)** 4 **10)** Yes **11)** 100; 25 **12)** 1 **13)** 0.004 **14)** 4 **15)** Yes

Review Set 14-3

1) 33; 19 **2)** 40; 42 **3)** 25; 32 **4)** 50; 90 **5)** 50; 40 **6)** 100; 100 **7)** 200; 76 **8)** 200; 122 **9)** 17; 21 **10)** 120; 112

SELECTED SOLUTIONS TO REVIEW SETS

Selected Solutions—Review Set 14-1

1) $\frac{D}{H} \times Q = \frac{1000 \cancel{\text{units}}/h}{\underset{25}{\cancel{25\,000}} \cancel{\text{units}}} \times \overset{1}{\cancel{1000}} \text{ mL} = \frac{\overset{40}{\cancel{1000}}}{\underset{1}{\cancel{25}}} \text{ mL/h}$

$= 40 \text{ mL/h}$

4) $\frac{D}{H} \times Q = \frac{1500 \cancel{\text{units}}/h}{\underset{80}{\cancel{40\,000}} \cancel{\text{units}}} \times \overset{1}{\cancel{500}} \text{ mL} = 18.7 \text{ mL/h}$

$= 19 \text{ mL/h}$

5) $\frac{D}{H} \times Q = \frac{1200 \cancel{\text{units}}/h}{\underset{25}{\cancel{25\,000}} \cancel{\text{units}}} \times \overset{1}{\cancel{1000}} \text{ mL} = 48 \text{ mL/h}$

The IV is infusing too rapidly. The prescriber should be called immediately for further action.

6) $\frac{D}{H} \times Q = \frac{800 \cancel{\text{units}}/h}{\underset{50}{\cancel{25\,000}} \cancel{\text{units}}} \times \overset{1}{\cancel{500}} \text{ mL} = \frac{\overset{16}{\cancel{800}}}{\underset{1}{\cancel{50}}} \text{ mL/h}$

$= 16 \text{ mL/h}$

7) 165 lb divided by 2.2 lb/kg = 75 kg

Initial heparin bolus: 80 units/~~kg~~ × 75 ~~kg~~

= 6000 units

$\frac{D}{H} \times Q = \frac{6000 \cancel{\text{units}}}{1000 \cancel{\text{units}}} \times 1 \text{ mL} = 6 \text{ mL}$

Initial heparin infusion rate: 18 units/~~kg~~/h × 75 ~~kg~~

= 1350 units/h

$\frac{D}{H} \times Q = \frac{1350 \cancel{\text{units}}/h}{\underset{100}{\cancel{25\,000}} \cancel{\text{units}}} \times \overset{1}{\cancel{250}} \text{ mL} = 13.5 \text{ mL/h}$

$= 14 \text{ mL/h}$

8) Rebolus: 80 units/~~kg~~ × 75 ~~kg~~ = 6000 units

$\frac{D}{H} \times Q = \frac{6000 \cancel{\text{units}}}{1000 \cancel{\text{units}}} \times 1 \text{ mL} = 6 \text{ mL}$

Reset infusion rate: 4 units/~~kg~~/h × 75 ~~kg~~

= 300 units/h (increase)

$\frac{300 \cancel{\text{units}}/h}{\underset{100}{\cancel{25000}} \cancel{\text{units}}} \times \overset{1}{\cancel{250}} \text{ mL} = 3 \text{ mL/h}$

14 mL/h + 3 mL/h = 17 mL/h

9) Rebolus: 40 units/~~kg~~ × 75 ~~kg~~ = 3000 units

$\frac{D}{H} \times Q = \frac{3000 \cancel{\text{units}}}{1000 \cancel{\text{units}}} \times 1 \text{ mL} = 3 \text{ mL}$

Reset infusion rate: 2 units/~~kg~~/h × 75 ~~kg~~

= 150 units/h (increase)

$\frac{150 \cancel{\text{units}}/h}{\underset{100}{\cancel{25\,000}} \cancel{\text{units}}} \times \overset{1}{\cancel{250}} \text{ mL} = 1.5 = 2 \text{ mL/h}$

17 mL/h + 2 mL/h = 19 mL/h

14) 8 units/h/100 units × 100 mL = 8 mL/h

Selected Solutions—Review Set 14-2

1) $\frac{D}{H} \times Q = \frac{4\ \cancel{mg}/min}{\underset{2}{\cancel{2000}}\ \cancel{mg}} \times \overset{1}{\cancel{1000}}\ mL = \frac{\overset{2}{\cancel{4}}}{\underset{1}{\cancel{2}}}\ mL/min$

$= 2\ mL/min$

$2\ mL/\cancel{min} \times 60\ \cancel{min}/h = 120\ mL/h$

2) $\frac{D}{H} \times Q = \frac{2\ \cancel{mg}/min}{\underset{2}{\cancel{500}}\ \cancel{mg}} \times \overset{1}{\cancel{250}}\ mL = \frac{\overset{1}{\cancel{2}}}{\underset{1}{\cancel{2}}}\ mL/min$

$= 1\ mL/min$

$1\ mL/\cancel{min} \times 60\ \cancel{min}/h = 60\ mL/h$

3) $\frac{D}{H} \times Q = \frac{6\ \cancel{mcg}/min}{\underset{4}{\cancel{2000}}\ \cancel{mcg}} \times \overset{1}{\cancel{500}}\ mL = \frac{6}{4}\ mL/min$

$= 1.5\ mL/min$

$1.5\ mL/\cancel{min} \times 60\ \cancel{min}/h = 90\ mL/h$

4) $4\ mcg/\cancel{kg}/min \times 90\ \cancel{kg} = 360\ mcg/min$

$450\ mg = 450 \times 1000 = 450\ 000\ mcg$

$\frac{D}{H} \times Q = \frac{360\ \cancel{mcg}/min}{\underset{900}{\cancel{450\ 000}}\ \cancel{mcg}} \times \overset{1}{\cancel{500}}\ mL = \frac{36}{90}\ mL/min$

$= 0.4\ mL/min$

$0.4\ mL/\cancel{min} \times 60\ \cancel{min}/h = 24\ mL/h$

5) $15\ mcg/\cancel{kg}/min \times 70\ \cancel{kg} = 1050\ mcg/min$

$800\ mg = 800 \times 1000 = 800\ 000\ mcg$

$\frac{D}{H} \times Q = \frac{1050\ \cancel{mcg}/min}{\underset{1600}{\cancel{800\ 000}}\ \cancel{mcg}} \times \overset{5}{\cancel{500}}\ mL = \frac{105}{160}\ mL/min$

$= 0.656\ mL/min = 0.66\ mL/min$

$0.66\ mL/\cancel{min} \times 60\ \cancel{min}/h = 39.6\ mL/h$

6) Minimum: $2.5\ mcg/\cancel{kg}/min \times 56.8\ \cancel{kg}$

$= 142\ mcg/min$

Maximum: $10\ mcg/\cancel{kg}/min \times 56.8\ \cancel{kg}$

$= 568\ mcg/min$

7) Minimum: $142\ mcg/min = 142 \div 1000$

$= 0.14\ mg/min$

Maximum: $568\ mcg/min = 568 \div 1000$

$= 0.57\ mg/min$

8) $\frac{500\ mg}{500\ mL} \rightleftarrows \frac{X\ mg/h}{15\ mL/h}$

$500X = 7500$

$\frac{500X}{500} = \frac{7500}{500}$

$X = 15\ mg/h$

$\frac{15\ mg/\cancel{h}}{60\ min/\cancel{h}} = 0.25\ mg/min$

Yes, the order is within the safe range of $0.14-0.57\ mg/min$.

9) $\frac{D\ mg/h}{\underset{4}{\cancel{2000}}\ mg} \times \overset{1}{\cancel{500}}\ mL = \frac{60\ mL}{h}$

$\frac{D}{4} = \frac{60}{h}$

$D = 240\ mg/h$

$\frac{240\ mg/\cancel{h}}{60\ min/\cancel{h}} = 4\ mg/min$

The dose is between 2 mg/min and 6 mg/min so the dose is safe.

11) Bolus:

$\frac{D}{H} \times Q = \frac{\overset{2}{\cancel{60}}\ \cancel{min}}{\underset{1}{\cancel{30}}\ \cancel{min}} \times 2\ g = 4\ g$ (per 60 min, or 4 g/h)

$\frac{D}{H} \times Q = \frac{4\ g/h}{20\ g} \times 500\ mL = 100\ ml/h$

Bolus rate $= 100\ mL/h$

Continuous:

$\frac{D}{H} \times Q = \frac{1\ g/h}{20\ g} \times 500\ mL = 25\ ml/h$

Continuous infusion $= 25\ mL/h$

12) $1\ milliunit/min \times 60\ seconds = 60\ milliunits/h$

$\frac{D}{H} \times Q = \frac{60\ \cancel{milliunits}/h}{150\ 00\ \cancel{milliunits}} \times 250\ mL$

$= 0.017\ mL/min$

$0.017\ mL/\cancel{min} \times 60\ \cancel{min}/h = 1.02\ mL/h = 1\ mL/h$

13) $\frac{D\ mg/h}{\underset{1}{\cancel{4}}\ mg} \times \overset{250}{\cancel{1000}}\ mL = \frac{60\ mL}{h}$

$D = 0.24\ mg$

Therefore, $0.24\ mg/h \div 60\ min/h = 0.004\ mg/min$

14) $0.004\ mg/min \times 1000 = 4\ mcg/min$

Selected Solutions—Review Set 14-3

1) Step 1. IVPB rate: $\frac{V}{T} \times C = \frac{100 \cancel{mL}}{\cancel{30}_{3} \text{ min}} \times \cancel{10}^{1} \text{ gtt}/\cancel{mL} = \frac{100}{3} \text{ gtt/min} = 33.3 \text{ gtt/min} = 33 \text{ gtt/min}$

Step 2. Total IVPB time: q4h × 30 min = 6 × 30 min = 180 min = 180 ÷ 60 = 3 h

Step 3. Total IVPB volume: 6 × 100 mL = 600 mL

Step 4. Total Regular IV volume: 3000 mL − 600 mL = 2400 mL

Step 5. Total Regular IV time: 24 h − 3 h = 21 h

Step 6. Regular IV rate:

$\frac{2400 \text{ mL}}{21 \text{ h}} = 114 \text{ mL/h}$

$\frac{\text{mL/h}}{\text{drop factor constant}} = \text{gtt/min}; \frac{114 \text{ mL/h}}{6} = 19 \text{ gtt/min}$

2) Step 1. IVPB rate: When drop factor is 60 gtt/mL, then mL/h = gtt/min. Rate is 40 gtt/min.

Step 2. Total IVPB time: qid × 1 h = 4 × 1 h = 4 h

Step 3. Total IVPB volume: 4 × 40 mL = 160 mL

Step 4. Total regular IV volume: 1000 mL − 160 mL = 840 mL

Step 5. Total regular IV time: 24 h − 4 h = 20 h

Step 6. Total regular IV rate: mL/h = $\frac{840 \text{ mL}}{20 \text{ h}}$ = 42 mL/h. When drop factor is 60 gtt/mL, then mL/h = gtt/min. Rate is 42 gtt/min.

3) Step 1. IVPB rate: $\frac{v}{T} \times C = \frac{50 \cancel{mL}}{\cancel{30}_{2} \text{ min}} \times \cancel{15}^{1} \text{ gtt}/\cancel{mL} = \frac{50}{2} \text{ gtt/min} = 25 \text{ gtt/min}$

Step 2. Total IVPB time: q6h × 30 min = 4 × 30 min = 120 min = 120 ÷ 60 = 2 h

Step 3. Total IVPB volume: 4 × 50 mL = 200 mL

Step 4. Total regular IV volume: 3000 mL − 200 mL = 2800 mL

Step 5. Total regular IV time: 24 h − 2 h = 22 h

Step 6. Total regular IV rate:

$\frac{2800 \text{ mL}}{22 \text{ h}} = 127 \text{ mL/h}$

$\frac{\text{mL/h}}{\text{drop factor constant}} = \text{gtt/min}; \frac{127 \text{ mL/h}}{4} = 31.7 \text{ gtt/min} = 32 \text{ gtt/min}$

4) Step 1. IVPB rate: 50 mL/h or 50 gtt/min (because drop factor is 60 gtt/mL)

Step 2. Total IVPB time: q6h × 1 h = 4 × 1 h = 4 h

Step 3. Total IVPB volume: 4 × 50 mL = 200 mL

Step 4. Total regular IV volume: 2000 mL − 200 mL = 1800 mL

Step 5. Total regular IV time: 24 h − 4 h = 20 h

Step 6. Regular IV rate: $\frac{1800 \text{ mL}}{20 \text{ h}}$ = 90 mL/h or 90 gtt/min (because drop factor is 60 gtt/mL)

5) Step 1. IVPB rate: 50 mL/h or 50 gtt/min (because drop factor is 60 gtt/mL)

Step 2. IVPB time: q8h × 1 h = 3 × 1 h = 3 h

Step 3. IVPB volume: 3 × 50 mL = 150 mL

Step 4. Total regular IV volume: 1000 mL − 150 mL = 850 mL

Step 5. Total regular IV time: 24 h − 3 h = 21 h

Step 6. Regular IV rate: $\frac{850 \text{ mL}}{21 \text{ h}}$ = 40.4 mL/h = 40 gtt/min (because drop factor is 60 gtt/mL)

6) Step 1. IVPB rate

$$\frac{50 \text{ mL}}{30 \text{ min}} \times \frac{X \text{ mL}}{60 \text{ min}}$$

$$30 X = 3000$$

$$\frac{30 X}{30} = \frac{3000}{30}$$

$$X = 100 \text{ mL}; 100 \text{ mL}/60 \text{ min} = 100 \text{ mL/h}$$

Step 2. IVPB time: q6h × 30 min = 4 × 30 min = 120 min = 120 ÷ 60 = 2 h

Step 3. IVPB volume: 4 × 50 mL = 200 mL

Step 4. Total regular IV volume: 2400 mL − 200 mL = 2200 mL

Step 5. Total regular IV time: 24 h − 2 h = 22 h

Step 6. Regular IV rate: $\frac{2200 \text{ mL}}{22 \text{ h}} = 100 \text{ mL/h}$

7) Step 1. IVPB rate:

$$\frac{100 \text{ mL}}{30 \text{ min}} \times \frac{X \text{ mL}}{60 \text{ min}}$$

$$30 X = 6000$$

$$\frac{30 X}{30} = \frac{6000}{30}$$

$$X = 200 \text{ mL}; 200 \text{ mL}/60 \text{ min} = 200 \text{ mL/h}$$

Step 2. IVPB time: q8h × 30 min = 3 × 30 min = 90 min = 90 ÷ 60 = $1\frac{1}{2}$ h

Step 3. IVPB volume: 3 × 100 mL = 300 mL

Step 4. Total regular IV volume: 2000 mL − 300 mL = 1700 mL

Step 5. Total regular IV time: 24 h − $1\frac{1}{2}$ h = $22\frac{1}{2}$ h

Step 6. Regular IV rate: $\frac{1700 \text{ mL}}{22.5 \text{ h}} = 75.5 \text{ mL/h} = 76 \text{ mL/h}$

8) Step 1. IVPB rate

$$\frac{50 \text{ mL}}{15 \text{ min}} \times \frac{X \text{ mL}}{60 \text{ min}}$$

$$15 X = 3000$$

$$\frac{15 X}{5} = \frac{3000}{15}$$

$$X = 200 \text{ mL}; 200 \text{ mL}/60 \text{ min} = 200 \text{ mL/h}$$

Step 2. IVPB time: q6h × 15 min = 4 × 15 min = 60 min = 1 h

Step 3. IVPB volume: 4 × 50 mL = 200 mL

Step 4. Total regular IV volume: 3000 mL − 200 mL = 2800 mL

Step 5. Total regular IV time: 24 h − 1 h = 23 h

Step 6. Regular IV rate: $\frac{2800 \text{ mL}}{23 \text{ h}} = 121.7 \text{ mL/h} = 122 \text{ mL/h}$

Chapter 12: Intravenous Solutions, Equipment, and Calculations

1. Which of the following IV solutions is normal saline?
   ________ 0.45% NaCl ________ 0.9% NaCl ________ D_5W
2. What are the solute and concentration of 0.9% NaCl? ________
3. What are the solute and concentration of 0.45% NaCl? ________

Use the following information to answer questions 4 and 5.

Order: *D_5 0.45% NaCl 1000 mL IV solution*

4. The IV solution contains ________ g dextrose.
5. The IV solution contains ________ g sodium chloride.
6. Order: *0.45% NaCl 500 mL IV q6h*. The IV solution contains ________ g sodium chloride.

Refer to the following order for questions 7 and 8.

Order: *D_5 0.9% NaCl 750 mL IV q8h*

7. The IV solution contains ________ g dextrose.
8. The IV solution contains ________ g sodium chloride.
9. Are most electronic infusion devices calibrated in gtt/min, mL/h, mL/min, or gtt/mL?
   ____

Use the following information to answer questions 10 and 11. Mrs. Wilson has an order to receive *2000 mL of D_5NS IV over 24 h*. The IV tubing is calibrated for a drop factor of 15 gtt/mL.

10. Calculate the watch count flow rate for Mrs. Wilson's IV. ________ gtt/min
11. An electronic infusion pump calibrated to deliver whole mL/h becomes available, and you decide to use it to regulate Mrs. Wilson's IV. Set the controller at ________ mL/h.
12. Mrs. Hawkins returns from the delivery room at 1530 with 400 mL D_5LR infusing at 24 gtt/min with the hospital's standard macrodrop infusion control set calibrated at 15 gtt/mL. Mrs. Hawkins's IV will be complete at ________ (hours).
13. The nurse starts a shift at 1500. On the nursing assessment rounds, the nurse finds that Mr. Johnson has an IV of $D_5 \frac{1}{2}$ NS infusing at 32 gtt/min. The tubing is calibrated for 10 gtt/mL. Mr. Johnson will receive ________ mL during the nurse's 8-hour shift.

Use the following information to answer questions 14 through 16. As you do your rounds, you find Mr. Boyd with an infiltrated IV. You decide to restart it and regulate it on an electronic infusion pump. The orders specify

NS 1000 mL IV with 20 mEq KCl q8h
cefazolin sodium 250 mg IVPB per 100 mL NS q8h over 30 min
Limit IV total fluids to 3000 mL daily

14. Interpret Mr. Boyd's IV and medication order. ____
    ____

15. Regulate the electronic infusion pump for Mr. Boyd's standard IV at ________ mL/h.
16. Regulate the electronic infusion pump for Mr. Boyd's IVPB at ________ mL/h.
17. Order: *D_5LR 1200 mL IV at 100 mL/h.* You start this IV at 1530 and regularly observe the IV and the patient. The IV has been infusing as scheduled, but during your nursing assessment at 2200, you find 650 mL remaining. The flow rate is 100 gtt/min using a microdrip infusion set. Describe your action now. ________________________________

____

Chapter 13: Body Surface Area and Advanced Pediatric Calculations

Calculate the hourly maintenance IV rate for the two pediatric patients described in questions 18 through 21. Use the following recommendations:

First 10 kg of body weight: 100 mL/kg/day

Second 10 kg of body weight: 50 mL/kg/day

Each additional kilogram over 20 kg of body weight: 20 mL/kg/day

18. A child who weighs 18.2 kg requires ________ mL/day for maintenance IV fluids.
19. The infusion rate is ________ mL/h.
20. An infant who weighs 1185 g requires ________ mL/day for maintenance IV fluids.
21. The infusion rate is ________ mL/h.

Use the BSA formula method (next page) to answer questions 22 and 23.

22. Height: 76 cm Weight: 11 kg BSA: ________ m^2
23. Height: 155 cm Weight: 39 kg BSA: ________ m^2

Questions 24 through 30 refer to the following situation. A child who is 71 cm tall and weighs 11.4 kg will receive one dosage of cisplatin IV. The recommended dosage is 37 to 75 mg/m^2 once every 2 to 3 weeks. Order: *cisplatin 18.5 mg IV at 1 mg/min today at 1500.* Available: a 50-mg vial of cisplatin. Reconstitution directions: add 50 mL of sterile water to yield 1 mg/mL. Minimal dilution instructions require 2 mL of IV solution for every 1 mg of cisplatin.

24. According to the nomogram on the next page, the child's BSA is ________ m^2.
25. The safe dosage range for this child is ________ to ________ mg.
26. Is this dosage safe? ________
27. If safe, you will prepare ________ mL. If not, describe your action. ________________

____

28. How many mL of IV fluid are required for safe dilution of the cisplatin? ________ mL
29. Given the ordered rate of 1 mg/min, set the infusion pump at ________ mL/h.
30. How long will this infusion take? ________ min

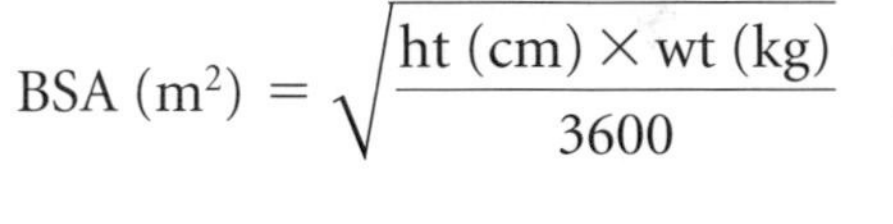

$$BSA\ (m^2) = \sqrt{\frac{ht\ (cm) \times wt\ (kg)}{3600}}$$

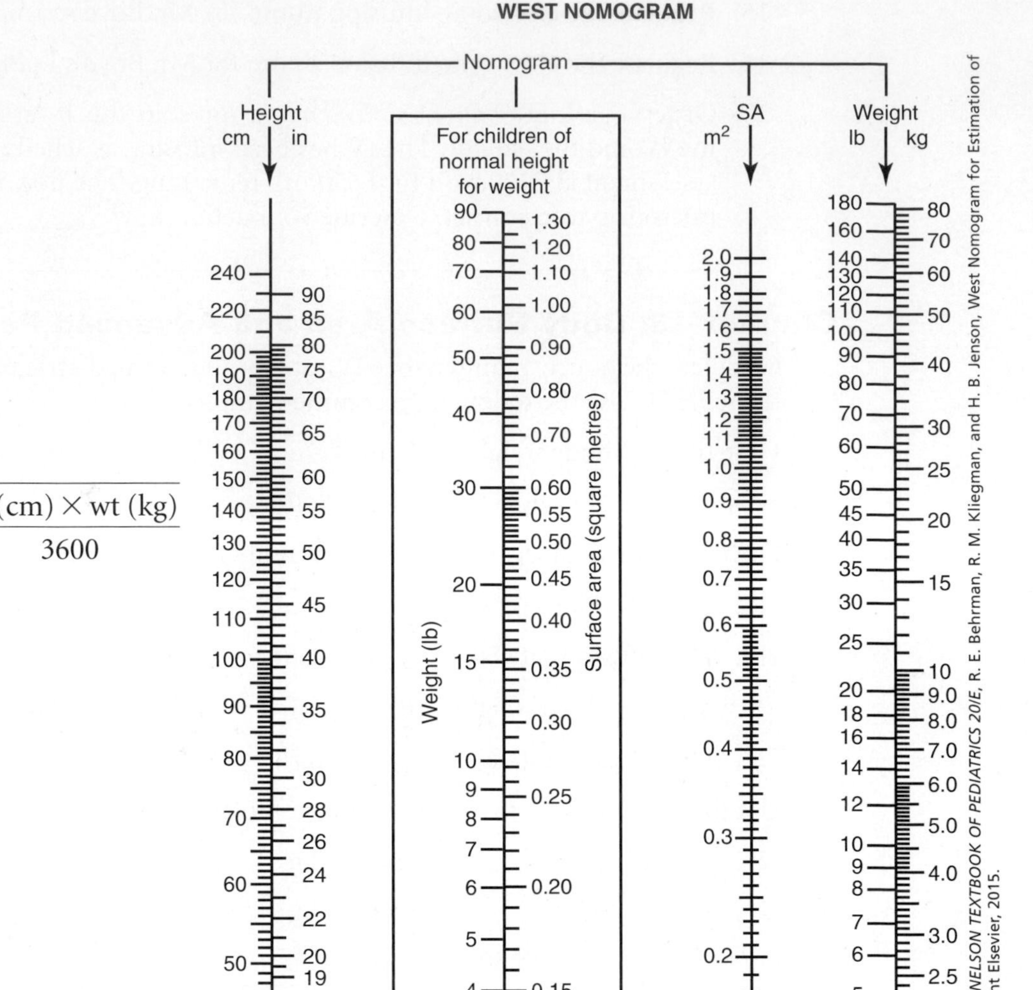

West Nomogram for Estimation of Body Surface Area

Questions 31 through 34 refer to the following situation. Order: *vincristine sulfate 1.6 mg IV stat*. The child is 127 cm tall and weighs 18.2 kg. The label on page 471 is from the vincristine sulfate solution available. The recommended initial dosage of vincristine sulfate is 2 mg/m^2 daily.

31. According to the nomogram, the child's BSA is ________ m^2.
32. The recommended safe dosage for this child is ________ mg.
33. Is the dosage ordered safe? ________
34. If safe, the nurse will prepare ________ mL vincristine sulfate to add to the IV. If not safe, describe the nurse's action. ____

____

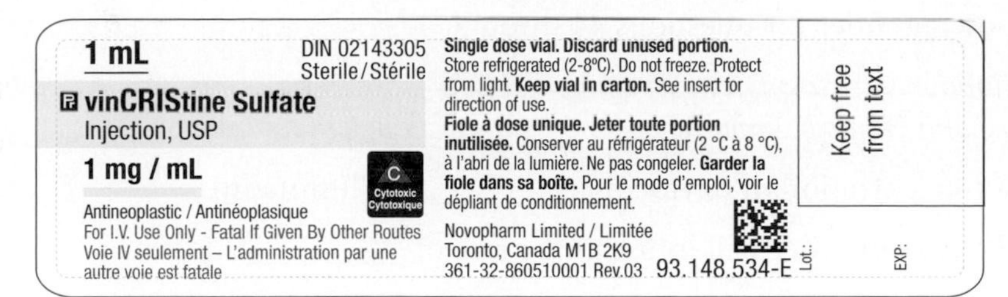

The product labels and intellectual property of Teva Canada Limited are reproduced with the permission of Teva Canada Limited and used herein for educational purposes only.

35. Order: *NS IV for continuous infusion at 40 mL/h with cefazolin sodium 250 mg IV q8h over 30 min by volume control set*

    Available: cefazolin sodium 125 mg/mL

    Add ________ mL of cefazolin sodium to the chamber and fill the chamber to ________ mL with NS and infuse at 40 mL/h.

36. Order: *metoclopramide hydrochloride 300 mcg/kg IV* once for a child who weighs 25 kg undergoing gastric intubation. Metoclopramide hydrochloride is available as a 2-mL vial with a concentration of 5 mg/mL.

    Calculate the dosage of metoclopramide hydrochloride. ________ mg

37. Order: *ticarcillin disodium/clavulanate potassium 750 mg IV q6h.* Recommended minimal dilution (maximal concentration) is 100 mg/mL. Calculate the mL to be used for minimal dilution of the ticarcillin disodium/clavulanate potassium ordered. ________ mL

Chapter 14: Advanced Adult Intravenous Calculations

Use the following information to answer questions 38 through 41. Mr. Amar is on restricted fluids. His IV order is *NS 1500 mL IV q24h with 300 000 units penicillin G sodium IVPB 100 mL NS q4h over 30 min*. The infusion set is calibrated at 60 gtt/mL.

38. Set Mr. Amar's regular IV at ________ gtt/min.

39. Set Mr. Amar's IVPB at ________ gtt/min.

40. Later, an electronic infusion pump becomes available. You decide to use it to regulate Mr. Amar's IVs. Regulate Mr. Amar's regular IV at ________ mL/h.

41. Regulate Mr. Amar's IVPB at ________ mL/h.

42. Order: *potassium chloride 40 mEq/L D_5W IV at 2 mEq/h*

    Regulate the infusion pump at ________ mL/h.

43. Order: *nitroglycerin 25 mg/L D_5W IV at 5 mcg/min*

    Regulate the infusion pump at ________ mL/h.

Refer to the following order for questions 44 through 47.

Order: *Induce labour with oxytocin 15 units/L LR IV continuous infusion at 2 milliunits/min; increase by 1 milliunit/min q30 min to a maximum of 20 milliunits/min*

44. The initial concentration of oxytocin is ________ milliunits/mL.
45. The initial oxytocin order will infuse at the rate of ________ mL/min.
46. Regulate the electronic infusion pump at ________ mL/h to initiate the order.
47. The infusion pump will be regulated at a maximum of ________ mL/h to infuse the maximum of 20 milliunits/min.

Use the following information to answer questions 48 and 49.

Order for Ms. Popovich, who weighs 68 kg: *dopamine hydrochloride 400 mg/0.5 L D_5W at 4 mcg/kg/min titrated to 12 mcg/kg/min to stabilize blood pressure*

48. Regulate the electronic infusion pump for Ms. Popovich's IV at ________ mL/h to initiate the order.
49. Anticipate that the maximum flow rate for Ms. Popovich's IV to achieve the maximum safe titration would be ________ mL/h.
50. Mr. Cara has a new order for *heparin sodium 10 000 units in 500 mL NS IV at 750 units/h*. Regulate the infusion pump at ________ mL/h.

After completing these problems, refer to the Answer section to check your answers. Give yourself 2 points for each correct answer.

Perfect score = 100% My score = ________

Mastery score = 86 or higher (43 or more correct)

Essential Skills Evaluation

This evaluation is designed to assess your mastery of essential dosage calculation skills. It excludes the advanced calculation skills presented in Chapters 13 and 14.

You are assigned to give the medications on a busy adult medical unit. The following labels represent the medications available in the medication cart to fill the orders given in questions 1 through 17. Calculate the amount you will administer for one dose. Assume that all tablets are scored. Draw an arrow on the appropriate syringe to indicate how much you will prepare for parenteral medications.

1. Order: *pencillin V potassium 250 mg PO q4h*

   Give: ______ mL

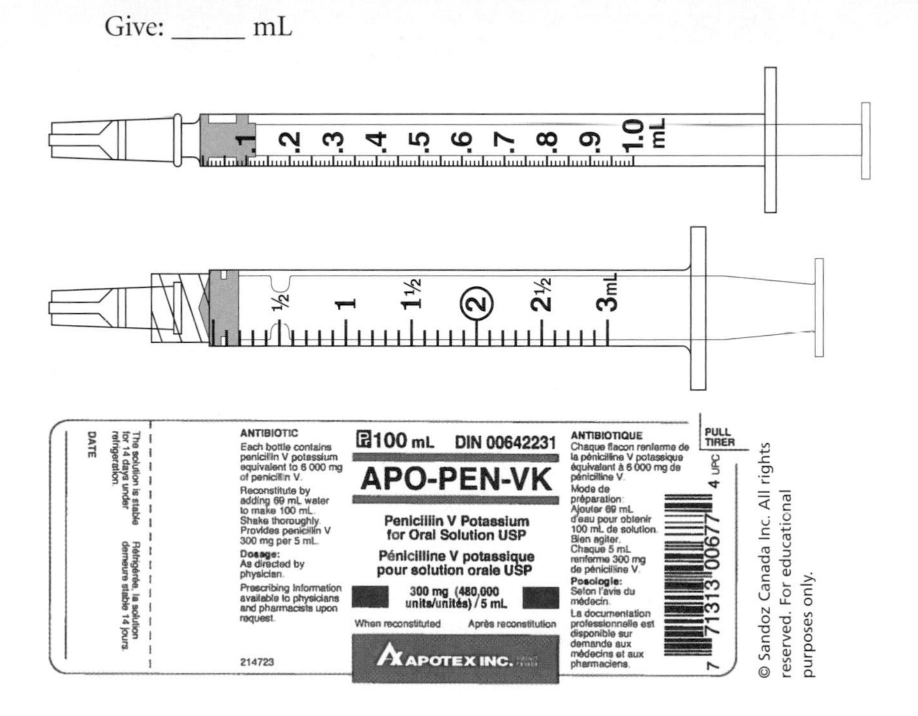

.1 .2 .3 .4 .5 .6 .7 .8 .9 1.0 mL
½ 1 1½ 2 2½ 3mL
ANTIBIOTIC
100 mL DIN 00642231
APO-PEN-VK
Penicillin V Potassium for Oral Solution USP
Pénicilline V potassique pour solution orale USP
300 mg (480,000 units/unités) / 5 mL
When reconstituted Après reconstitution
APOTEX INC.
ANTIBIOTIQUE
PULL TIRER

2. Order: *clindamycin 100 mg IM stat*

   Give: ______ mL

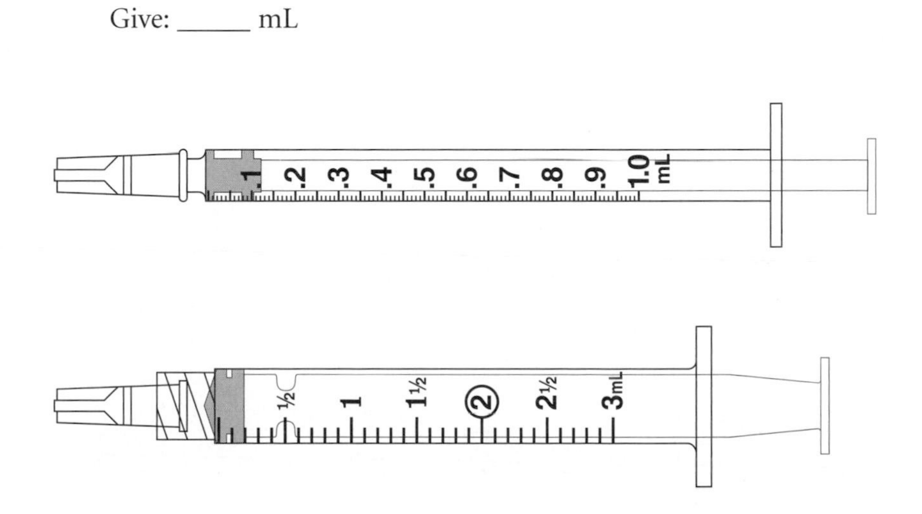

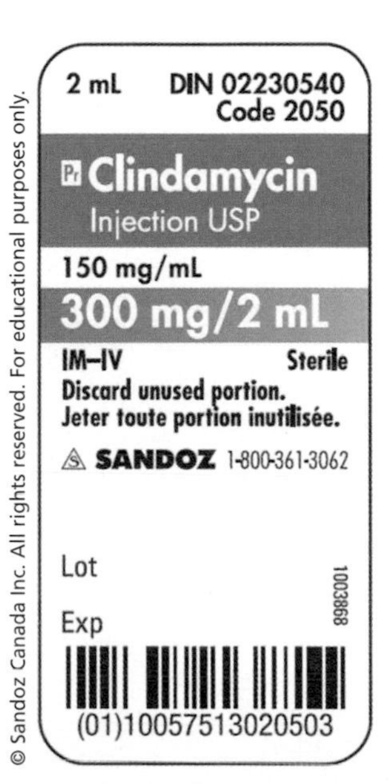

3. Order: *diazepam 7.5 mg direct IV (administer slowly, at 5 mg/min)*

   Give: _____ mL at _____ mL/min or _____ mL/15 sec

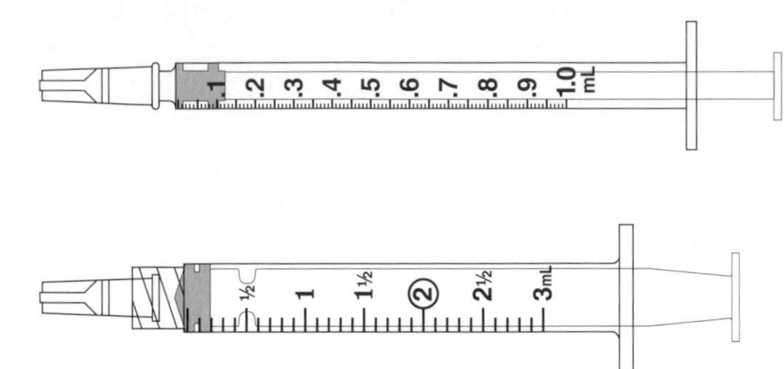

2 mL DIN 02386143
Code 44045980
Diazepam
Injection SDZ
Diazepam Injection BP
10 mg/2 mL
5 mg/mL
IM–Slow IV Sterile
SANDOZ 1-800-361-3062
(01)10057513214810
Lot
Exp.
46108335
Hameln

4. Order: *glycopyrrolate 200 mcg IV stat*

   Give: _____ mL

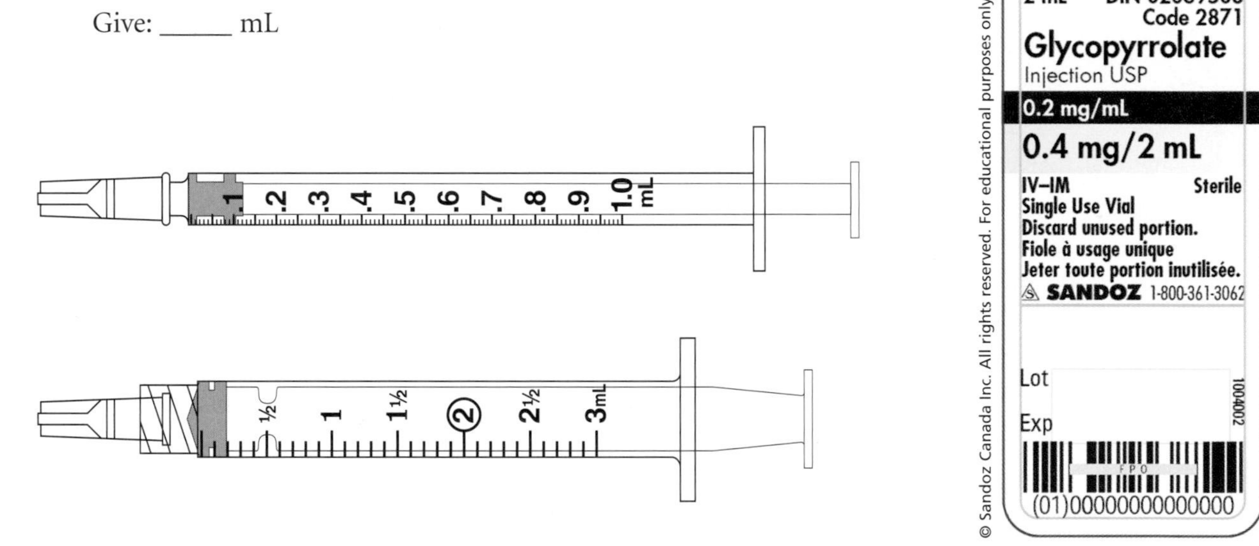

5. Order: *oxycodone hydrochloride 5 mg and acetaminophen 325 mg PO q3h prn, pain*

   Dosage is based on oxycodone hydrochloride.

   Give: _____ tablet(s)

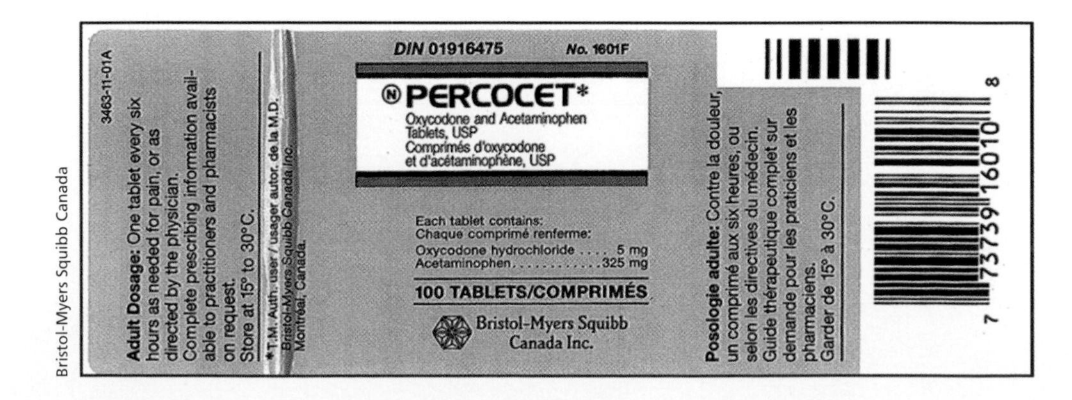

6. Order: *digoxin 0.125 mg IV daily at 0800*

   Give: ______ mL

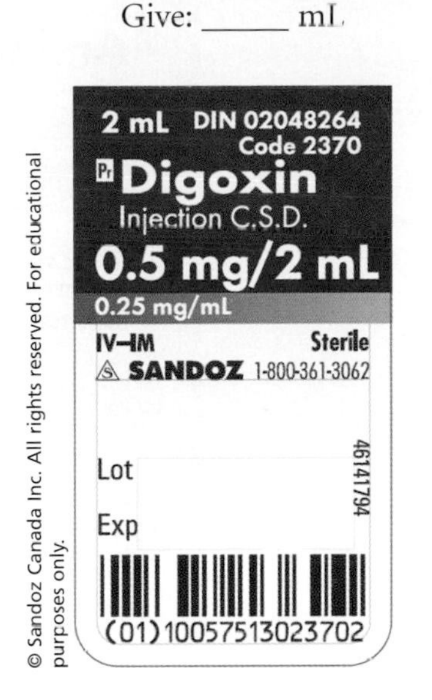

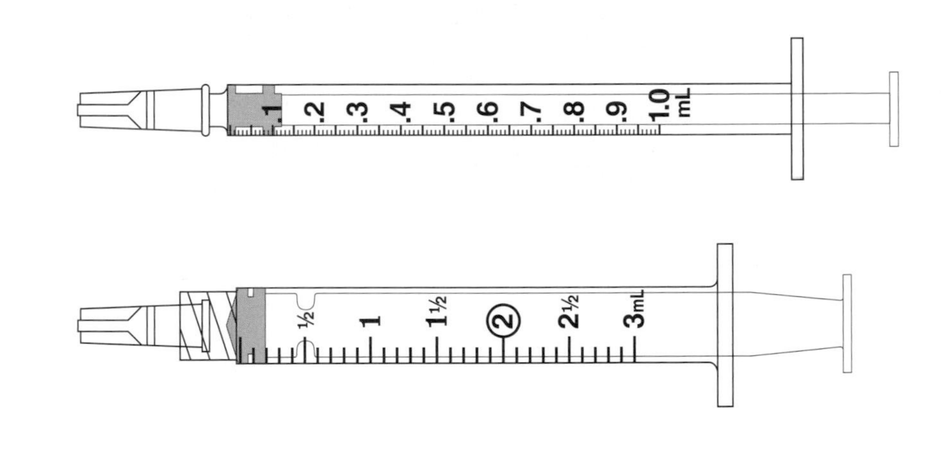

7. Order: *dilantin 187.5 mg PO TID*

   Give: ______ mL

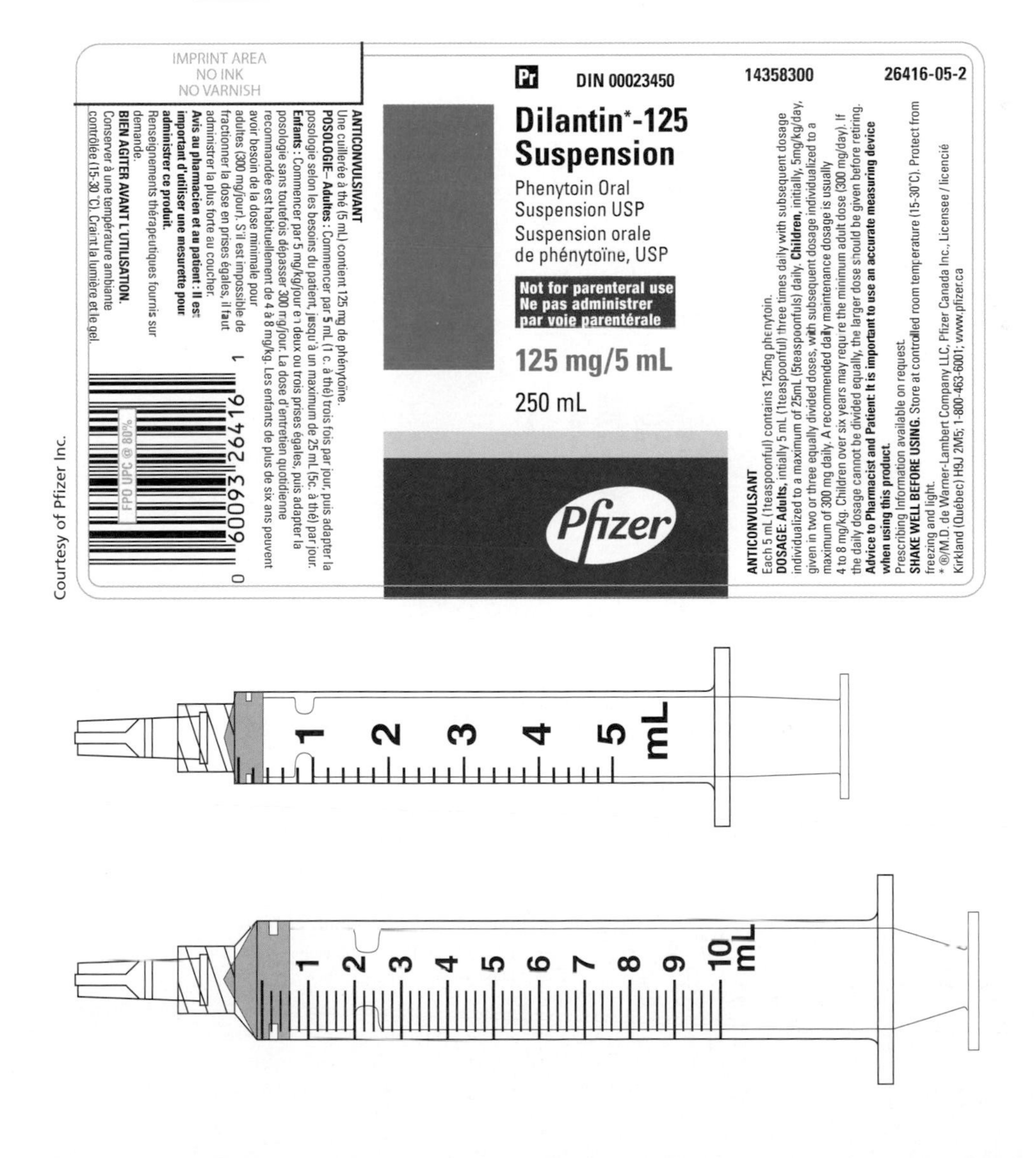

8. Order: *amikacin sulfate 350 mg IM BID*

   Give: _____ mL

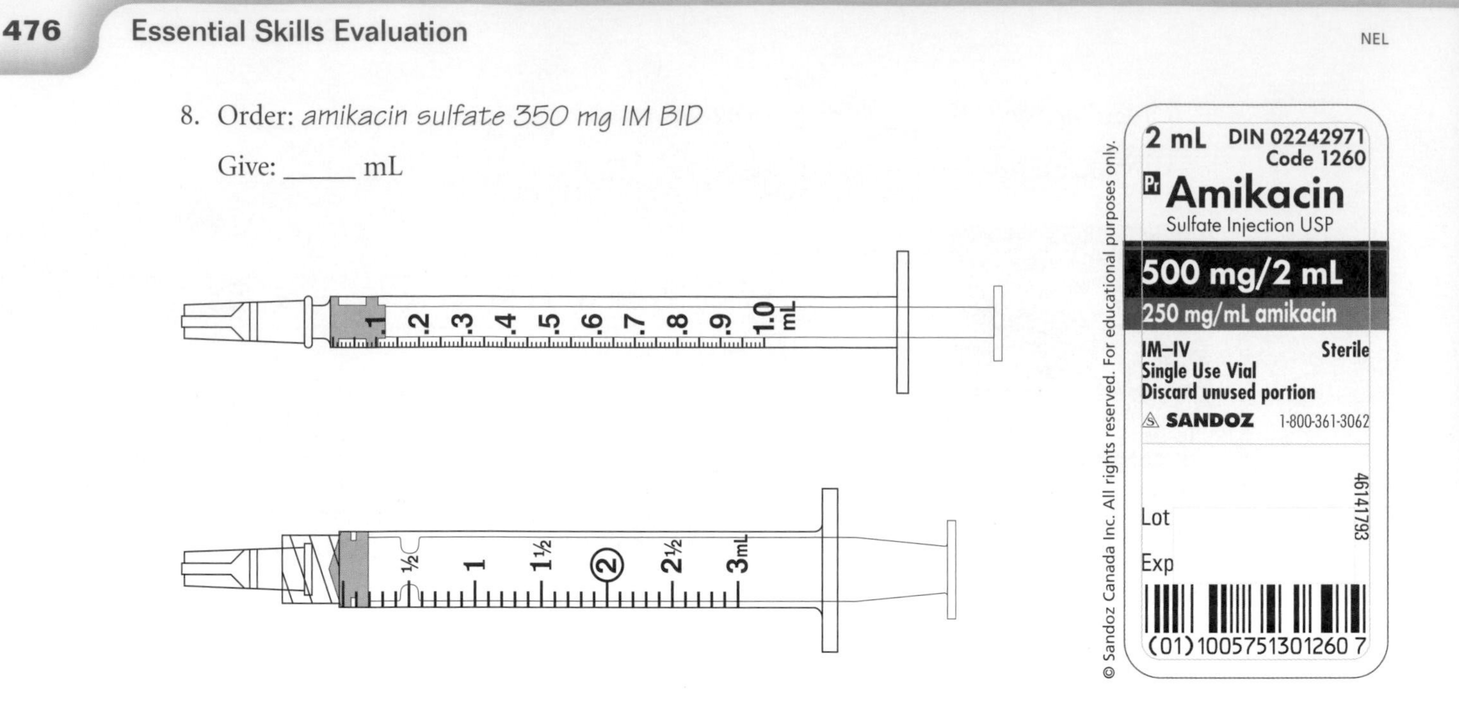

9. Order: *Humulin N insulin 46 units with Humulin R insulin 22 units subcut stat*

   You will give _____ units total.

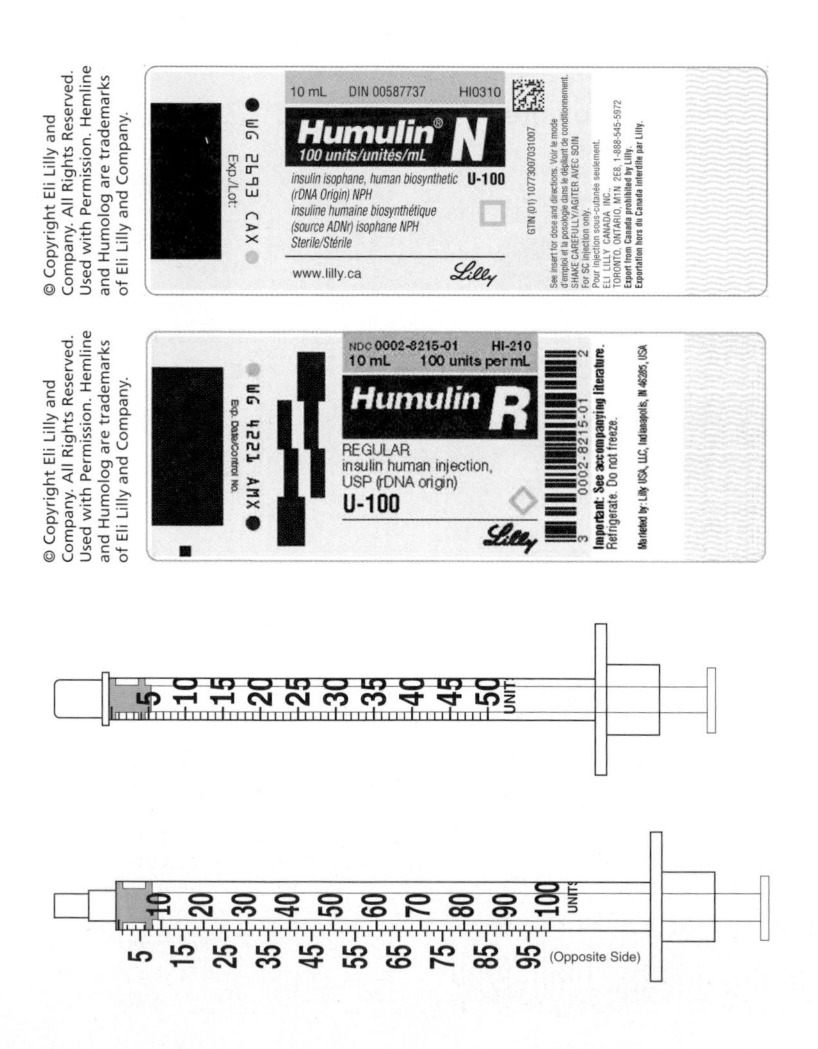

.1 .2 .3 .4 .5 .6 .7 .8 .9 1.0 mL

10. Order: *levothyroxine sodium 0.3 mg PO qAM*

    Give: _____ tablet(s)

Pharmacist should not dispense if seal is broken.
Each tablet contains : levothyroxine sodium 150 mcg.
DOSAGE : 50 to 300 mcg per day. Protect from light. Product Monograph available to physicians and pharmacists on request.
Pharmacien : ne pas remettre si le sceau de sécurité est brisé.
Chaque comprimé contient : 150 mcg de lévothyroxine sodique.
POSOLOGIE : 50 à 300 mcg par jour. Garder à l'abri de la lumière. Monographie de produit fournie sur demande aux médecins et aux pharmaciens.

DIN 02213214
500 TABLETS/COMPRIMÉS
Eltroxin®
levothyroxine sodium tablets USP
comprimés de lévothyroxine sodique USP
150 mcg
THYROID HORMONE/HORMONE THYROÏDIENNE
aspen TRITON PHARMA INC.

1 84814 00015 6
® used under license by / utilisée sous licence par Aspen.
TRITON Pharma inc.
Concord (Ontario) L4K 3T8
A082826

TRITON PHARMA INC.

11. Order: *verapamil hydrochloride SR 240 mg each morning plus 120 mg each evening, with food*

    Give: _____ tablet(s) for the morning dose and _____ for the evening dose

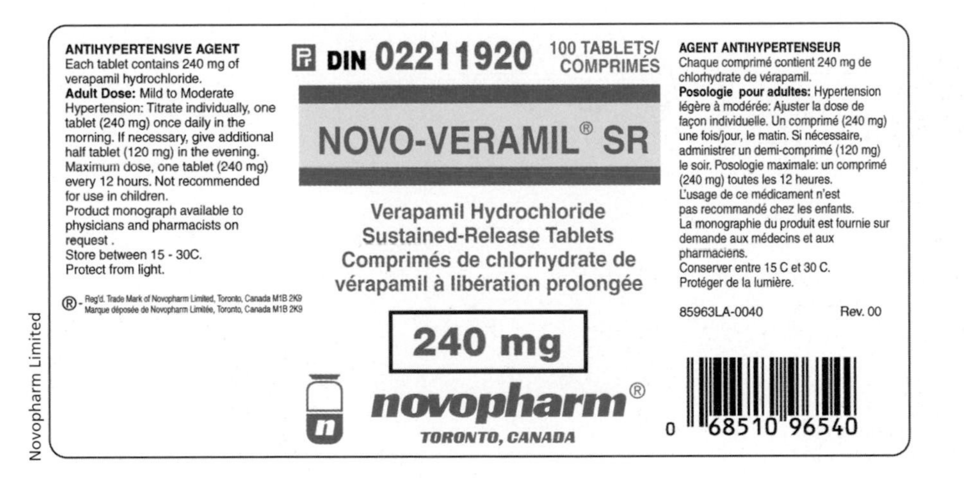
ANTIHYPERTENSIVE AGENT
Each tablet contains 240 mg of verapamil hydrochloride.
Adult Dose: Mild to Moderate Hypertension: Titrate individually, one tablet (240 mg) once daily in the morning. If necessary, give additional half tablet (120 mg) in the evening. Maximum dose, one tablet (240 mg) every 12 hours. Not recommended for use in children.
Product monograph available to physicians and pharmacists on request.
Store between 15 - 30C.
Protect from light.
DIN 02211920
100 TABLETS/COMPRIMÉS
NOVO-VERAMIL® SR
Verapamil Hydrochloride Sustained-Release Tablets
Comprimés de chlorhydrate de vérapamil à libération prolongée
240 mg
novopharm®
TORONTO, CANADA
AGENT ANTIHYPERTENSEUR
Chaque comprimé contient 240 mg de chlorhydrate de vérapamil.
Posologie pour adultes: Hypertension légère à modérée: Ajuster la dose de façon individuelle. Un comprimé (240 mg) une fois/jour, le matin. Si nécessaire, administrer un demi-comprimé (120 mg) le soir. Posologie maximale: un comprimé (240 mg) toutes les 12 heures.
L'usage de ce médicament n'est pas recommandé chez les enfants.
La monographie du produit est fournie sur demande aux médecins et aux pharmaciens.
Conserver entre 15 C et 30 C.
Protéger de la lumière.
85963LA-0040 Rev. 00
0 68510 96540
Novopharm Limited

12. Order: *naproxen 500 mg PO BID*

    Give: _____ tablet(s)

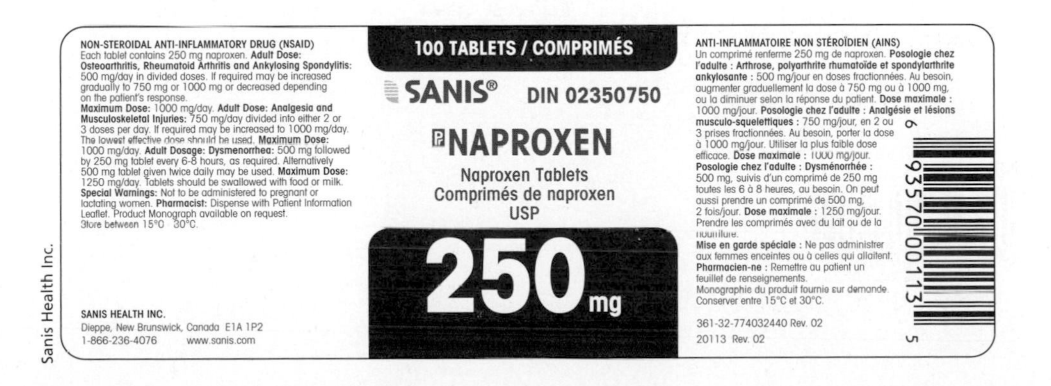
NON-STEROIDAL ANTI-INFLAMMATORY DRUG (NSAID)
Each tablet contains 250 mg naproxen.
100 TABLETS / COMPRIMÉS
SANIS® DIN 02350750
NAPROXEN
Naproxen Tablets
Comprimés de naproxen USP
250 mg
ANTI-INFLAMMATOIRE NON STÉROÏDIEN (AINS)
Un comprimé renferme 250 mg de naproxen.
SANIS HEALTH INC.
Dieppe, New Brunswick, Canada E1A 1P2
1-866-236-4076 www.sanis.com
361-32-774032440 Rev. 02
20113 Rev. 02
Sanis Health Inc.

13. Order: *famotidine 20 mg IV q12h*

Give: ______ mL

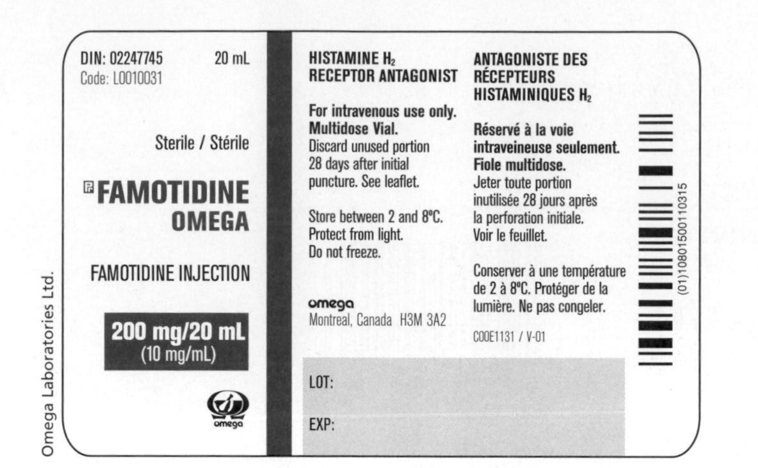

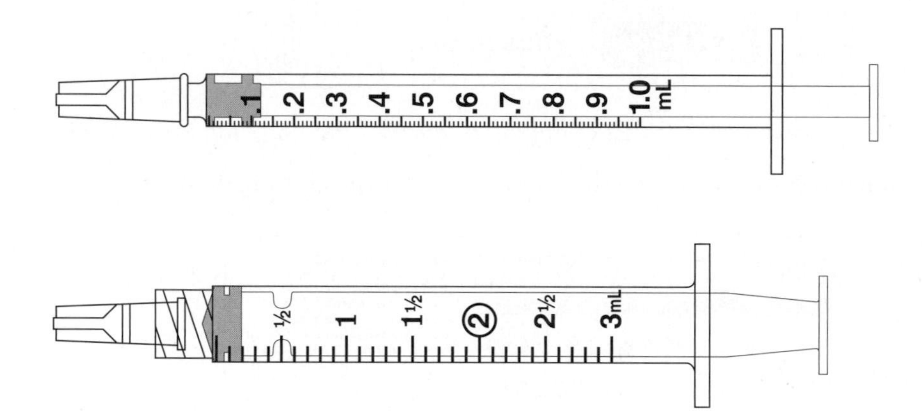

14. Order: *morphine sulfate 15 mg IV q4h*

Give: ______ mL

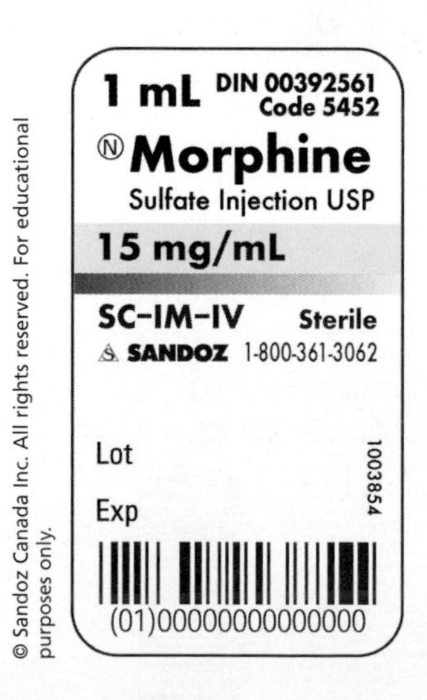

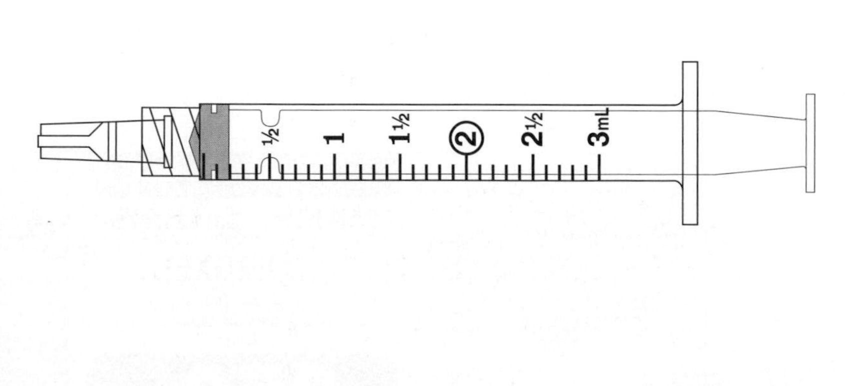

15. Order: *amoxicillin/clavulanate potassium 100 mg (based on amoxicllin) PO q8h*

    Give: _____ mL

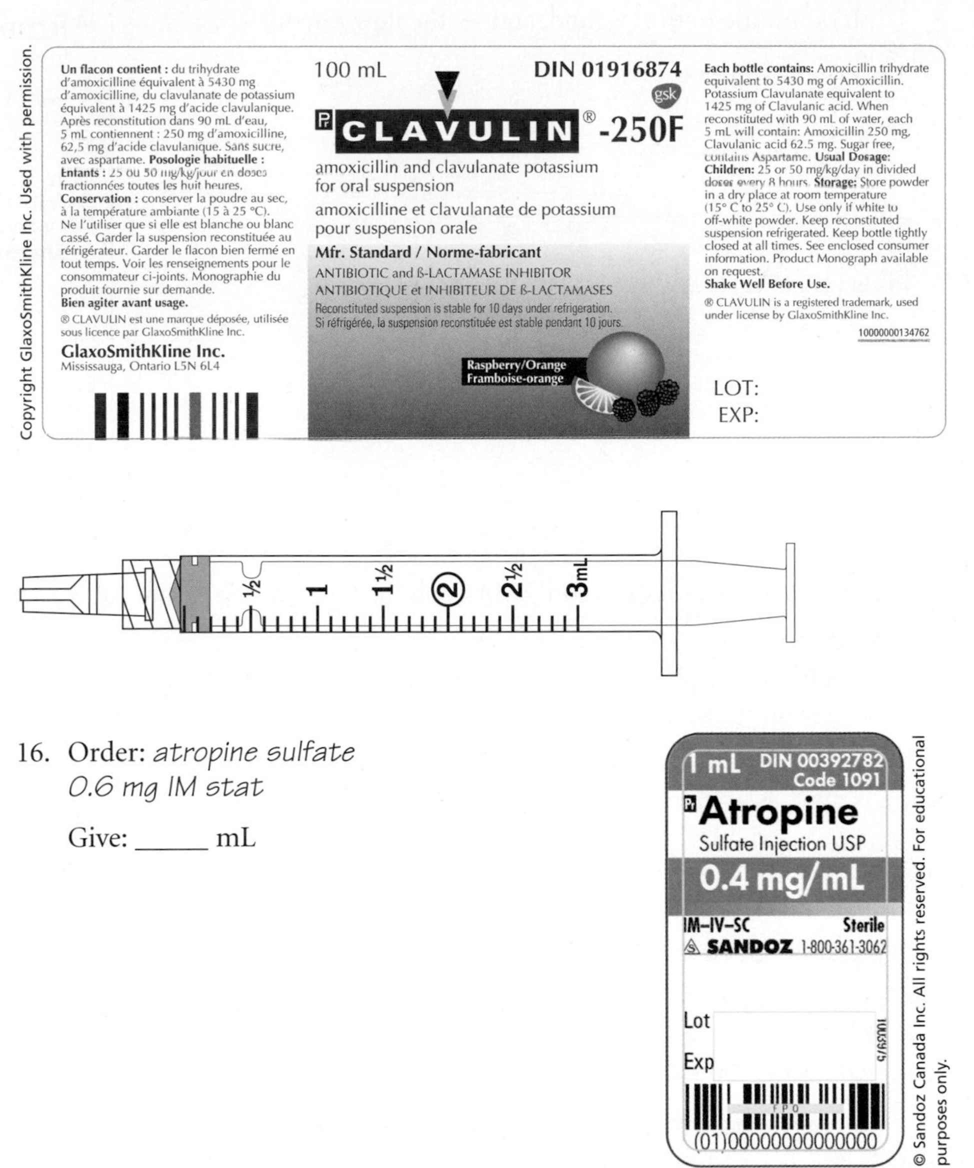

16. Order: *atropine sulfate 0.6 mg IM stat*

    Give: _____ mL

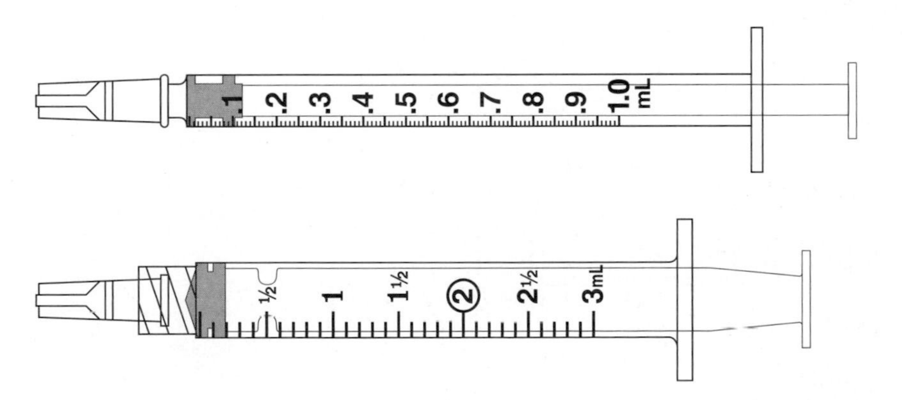

17. Order: *ranitidine hydrochloride 35 mg in 100 mL D_5W IVPB over 20 min* (drop factor: 15 gtt/mL)

    Add _____ mL ranitidine to the IV fluid, and set the flow rate to _____ gtt/min.

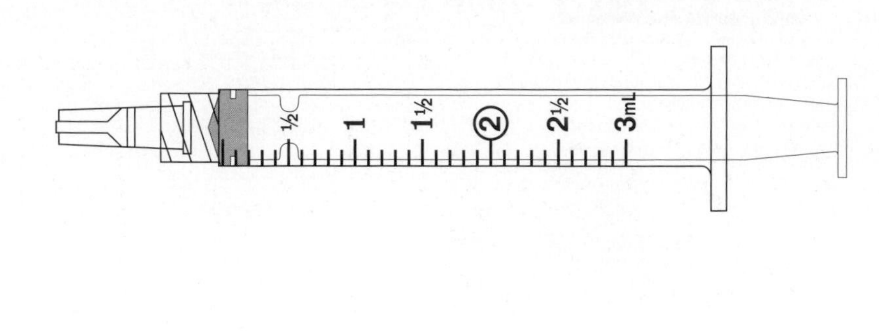

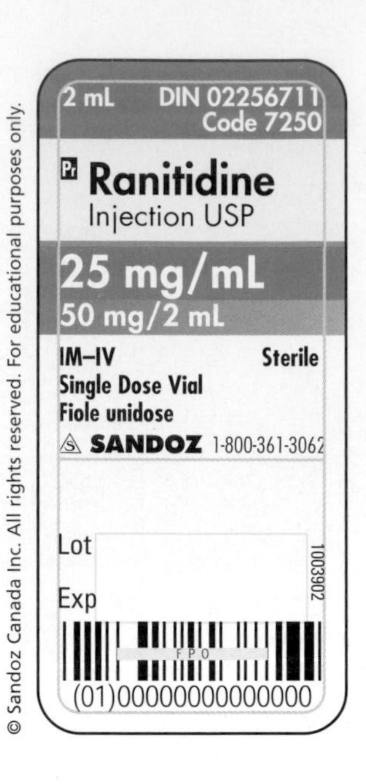

Refer to the medication administration record (MAR) on the next page to answer questions 18 through 22.

Mrs. Anjali Mohan in Room 217A is assigned to your team. She is hospitalized with osteoarthritis. The medications available from the pharmacy are noted on the MAR.

18. Mrs. Mohan had her last dose of acetaminophen at 2110. It is now 0215, and the patient's temperature is 39°C. Is acetaminophen indicated? _____

    Explain: ____

    ____

19. How much acetaminophen should Mrs. Mohan receive for each dose? _____ tablet(s)

20. Mrs. Mohan had 60 mg IM of ketorolac tromethamine at 1500. At 2130, the patient reports severe pain again. How much ketorolac tromethamine will you give the patient now? Available is ketorolac tromethamine injection 30 mg/mL. Give _____ mL.

21. Mrs. Mohan is reporting itching. What prn medication would you select, and how much will you administer? Select _____, and give _____ capsule.

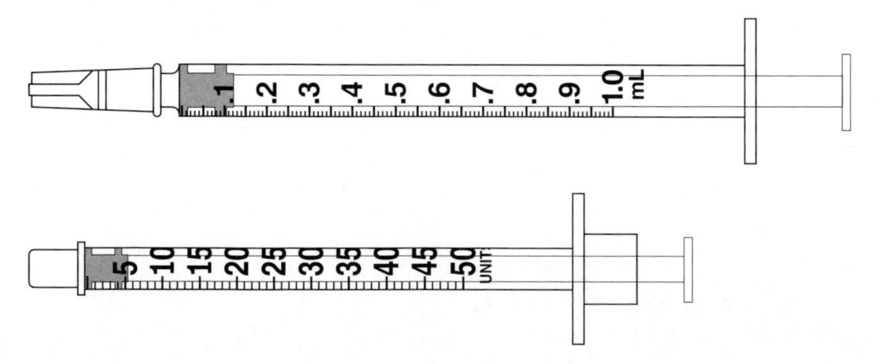

15/09/xx
18:26
CHECKED BY: ______________

MEDICATION ADMINISTRATION RECORD

PAGE: 1
REPT: PHR20B

2ND 241
217A 532729
Mohan, Anjali

DIAGNOSIS: 71590
ALLERGIES: NKA
NOTES:

DIET: Regular
ADMIT: 15/09/xx
WT: 70 kg

DX: OSTEOARTHRITIS-UNSPEC

ADMINISTRATION PERIOD: 0730 15/09/xx TO 0729 16/09/xx

ORDER # DRUG NAME, STRENGTH, DOSAGE FORM DOSE RATE ROUTE SCHEDULE	START	STOP	TIME PERIOD 0730 to 1529	TIME PERIOD 1530 to 2329	TIME PERIOD 2330 to 0729
NURSE:					
• • • PRN's FOLLOW • • •			• • • PRN's FOLLOW • • •		
264077 acetaminophen 325 mg TABLET PRN **650 mg** ORAL Q4H/PRN FOR TEMP over 38.3 C	0930 15/09/xx		0930 BS	2110 BS	
264147 ketorolac tromethamine 60 mg PRN **60 mg** IM PRN GIVE 60 mg FOR BREAKTHROUGH PAIN X1 DOSE THEN 30 mg Q6H/PRN	1500 15/09/xx		60 mg 1500 MK		
264148 ketorolac tromethamine 60 mg PRN **30 mg** IM Q6H/PRN GIVE 6 HOURS AFTER 60 mg DOSE FOR BREAK-THROUGH PAIN.	1500 15/09/xx				
264151 droperidol 2.5 mg/mL AMPOULE PRN **SEE NOTE** IV Q6H/PRN DOSE IS 0.625 mg TO 1.25 mg (0.5-1.0 mL) FOR NAUSEA	1500 15/09/xx				
264152 diphenhydramine 50 mg CAPSULE PRN **50 mg** ORAL Q4H/PRN FOR ITCHING	1500 15/09/xx				
264153 naloxone hydrochloride 0.4 mg/mL AMPOULE PRN **0.4 mg** IV PRN FOR RR less than 8 AND IF PATIENT IS UNAROUSABLE	1500 15/09/xx				
NURSE:					
NURSE:					

INITIALS	SIGNATURE	INITIALS	SIGNATURE	NOTES	
BS	B. Swart, RN				
MK	M. Kerrigan, RN				

217A Anjali Mohan AGE: 73 SEX: F PHYSICIAN: J. Physician, MD

22. Mrs. Mohan's respiratory rate is 7, and she is difficult to arouse. What medication is indicated? ______________. Draw an arrow on the syringe to indicate how much of this medication you will give.

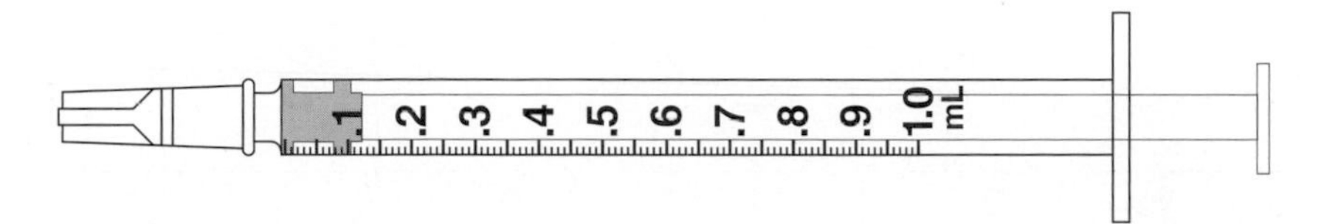

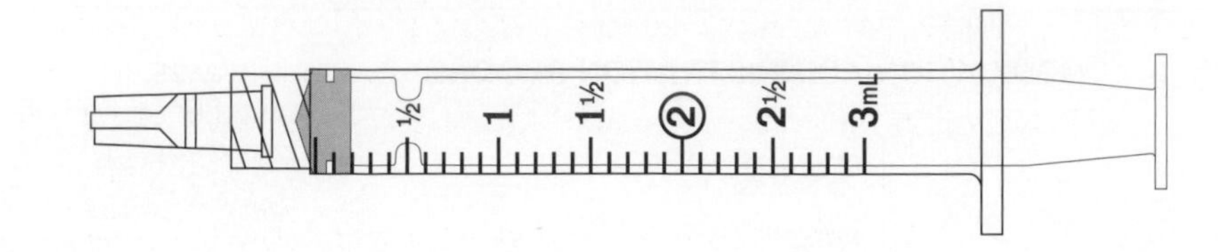

Refer to the following MAR to answer questions 23 through 27.

PAGE ____ of ____

MEDICATION ADMINISTRATION RECORD

ORIGINAL ORDER DATE	DATE STARTED/RENEWED	MEDICATION - DOSAGE	ROUTE	SCHEDULE 2300–0700	SCHEDULE 0700–1500	SCHEDULE 1500–2300	DATE 10-03-xx 2300–0700	10-03-xx 0700–1500	10-03-xx 1500–2300	DATE 10-04-xx 2300–0700	10-04-xx 0700–1500	10-04-xx 1500–2300	DATE 10-05-xx 2300–0700	10-05-xx 0700–1500	10-05-xx 1500–2300	DATE 10-06-xx 2300–0700	10-06-xx 0700–1500	10-06-xx 1500–2300
10-03-xx	10-3	theophylline 300 mg q12h	PB	0800		2000		BS 0800	MK 2000									
10-03-xx	10-3	hydrocortisone 125 mg q8h	IV	0600	1200	1800	BS 0600	BS 1200	MK 1800	AA0600								
10-03-xx	10-3	sucralfate 1 g qid 30 minutes before meals	PO		0730 1130	17 21430		BS0730 BS1130	MK11730 MS2130									
10-03-xx	10-3	Humulin R	SUB-CUT		0730 1130	1730		BS0730 BS1130	MK1730									
		per sliding scale: Blood glucose Units																
		0-8 0 units																
		8.1-12 2 units																
		12.1-14 4 units																
		14.1-16 6 units																
		16.1-18 8 units																
		18.1-20 10 units																
		more than 20 call prescriber stat																

PRN

INJECTION SITES

B - RIGHT ARM
C - RIGHT ABDOMEN
D - RIGHT ANTERIOR THIGH
G - LEFT ARM
H - LEFT ABDOMEN
J - LEFT ANTERIOR THIGH
L - LEFT BUTTOCKS
M - RIGHT BUTTOCKS

DATE GIVEN	TIME	INT.	ONE - TIME MEDICATION - DOSAGE	RT.

SIGNATURE OF NURSE ADMINISTERING MEDICATIONS — SCHEDULE	DATE 10-03-xx	DATE 10-04-xx	DATE 10-05-xx	DATE 10-06-xx
2300–0700		AA A. Azaryev LPN		
0700–1500	BS B. Swart, RN			
1500–2300	MK M. Kelly, RN			

LITHO IN U.S.A. K6508 (7-92) D395538

DATE GIVEN	TIME	INT.	MEDICATION-DOSAGE-CONT.	RT.
			RECOPIED BY:	
			CHECKED BY:	

Kular, Amanjet
ID #76834-21

ALLERGIES:

602-31 (7-xx) (MPC# 1355)

1 ORIGINAL COPY

PRINTED BY STANDARD REGISTER U.S.A. ZIPSET ®

Amanjet Kular, 19 years old, has diabetes and is admitted to the medical unit with asthma. The nurse is administering his medications. The MAR on page 482 is in the medication notebook on the medication cart. The label represents the infusion set available. Questions 23 through 27 refer to Mr. Kular.

23. Theophylline is available in 100-, 200-, and 300-mg extended-release tablets. Which dosage of tablet would be preferred, and how many tablets are administered? ______ tablet(s)

24. Theophylline is an extended-release tablet. What does this mean? Can an extended-release tablet be divided?

25. Reconstitute the hydrocortisone sodium succinate with _____ mL diluent, and give _____ mL.

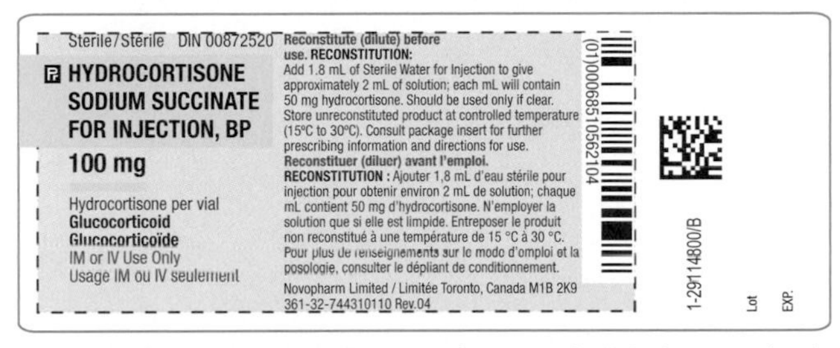

The product labels and intellectual property of Teva Canada Limited are reproduced with the permission of Teva Canada Limited and used herein for educational purposes only.

26. Mealtimes and bedtime are 0800, 1200, 1800, and 2200. Administer _____ tablet(s) of Apo-sucralfate per dose each day at _____, _____, _____, and _____ hours.

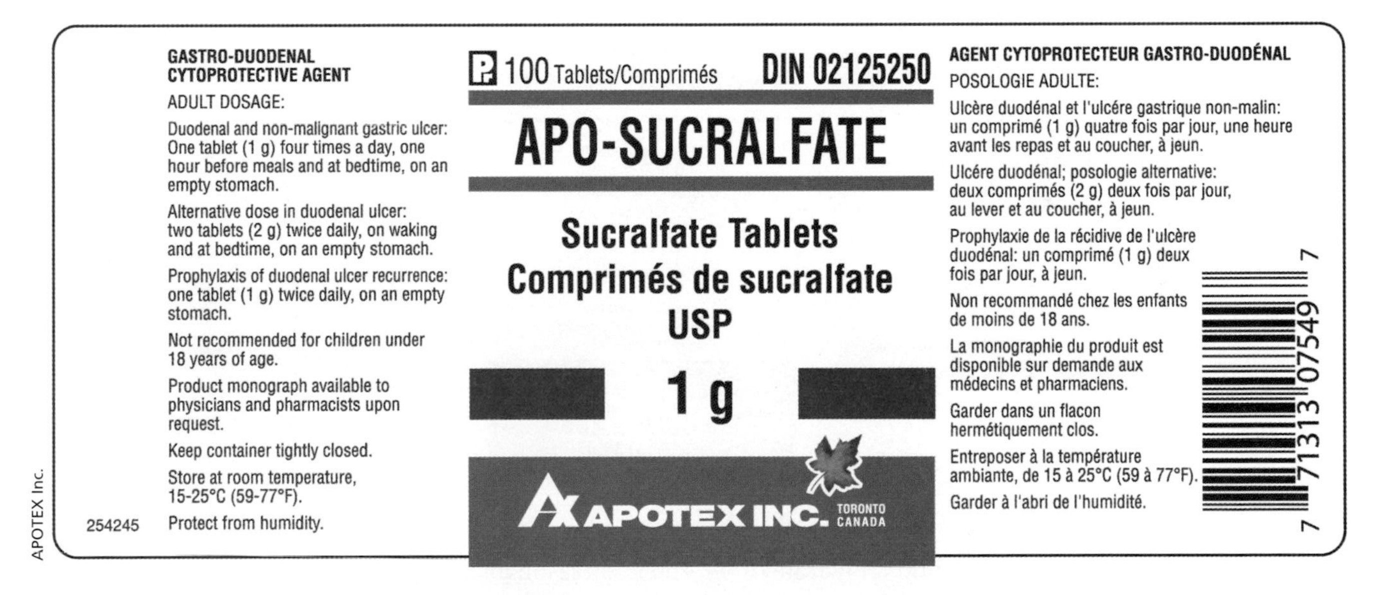

27. At 0730, Mr. Kular blood glucose is 20 mmol/L. You will give him _____ units of insulin by the _____ route. Draw an arrow on the appropriate syringe to indicate the correct dosage.

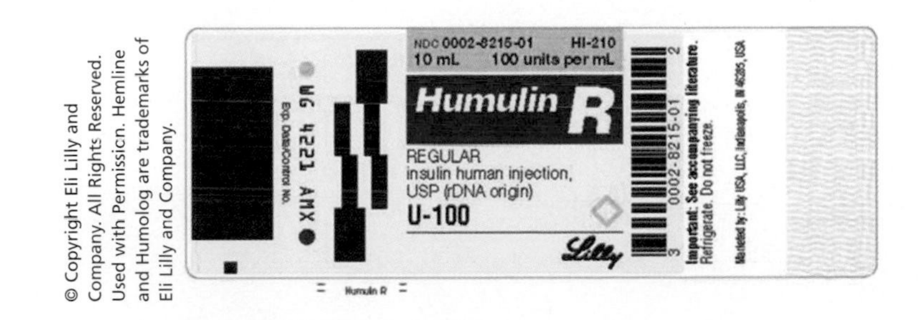

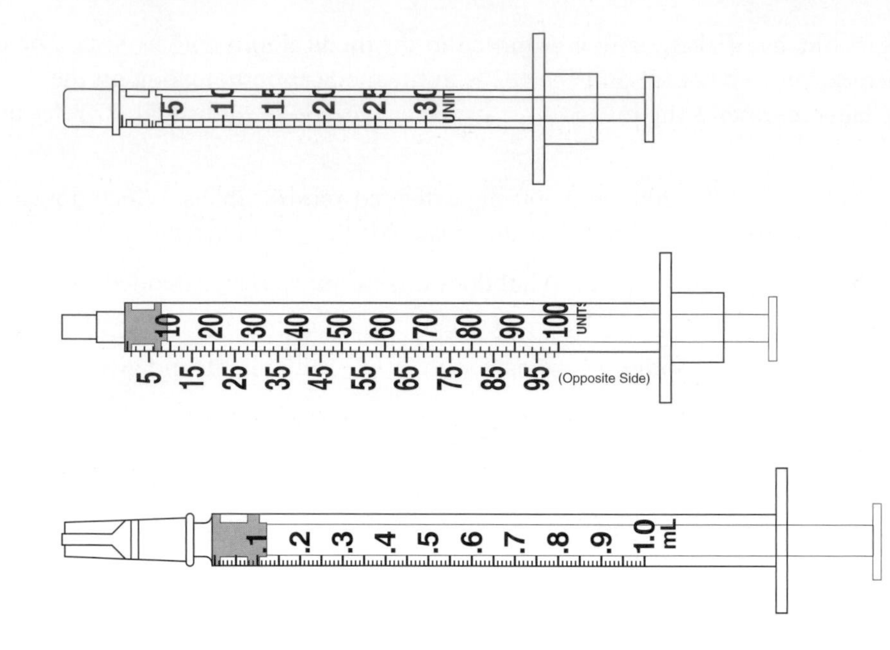

Suad is brought to the clinic. The patient weighs 6.8 kg and has an ear infection. Questions 28 through 31 refer to Suad.

28. The prescriber orders *amoxicillin trihydrate 91 mg PO q8h* for Suad. See the label for the recommended dose.

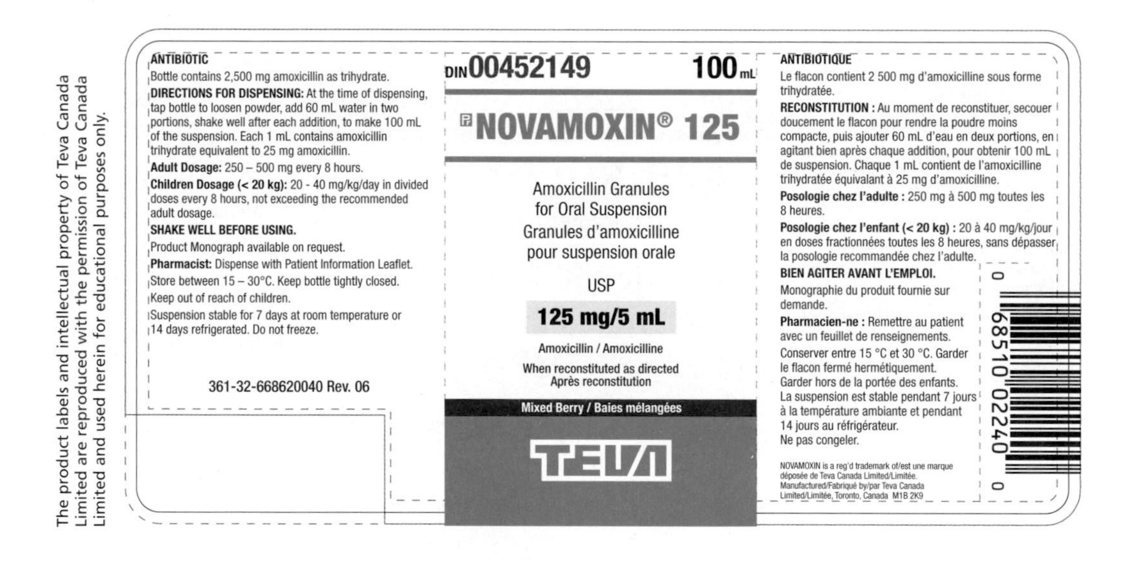

Is Suad's amoxicillin trihydrate order safe and reasonable? ________________

Explain: ____

29. The prescriber asks the nurse to give Suad one dose of the amoxicillin trihydrate stat. How many mL of water will be used to reconstitute the solution? ______mL
30. Once reconstituted, the nurse would administer ______mL to Suad.
31. The prescriber also asks the nurse to instruct Suad's mother about administering the medication at home. The nurse tells Suad's mother to give the baby medication up to the ______ mL line of the oral syringe for each dose. How often will she give Suad her dose?

    ____

32. Alda Chow is a 16-year-old who weighs 50 kg and has a duodenal ulcer and abdominal pain. Order: *ranitidine hydrochloride 50 mg q6h in 50 mL D_5W to be infused in 20 min*

    The recommended ranitidine hydrochloride dosage is 2 to 6 mg/kg/day in 4 divided doses. The label below represents the infusion set available.

    What is the safe single dosage range for Alda? ______ mg/dose to ______ mg/dose. Is this ordered dosage safe? ______

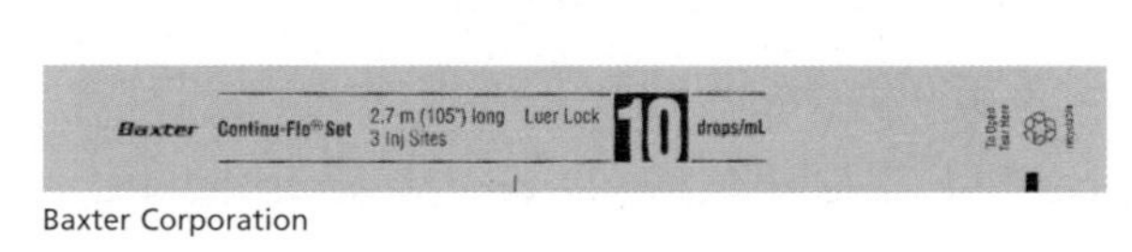

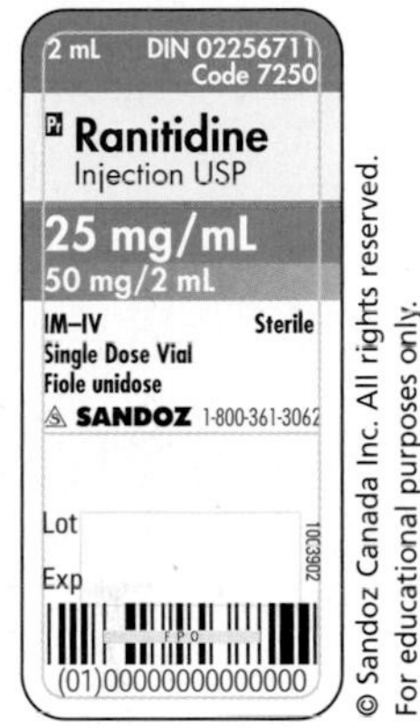

    If safe, add ______ mL ranitidine hydrochloride, and set the flow rate at ______ gtt/min.

33. The prescriber writes a new patient care order for strict intake and output assessment for a child. During the nurse's 8-hour shift, in addition to the IV fluids of 200 mL D_5NS, the child consumed the following oral fluids:

    gelatin—120 mL

    water—90 mL × 2

    apple juice—500 mL

    What is the child's total fluid intake during the nurse's shift? ______ mL

Use the following information to answer questions 34 through 36.

Order for a child with severe otitis media (inner ear infection) who weighs 18.2 kg: *amoxicillin/clavulanate potassium 240 mg PO q8h.* The following amoxicillin/clavulanate potassium label represents the dosage available. See the label for amoxicillin/clavulanate potassium recommended dosages.

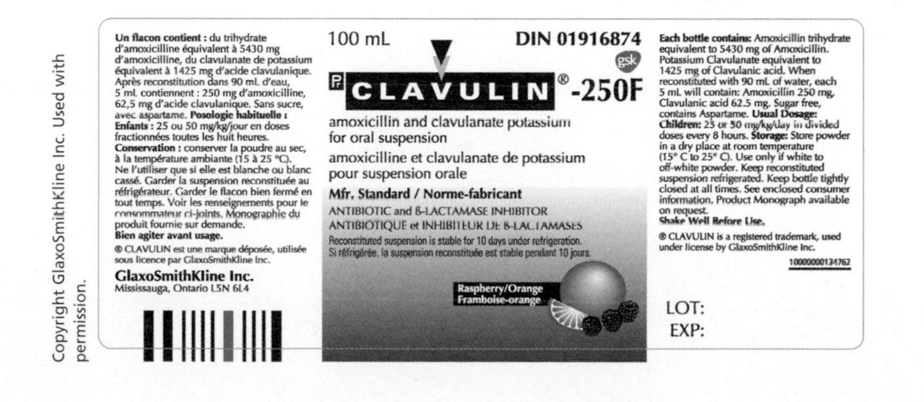

34. Is the ordered dosage safe? _____

35. If it is safe, how much would you administer to the child? _____ mL per dose. If it is not safe, what would you do next? ____________________

36. The prescriber has ordered *washed, packed red blood cells 2 units (600 mL) IV to infuse in 4 h.* The IV tubing has a drop factor of 15 gtt/mL. The nurse will regulate the IV infusion rate at _____ gtt/min.

Use the following information to answer questions 37 and 38.

A child who weighs 28 kg has an elevated temperature. For hyperthermia in children, the recommended dosage of acetaminophen is 10 to 15 mg/kg PO q4h, not to exceed 5 doses per day.

37. What is the safe single dosage range of acetaminophen for this child?
_____ mg/dose to _____ mg/dose

38. If the prescriber orders the maximum safe dosage and acetaminophen is available as a suspension of 160 mg/5 mL, how many millilitres will the nurse give per dose? _____ mL

Use the following information to answer questions 39 and 40 for a child who weighs 23.6 kg.

Order: *diphenhydramine hydrochloride 25 mg IV q6h*

Supply: diphenhydramine hydrochloride 50 mg/mL

Recommended dosage: 5 mg/kg/day in 4 divided doses

39. A safe single dosage for this child is _____ mg/dose. Is the order safe? _____

40. If safe, administer _____ mL. If not safe, what should you do? ____________________

____

Use the following information to answer questions 41 through 44.

At 1430, a patient is started on *morphine sulfate PCA IV pump at 5 mg q10 min with an hourly maximum of 10 mg.* The morphine sulfate syringe in the pump contains 150 mg/30 mL.

41. The patient can receive _____ mL every 10 minutes.

42. If the patient attempts 5 doses this hour, he would receive _____ mg and _____ mL of morphine sulfate.

43. Based on the amount of morphine sulfate in the syringe in the patient-controlled analgesia pump, how many total doses can the patient receive? _____ dose(s)

44. If the patient receives 5 doses every hour, the morphine sulfate will be empty at _____ hours.

45. Order: *sodium nitroprusside 100 mg stat in 250 mL D_5W IVPB to infuse over 30 min*

    Regulate the infusion pump at _____ mL/h.

Use the following information to answer questions 46 through 49.

Order: *ceftazidime 0.5 g IV q8h*

The following label represents the drug available. You reconstitute the drug at 1400 on 30/01/xx.

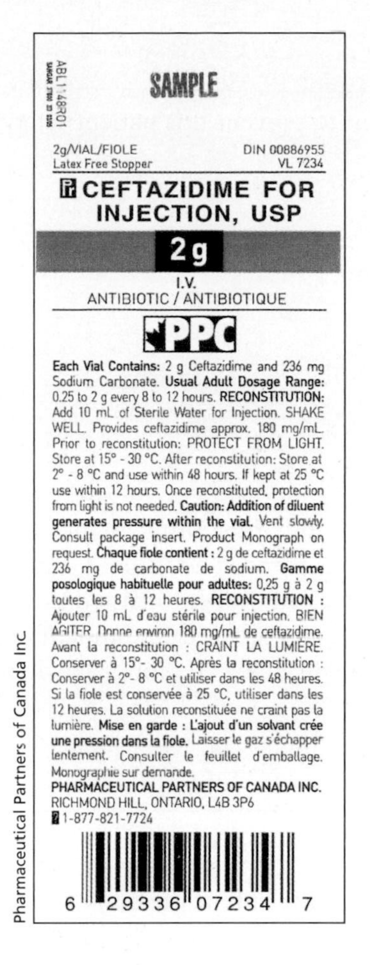

46. The total volume of ceftazidime after reconstitution is _____ mL.
47. The resulting dosage strength of ceftazidime is _____ mg/mL.
48. Give _____ mL of ceftazidime.
49. Prepare a reconstitution label for ceftazidime.

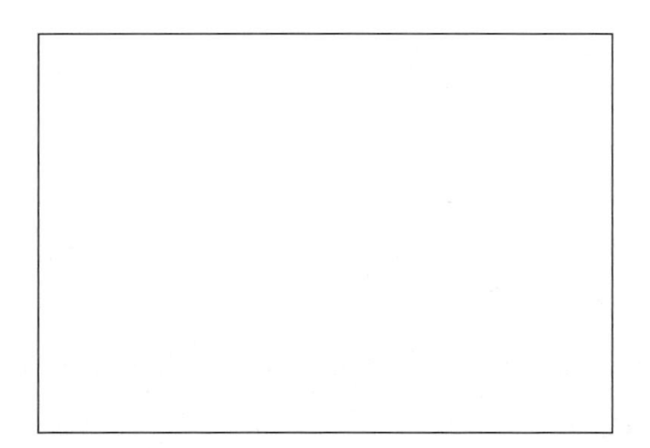

APPLICATION OF CLINICAL REASONING

ESE-1 Describe the clinical reasoning that you would implement to prevent this patient safety incident.

Possible Scenario

Order: *dexamethasone sodium phosphate 4 mg IV q6h*

Day 1 Supply: dexamethasone sodium phosphate 4 mg/mL

Student nurse prepared and administered 1 mL.

Day 2 Supply: dexamethasone sodium phosphate 10 mg/mL

Student nurse prepared 1 mL.

Potential Outcome

Day 2, the student's instructor asked the student to recheck the order, think about the action, check the calculation, and provide the rationale for the amount prepared. The student was alarmed at the possibility of administering 2.5 times the prescribed dosage. The student insisted that the pharmacy should consistently supply the same unit dosage. The instructor advised the student of the possibility that different pharmacy technicians could be involved, or possibly the original supply dosage was not available.

Prevention

____

____

After completing these problems, see the Answers section at the end of the book to check your answers. Give yourself 2 points for each correct answer.

Perfect score = 100 My score = _____

Mastery score = 90 or higher (45 or more correct)

Check your work! Answers to all Application of Clinical Reasoning Problems are provided at the end of each chapter.

Comprehensive Skills Evaluation

This evaluation is a comprehensive assessment of your mastery of the concepts presented in all 14 chapters of *Dosage Calculations*.

Mei Lam, a 46-year-old patient, has been admitted to the Telemetry Unit, reporting an irregular heartbeat, shortness of breath, and chest pain relieved by nitroglycerin. Mrs. Lam weighs 50 kg. Questions 1 through 14 refer to the admitting orders on the next page for Mrs. Lam. The labels shown below represent the available medications and infusion set.

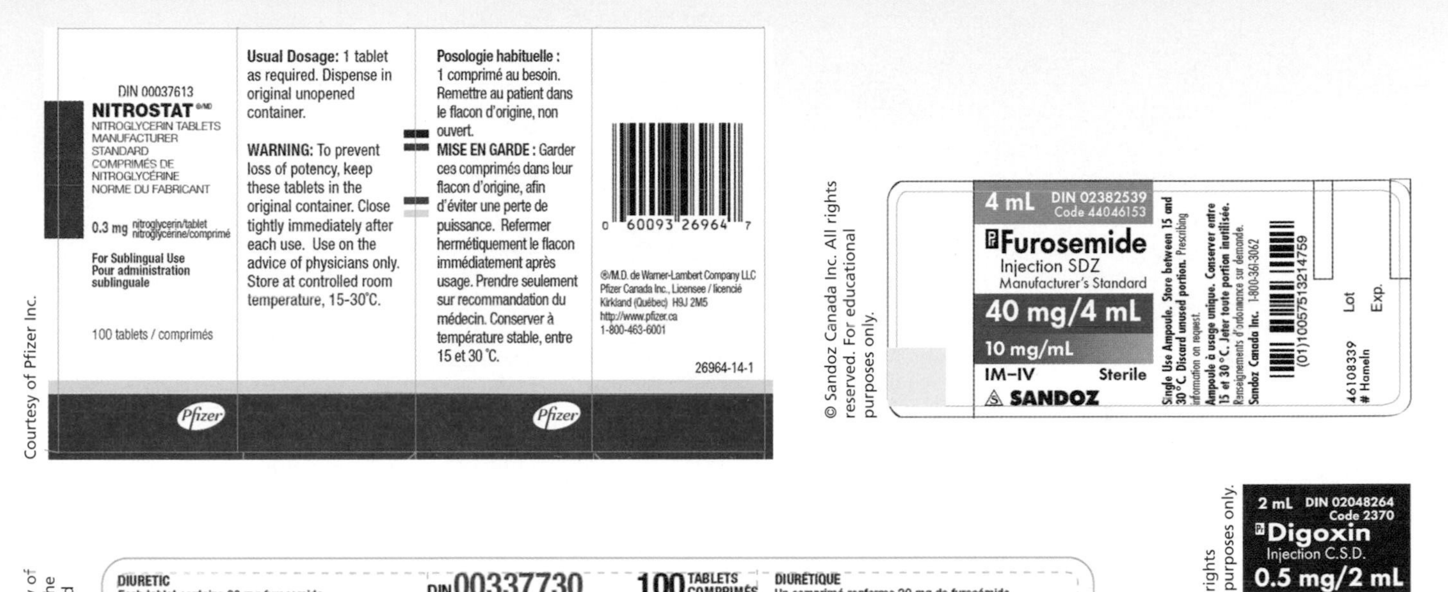

Courtesy of Pfizer Inc.

© Sandoz Canada Inc. All rights reserved. For educational purposes only.

The product labels and intellectual property of Teva Canada Limited are reproduced with the permission of Teva Canada Limited and used herein for educational purposes only.

© Sandoz Canada Inc. All rights reserved. For educational purposes only.

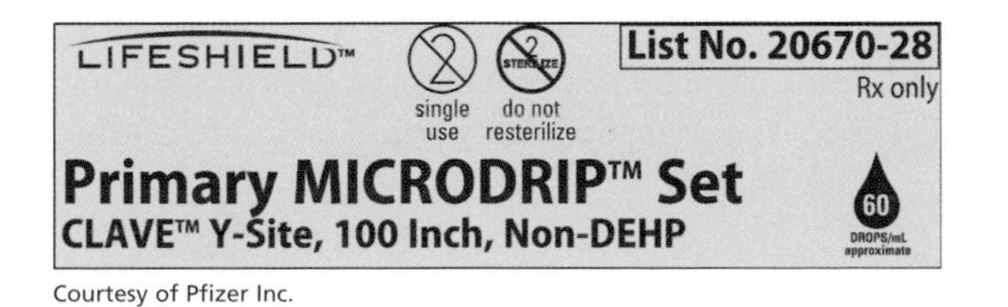

Courtesy of Pfizer Inc.

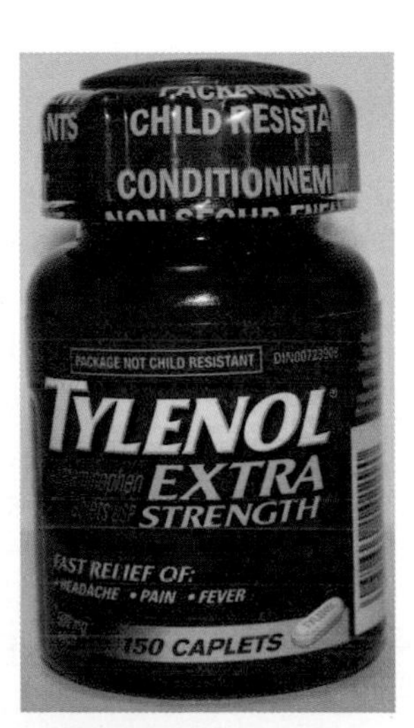

Natalie Barrington

ENTERED	FILLED	CHECKED	VERIFIED
			—

NOTE: A NON-PROPRIETARY DRUG OF EQUAL QUALITY MAY BE DISPENSED - IF THIS COLUMN IS NOT CHECKED!

DATE	TIME WRITTEN	PLEASE USE BALL POINT - PRESS FIRMLY	✓	TIME NOTED	NURSES SIGNATURE
03/09/xx	1600	Admit to telemetry unit	✓		
		Bedrest with bathroom privileges	✓		
		nitroglycerin 0.3 mg SL q8h stat followed by 0.3 mg q5 min X	✓		
		2 doses for angina pain	✓		
		furosemide 20 mg direct IV stat, then 20 mg PO bid	✓	1610 BS	
		digoxin 0.25 mg direct IV stat then 0.125 mg PO daily			
		D5 1/2 NS with KCl 10 mEq at 80 mL/h	✓		
		acetaminophen 1 g q4h prn for headache	✓		
		Electrolytes and CBC in am	✓		
		Soft diet, advance as tolerated	✓		
		Dr. J. Prescriber			

AUTO STOP ORDERS: UNLESS REORDERED, FOLLOWING WILL BE D/C'D AT 0800 ON:

DATE	ORDER		
		☐ CONT ☐ D/C	PHYSICIAN SIGNATURE
		☐ CONT ☐ D/C	PHYSICIAN SIGNATURE
		☐ CONT ☐ D/C	PHYSICIAN SIGNATURE

CHECK WHEN ANTIBIOTICS ORDERED ☐ Prophylactic ☐ Empiric ☐ Therapeutic

Allergies: None Known

CLIENT DIAGNOSIS: Chest Pain

HEIGHT 152 cm WEIGHT 50 kg

Lam, Mei
ID #257-226-3

FORM 959-708 (8-XX) PHYSICIANS ORDER Reynolds + Reynolds LITHO IN U.S.A. K41814 (7-90) D339080

1

1. The Telemetry Unit has no available IV pumps. The nurse implements a backup plan and starts a straight gravity-flow IV on Mrs. Lam at 1630. Calculate the watch-count flow rate for the IV fluid ordered. __________ gtt/min
2. Estimate the length of time and date when the nurse should plan to hang the next dose of $D_5\frac{1}{2}NS$. __________ hours on __________ (date)
3. At the present infusion rate, how much $D_5\frac{1}{2}NS$ will Mrs. Lam receive in a 24-hour period?
4. How many mEq of KCl will Mrs. Lam receive per hour and per day? __________ mEq/h and __________ mEq/day

5. Both furosemide and digoxin are ordered stat.

   a. What does this mean? ______________________________

   ____

   b. How frequently should the nurse administer the stat order? ______________

6. Prior to administering the IV digoxin, the nurse consults the drug guide. The recommended rate for direct IV administration of digoxin is 0.25 mg in 4 mL NS administered at the rate of 0.25 mg/minute.

   How much digoxin should the nurse administer for the stat IV order? At what rate?
   Prepare __________ mL digoxin, and add __________ mL NS for a total of __________ mL.
   Administer at the rate of __________ mL/minute or __________ mL/15 seconds.

7. Draw an arrow on the appropriate syringe to indicate how much digoxin to prepare.

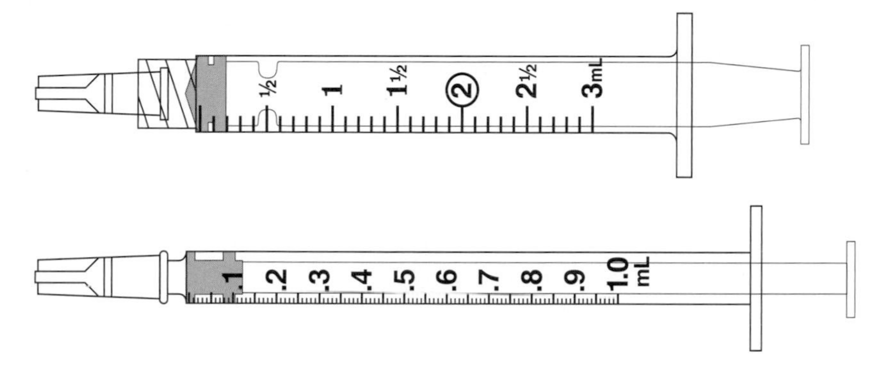

8. The nurse consults the drug guide for more information about the furosemide ordered. The recommended rate for direct IV administration is 40 mg/2 minutes.

   a. How much furosemide should the nurse administer for Mrs. Lam's stat dose? At what rate?

   Give: __________ mL at the rate of __________ mL/min or __________ mL/15 seconds

   b. Draw an arrow on the appropriate syringe to indicate how much furosemide to prepare.

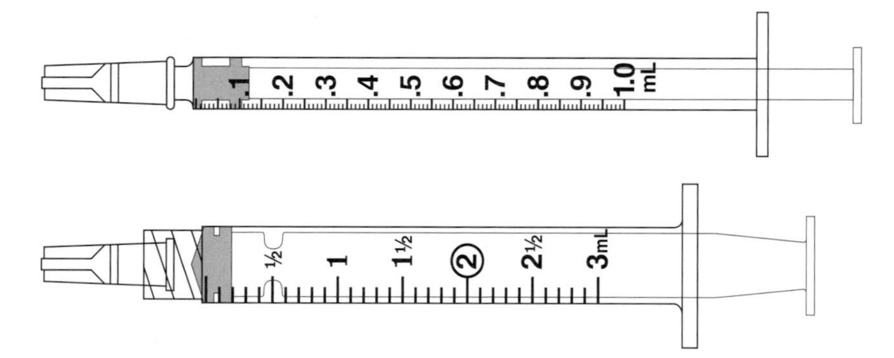

9. Digoxin tablets are available in 0.625-mg and 0.125-mg dosages. How many digoxin tablets will Mrs. Lam require for a 24-hour period for the PO digoxin order? Select __________ dosage and administer __________ tablet(s)

10. After the initial dose of furosemide, how many tablets should the nurse give Mrs. Lam for each subsequent dose? __________ tablet(s)

11. How much nitroglycerin should the nurse give Mrs. Lam for each subsequent dose? __________ tablet(s)

12. Mrs. Lam has a headache.

    a. How much acetaminophen should the nurse give Mrs. Lam for one dose? __________ tablet(s)

    b. When should the nurse give Mrs. Lam the next dose? __________

13. Compare the drug labels for Mrs. Lam, and identify the drug(s) that is (are) supplied by their generic name(s). ______________________

14. An IV infusion pump that is programmable in whole millilitres becomes available for Mrs. Lam. At what rate should the nurse now set the IV pump for continuous infusion? __________ mL/h

Despite excellent care, Mrs. Lam's condition worsens and she is transferred into the coronary care unit (CCU) with the medical orders as given below. CCU IV infusion pumps are programmable in tenths of a millilitre. Questions 15 through 20 refer to these orders.

ENTERED	FILLED	CHECKED	VERIFIED
			—

NOTE: A NON-PROPRIETARY DRUG OF EQUAL QUALITY MAY BE DISPENSED - IF THIS COLUMN IS NOT CHECKED!

DATE	TIME WRITTEN	PLEASE USE BALL POINT - PRESS FIRMLY	✓	TIME NOTED	NURSES SIGNATURE
04/09/xx	2230	Transfer to CCU	✓	2235 B.S.	
		NPO	✓		
		Discontinue nitroglycerin	✓		
		Lidocaine hydrochloride bolus 50 mg IV stat, then	✓		
		begin lidocaine hydrochloride drip 2 g in 500 mL D_5W			
		(premixed solution) at 2 mg/min by infusion pump			
		Increase lidocaine hydrochloride to 4 mg/min if PVCs	✓		
		(premature ventricular contractions)			
		persist			
		dopamine hydrochloride 400 mg	✓		
		IVPB in 250 mL D_5W (premixed solution)			
		at 500 mcg/kg/min by infusion pump			
		Increase KCl to 20 mEq per L D_5W 1/2 NS	✓		
		IV at 50 mL/h			
		Increase furosemide to 40 mg IV q12h	✓		
		O_2 at 30% after ABGs (arterial blood gases)	✓		
		Electrolytes stat and in am and	✓		
		ABGs stat and prn			
		Dr. J. Prescriber			

AUTO STOP ORDERS: UNLESS REORDERED, FOLLOWING WILL BE D/C^D AT 0800 ON:

DATE	ORDER		PHYSICIAN SIGNATURE
		☐ CONT ☐ D/C	
		☐ CONT ☐ D/C	
		☐ CONT ☐ D/C	

CHECK WHEN ANTIBIOTICS ORDERED ☐ Prophylactic ☐ Empiric ☐ Therapeutic

Allergies: None Known

Chest Pain
CLIENT DIAGNOSIS

HEIGHT 152 cm WEIGHT 50 kg

Lam, Mei
ID #257-226-3

FORM 959-708 (8-XX) PHYSICIANS ORDER Reynolds • Reynolds LITHO IN U.S.A. K41814 (7-00) D339080

1

15. Lidocaine hydrochloride is supplied in 10 mg/mL dosage strength. The nurse is familiar with lidocaine hydrochloride and knows the order is safe.

    a. How much lidocaine hydrochloride will you give for the bolus?

    b. Draw an arrow on the appropriate syringe to indicate the amount to prepare.

    How much lidocaine hydrochloride should the nurse administer for the bolus. __________ mL

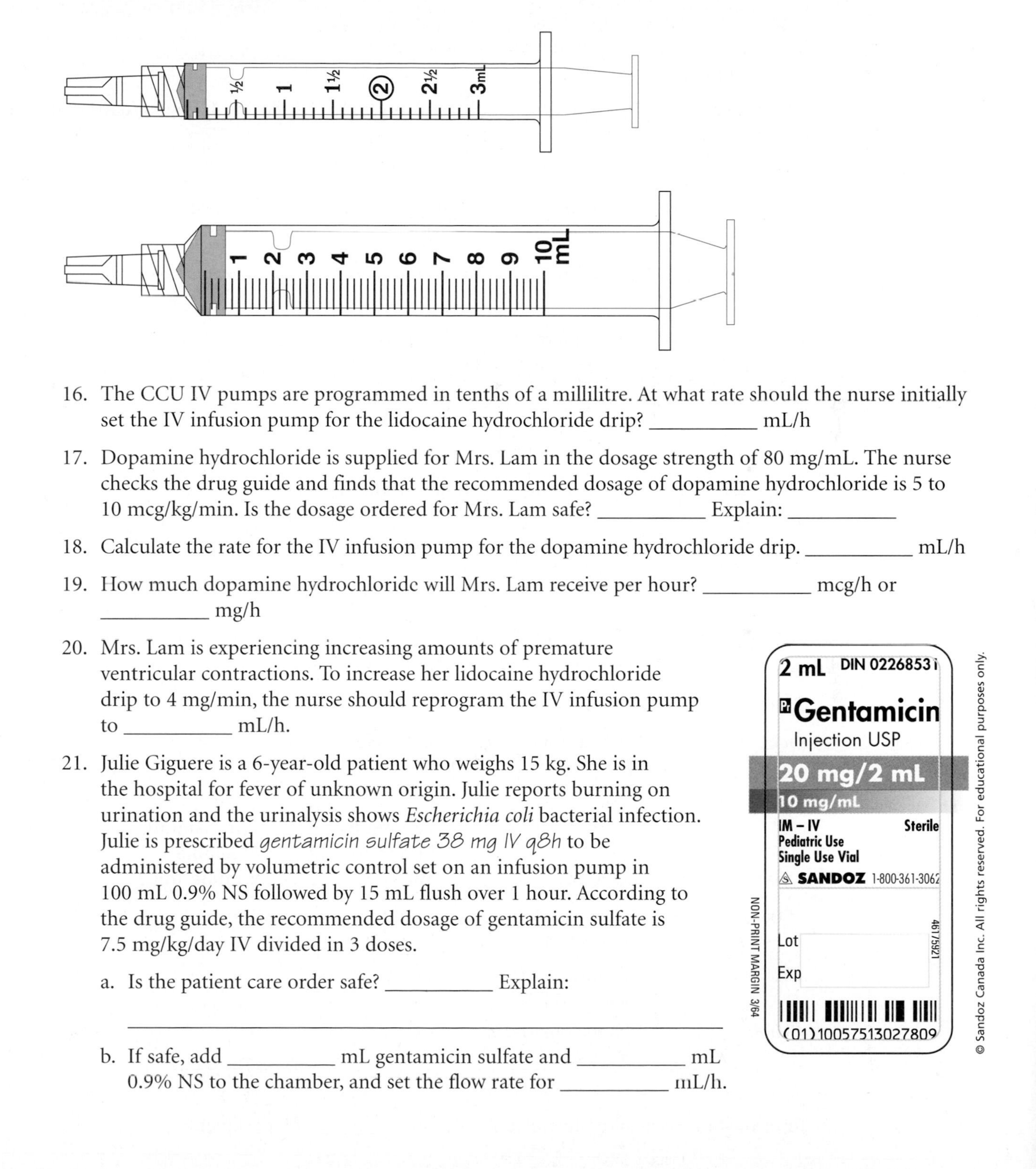

16. The CCU IV pumps are programmed in tenths of a millilitre. At what rate should the nurse initially set the IV infusion pump for the lidocaine hydrochloride drip? __________ mL/h

17. Dopamine hydrochloride is supplied for Mrs. Lam in the dosage strength of 80 mg/mL. The nurse checks the drug guide and finds that the recommended dosage of dopamine hydrochloride is 5 to 10 mcg/kg/min. Is the dosage ordered for Mrs. Lam safe? __________ Explain: __________

18. Calculate the rate for the IV infusion pump for the dopamine hydrochloride drip. __________ mL/h

19. How much dopamine hydrochloride will Mrs. Lam receive per hour? __________ mcg/h or __________ mg/h

20. Mrs. Lam is experiencing increasing amounts of premature ventricular contractions. To increase her lidocaine hydrochloride drip to 4 mg/min, the nurse should reprogram the IV infusion pump to __________ mL/h.

21. Julie Giguere is a 6-year-old patient who weighs 15 kg. She is in the hospital for fever of unknown origin. Julie reports burning on urination and the urinalysis shows *Escherichia coli* bacterial infection. Julie is prescribed *gentamicin sulfate 38 mg IV q8h* to be administered by volumetric control set on an infusion pump in 100 mL 0.9% NS followed by 15 mL flush over 1 hour. According to the drug guide, the recommended dosage of gentamicin sulfate is 7.5 mg/kg/day IV divided in 3 doses.

    a. Is the patient care order safe? __________ Explain:

    ____

    b. If safe, add __________ mL gentamicin sulfate and __________ mL 0.9% NS to the chamber, and set the flow rate for __________ mL/h.

Jamie Mukulu is hospitalized with a staphylococcal bone infection. He weighs 30 kg. The nurse intends to use an IV pump for Jamie. The pump is programmable in tenths of a millilitre. Questions 22 through 24 refer to Jamie.

Orders: *$D_5 \frac{1}{2}$ NS IV at 50 mL/h for continuous infusion*

vancomycin hydrochloride 300 mg IV q6h

Supply: vancomycin hydrochloride 500 mg/10 mL with instructions to "add to volumetric control set and infuse over 60 min."

10 x 10 mL Single-Use Vials/ Flacons uniservices Sterile/ Stérile DIN 02230191 Nº M109D001
Sterile Vancomycin Hydrochloride USP
Chlorhydrate de vancomycine stérile USP
500 mg Vancomycin / vial de vancomycine / flacon
Antibiotic for Intravenous Infusion Only / Antibiotique pour perfusion intraveineuse seulement

Courtesy of Pfizer Inc.

Recommended dosage from drug guide: vancomycin hydrochloride 40 mg/kg/day IV in 4 equally divided doses

22. a. Is this patient care order safe? ____________ Explain: ____________________________

    b. If safe, how much vancomycin hydrochloride will the nurse add to the chamber? ____________ mL

23. a. How much IV fluid will the nurse add to the chamber with the vancomycin hydrochloride? ____________ mL

    b. How much IV fluid will Jamie receive in 24 hours? ____________ mL

24. Use the following recommendations to calculate the hourly maintenance IV rate for Jamie.

    First 10 kg of body weight: 100 mL/kg/day

    Second 10 kg of body weight: 50 mL/kg/day

    Each additional kg over 20 kg of body weight: 20 mL/kg/day

    a. Jamie requires ____________ mL/day for maintenance IV fluids.

    b. The infusion rate should be set at ____________ mL/h

    c. Does the recommended rate match the ordered rate? ____________________________

Use the following related orders and labels to answer questions 25 through 29. Select and mark the dose volume on the appropriate syringe, as indicated.

25. Order: *cefazolin sodium 500 mg IV q6h in 50 mL D_5W IV by volumetric control set over 30 min.*

    Package insert directions are shown in the table below:

Vial Size (mg)	Diluent	Volume to Be Added to Vial (mL)	Approximate Available Volume (mL)	Nominal Concentration (mg/mL)
500	0.9% Sodium chloride injection	2	2.2	225
500	Sterile water for injection	3.8	4.0	125
1000	Sterile water for injection	2.5	3.0	334

To reconstitute cefazolin, the nurse should add __________ mL of diluent.

26. If necessary, prepare a reconstitution label for the cefazolin sodium.

PF320021 DIN 02237138
Latex Free Stopper
CEFAZOLIN
for Injection, USP
1 g
Vial/Fiole
Sterile/Stérile
Antibiotic/Antibiotique
IM/IV
PPC
SAMPLE
LOT:
EXP.:
Single Dose Vial: Discard unused portion.
Each vial contains: Cefazolin (as sodium) 1 g and 48 mg sodium. **Reconstitution: IM.:** add **2.5 mL** SWFI. Provides 334 mg/mL. Shake well. **I.V.:** see package insert. Stable for 24 hours at 25°C and 72 hours at 2 - 8°C. **Usual Adult Dosage:** 250 mg to 1 g every 6 - 12 hours. Store dry powder between 15°C - 30°C. Protect from light.
Fiole unidose : Jeter toute portion inutilisée.
Conserver la poudre sèche entre 15 °C - 30 °C. Protéger de la lumière.
85015/A
PHARMACEUTICAL PARTNERS OF CANADA INC.
Richmond Hill, ON L4B 3P6 1-877-821-7724
6 29336 32021 9

Pharmaceutical Partners of Canada Inc.

27. To prepare the IVPB for administration, the nurse should add __________ cefazolin to the 50 mL D5W IVPB. Choose and mark the appropriate syringe.

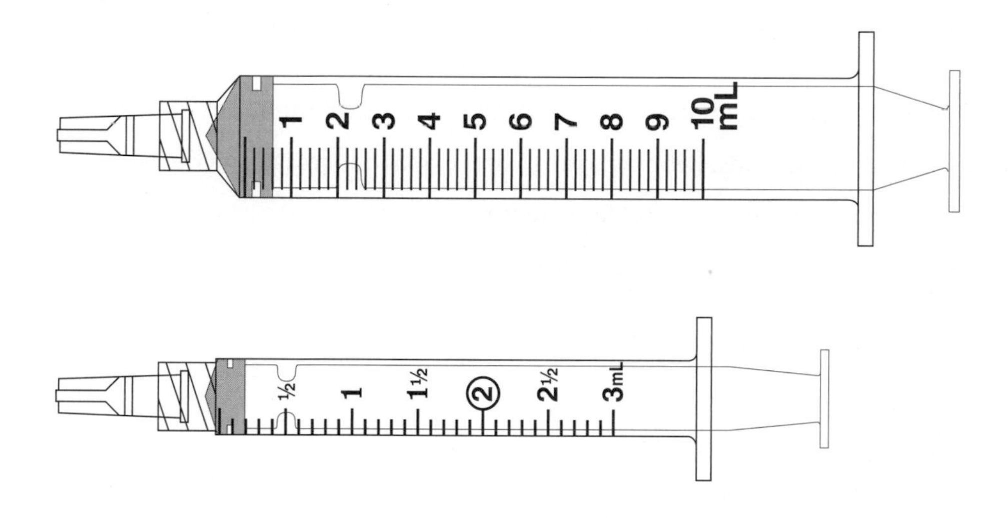

28. The IV cefazolin sodium is regulated on an IV infusion pump. The nurse should set the flow rate at __________ mL/h.

29. Order: *heparin sodium 10 000 units IV in 500 mL D_5W to infuse at 1200 units/h*

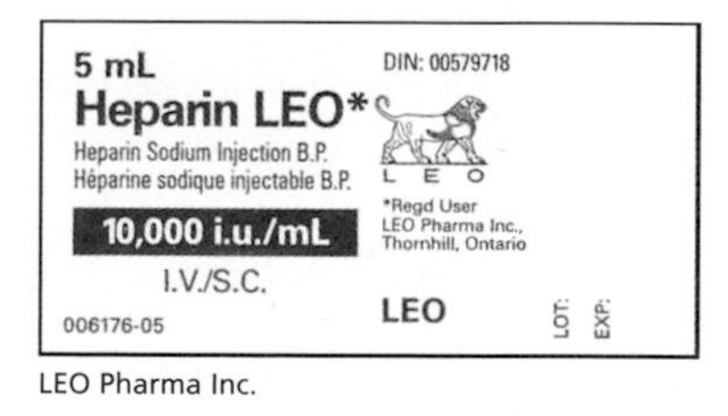

LEO Pharma Inc.

a. Add __________ mL heparin sodium to the IV solution. Mark the dose amount on the syringe.

b. Set the flow rate to __________ mL/h on an IV infusion pump.

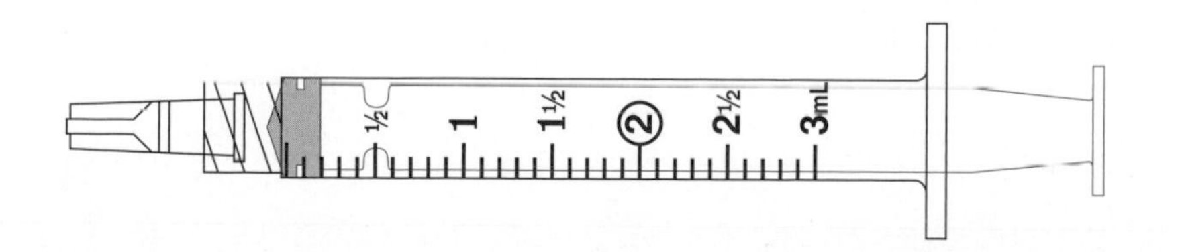

Questions 30 and 31 refer to a patient who weighs 56.8 kg and is receiving IV heparin sodium therapy.

30. Use the Weight-Based Heparin Sodium Protocol below to calculate bolus dosage and infusion rate. The IV pump delivers tenths of a millilitre.

    a. Calculate the initial heparin sodium bolus dosage: __________ units

    b. Calculate the bolus dose: __________ mL

    c. Calculate the initial heparin sodium infusion rate: __________ units/h or __________ mL/h

Weight-Based Heparin Sodium Protocol:

Heparin sodium IV infusion: *heparin sodium 25 000 units in 250 mL of $\frac{1}{2}$ NS*

IV boluses: Use heparin sodium 1000 units/mL

Bolus with heparin sodium 80 units/kg. Then initiate heparin sodium drip at 18 units/kg/h. Obtain aPTT every 6 hours, and adjust dosage and rate as follows:

If aPTT is less than 35 seconds: Rebolus with 80 units/kg and increase rate by 4 units/kg/h

If aPTT is 36 to 44 seconds: Rebolus with 40 units/kg and increase rate by 2 units/kg/h

If aPTT is 45 to 75 seconds: Continue current rate

If aPTT is 76 to 90 seconds: Decrease rate by 2 units/kg/h

If aPTT is greater than 90 seconds: Hold heparin sodium for 1 hour and then decrease rate by 3 units/kg/h

31. At 0930, the patient's aPTT is 77 seconds.

    a. According to the protocol, what action should the nurse take?

    ____

    ____

    b. The nurse should decrease the infusion rate by __________ units/h or __________ mL/h.

    c. The nurse should reset the infusion rate to __________ mL/h.

32. Order: *Humulin R regular insulin subcut as per sliding scale and blood glucose level.* The patient's blood glucose at 1730 h is 13.2 mmol/L.

Sliding Scale	Insulin Dosage
Blood glucose: 0 to 8	0 units
Blood glucose: 8.1 to 14	8 units
Blood glucose: 14.1 to 19	13 units
Blood glucose: 19.1 to 22	18 units
Blood glucose: greater than 22.1	Call Prescriber

Give: __________ units. (Mark dose on appropriate syringe.)

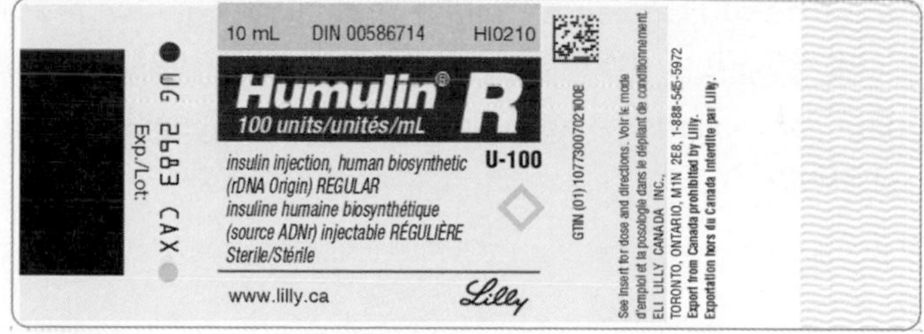

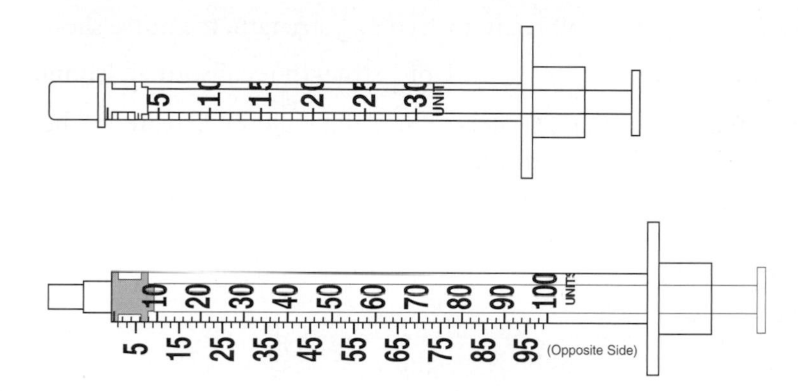

33. Order: *Humulin R regular insulin 15 units with Humulin N NPH insulin 45 units subcut at 0730*

 a. The nurse should give a total of __________ units insulin. (Remember, the nurse will get independent verification after drawing up each insulin.)

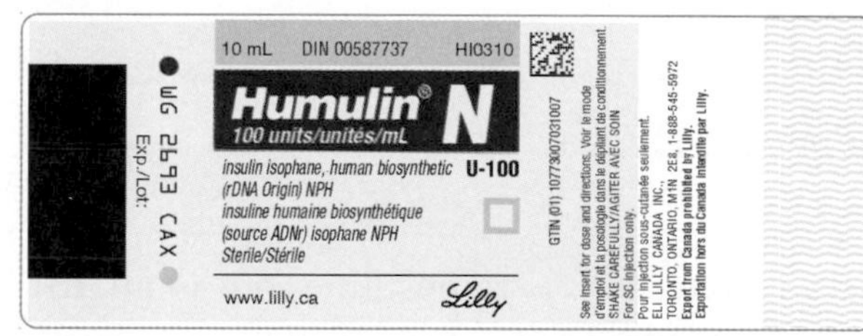

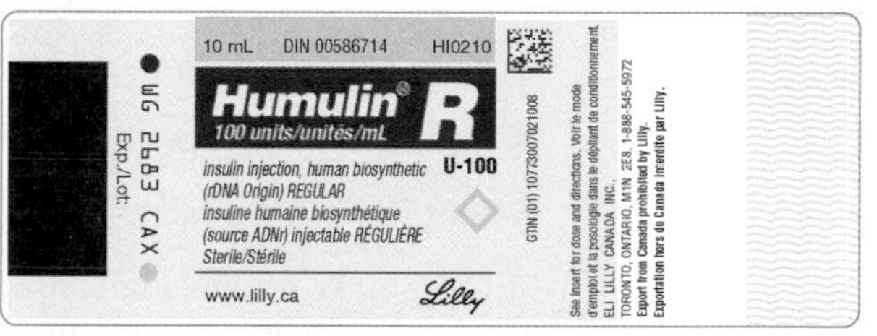

 b. Mark the dose on the appropriate syringe, designating measurement of both regular and NPH insulin.

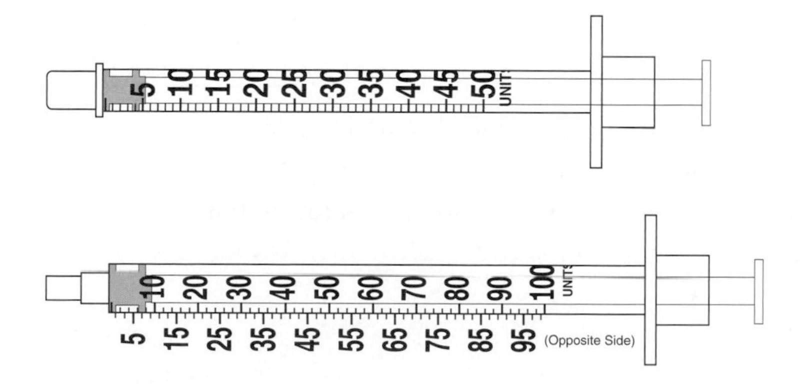

34. A patient is receiving an insulin drip of *Humulin R regular insulin 300 units in 150 mL NS infusing at 10 mL/h.* How many units/h of insulin is this patient receiving? __________ units/h

Questions 35 and 36 refer to an infant who weighs 7.3 kg and is admitted to the pediatric unit with vomiting and diarrhea of 3 days' duration.

Order: *$\frac{1}{4}$ strength Isomil 80 mL q3h for four feedings; if tolerated, increase Isomil to $\frac{1}{2}$ strength 80 mL q3h for four feedings*

Supply: Isomil ready-to-feed formula in 235-mL cans

35. To reconstitute a full 235-mL can of Isomil ready-to-feed to $\frac{1}{4}$ strength, the nurse should add __________ mL water for a total of __________ mL of $\frac{1}{4}$ strength reconstituted Isomil.

36. The child is not tolerating the oral feedings. Calculate this child's allowable daily and hourly IV maintenance fluids using the following recommendation.

    Daily rate of pediatric maintenance IV fluids:

    100 mL/kg for first 10 kg of body weight

    50 mL/kg for next 10 kg of body weight

    20 mL/kg for each kilogram above 20 kg of body weight

    Allowance: __________ mL/day or __________ mL/h

Use the following information and order to answer questions 37 through 39.

$$\text{BSA (m}^2) = \sqrt{\frac{\text{ht (cm)} \times \text{wt (kg)}}{3600}}$$

Order: *mitomycin 28 mg direct IV stat*

Recommended dosage is 10 to 20 mg/m²/single IV dose.

Patient is 157.5 cm tall and weighs 46.8 kg.

Mitomycin is available in a 20-mg vial with directions to reconstitute with 40 mL sterile water for injection to make a final volume of 40 mL and inject slowly over 10 minutes.

37. The patient's BSA is __________ m².

38. a. What is the recommended dosage range of mitomycin for this patient?

    __________ mg to __________ mg

    b. Is the ordered dosage safe? __________ Explain: ______________________________

39. a. What is the concentration of mitomycin after reconstitution? __________ mg/mL

    b. If the order is safe, administer __________ mL mitomycin at the rate of __________ mL/min or __________ mL/15 sec.

40. A child's IV is *1 L D_5 0.45% NaCl*. Calculate the amount of solute in this IV solution.

    __________ g dextrose and _____ g NaCl.

Use the following order and vancomycin label for the available drug to answer questions 41 and 42.

Order: *vancomycin hydrochloride 500 mg IV q6h in IV fluid for total volume of 100 mL to infuse over 1 h via volume control set.* According to the package insert: For IV administration, reconstitute 500-mg vial with 10 mL sterile water for injection for a concentration of 50 mg/mL.

10 x **10 mL** Single-Use Vials/ Flacons uniservices Sterile/ Stérile DIN 02230191 N° M109D001

Sterile Vancomycin Hydrochloride USP
Chlorhydrate de vancomycine stérile USP

500 mg Vancomycin / vial de vancomycine / flacon

Antibiotic for Intravenous Infusion Only / Antibiotique pour perfusion intraveineuse seulement

Courtesy of Pfizer Inc.

41. The nurse should add __________ mL vancomycin hydrochloride and __________ mL IV fluid to the chamber.

42. According to the package insert, the minimal dilution (maximal concentration) of vancomycin hydrochloride is 10 mg/mL. Is the ordered amount of IV fluid sufficient to safely dilute the vancomycin hydrochloride? __________ Explain: ______________________________

____

____

Use the following information to answer questions 43 and 44.

Order: *penicillin G sodium 400 000 units IVPB q6h* for a child who weighs 10 kg. Recommended dosage for children: Give penicillin G sodium 100 000 to 400 000 units/kg/day in divided doses q6h; dilute with 50 mL NS and infuse over 30 minutes.

Pharmaceutical Partners of Canada Inc.

LOT : 302081
EXP. : 2005 FE

15 mL DIN 02220288
PF370070

PENICILLIN G
Sodium for Injection USP

5 million IU
per Vial/par fiole

IM/IV
Sterile/Stérile
Antibiotic / Antibiotique

Usual adult dose:
1,000,000 to 5,000,000 IU every 4 to 6 hours.
For full prescribing information, see package insert.
Reconstitution: Use Sterile Water for Injection, USP or other recommended diluent.

Volume of diluent	Approximate Concentration/mL	Withdrawable Volume
3.1 mL	1,000,000 IU	5 mL
8.2 mL	500,000 IU	10 mL

Reconstituted solution is stable for 5 days refrigerated or 24 hours room temperature.

Pharmaceutical Partners of Canada Inc.
Richmond Hill, Ontario L4C 9S6
1-877-821-7724

Dose habituelle pour adultes :
1 000 000 à 5 000 000 UI toutes les 4 à 6 heures.
Pour les renseignements posologiques complets, consulter le feuillet d'emballage.
Reconstitution : Utiliser de l'eau stérile pour préparations injectables USP ou un autre diluant recommandé.

Volume de diluant	Concentration approximative/mL	Volume obtenu
3,1 mL	1 000 000 UI	5 mL
8,2 mL	500 000 UI	10 mL

La solution reconstituée est stable pendant 5 jours au réfrigérateur ou pendant 24 heures à la température ambiante.

85009/A

6 29336 37070 2

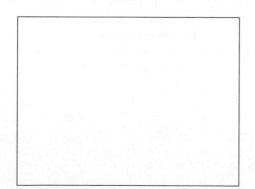

43. a. How many units per day of penicillin G sodium is this child ordered to receive? __________ units/day

    b. Is the ordered dosage safe? __________ Explain: ______________________________

    c. If safe, reconstitute with __________ mL diluent for a concentration of __________ units/mL, and prepare a reconstitution label.

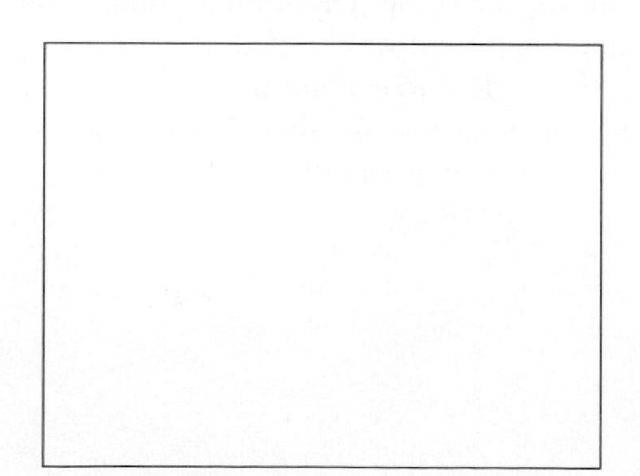

d. Prepare to give __________ mL.

e. If the order is not safe, what should the nurse do? ______________________________

44. The child's IV is infusing on an IV pump programmable in whole millilitres. If the dosage is safe, set the IV flow rate at __________ mL/h.

Use the following patient situation to answer questions 45 through 47.

A patient has been admitted to the hospital with fever and chills, productive cough with yellow-green sputum, shortness of breath, malaise, and anorexia. Laboratory tests and X-rays confirmed a diagnosis of pneumonia. The patient is reporting nausea. The prescriber writes the following orders. The labels represent the drugs you have available.

NS 1000 mL IV at 125 mL/h

ceftazidime 1500 mg IVPB q8h in 100 mL NS over 30 min

45. The nurse starts the primary IV at 1315 on an IV infusion pump. When will the primary IV be completely infused and have to be replaced? __________ hours

46. Calculate one dose of ceftazidime. __________ mL

47. Calculate the IVPB flow rate for each dose of ceftazidime at __________ mL/h.

48. A patient is to receive a single dose of ondansetron hydrochloride dihydrate 4 mg direct IV at 2 mg/min for established post-operative nausea and vomiting, The nurse should give __________ mL/min of ondansetron hydrochloride dihydrate at the rate of __________ or __________ every 15 seconds.

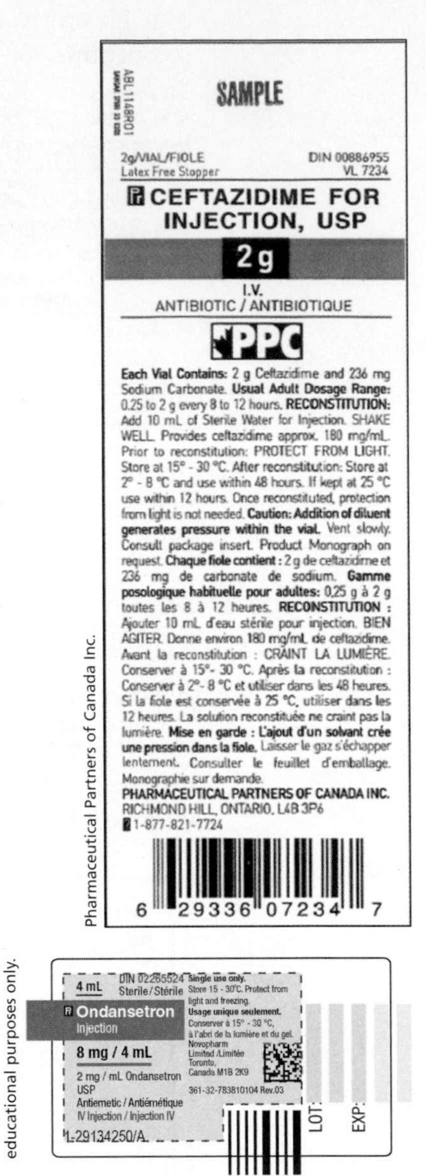

APPLICATION OF CLINICAL REASONING

CSE-1 Describe the clinical reasoning that you would implement to prevent this patient safety incident.

Possible Scenario

A student nurse was preparing for medication administration. One of the orders on the medication administration record was written as *digoxin 0.125 mg OD*. The student nurse crushed the digoxin tablet. Prior to giving the medication, the nursing instructor checked the medications that the student had prepared. The instructor asked the student to explain the rationale for crushing the digoxin tablet. The student explained to the instructor that the digoxin order was for the right eye and the student planned to add a small amount of sterile water to the crushed tablet and put it in the patient's eye.

Potential Outcome

What is wrong with the digoxin order? ____________________

What could be the result? ____________________

Prevention

____

____

CSE-2 Describe the clinical reasoning that you would implement to prevent this patient safety incident.

Possible Scenario

Order: *quinine sulfate 300 mg PO bedtime*

Supply: quinidine sulfate 300 mg tablets

A student nurse administering medications noted the difference between the order and the supply drug, and queried the staff nurse about the order and what had been administered. The staff nurse at first dismissed it as only the brand name versus the generic name of the drug. Later, the staff nurse realized that the student nurse was exactly right to question the order and the drug supplied, and admitted to the student that the patient had been receiving the wrong drug all week.

Potential Outcome

The student referred to a drug reference book and compared the therapeutic and adverse effects of both drugs. The quinine sulfate was correctly ordered for leg cramps. Quinidine sulfate is an anti-dysrhythmic heart medication. The student reviewed the patient's record and noted that the patient had been experiencing serious hypotension (an adverse effect of quinidine) for the past several days.

Prevention

____

____

After completing these problems, see the Answers section at the end of the book to check your answers. Give yourself 2 points for each correct answer.

Perfect score = 100 My score = __________

Mastery score = 90 or higher (45 or more correct)

Check your work! Answers to all Application of Clinical Reasoning Problems are provided at the end of each chapter.

APPENDIX A

Answers

Answers to Practice Problems—Chapter 1

1) $\frac{7}{20}$ **2)** 0.375 **3)** LCD = 21 **4)** LCD = 55 **5)** LCD = 18 **6)** LCD = 15 **7)** $3\frac{7}{15}$ **8)** $7\frac{29}{60}$ **9)** $\frac{1}{2}$ **10)** $2\frac{7}{24}$ **11)** $\frac{7}{27}$ **12)** $10\frac{1}{8}$ **13)** $4\frac{4}{17}$ **14)** $\frac{39}{80}$ **15)** $5\frac{1}{55}$ **16)** $5\frac{5}{18}$ **17)** $2\frac{86}{87}$ **18)** $\frac{3}{20}$ **19)** $\frac{1}{3125}$ **20)** $\frac{1}{4}$ **21)** $1\frac{5}{7}$ **22)** $16\frac{1}{32}$ **23)** 60.27 **24)** 66.74 **25)** 42.98 **26)** 4833.92 **27)** 190.8 **28)** 19.17 **29)** 9.48 **30)** 7.7 **31)** 42.75 **32)** 300 **33)** 12 930.43 **34)** 3200.63 **35)** 2 **36)** 150.96 **37)** 9.716. **38)** 0.50.25 **39)** 0.25. = 25 **40)** 5.750. = 5750 **41)** .0.25 = 0.025 **42)** 11.5.25 = 115.25 **43)** 0.16 mg **44)** $\frac{1}{8}$ **45)** 0.35 mg **46)** \$915.08 **47)** \$1.46 **48)** 2.5 tablets **49)** 800 mL **50)** 2.95 kg

Selected Solutions to Practice Problems—Chapter 1

43) $4 \text{ tab} \times \frac{0.4 \text{ mg}}{1 \text{ tab}} = 0.16 \text{ mg}$

44) $\left(1 \text{ assignment} - \frac{1}{2} \text{ assignment completed}\right) = \frac{1}{2} \text{ assignment remaining}$

$\frac{1}{2} \text{ assignment remaining} \div 4 \text{ students} = \frac{1}{2} \text{ assignment} \times \frac{1}{4 \text{ students}} = \frac{1}{8} \text{ assignment remaining per student}$

45) $\frac{0.1 \text{ mg}}{\text{tab}} \times 3.5 \text{ tab} = 0.35 \text{ mg}$

46) (\$17.43/h × 40 h) + (6.25 h × \$17.43 × 2)

= \$697.20 + \$217.875 (round off routinely)

= \$697.20 + \$217.88 = \$915.08

47) \$98.76/12 catheters = \$8.23 per catheter

$\$975 \div (12 \times 12) = \frac{\$975}{144} = \$6.77$ per catheter

\$8.23 − \$ 6.77 = \$1.46 is saved per catheter

48) $1.25 \text{ mg} \div \frac{0.5 \text{ mg}}{\text{tablet}} = 1.25 \text{ mg} \times \frac{1 \text{ tablet}}{0.5 \text{ mg}} = 2.5 \text{ tablets or } 2\frac{1}{2} \text{ tablets}$

49) $\frac{2}{\cancel{3}_1}$ of $\overset{400}{\cancel{1200}}$ mL = 2 × 400 mL = 800 mL

50)
$$\begin{array}{r} 6.65 \text{ kg} \\ -\ 3.70 \text{ kg} \\ \hline 2.95 \text{ kg} \end{array}$$

Answers to Practice Problems—Chapter 2

1) 0.4, 40%, 2:5 **2)** $\frac{1}{20}$, 5%, 1:20 **3)** 0.17, $\frac{17}{100}$, 17:100 **4)** 0.25, $\frac{1}{4}$, 25% **5)** 0.06, $\frac{3}{50}$, 3:50 **6)** 0.17, 17%, 1.6 **7)** 0.5, $\frac{1}{2}$, 1:2 **8)** 0.01, $\frac{1}{100}$, 1% **9)** $\frac{9}{100}$, 9%, 9:100 **10)** 0.38, 38%, 3:8 **11)** 0.67, $\frac{2}{3}$, 67% **12)** 0.33, 33%, 1:3 **13)** $\frac{13}{25}$, 52%, 13:25 **14)** 0.45, $\frac{9}{20}$, 45% **15)** 0.86, 86%, 6:7 **16)** 0.3, $\frac{3}{10}$, 30% **17)** 0.02, 2%, 1:50 **18)** $\frac{3}{50}$, 6%, 3:50 **19)** $\frac{1}{25}$, 4%, 1:25 **20)** 0.1, $\frac{1}{10}$, 1:10 **21)** 0.04 **22)** 1:40 **23)** 7.5% **24)** $\frac{1}{2}$ **25)** 3:4 **26)** 262.5 **27)** 3.64 **28)** 1.99 **29)** 1:4 **30)** $\frac{1}{10}$ **31)** 84 **32)** 16 **33)** 1 **34)** 1.1 **35)** 100 **36)** 35.33 **37)** 0.75 **38)** 21 **39)** 120 **40)** 90 **41)** 138 nurses; 46 maintenance/cleaners; 92 technicians; 92 others **42)** 25 g protein; 6.25 g fat **43)** 231 points **44)** 60 min **45)** 50 mL **46)** 27 mg **47)** 283.5 mg **48)** 3 kg **49)** \$10.42 **50)** 6 total doses

Selected Solutions to Practice Problems—Chapter 2

41) $\frac{3}{8} \times 368 = 138$ nurses

$\frac{1}{8} \times 368 = 46$ maintenance/cleaners

$\frac{1}{4} \times 368 = 92$ technicians and 92 others

42) $125 \times 0.2 = 25$ g protein

$125 \times 0.05 = 6.25$ g fat

$$\begin{array}{r} 125 \\ \times 0.2 \\ \hline 25.0 \end{array} = 25$$

$$\begin{array}{r} 125 \\ \times 0.05 \\ \hline 6.25 \end{array} = 6.25$$

44) $\frac{27 \text{ minutes}}{\cancel{90}_{9} \cancel{\text{calories}}} \times \cancel{200}^{20} \cancel{\text{calories}} =$

$\frac{540 \text{ minutes}}{9} = 60$ min

46) $60 \times 0.45 = 27$ mg

$$\begin{array}{r} 60 \\ \times 0.45 \\ \hline 300 \\ 240 \\ \hline 27.00 \end{array} = 27$$

47) $\frac{6.75 \text{ mg}}{1 \cancel{\text{min}}} \times 42 \cancel{\text{min}} =$

$6.75 \text{ mg} \times 42 = 283.5$ mg of medication

48) $60 \text{ kg} \times 0.05 = 3$ kg

49) $0.17 \times \$12.56 = 2.14$;

$$\begin{array}{r} \$12.56 \\ -2.14 \\ \hline \$10.42 \end{array}$$

50) 10% of 150 $= 0.10 \times 150 = 15$;

$$\begin{array}{rl} 150 & \text{mg first dose} \\ -15 & \\ \hline 135 & \text{mg second dose} \\ -15 & \\ \hline 120 & \text{mg third dose} \\ -15 & \\ \hline 105 & \text{mg fourth dose} \\ -15 & \\ \hline 90 & \text{mg fifth dose} \\ -15 & \\ \hline 75 & \text{mg sixth dose} \end{array}$$

6 total doses

Answers to Practice Problems—Chapter 3

1) milli **2)** micro **3)** centi **4)** kilo **5)** 1 milligram **6)** 1 kilogram **7)** 1 microgram **8)** 1 centimetre **9)** metre **10)** gram **11)** litre **12)** milligram **13)** microgram **14)** unit **15)** milliequivalent **16)** millilitre **17)** kilometre **18)** millimetre **19)** gram **20)** centimetre **21)** litre **22)** metre **23)** kilogram **24)** millimole **25)** 500 mg **26)** 0.5 L **27)** 0.05 mg **28)** three hundred seventy-five units **29)** two and six tenths millilitres **30)** twenty milliequivalents **31)** four tenths of a litre **32)** seventeen hundredths of a milligram **33)** 250 mL **34)** 0.15 mg **35)** 1500 g **36)** 100 mg **37)** 1.5 cm **38)** 200 mcg **39)** 500 mL **40)** 0.256g **41)** 150 mg **42)** 1330 **43)** 0004 **44)** 2400 or 0000 **45)** 0620 **46)** zero zero forty-one hours **47)** eleven fifteen hours **48)** zero six twenty-three hours

Answers to Application of Clinical Reasoning

3-1) This type of patient safety incident can be prevented by avoiding the use of a decimal point or extra zero when not necessary. In this instance, the decimal point and zero serve no purpose and can easily be misinterpreted, especially if the decimal point is difficult to see. Question any order that appears unclear or unreasonable.

3-2) This was an example of a "near miss" patient safety incident. The original nurse may have prevented the near miss by carefully comparing the order and the stock solution. If the nurse transcribed the units as part of the calculation process, the confusion between *mg* and *mL* may have been noticed earlier. When using stock supplies, extra diligence by the nurse is frequently required. The nurse always should follow up on any sense of "it does not seem reasonable" and question any order that appears out of the ordinary. In addition to double-checking calculations with a colleague when the policy of the institution requires it, the nurse should also double-check calculations with a colleague when the nurse feels uncertain.

Answers to Practice Problems—Chapter 4

1) 45 **2)** 2 **3)** 2 **4)** 2.5 **5)** 0.5 **6)** 16 **7)** 1.4 **8)** 0.7 **9)** 2.3 **10)** 0.25 **11)** 1.6 **12)** 1.5 **13)** 2 **14)** 2.5 **15)** 9 **16)** 7.5 **17)** 8 **18)** 2 **19)** 8 **20)** 3 **21)** 1.4 **22)** 15 **23)** 12

Answers to Application of Clinical Reasoning

4-1) This type of calculation error occurred because the nurse used the formula method to calculate the amount but mixed up the desired strength and the medication strength. If done correctly by the formula method, it would had been set up like this: $\frac{50 \text{ mg}}{125 \text{ mg}} \times 5 \text{ mL}$. This type of error can be avoided by using the dimensional analysis method of medication calculation. For example,

$$\text{mL} = 50 \cancel{\text{mg}} \times \frac{5 \text{ mL}}{125 \cancel{\text{mg}}}$$

$$= \frac{\overset{2}{\cancel{50}} \times 5 \text{ mL}}{\underset{5}{\cancel{125}}}$$

$$= 2 \text{ mL}$$

The child should receive 2 mL of amoxicillin suspension.

4-2) The nurse did not set up the problem correctly with all the information needed. If the nurse were to use the equation $\frac{D}{H} \times Q$, the nurse would have written $\frac{2 \text{ g}}{1000 \text{ mg}} \times 10 \text{ mL}$. Then the nurse could have added the conversion factor to convert grams to milligrams. The problem would then look like this: $\frac{2 \cancel{\text{g}}}{1000 \cancel{\text{mg}}} \times 10 \text{ mL} \times \frac{1000 \cancel{\text{mg}}}{1 \cancel{\text{g}}}$. Then the nurse could have easily seen that the answer would correctly result with *mL* as the units left when the other units cancel out each other. Then the arithmetic could have been completed and the answer found to be 10 mL.

The nurse could then double-check by asking the question, "Is this dosage reasonable?" Since the nurse knows there are *1000 mg in 1 g* and that the dosage required is 2 g, then it is obvious that more than one vial of the medication will be necessary for this prescribed dose.

Selected Solutions to Practice Problems—Chapter 4

1) $\text{mL} = \frac{1 \text{ mL}}{667 \text{ mg}} \times \frac{1000 \text{ mg}}{1 \text{ g}} \times \frac{30 \text{ g}}{1 \text{ dose}} = \frac{30\,000}{667} = 45 \text{ mL/dose}$

2) $\text{mL} = \frac{20 \text{ mL}}{5\,000\,000 \cancel{\text{units}}} \times \frac{500\,000 \cancel{\text{units}}}{1 \text{ dose}} = 2 \text{ mL/dose}$

6) $\text{mL} = \frac{5 \text{ mL}}{12.5 \cancel{\text{mg}}} \times \frac{40 \cancel{\text{mg}}}{1 \text{ dose}} = 16 \text{ mL/dose}$

7) $\text{mL} = \frac{2 \text{ mL}}{500\,000 \cancel{\text{units}}} \times \frac{350\,000 \cancel{\text{units}}}{1 \text{ dose}} = 1.4 \text{ mL /dose}$

8) $\text{mL} = \frac{1 \text{ mL}}{5 \cancel{\text{mg}}} \times \frac{3.5 \cancel{\text{mg}}}{1 \text{ dose}} = 0.7 \text{ mL/dose}$

9) $\text{mL} = \frac{2 \text{ mL}}{80 \cancel{\text{mg}}} \times \frac{90 \cancel{\text{mg}}}{1 \text{ dose}} = 2.25 \text{ mL/dose} = 2.3 \text{ mL/dose}$

13) $\frac{1 \text{ mL}}{250 \text{ mg}} \times \frac{500 \text{ mg}}{1 \text{ dose}} = 2 \text{ mL}$

16) $\frac{5 \text{ mL}}{8 \cancel{\text{mmol}}} \times \frac{12 \cancel{\text{mmol}}}{1 \text{ dose}} = 7.5 \text{ mL}$

18) $\text{tablets} = \frac{1 \text{ tablet}}{0.075 \cancel{\text{mg}}} \times \frac{1 \cancel{\text{mg}}}{1000 \cancel{\text{mcg}}} \times \frac{150 \cancel{\text{mcg}}}{1 \text{ dose}} = 2 \text{ tablets/dose}$

Answers to Section 1—Self-Evaluation

1) 3.05 **2)** 4002.5 **3)** LCD = 12 **4)** LCD = 110 **5)** $\frac{11}{12}$ **6)** $\frac{47}{63}$ **7)** 1 **8)** $\frac{1}{2}$ **9)** 45.78 **10)** 0.02 **11)** 59.24 **12)** 0.09 **13)** $\frac{2}{3}$ **14)** $\frac{1}{2}$ **15)** 0.64 **16)** $\frac{1}{10}, \frac{1}{6}, \frac{1}{5}, \frac{1}{3}, \frac{1}{2}$ **17)** 0.009, 0.125, 0.1909, 0.25, 0.3 **18)** 1:3 **19)** 0.01 **20)** 0.04 **21)** 0.9% **22)** $\frac{1}{3}$ **23)** $\frac{1}{20}$ **24)** 1:200 **25)** $\frac{2}{3}$ **26)** 75% **27)** 40% **28)** 1.21 **29)** 1.3 **30)** 4 **31)** 20 000 **32)** 3.3 **33)** 0.5 mL **34)** four hundred fifty milligrams **35)** twenty-five hundredths of a litre **36)** (7.13 kg) = 7130 g = 7 130 000 mg = 7 130 000 000 mcg **37)** 0.000 000 925 kg = 0.000 925 g = 0.925 mg = (925 mcg) **38)** 0.000 125 kg = 0.125 g = (125 mg) = 125 000 mcg **39)** 0.0164 kg = (16.4 g) = 16 400 mg = 16 400 000 mcg **40)** 0.02 g **41)** 5.62 cm **42)** 11 590 g **43)** 6 **44)** 2335 h **45)** 6:44 PM **46)** 1 capsule **47)** 0.8 mL **48)** 20 mL **49)** 0.5 mL **50)** 0.5 mL

Selected Solutions to Section 1—Self-Evaluation

13) $\frac{1}{150} \div \frac{1}{100} = \frac{1}{150} \times \frac{100}{1} = \frac{\overset{2}{\cancel{100}}}{\underset{3}{\cancel{150}}} = \frac{2}{3}$

15) $\frac{16\%}{\frac{1}{4}} = 16\% \times \frac{4}{1} = 0.16 \times 4 = 0.64$

26) $3{:}4 = \frac{3}{4} = 4\overline{)3.0}^{\,0.75} = 75\%$

29) $\frac{0.3}{2.6} \rightleftarrows \frac{0.15}{X}$

$0.3X = 2.6 \times 0.15$

$0.3X = 0.39$

$\frac{\cancel{0.3}X}{\cancel{0.3}} = \frac{0.39}{0.3}$

$X = 1.3$

31) $\frac{10\%}{\frac{1}{2}\%} \times 1000 = X$

$\frac{0.1}{0.005} \times \frac{1000}{1} = X$

$\frac{100}{0.005} = X$

$X = 20\ 000$

47) $\text{mL} = 60\ \cancel{\text{mg}} \times \frac{1\ \text{mL}}{75\ \cancel{\text{mg}}}$

$= \frac{60\ \text{mL}}{75}$

$= \frac{4\ \text{mL}}{5}$

$= 0.8\ \text{mL}$

Answers to Practice Problems—Chapter 5

1) 1 **2)** hundredths or 0.01 **3)** No. The tuberculin syringe has a maximum capacity of 1 mL. **4)** Round to 1.3 mL and measure at 1.3 mL. **5)** 30 mL **6)** 1 mL; if drug is ordered by mouth, an oral syringe or calibrated oral device should be used. **7)** 5-mL oral syringe or medicine cup depending on institution policy **8)** False **9)** False **10)** True **11)** To prevent accidental needlesticks during intravenous administration **12)** top ring **13)** 10 **14)** True **15)** standard 3-mL, 1-mL, and insulin

16)

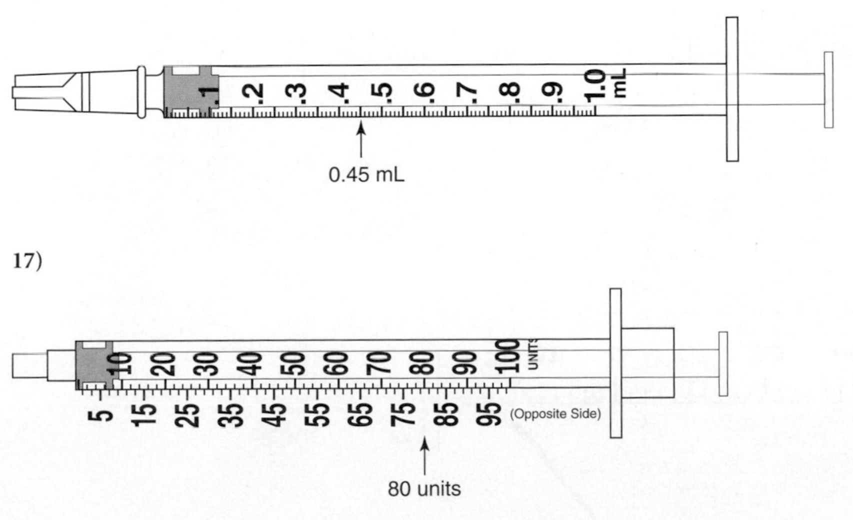

17)

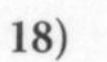
18)

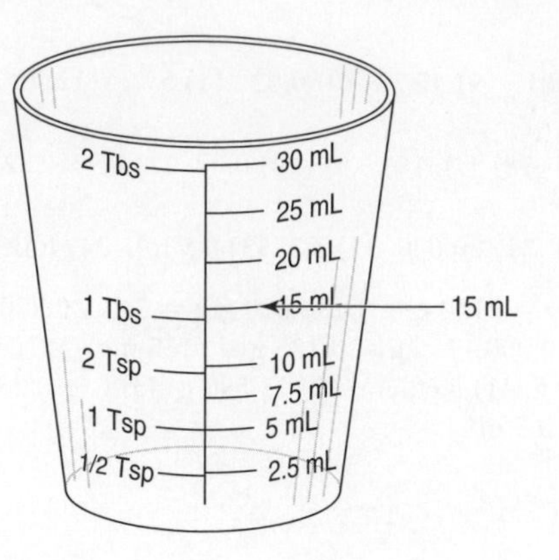
2 Tbs
30 mL
25 mL
20 mL
1 Tbs
15 mL
15 mL
2 Tsp
10 mL
7.5 mL
1 Tsp
5 mL
1/2 Tsp
2.5 mL

19)

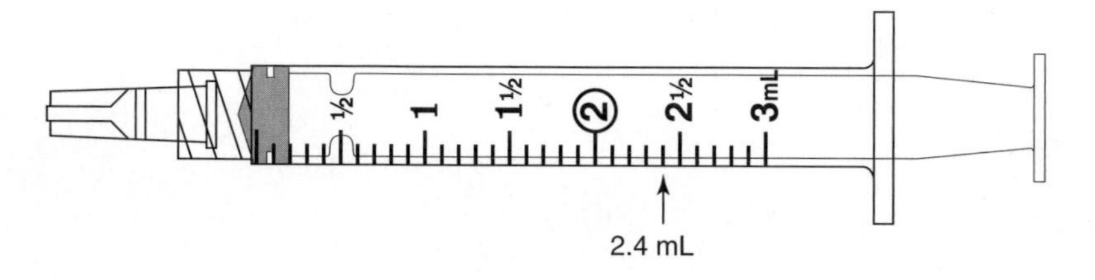
½
1
1½
2
2½
3mL
2.4 mL

20)

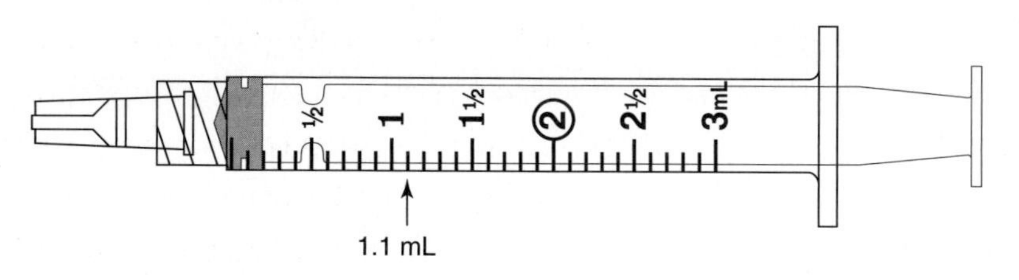
½
1
1½
2
2½
3mL
1.1 mL

21)

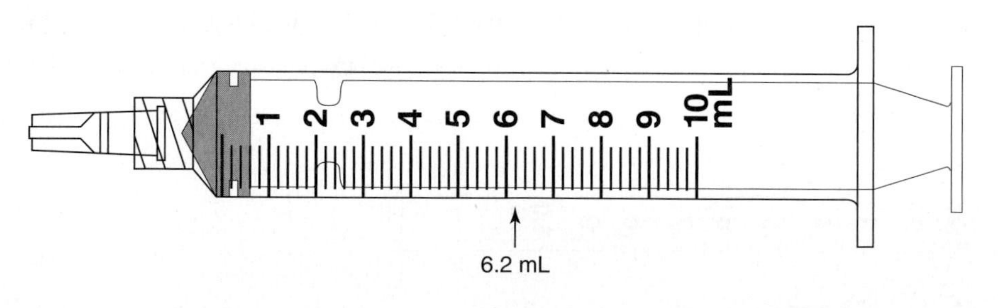
1
2
3
4
5
6
7
8
9
10
mL
6.2 mL

22)

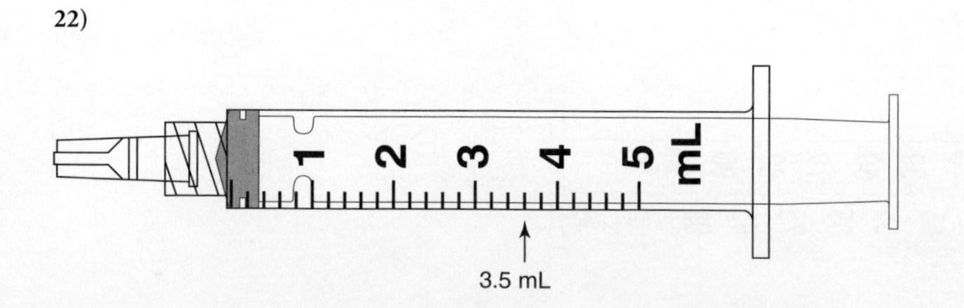
1
2
3
4
5
mL
3.5 mL

23)

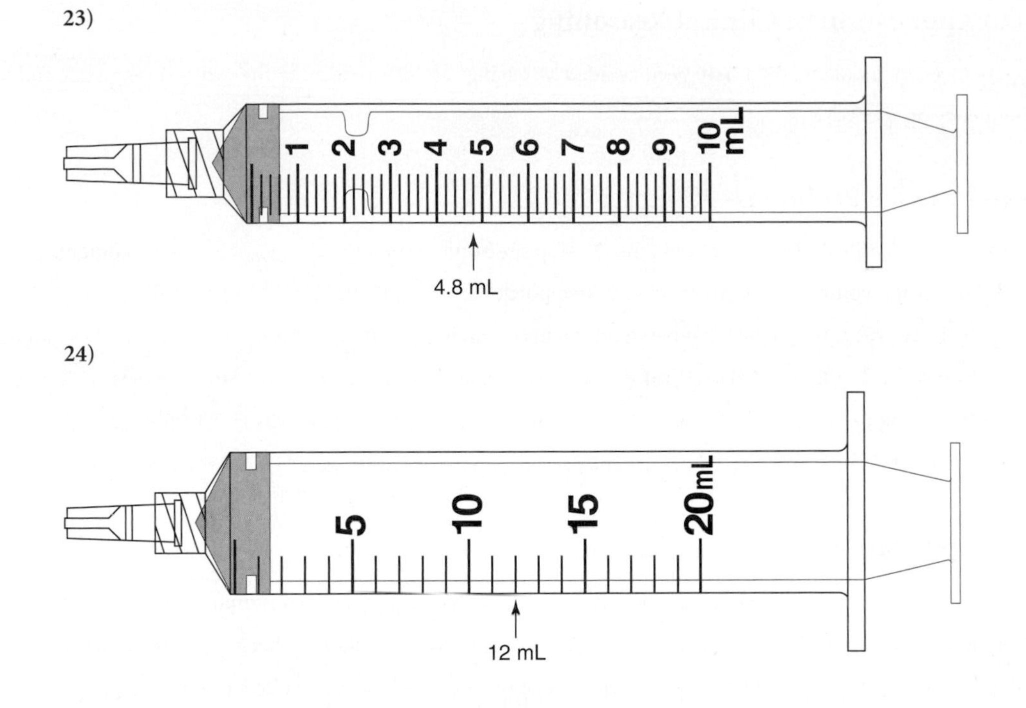

24)

Answers to Application of Clinical Reasoning

5-1) This patient safety incident could have been avoided by following the principle of not putting oral drugs in syringes intended for injection. Instead, place the medication in an oral syringe to which a needle cannot be attached. In addition, the medication should have been labelled for oral use only. The medication was ordered orally, not by injection. The alert nurse would have noticed the discrepancy. Finally, but certainly as important, a medication should be prepared just before administration and should be administered only by the nurse who prepared it.

5-2) The nurse needs to recognize the difference between an oral and a parenteral syringe. Look at the syringe markings that are typically for oral measurement and the absence of the Luer-Lok hub, found on parenteral injection syringes. The nurse must remove the cap on the oral syringe prior to administering the medication, so that the child cannot choke on the cap.

Answers to Practice Problems—Chapter 6

1) nasogastric **2)** per rectum **3)** before meals **4)** sublingual **5)** 3 times a day **6)** every 4 hours **7)** when necessary **8)** by mouth, orally **9)** tablet **10)** immediately **11)** freely, as desired **12)** intramuscular **13)** after meals **14)** NPO **15)** gtt **16)** mL **17)** hs **18)** g **19)** QID **20)** qh **21)** subcut **22)** IV **23)** BID **24)** q3h **25)** q12h **26)** cap **27)** kg **28)** SR **29)** EC **30)** LA **31)** IR **32)** Give 60 milligrams of keterolac tromethamine intramuscularly immediately and every 6 hours. **33)** Give 300 000 units of procaine penicillin G intramuscularly 4 times a day. **34)** Give 1 tablet of Mylanta orally 1 hour before and 1 hour after meals, at bedtime, and every 2 hours during the night as needed for gastric upset. **35)** Give 25 milligrams of chlordiazepoxide orally every 6 hours when necessary for agitation. **36)** Give 5000 units of heparin sodium subcutaneously immediately. **37)** Give 150 milligrams (1 tablet) of codeine controlled release every 12 hours for pain. **38)** Give 0.25 milligram of digoxin orally every day. **39)** Give 2 drops of Optimyxin Plus ophthalmic to the left eye 4 times a day. **40)** Give 40 milligrams of furosemide intramuscularly immediately. **41)** Give 4 milligrams of betamethasone intravenously twice a day. **42)** 20 units **43)** Subcut, subcutaneously **44)** Give 500 milligrams of ciprofloxacin hydrochloride orally every 12 hours. **45)** 0800, 1200, 1800 **46)** digoxin (Lanoxin) 0.125 mg PO **47)** Give 150 milligrams of ranitidine tablets orally twice daily with breakfast and supper. **48)** Vancomycin **49)** 12 h

Answers to Application of Clinical Reasoning

6-1) This patient safety incident could have been avoided by paying careful attention to the ordered frequency and by writing the frequency on the MAR.

Answers to Practice Problems—Chapter 7

1) 125 mg/5 mL **2)** 02250896 **3)** 237 mL **4)** cefixime **5)** "Tap the bottle several times to loosen powder contents prior to reconstitution. Add a total volume of 33 mL of water in two portions. Mix well after each addition." **6)** Sanofi **7)** 2 mL **8)** 50 mg/2 mL **9)** 1 mL **10)** multiple doses; if based on the maximal dose of 80 mg, it would be 15 doses. **11)** tobramycin **12)** 00533688 **13)** syrup **14)** 500 mL **15)** oral **16)** Pfizer **17)** extended-release capsules **18)** Store between 15°C and 30°C (as per label) **19)** 0.15 mg per pen (0.3 mL) **20)** 0.3 mg per pen (0.3 mL) **21)** I **22)** H **23)** H **24)** oral **25)** 50 mg of each **26)** 2% **27)** 2 g per 100 mL, or 20 mg per mL **28)** oral liquid; children under the age of 12 **29)** 6.25 mg/5 mL

Answers to Application of Clinical Reasoning

7-1) The nurse should have recognized that the patient was still experiencing signs and symptoms that the medication had been ordered to treat. If the order was difficult to read, the prescriber should have been called to clarify the order. Was the dosage of 100 mg a usual dosage for Celexa? The nurse should have consulted a drug guide to ensure that the dosage was appropriate. Also, if the patient was not diagnosed with depression, the nurse should have questioned why Celexa, an antidepressant, was ordered.

Answers to Section 2—Self-Evaluation

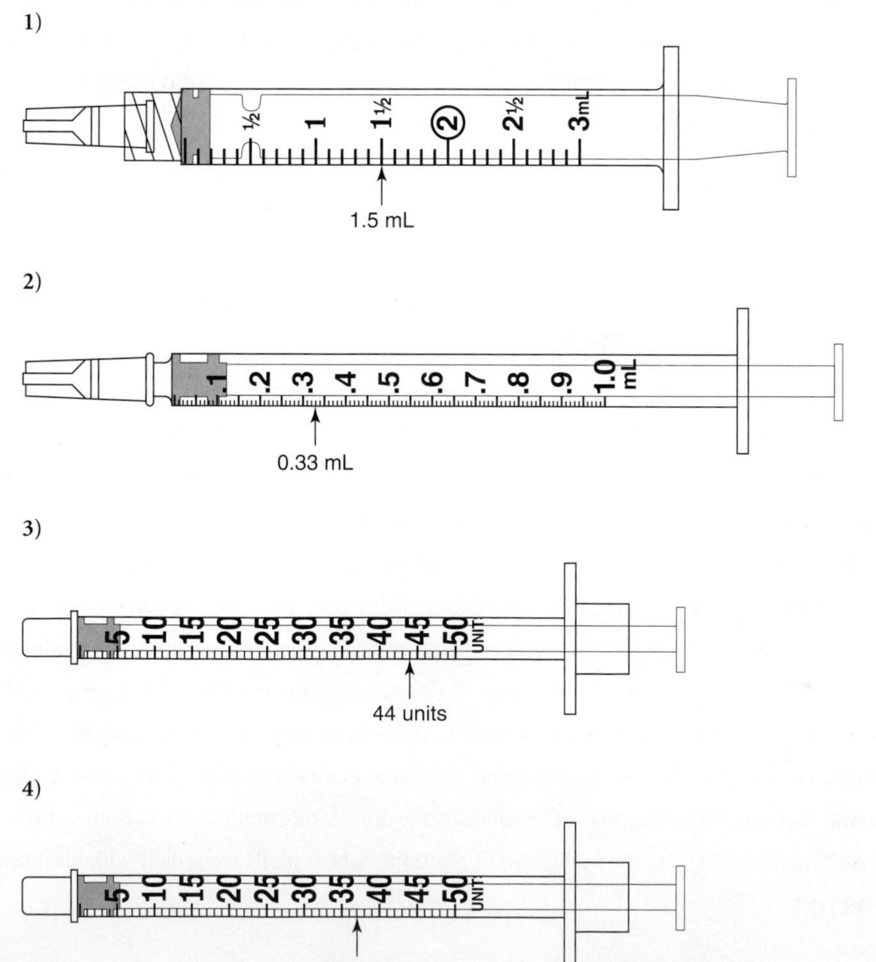

5)

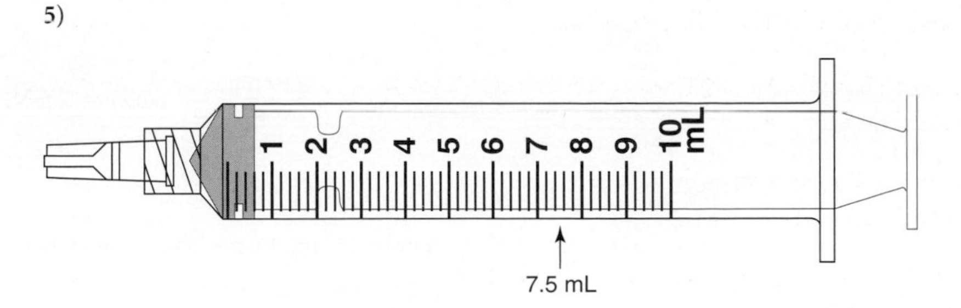

6) framycetin, gramicidin, and dexamethasone **7)** Use in ears and eyes. **8)** 8 mL **9)** Give 2 drops of Sofracort otic/ophthalmic solution in each ear every 15 minutes for 3 doses. **10)** 250 mg/tablet **11)** 02350750 **12)** Give 1 tablet of naproxen orally 3 times a day. **13)** Novo-Trimel **14)** 200 mg of sulfamethoxazole and 40 mg of trimethoprim in every 5 mL

15) a. 2.5 mL

b.

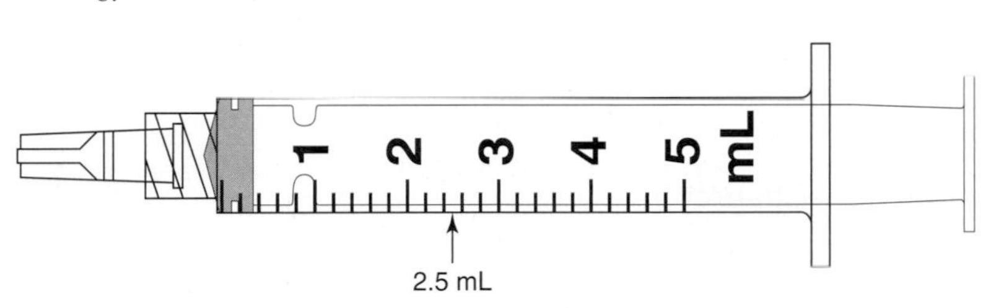

16) Give 250 mg of amoxicillin by mouth every 8 hours **17)** prednisone 50 mg PO daily. **18)** hydrochlorothiazide 50 mg PO BID **19)** Novolin regular insulin 30 units subcut daily **20)** Pen VK would be the only product that could be given by NG tube as it is a solution and the others are CD or SR products that cannot be crushed

Answers to Practice Problems—Chapter 8

1) $\frac{1}{2}$ **2)** 3 **3)** $\frac{1}{2}$ **4)** 10 **5)** 10 **6)** 2 **7)** 8 mL **8)** $1\frac{1}{2}$ **9)** 2 **10)** $\frac{1}{2}$ **11)** $1\frac{1}{2}$ **12)** 1 **13)** $1\frac{1}{2}$ **14)** 1 **15)** 5; $1\frac{1}{2}$ **16)** 7.5 **17)** $1\frac{1}{2}$ **18)** 2 **19)** 0.5 **20)** 0.75; 1 **21)** $\frac{1}{2}$ **22)** 2 **23)** 2 **24)** 2 **25)** 2 **26)** 15 and 30; one of each or 3 of 15 mg or $1\frac{1}{2}$ of 30 mg **27)** 7.5 **28)** 2 **29)** 3 **30)** B, 1 tablet **31)** A; 1 tablet **32)** C; 1 tablet **33)** G; 2 tablets **34)** D, 2 tablets **35)** F; 2 tablets **36)** E; 1 tablet **37)** K; 4 tablets **38)** H; $\frac{1}{2}$ tablet **39)** L; 2 tablets **40)** J; 2 tablets **41)** I; 2 tablets **42)** M; 1 tablet **43)** O; 2 tablets **44)** N; 2 tablets **45)** P; 1 tablet **46)** Q; 15 mL

Answers to Application of Clinical Reasoning

8-1) This patient safety incident could have been prevented if the nurse had carefully read both the patient care order and the medication label. The patient care order may have misled the nurse by placing the volume first and then the drug dosage. If confused by the order, the nurse should have clarified the intent with the prescriber. By focusing on the volume, the nurse failed to follow the steps in dosage calculation. Had the nurse noted 250 mg as the desired dosage and the supply (or on-hand) dosage as 125 mg per 5 mL, the correct amount to be administered would have been clear. Slow down and take time to compare the order with the labels. Calculate each dose carefully before preparing and administering both solid- and liquid-form medications.

Selected Solutions to Practice Problems—Chapter 8

2) Order: 45 mg

Supply: 15 mg/tablet

$$\frac{D}{H} \times Q = \frac{\overset{3}{\cancel{45}}\text{ mg}}{\underset{1}{\cancel{15}}\text{ mg}} \times 1 \text{ tablet} = 3 \text{ tablets}$$

3) Order: 0.075 mg = 0.075 × 1000 = 75 mcg

Supply: 150 mcg/tablet

$$\frac{D}{H} \times Q = \frac{\overset{1}{\cancel{75\text{ mcg}}}}{\underset{2}{\cancel{150\text{ mcg}}}} \times 1 \text{ tablet} = \frac{1}{2} \text{ tablet}$$

8) Order: 120 mg

Supply: 80 mg/tablet

$$\frac{D}{H} \times Q = \frac{\overset{3}{\cancel{120}}\text{ mg}}{\underset{2}{\cancel{80}}\text{ mg}} \times 1 \text{ tablet} = 1\frac{1}{2} \text{ tablets}$$

18) Order: 0.25 mg = 0.250 mg

Supply: 0.125 mg/tablet

$$\frac{D}{H} \times Q = \frac{\overset{2}{\cancel{0.250\text{ mg}}}}{\underset{1}{\cancel{0.125\text{ mg}}}} \times 1 \text{ tablet} = 2 \text{ tablets}$$

26) Order: 45 mg

Supply: 10-mg, 15-mg, and 30-mg tablets

Select: One 15-mg tablet and one 30-mg tablet for 45 mg total

Alternative choices: give 3 of the 15 mg tablets OR give $1\frac{1}{2}$ of the 30 mg tablets to provide 45 mg total

Remember: If you have a choice, give whole tablets and as few as possible.

Answers to Practice Problems—Chapter 9

1) 0.4; 1 mL
2) 1.5; 3 mL
3) 0.5; 1 mL
4) 0.4; 1 mL
5) 2; 3 mL
6) 0.75; 1 mL
7) 0.67; 1 mL
8) 1; 3 mL
9) 4 mL; 10 mL
10) 1; 3 mL
11) 1; 3 mL
12) 1; 3 mL
13) 0.6; 1 mL or 3 mL
14) 1.9; 3 mL
15) 2.4; 3 mL
16) 1; 1 mL or 3 mL
17) 0.13; 1 mL
18) 0.8; 1 mL
19) 0.3; 1 mL
20) 0.2; 1 mL
21) 0.75; 1 mL
The route is IM; the needle may need to be changed to an appropriate gauge and length.
22) 1.5; 3 mL
23) 0.7; 1 mL or 3 mL
24) 1; 1 mL or 3 mL
25) 0.75; 1 mL
26) 0.5; 1 mL
27) 6; 10 mL
28) 0.8; 1 mL or 3 mL
29) 1.5; 3 mL
30) 2.5; 3 mL
31) 1; 1 mL or 3 mL
32) 2; 3 mL
33) 0.5; 1 mL or 3 mL
34) 0.5; 1 mL or 3 mL
35) 16; 30 units lo-dose insulin
36) 25; 50 units lo-dose insulin

37) 0.3

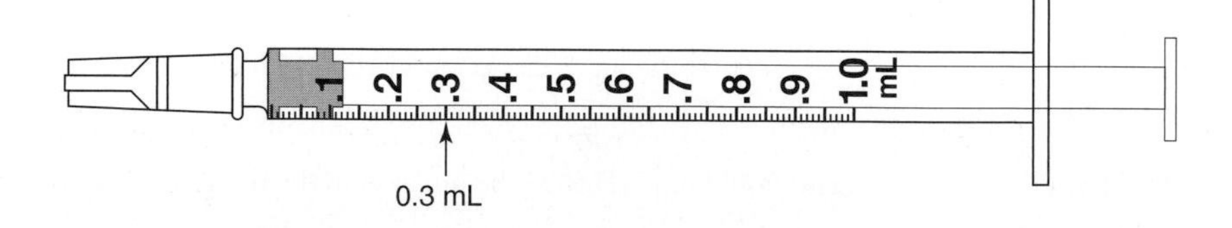

38) 6 mL

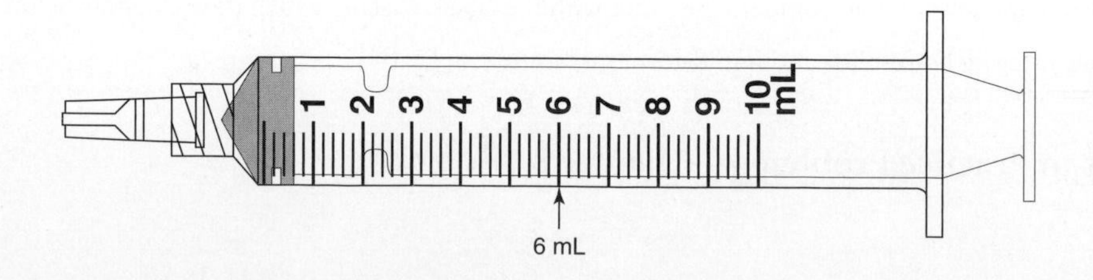

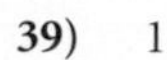

39) 1

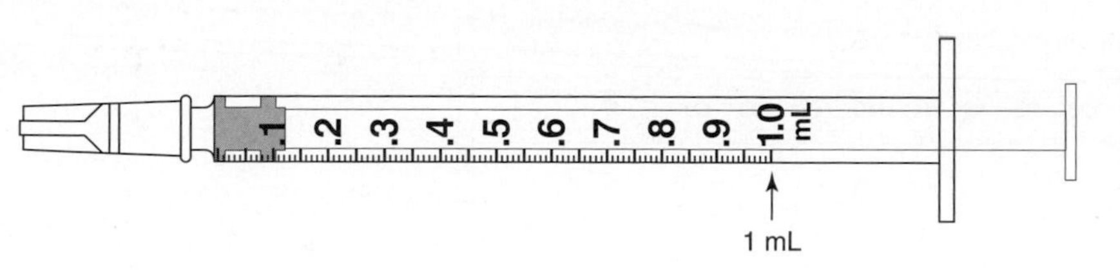

40) 2

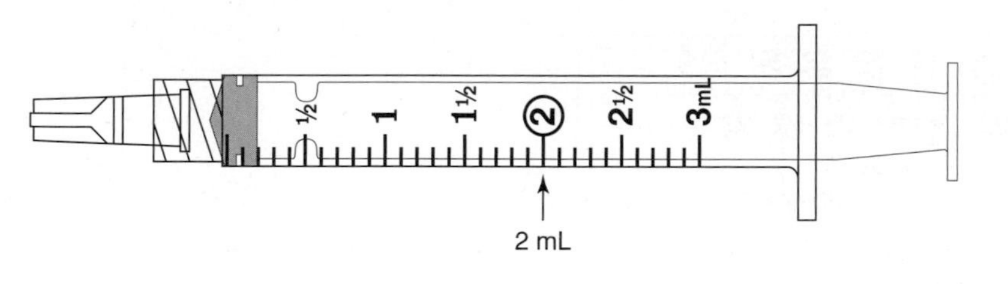

41) 1.2

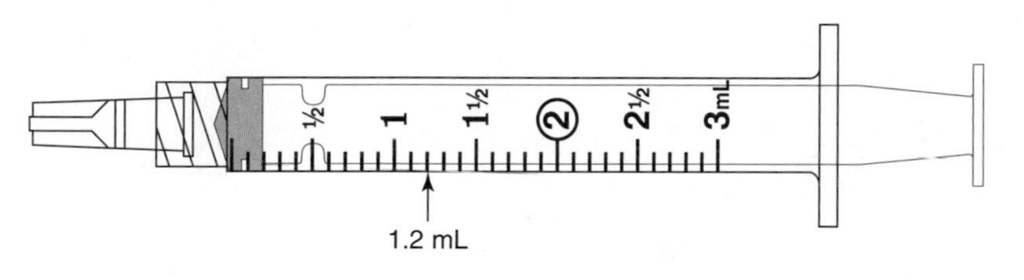

42) 22

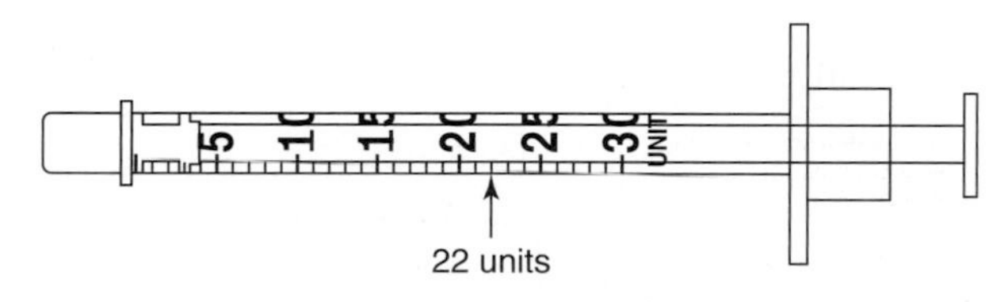

43) 0.9

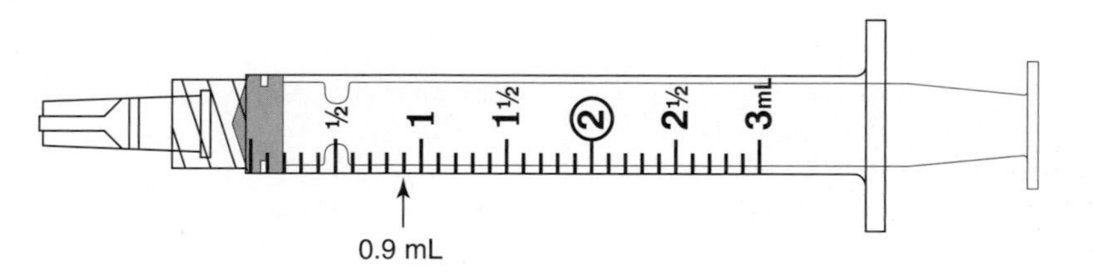

44) 0.5 mL

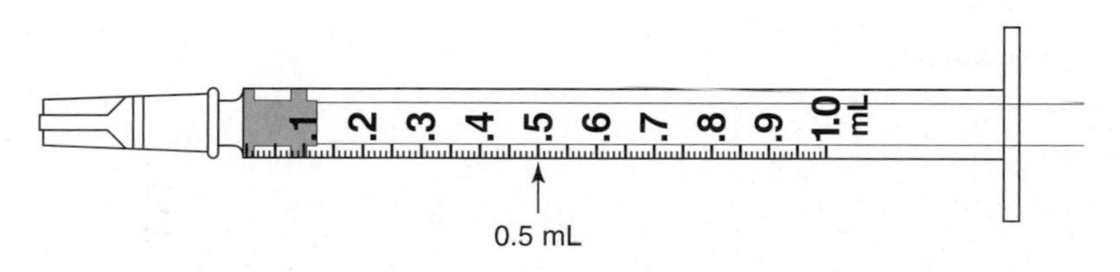

45) 1.4

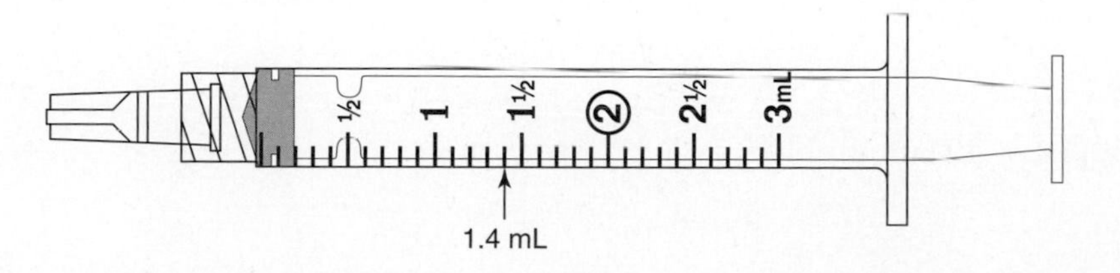

46) 0.75

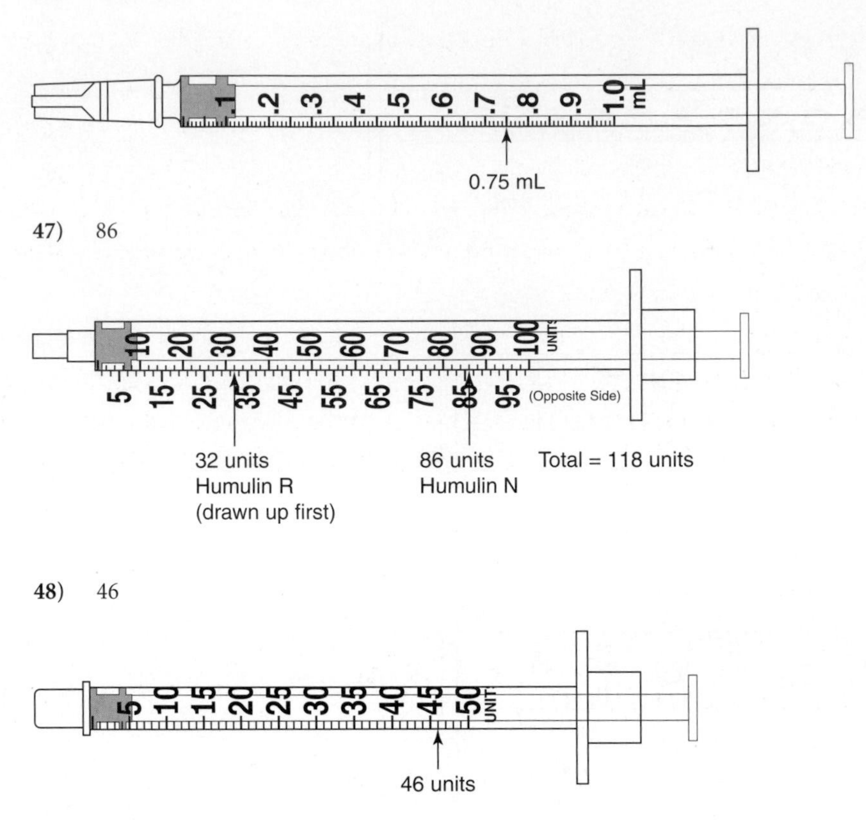

47) 86

48) 46

Selected Solutions to Practice Problems—Chapter 9

3) Order: 2.5 mg

Supply: 5 mg/mL

$$\frac{D}{H} \times Q = \frac{20 \text{ mg}}{50 \text{ mg}} \times 1 \text{ mL} = \frac{2.5 \cancel{\text{mg}}}{5 \cancel{\text{mg}}} \times 1 \text{ mL} = 0.5 \text{ mL}$$

4) Order: 20 mg

Supply: 50 mg/mL

$$\frac{D}{H} \times Q = \frac{\cancel{20} \cancel{\text{mg}}}{\cancel{50} \cancel{\text{mg}}} \times 1 \text{ mL} = \frac{2}{5} \times 1 \text{ mL} = 0.4 \text{ mL}$$

6) Order: 0.3 mg

Supply: 0.4 mg/mL

$$\frac{D}{H} \times Q = \frac{0.3 \cancel{\text{mg}}}{0.4 \cancel{\text{mg}}} \times 1 \text{ mL} = 0.75 \text{ mL}$$

14) Order: 75 mg

Supply: 80 mg/2 mL

$$\frac{D}{H} \times Q = \frac{75 \cancel{\text{mg}}}{\underset{40}{\cancel{80}} \cancel{\text{mg}}} \times \overset{1}{\cancel{2}} \text{ mL} = \frac{75}{40} \text{ mL} = 1.87 \text{ mL} = 1.9 \text{ mL}$$

15) Order: 0.6 mg

Supply: 0.25 mg/mL

$$\frac{D}{H} \times Q = \frac{0.6 \cancel{\text{mg}}}{0.25 \cancel{\text{mg}}} \times 1 \text{ mL} = 2.4 \text{ mL}$$

19) Order: 3 mg

Supply: 10 mg/mL

$$\frac{D}{H} \times Q = \frac{3 \cancel{\text{mg}}}{10 \cancel{\text{mg}}} \times 1 \text{ mL} = \frac{3}{10} \text{ mL} = 0.3 \text{ mL}$$

30) Order: 50 mg

Supply: 20 mg/mL

$$\frac{D}{H} \times Q = \frac{\overset{5}{\cancel{50}} \cancel{\text{mg}}}{\underset{2}{\cancel{20}} \cancel{\text{mg}}} \times 1 \text{ mL} = \frac{5}{2} \text{ mL} = 2.5 \text{ mL}$$

33) Order: 0.5 mg

Supply: 1 mg/mL

1000 mg/2000 mL = 0.5 mg/mL

$$\frac{D}{H} \times Q = \frac{0.5 \text{ mg}}{1 \text{ mg}} \times 1 \text{ mL} = 0.5 \text{ mL}$$

41) Order: 12 000 units

Supply: 10 000 units/mL

$$\frac{D}{H} \times Q = \frac{\cancel{12\,000} \cancel{\text{unit}}}{\cancel{10\,000} \cancel{\text{unit}}} \times 1 \text{ mL} = \frac{12}{10} \text{ mL} = 1.2 \text{ mL}$$

Answers to Application of Clinical Reasoning

9-1) This patient safety incident could have been avoided if the nurse had been more careful checking the label of the insulin vial and comparing the label to the order. The nurse should have checked the label 3 times. In addition, the nurse should have asked another nurse to double-check her as she was drawing up the insulin, as required. Such hospital policies and procedures are written to protect the patient and the nurse.

9-2) This insulin patient safety incident should never occur. It is obvious that the nurse did not use Step 2 of the Three-Step Approach. The nurse did not stop to think of the reasonable dosage. If so, the nurse would have realized that the supply dosage of 100-unit insulin is 100 units/mL, not 10 units/mL.

If you are unsure of what you are doing, you need to ask before you act. Insulin should be given only in an insulin syringe. The likelihood of the nurse needing to give insulin in a tuberculin syringe because an insulin syringe was unavailable is almost nonexistent today. The nurse chose the incorrect syringe. Whenever in doubt, the nurse should ask for help. Further, if the nurse had asked another nurse to double-check the dosage, as required, the patient safety incident could have been found before the patient received the wrong dosage of insulin. After giving the insulin, it is too late to rectify the patient safety incident.

Answers to Practice Problems—Chapter 10

1) 0.194.mL; 12.9; 20 mL or two syringes: 10 mL plus 3 mL; note that piperacillin sodium/tazobactam sodium is further diluted for intravenous administration **2)** 2; 3 mL **3)** 1.5; 3 mL **4)** 9.6; 100; 7.5; 1; 10 mL
5) 1.8; 3 mL; 2

> 06/02/XX, 0800, reconstituted as 280 mg/mL.
> Expires 09/02/XX, 0800. Keep refrigerated. B.S.

6) 10 and 5; 10 and 5 mL; 1 **7)** 2; 225; 1.3; 3 mL; 1; No **8)** 15.6; 62.5 mg/mL; 3.2; 10 mL; single-dose vial, no reconstitution label.
9) 2.5; 334; 1 mL; 3 mL; 2; Yes **10)** 9.8; 5000; 1.5; 3 mL; 6; Yes **11)** 10; 180; 6.9; 10 mL; 1; No
12) 30; 40; 1.5; 3 mL; potentially 8; however, this solution once reconstituted must be used within 8 h so no label.
13) 3.1; 1 000 000; 2; 3 mL; 2; Yes **14)** 1.8; 500 000; 2; 3 mL; 1; No **15)** 2; 225; 1.8; 3 mL; 1; No

16) 60 mL hydrogen peroxide + 420 mL normal saline = 480 mL $\frac{1}{8}$-strength solution

17) 120 mL hydrogen peroxide + 200 mL normal saline = 320 mL $\frac{3}{8}$-strength solution

18) 50 mL hydrogen peroxide + 30 mL normal saline = 80 $\frac{5}{8}$-strength solution

19) 360 mL hydrogen peroxide + 180 mL normal saline = 540 mL $\frac{2}{3}$-strength solution

20) 437.5 mL hydrogen peroxide + 62.5 mL normal saline = 500 mL $\frac{7}{8}$-strength solution

21) 250 mL hydrogen peroxide + 750 mL normal saline = 1000 mL (1 L) $\frac{1}{4}$-strength solution

22) 30 mL Enfamil + 90 mL water = 120 mL $\frac{1}{4}$-strength Enfamil; one 235-mL can. Discard 205 mL.

23) 270 mL Boost Plus + 90 mL water = 360 mL $\frac{3}{4}$-strength Boost Plus; two 237-mL bottles. Discard 204 mL.

24) 300 mL Ensure + 150 mL water = 450 mL $\frac{2}{3}$-strength Ensure; two 235-mL cans. Discard 170 mL.

25) 2880 mL Enfamil − 1800 mL water = 1080 mL $\frac{3}{8}$-strength Enfamil; five 235-mL cans. Discard 95 mL.

26) 20 mL Ensure + 140 mL water = 160 mL $\frac{1}{8}$-strength Ensure; one 235-mL can. Discard 215 mL.

27) 275 mL Ensure + 275 mL water = 550 mL $\frac{1}{2}$-strength Ensure; two 235-mL cans. Discard 195 mL.

28) Use 2 cans; 120 mL discarded.

29) 1050

Answers to Application of Clinical Reasoning

10-1) This type of patient safety incident could have been prevented had the nurse read the label carefully for the correct amount of diluent for the dosage of medication to be prepared. Had the nurse read the label carefully before the medication was prepared, the incorrect medication, loss of valuable time, misuse of healthcare resources, and potential harm to the patient would have been avoided.

Selected Solutions to Practice Problems—Chapter 10

1) Concentration is 0.194/mL

Order: 2.5 g

Supply: 0.194/mL

$$\frac{D}{H} \times Q = \frac{2.5\ \cancel{g}}{0.195\ \cancel{g}} \times 1\ \text{mL} = 12.88\ \text{mL} = 12.9\ \text{mL}$$

4) Order: 750 mg

Supply: 100 mg/mL

$$\frac{D}{H} \times Q = \frac{750\ \cancel{mg}}{100\ \cancel{mg}} \times 1\ \text{mL} = 7.5\ \text{mL}$$

Vial has 1 g ceftriaxone sodium. Order is for 750 mg/dose.

1 g = 1000 mg/vial; 1000 $\cancel{mg}$/vial ÷ 750 $\cancel{mg}$/dose = 1 full dose

9) Order: 350 mg

Supply: 334 mg/mL

$$\frac{D}{H} \times Q = \frac{350\ \cancel{mg}}{334\ \cancel{mg}} \times 1\ \text{mL} = 1.04\ \text{mL} = 1\ \text{mL}$$

1000 $\cancel{mg}$/vial ÷ 334 $\cancel{mg}$/dose = 2.9 doses/vial = 2 full doses/vial available.

14) Order: 1 000 000 units

Supply: 250 000 units/mL

$$\frac{D}{H} \times Q = \frac{\overset{4}{\cancel{1\,000\,000\ \text{units}}}}{\underset{1}{\cancel{250\,000\ \text{units}}}} \times 1\ \text{mL} = 4\ \text{mL}$$

(acceptable for IM dose)

Order: 1 000 000 units

Supply: 500 000 units/mL

$$\frac{D}{H} \times Q = \frac{\overset{2}{\cancel{1\,000\,000\ \text{units}}}}{\underset{1}{\cancel{500\,000\ \text{units}}}} \times 1\ \text{mL} = 2\ \text{mL}$$

(better for IM dose)

22) 12 mL every hour for 10 hours = 12 × 10 = 120 mL total;

$$D \times Q = \frac{1}{\underset{1}{\cancel{4}}} \times \overset{30}{\cancel{120}}\ \text{mL} = 30\ \text{mL Enfamil;}$$

120 mL (solution) − 30 mL (Enfamil) = 90 mL (water); one 235-mL can available

30 mL Enfamil required

205 mL discarded

28) $D \times Q = \frac{1}{4} \times 1400\ \text{mL} = 350\ \text{mL Enfamil.}$

Need 2 cans of 235 mL Enfamil; discard 470 ml − 350 mL = 120 mL

29) 1400 mL − 350 mL = 1050 mL water.

Answers to Practice Problems—Chapter 11

1) 5.5 **2)** 3.8 **3)** 1.6 **4)** 2.3 **5)** 15.5 **6)** 3 **7)** 23.6 **8)** 0.9 **9)** 240 **10)** 80 **11)** 19.5; 19.5; 39; Yes

12) Dose is safe. Give 4 mL.

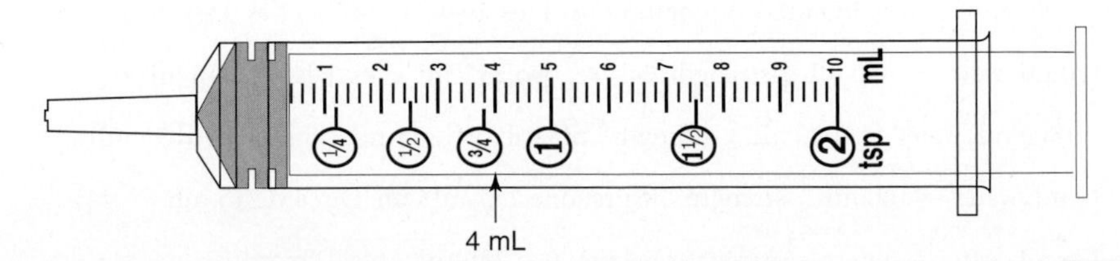

13) 7.3; 1.8; 3.6; No

14) Do *not* administer. It is *not* a safe dosage. The ordered amount is too high. Contact the prescriber to clarify the order.

15) 22.7; 90.8; 45.4; 181.6; 90.8; No (overdose)

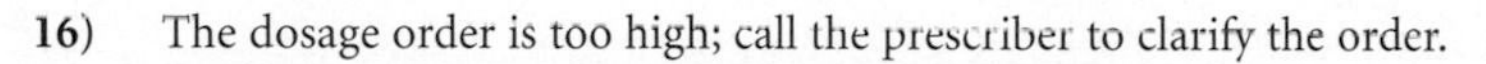

16) The dosage order is too high; call the prescriber to clarify the order.

17) 29.1; 291; 145.5; 436.5; 218.3; Yes

18) 3

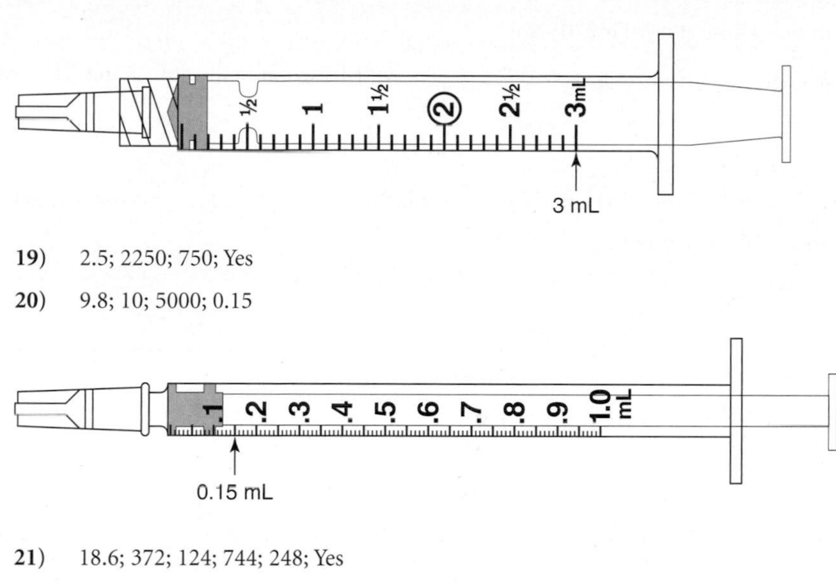

19) 2.5; 2250; 750; Yes

20) 9.8; 10; 5000; 0.15

21) 18.6; 372; 124; 744; 248; Yes

22) 6

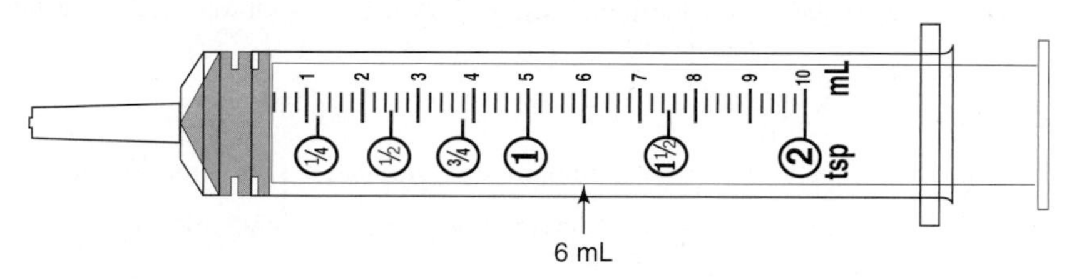

23) 9.3; 418.5; 139.5; 558; 186. Yes the dosage is reasonably safe.

24) 7.4

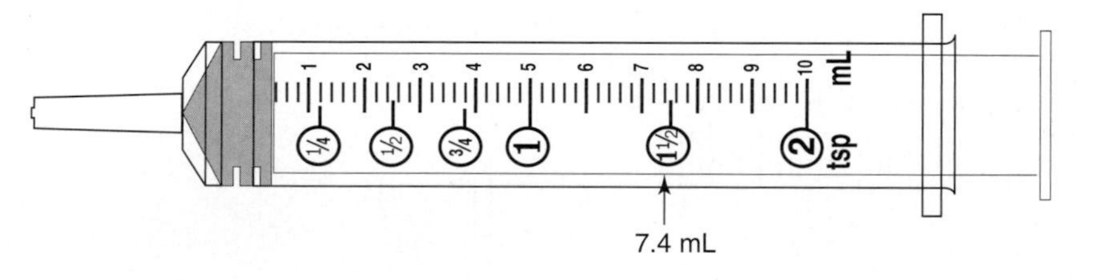

25) 10; 0.1; Yes

26) 0.25

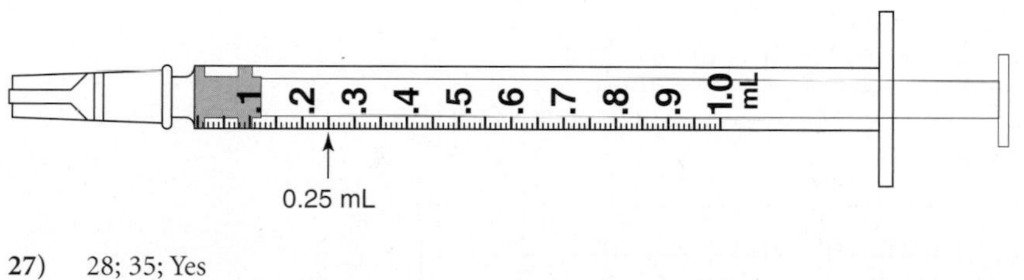

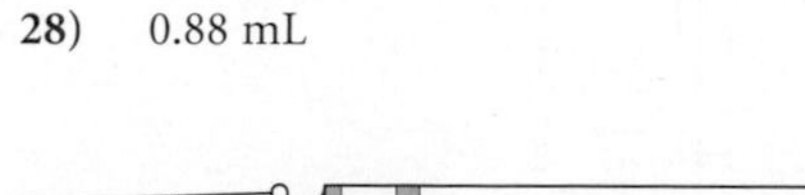

27) 28; 35; Yes

28) 0.88 mL

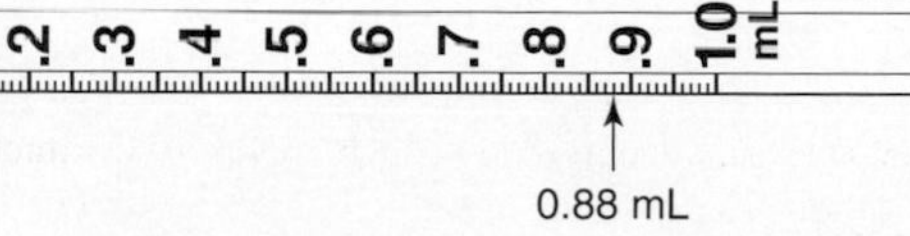

29) 9.1; 227.5; 341.3; No

30) The ordered dosage of 1 g is *not* safe. The recommended dosage range for a child of this weight is 227.5 to 341.3 mg/dose. Physician should be called for clarification.

31) 0.057; The maximum single dose allowed is 0.01; No

32) The dosage is *not* safe; ordered dose of 5 mg exceeds the recommended maximum dose of 3.6 mg. The order should be clarified with the prescriber.

33) 8.2; 82; 270.6; No

34) Dosage is *not* safe; recommended dose of 400 mg IV q8h exceeds the maximum recommended individual dose. The order should be clarified with the prescriber.

35) 20.5; 512.5; 1025; 171; 341; Yes

36) 4 mL

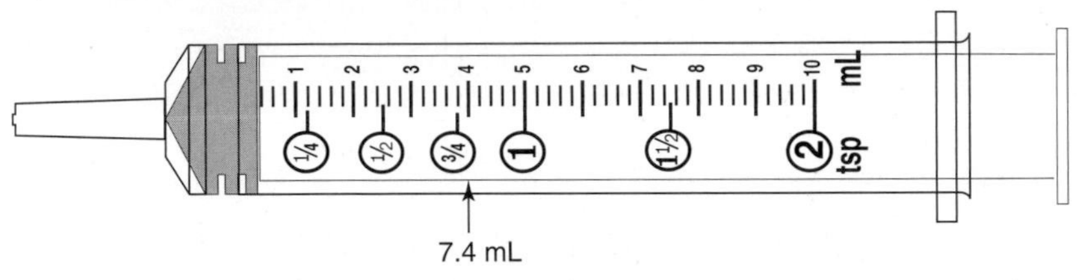

37) 8.2; 123; 61.5; No

38) Dosage ordered is *not* safe. Call prescriber for clarification, because ordered dosage is lower than the recommended dosage.

39) 20.5; 512.5; 128.1; 1025; 256.3; Yes

40) 5 mL (Note: the ordered dose is just slightly below the minimum recommended dose by 3 mg, but this is safe because it is an oral drug. The therapeutic effect between the two doses would not be significant enough to warrant contacting the prescriber.)

41) 23.2; 348; 174; Yes, dosage is reasonably safe. It is 1 mg above the recommended dose.

42) 7

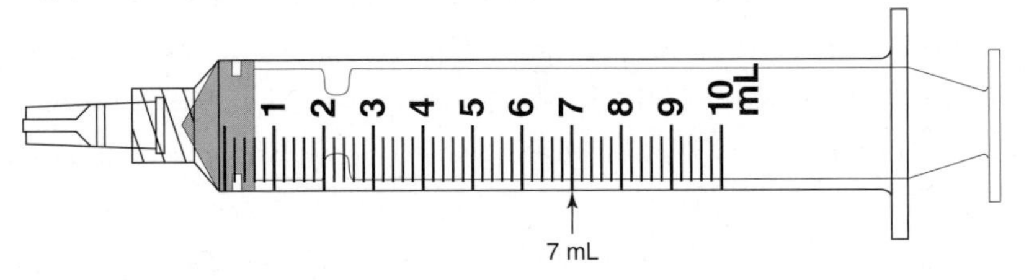

43) The dose is safe. The prescribed dose of 40 mg per day is greater than the minimum required of 21.6 mg/day. Administer 0.25 mL.

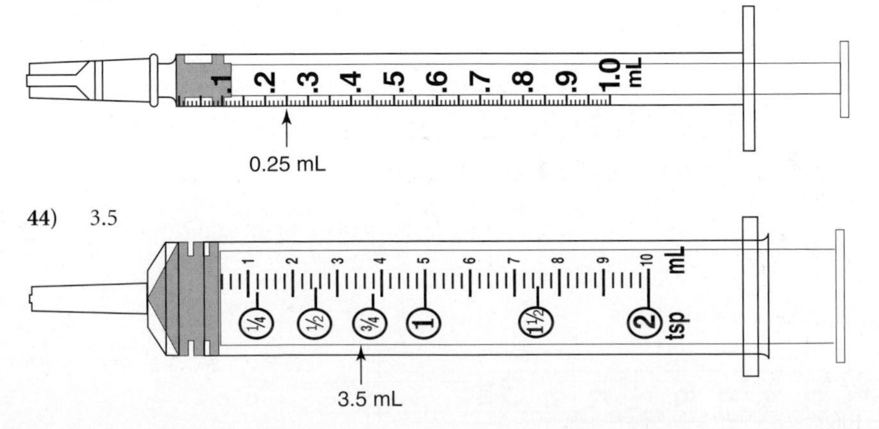

45) 500 000; 0.9

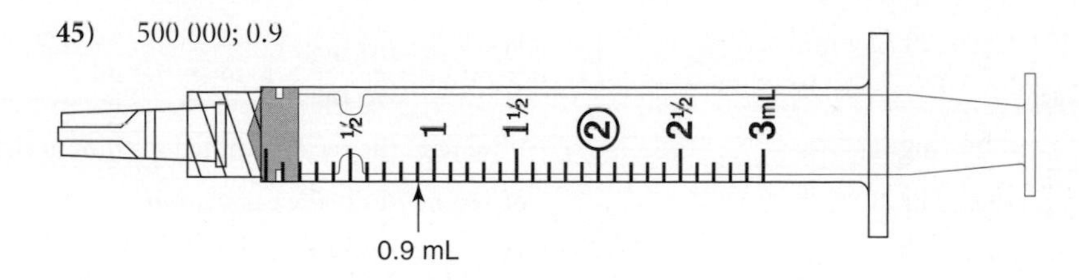

46) Dosage is not safe (overdose). The dose of 1 mg is above the safe range of 0.13 mg to 0.38 mg per dose for this child. Contact the prescriber.

47) The ordered dosage of 20 mg q3 to 4h prn is too high when compared to the recommended dosage range of 9 to 14.8 mg per dose for a child of this weight. The order should be clarified with the prescriber.

48) 0.75

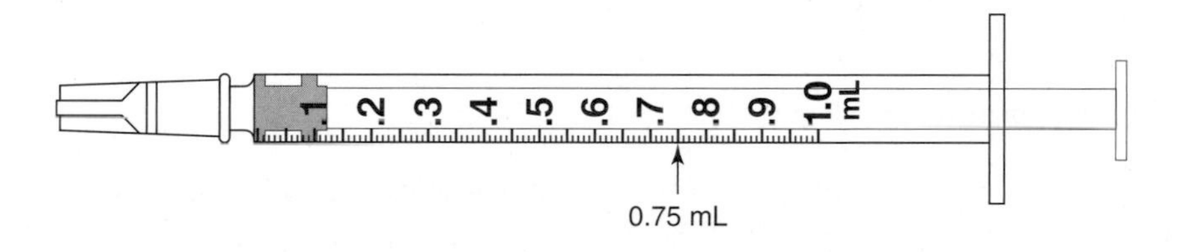

49) #45 (penicillin G sodium) and #48 (cefazolin sodium). (Note: #43 methylprednisolone is a single-dose vial. Check package insert to determine whether storage after mixing is safe.)

Answers to Application of Clinical Reasoning

11-1) The child should have received 75 mg a day and no more than 25 mg per dose. The child received more than 4 times the safe dosage of tobramycin sulfate. Had the nurse calculated the safe dosage, the patient safety incident would have been caught sooner, the resident consulted, and the dosage could have been adjusted before the child ever received the first dose. The pharmacist also should have caught the patient safety incident but did not. In this scenario, the resident, pharmacist, and nurse all contributed to the patient safety incident. If the resident had not noticed the patient safety incident, one can only wonder how many doses the child would have received. The nurse is the last safety net for the child when it comes to a dosage patient safety incident, because the nurse administers the drug.

In addition, the nurse needs to reconcile the fact that she actually gave the overdose. The nurse is responsible for whatever dosage is administered and must verify the safety of the order and the patient's rights. Nurses are held accountable for their actions. Taking shortcuts in administering medications to children can be disastrous. The time the nurse saved by not calculating the safe dosage was more than lost in the extra monitoring, not to mention the cost of followup to the medication patient safety incident, *and most importantly*, the risk to the child.

Selected Solutions to Practice Problems—Chapter 11

1) 1 kg = 2.2 lb; smaller → larger: (÷)

$12 \text{ lb} = 12 \div 2.2 = 5.45 \text{ kg} = 5.5 \text{ kg}$

2) $8 \text{ lb } 4 \text{ oz} = 8\frac{4}{16} \text{ lb} = 8\frac{1}{4} \text{ lb} = 8.25 \text{ lb}$

$8.25 \text{ lb} = 8.25 \div 2.2 = 3.75 \text{ kg} = 3.8 \text{ kg}$

3) $1570 \text{ g} = 1570 \div 1000 = 1.57 \text{ kg} = 1.6 \text{ kg}$

6) $1 \text{ lb} = 16 \text{ oz}; 10 \text{ oz} = 10 \div 16 = \frac{5}{8} \text{ lb}$

$6 \text{ lb } 10 \text{ oz} = 6\frac{5}{8} \text{ lb} = 6.625 \text{ lb}$

$6.625 \text{ lb} = 6.625 \div 2.2 = 3.01 \text{ kg} = 3 \text{ kg}$

17) 64 lb = 64 ÷ 2.2 = 29.09 kg = 29.1 kg

Minimum daily dosage:

10 mg/$\cancel{kg}$/day × 29.1 $\cancel{kg}$ = 291 mg/day

Minimum single dosage: (based on BID)

291 mg/2 doses = 145.5 mg/dose

Maximum daily dosage:

15 mg/$\cancel{kg}$/day × 29.1 $\cancel{kg}$ = 436.5 mg/day

Maximum single dosage: (based on BID)

436.5 mg ÷ 2 doses = 218.25 = 218.3 mg/dose

Dosage ordered is safe. Child will receive 300 mg in a 24-hour period in divided doses of 150 mg BID. This falls within the recommended dosage range of 145.5 mg/dose to 218.3 mg/dose and does not exceed the maximum recommended single-dosage allowance of 250 mg/dose.

18) $\frac{D}{H} \times Q = \frac{\overset{3}{\cancel{150\text{ mg}}}}{\underset{1}{\cancel{5\text{ mg}}}} \times 1\text{ mL} = \frac{3}{\cancel{1}} \times \cancel{1}\text{ mL} = 3\text{ mL}$

19) 2500 g = 2500 ÷ 1000 = 2.5 kg

Recommended daily dosage:

900 units/$\cancel{kg}$/day × 2.5 $\cancel{kg}$ = 2250 units/day

Recommended single dosage:

2250 units ÷ 3 doses = 750 units/dose

Ordered dosage is safe.

23) 20.5 lb = 20.5 ÷ 2.2 = 9.31 kg = 9.3 kg

Recommended minimum daily dosage:

45 mg/$\cancel{kg}$/day × 9.3 $\cancel{kg}$ = 418.5 mg/day

Recommended minimum single dosage:

418.5 mg ÷ 3 doses = 139.5 mg/dose

Recommended maximum daily dosage:

60 mg/kg/day × 9.3 kg = 558 mg

Recommended maximum single dosage:

558 mg ÷ 3 doses = 186 mg

The ordered dosage of 185 mg PO is safe for this child.

24) $\frac{D}{H} \times Q = \frac{\overset{1}{\cancel{187\text{ mg}}}}{\underset{1}{\cancel{125\text{ mg}}}} \times 5\text{ mL} = 7.4\text{ mL}$

If we used the recommended maximum single dosage of 186 mg/dose, the calculation would be

$\frac{D}{H} \times Q = \frac{186\ \cancel{\text{mg}}}{125\ \cancel{\text{mg}}} \times 5\text{ mL} = 7.44\text{ mL};$

which is rounded to 7.4 mL to measure in the pediatric oral syringe; therefore, as indicated above, the ordered dosage is safe.

25) 22 lb = 22 ÷ 2.2 = 10 kg

0.01 mg/$\cancel{kg}$/dose 10 $\cancel{kg}$ = 0.1 mg/dose

0.1 mg = 0.1 × 1000 = 100 mcg

Ordered dosage is safe.

29) 20 lb = 20 ÷ 2.2 = 9.1 kg

Recommended minimum daily dosage:

25 mg/$\cancel{kg}$/day × 9.1 $\cancel{kg}$ = 227.5 mg/day

Recommended maximum daily dosage:

375 mg/$\cancel{kg}$/day × 9.1 $\cancel{kg}$ = 341.3 mg/day

The dosage ordered (1 g q12h) is *not* safe. The recommended dosage range for a child of this weight is 227.5 to 341.3 mg/dose. The prescriber should be called for clarification.

41) 51 lb = 51 ÷ 2.2 = 23.2 kg

Recommended daily dosage:

15 mg/$\cancel{kg}$/day × 23.2 $\cancel{kg}$ = 348 mg/day

Recommended single dosage:

348 mg ÷ 2 doses = 174 mg/dose

Ordered dosage of 175 mg is reasonably safe as an oral medication and should be given.

43) 95 lb = 95 ÷ 2.2 = 43.2 kg

0.5 mg/$\cancel{kg}$/day × 43.2 $\cancel{kg}$ = 21.6 mg/day

21.6 mg ÷ 4 doses = 5.4 mg per dose.

Since the dose should be not less than 5.4 mg, the dose of 10 mg is safe.

Answers to Section 3—Self-Evaluation

1) C; 2 **2)** A; 2 F; 1/2 **3)** J; 2 or G; 1/2 **4)** B; 7.5 **5)** H; 9 **6)** D; 2.5 **7)** E; 3 **8)** K; 1.5 **9)** M; 1.25 **10)** L; 3.5 **11)** E; 0.2 **12)** C; 0.5 **13)** G; 0.2 **14)** A; 4 **15)** D; 6 **16)** F; 7.5 **17)** B; 1.5 **18)** H; 0.75

19)

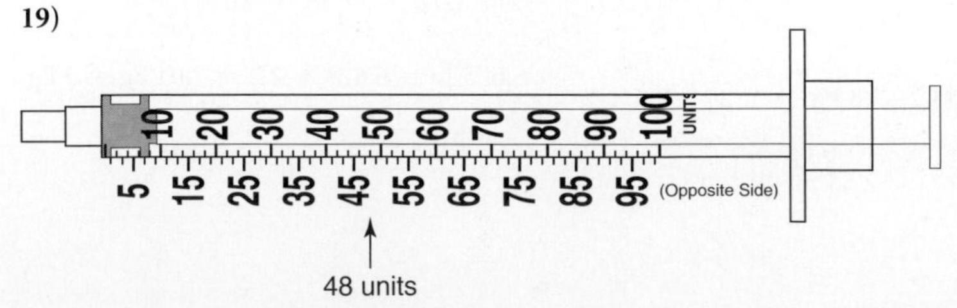

20)

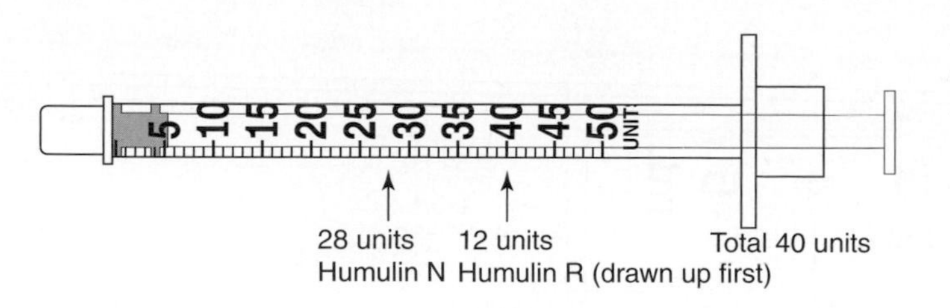

21) 4.8; 5; 100; 4

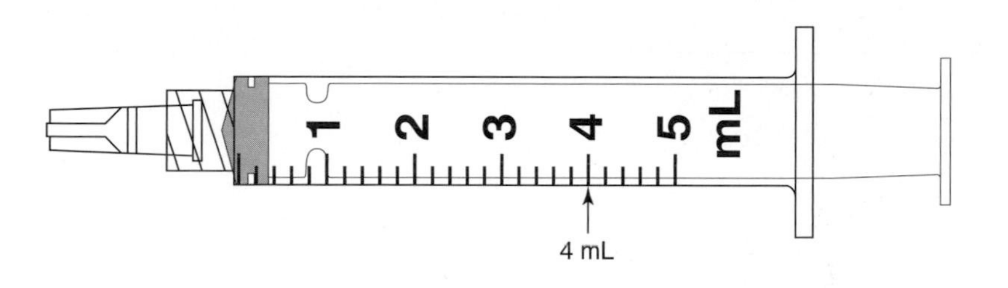

22) 10; 50; 10; 1

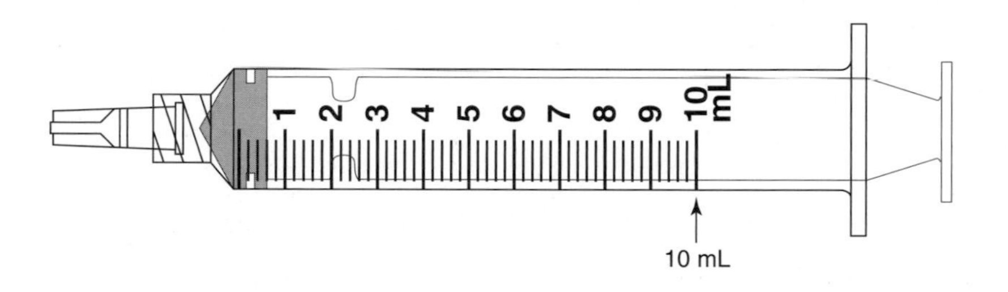

23) 3; 280; 0.71

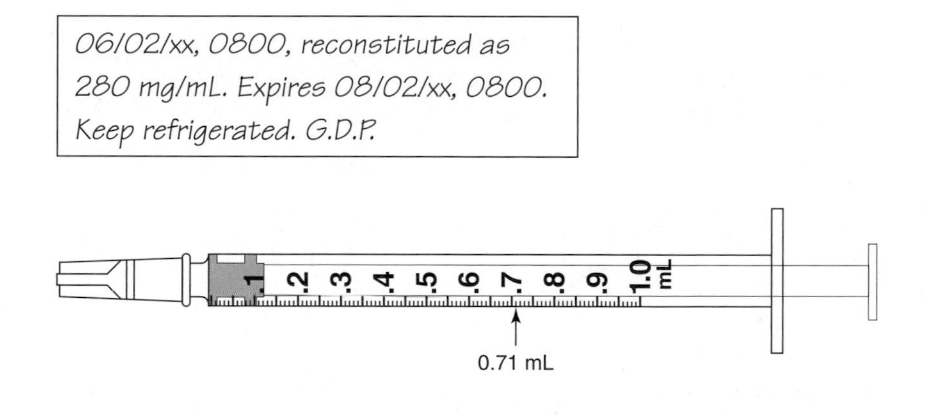

24) 2.5; 334; 2.2

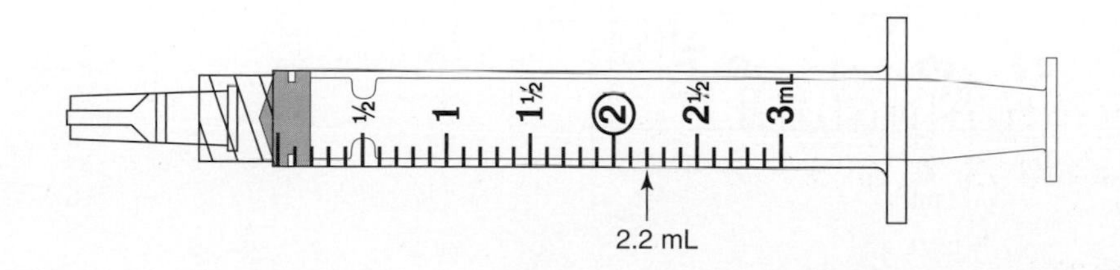

25) 7.8; 8; 62.5; 4; discard unused portion, no label required

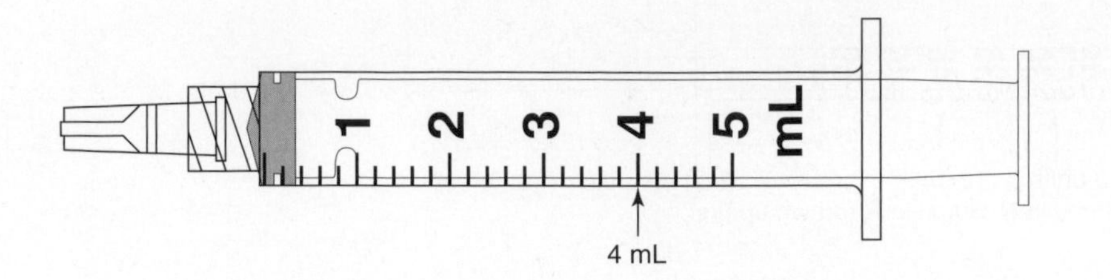

26) 30; 30; 40; 2.5

06/02/xx, 0800, reconstituted as 40 mg/mL. Expires 06/02/xx, 1600. Store at room temperature. B. S.

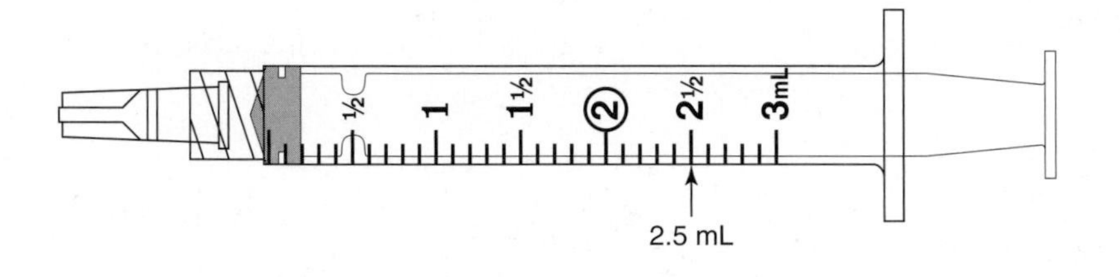

27) 12 doses are available, but the product is only good for 8 hours once reconstituted.

28) The medication will expire before all the doses are completed because the reconstituted vial of tobramycin is stable for only 8 hours at room temperature. The further diluted tobramycin within an IV infusion fluid is stable for 24 hours at room temperature or 36 hours refrigerated. Therefore, if the reconstituted tobramycin is added immediately to four different bags of the IV infusion liquid, the infusion fluid would be good for four doses if refrigerated.

29) 120; 240 **30)** 180; 60 **31)** 1280; 640 **32)** 6; 160 **33)** 3 **34)** 540

35) 1.2

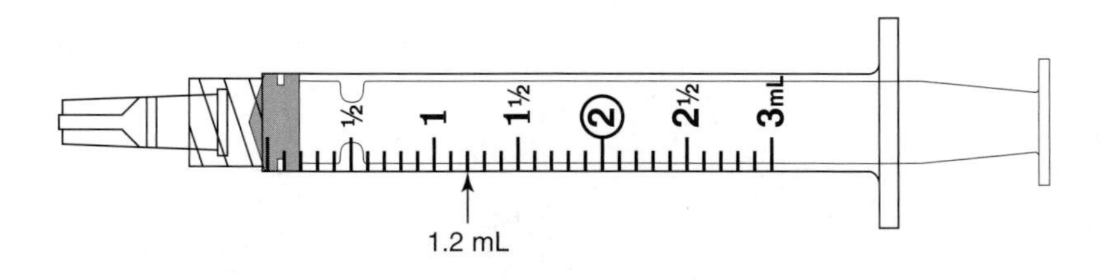

36) 45; 75; 25; 3

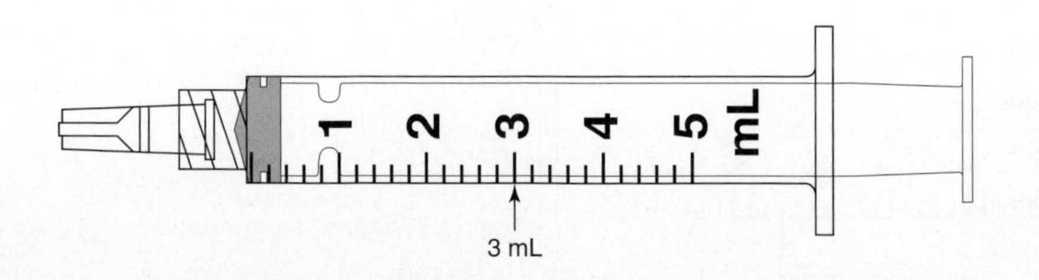

37) Order of 200 mg IV is insufficient for this child considering the circumstances. The prescriber should be called for clarification.

38) 33; 50; 20; 3

39) Order is too high and is *not* safe. The maximum recommended dosage for the child weighing 7.3 kg is 54.8 mg/day or 18.3 mg/dose. The prescriber should be called for clarification.

40) 250; 313

Selected Solutions to Section 3—Self-Evaluation

5) Order: 90 mg

Supply: 50 mg/5 mL

$$\frac{D}{H} \times Q = \frac{\overset{9}{\cancel{90}}\ \cancel{mg}}{\underset{\cancel{5}}{\cancel{50}}\ \cancel{mg}} \times \cancel{5}\ mL = 9\ mL$$

7) Order: 75 mg

Supply: 25 mg/tablet

$$\frac{D}{H} \times Q = \frac{\overset{3}{\cancel{75}}\ \cancel{mcg}}{\underset{1}{\cancel{25}}\ \cancel{mcg}} \times 1\ tablet = 3\ tablets$$

8) Order: 7.5 mg

Supply: 5 mg/tablet

$$\frac{D}{H} \times Q = \frac{\overset{1.5}{\cancel{7.5}}\ \cancel{mg}}{\underset{1}{\cancel{5}}\ \cancel{mg}} \times 1\ tablet = 1.5\ tablets$$

9) Order: 12.5 mg

Supply: 10 mg/mL

$$\frac{D}{H} \times Q = \frac{12.5\ \cancel{mg}}{10\ \cancel{mg}} \times 1\ mL = 1.25\ mL$$

Answer should be left at 1.25 mL because the dropper supplied with the medication will measure 1.25 mL.

35) Recommended dosage:

100 mcg/ $\cancel{kg}$ /dose × 30.5 $\cancel{kg}$ = 3050 mcg (minimum) = 3 mg

200 mcg/ $\cancel{kg}$ /dose × 30.5 $\cancel{kg}$ = 6100 mcg (maximum) = 6.1 mg

Order: 6.0 mg

This dosage is safe.

$$\frac{D}{H} \times Q = \frac{6\ \cancel{mg}}{5\ \cancel{mg}} \times 1\ mL = \frac{6}{5}\ mL = 1.2\ mL$$

36) Minimum daily dosage:

20 $\cancel{mg}$/kg/day × 6.8 $\cancel{mg}$ = 136 mg

Minimum single dosage:

136 mg ÷ 3 doses = 45.3 mg

Maximum daily dosage:

40 mg/$\cancel{kg}$/day × 6.8 $\cancel{kg}$ = 272 mg

Maximum single dosage:

272 mg ÷ 3 doses = 90.7 mg

Ordered dose is safe.

$$\frac{D}{H} \times Q = \frac{75\ \cancel{mg}}{125\ \cancel{mg}} \times 5\ mL = 3\ mL$$

37) Recommended dosage:

15 mg/ $\cancel{kg}$ /day × 20 $\cancel{kg}$ = 300 mg/day (minimum)

Order is insufficient to be effective. The prescriber should be contacted.

38) Recommended dosage:

8 mg/ $\cancel{kg}$ /day × 7.5 $\cancel{kg}$ = 60 mg/day

Ordered dosage of 60 mg is safe.

Reconstitute with 33 mL of water for 50 mL total volume. Concentration is 100 mg/5 mL or 20 mg/mL.

$$\frac{D}{H} \times Q = \frac{60\ \cancel{mg}}{20\ \cancel{mg}} \times 1\ mL = 3\ mL$$

39) Recommended dosage:

Minimum daily dosage:

6 mg/ $\cancel{kg}$ /day × 7.3 $\cancel{kg}$ = 43.8 mg/day;

43.8 mg/day ÷ 3 doses/day = 14.6 mg/dose

Maximum daily dosage:

7.5 mg/ $\cancel{kg}$ /day × 7.3 $\cancel{kg}$ = 54.75 = 54.8 mg/day

54.8 mg ÷ 3 doses = 18.28 = 18.3 mg/dose

Order is too high and is *not* safe. Recommended dosage is 14.6–18.3 mg/dose.

40) 7.5 mg/ $\cancel{kg}$ /day × 125 $\cancel{kg}$ = 937.5 mg/day (maximum)

divided by 3 = 313 mg/dose

6 mg/kg/day × 125 mg = 750 mg/day (minimum)

divided by 3 = 250 mg/dose

Dosage range for this person would be between 250 mg to 313 mg per dose (maximum of 1.5 g/day or 1500 mg/day).

Answers to Practice Problems—Chapter 12

1) 17 **2)** 42 **3)** 21 **4)** 8 **5)** 125 **6)** Assess the patient and the pump. If the pump is programmed at 125 mL/h and is plugged in, discontinue the IV pump and discuss your backup plan with the appropriate nurse leader. **7)** 31 **8)** 21 **9)** Assess patient. If stable, recalculate and reset to 50 gtt/min; observe patient closely. **10)** 3000 **11)** Abbott Laboratories **12)** 15 gtt/mL **13)** 4 **14)** 31 gtt/min **15)** 31 gtt/min **16)** 1930 **17)** 250 **18)** Recalculate 210 mL to infuse over remaining 2 hours. Reset IV to 26 gtt/min and observe patient closely. **19)** 125 **20)** 100 **21)** Dextrose 2.5% (2.5 g/100 mL) and NaCl 0.45% (0.45 g/100 mL) **22)** 25; 4.5 **23)** A central line is a special catheter inserted to access a large vein in the chest. **24)** A primary line is the IV tubing used to set up a primary IV infusion. **25)** The purpose of a saline lock is to administer IV medications when the patient does not require continuous IV fluids. **26)** 10; 5; 0.5; 0.13 **27)** The purpose of the PCA pump is to allow the patient to safely self-administer IV pain medication without having to call the nurse for a prn medication. **28)** Advantages of a syringe pump are that it can: (a) infuse medication directly from syringe; (b) deliver small volumes at a low rate; when drugs cannot be mixed with other fluids or medications or to reduce volume of diluent; and (c) deliver up to 16 different modes. **29)** Every 30 minutes to 1 h, according to institution policy **30)** This IV tubing has two spikes—one for blood, the other for saline—that join at a common drip chamber, or Y connection. **31)** 14 **32)** 21 **33)** 83 **34)** 17 **35)** 25 **36)** 100 **37)** 33 **38)** 50 **39)** 200 **40)** 8 **41)** 11 **42)** 45 **43)** 60; the IV bag will be empty before the nurse returns from lunch **44)** 1248 **45)** 2 h 48 min **46)** 11 gtt/min **47)** (a) 10 h 42 min; (b) select the macrodrip tubing, which is easier to count and provides sufficient flow in the vein; (c) 13 gtt/min **48)** (a) 30 gtt/min; 5 gtt/min; (b) 500-mL bag; select the microtubing, which would be easier to count and would provide sufficient flow in the vein; as well a 500-mL bag of solution is more economical as bags are changed every 24 h **49)** (a) 125 gtt/min; 21 gtt/min; (b) 1000 mL; select the macrodrip tubing, as the rate is sufficient to maintain flow; also the 1000-mL bag, as the amount per hour is such that the bag needs to be replaced every 8 h

Answers to Application of Clinical Reasoning

12-1) This error could have been prevented had the nurse carefully inspected the IV tubing package to determine the drop factor. Every IV tubing set has the drop factor printed on the package, so it is not necessary to memorize or guess the drop factor. The IV calculation should have looked like this:

$$\frac{125\ \cancel{mL}}{\underset{6}{\cancel{60}}\ min} \times \overset{1}{\cancel{10}}\ gtt/\cancel{mL} = \frac{125\ gtt}{6\ min} = 20.8\ gtt/min = 21\ gtt/min$$

With the infusion set of 10 gtt/mL, a flow rate of 21 gtt/min would infuse 125 mL/h. At the 125-gtt/min rate the nurse calculated, the patient received 6 times the IV fluid ordered hourly. Thus, the patient actually received 750 mL/h of IV fluids.

Selected Solutions to Practice Problems—Chapter 12

1) $$\frac{Total\ mL}{Total\ h} = \frac{200\ mL}{2\ h} = 100\ mL/h$$

$$\frac{V}{T} \times C = \frac{100\ \cancel{mL}}{\underset{6}{\cancel{60}}\ min} \times \overset{1}{\cancel{10}}\ gtt/\cancel{mL} = \frac{100\ gtt}{6\ min}$$

$$= 16.6\ gtt/min = 17\ gtt/min$$

2) $$\frac{Total\ mL}{Total\ h} = \frac{1000\ mL}{24\ h} = 41.6\ mL/h = 42\ mL/h$$

drop factor is 60 gtt/mL: 42 mL/h = 42 gtt/min

5) $$\frac{Total\ mL}{Total\ h} = \frac{1000\ mL}{8\ h} = 125\ mL/h$$

7) 1000 mL + 2000 mL = 3000 mL;

$$\frac{Total\ mL}{Total\ h} = \frac{3000\ mL}{24\ h} = 125\ mL/h$$

$$\frac{V}{T} \times C = \frac{125\ \cancel{mL}}{\underset{4}{\cancel{60}}\ min} \times \overset{1}{\cancel{15}}\ gtt/\cancel{mL} = \frac{125\ gtt}{4\ min}$$

$$= 31.3\ gtt/min = 31\ gtt/min$$

8) $$\frac{V}{T} \times C = \frac{125\ \cancel{mL}}{\underset{6}{\cancel{60}}\ min} \times \overset{1}{\cancel{10}}\ gtt/\cancel{mL} = \frac{125\ gtt}{6\ min}$$

$$= 20.6\ gtt/min = 21\ gtt/min$$

9) $\frac{\text{Total mL}}{\text{Total h}} = \frac{1000\text{ mL}}{6\text{ h}} = 166.6\text{ mL/h} = 167\text{ mL/h}$

$\frac{V}{T} \times C = \frac{167\ \cancel{\text{mL}}}{\underset{4}{\cancel{60}}\text{ min}} \times \overset{1}{\cancel{15}}\text{ gtt/}\cancel{\text{mL}} = \frac{167\text{ gtt}}{4\text{ min}}$

$= 41.7\text{ gtt/min} = 42\text{ gtt/min}$

$6\text{ h} - 2\text{ h} = 4\text{ h}$ remaining;

$\frac{\text{Total mL}}{\text{Total h}} = \frac{\overset{200}{\cancel{800}}\text{ mL}}{\underset{1}{\cancel{4}}\text{ h}} = 200\text{ mL/h}$

$\frac{V}{T} \times C = \frac{200\ \cancel{\text{mL}}}{\underset{4}{\cancel{60}}\text{ min}} \times \overset{1}{\cancel{15}}\text{ gtt/}\cancel{\text{mL}} = \frac{\overset{50}{\cancel{200}}\text{ gtt}}{\underset{1}{\cancel{4}}\text{ min}}$

$= 50\text{ gtt/min}$

$\frac{\text{Adjusted gtt/min} - \text{Ordered gtt/min}}{\text{Ordered gtt/min}} = \%\text{ variation:}$

$\frac{50 - 42}{42} = \frac{8}{42} = 0.19 = 19\%$ increase;

within safe limits of 25% variance

Reset infusion rate to 50 gtt/min.

10) q4h = 6 times/24 h; $6 \times 500\text{ mL} = 3000\text{ mL}$

13) $\frac{60}{15} = 4$

14) $\text{mL/h} = \frac{500\text{ mL}}{4\text{ h}} = 125\text{ mL/h}$

$\frac{\text{mL/h}}{\text{drop factor constant}} = \text{gtt/min:}$

$\frac{125\text{ mL/h}}{4} = 31.2\text{ gtt/min} = 31\text{ gtt/min}$

15) $\frac{V}{T} \times C = \frac{125\ \cancel{\text{mL}}}{\underset{4}{\cancel{60}}\text{ min}} \times \overset{1}{\cancel{15}}\text{ gtt/}\cancel{\text{mL}}$

$= \frac{125\text{ gtt}}{4\text{ min}} = 31.3\text{ gtt/min} = 31\text{ gtt/min}$

16) $1530 + 4\text{ h} = 1530 + 0400 = 1930$

17) $\frac{\text{Total mL}}{\text{Total h}} = \frac{500\text{ mL}}{4\text{ h}} = 125\text{ mL/h}$

$125\text{ mL/}\cancel{\text{h}} \times 2\ \cancel{\text{h}} = 250\text{ mL}$

18) $\frac{\text{Total mL}}{\text{Total h}} = \frac{210\text{ mL}}{2\text{ h}} = 105\text{ mL/h}$

$\frac{V}{T} \times C = \frac{105\ \cancel{\text{mL}}}{\underset{4}{\cancel{60}}\text{ min}} \times \overset{1}{\cancel{15}}\text{ gtt/}\cancel{\text{mL}} = \frac{105\text{ gtt}}{4\text{ min}}$

$= 26.2\text{ gtt/min} = 26\text{ gtt/min}$

$\frac{\text{Adjusted gtt/min} - \text{Ordered gtt/min}}{\text{Ordered gtt/min}} = \%\text{ variation:}$

$\frac{26 - 31}{31} = \frac{-5}{31} = 0.16 = -16\%$ decrease; within safe limits

Reset infusion rate to 26 gtt/min.

19) $\frac{\text{Total mL}}{\text{Total h}} = \frac{500\text{ mL}}{4\text{ h}} = 125\text{ mL/h}$

20) $\frac{50\text{ mL}}{30\text{ min}} \times \frac{X\text{ mL}}{60\text{ min}}$

$30X = 3000$

$\frac{30X}{30} = \frac{3000}{30}$

$X = 100\text{ mL/h}$

22) Dextrose 5% = 5 g/100 mL NaCl 0.9% = 0.9 g/100 mL

Dextrose:

$\frac{5\text{ g}}{100\text{ mL}} \times \frac{X\text{ g}}{500\text{ mL}}$

$100X = 2500$

$\frac{100X}{100} = \frac{2500}{100}$

$X = 25\text{ g}$

NaCl:

$\frac{0.9\text{ g}}{100\text{ mL}} \times \frac{X\text{ g}}{500\text{ mL}}$

$100X = 450$

$\frac{100X}{100} = \frac{450}{100}$

$X = 4.5\text{ g}$

26) $\frac{5\text{ mg}}{1\text{ min}} \times \frac{50\text{ mg}}{X\text{ min}}$

$5X = 50$

$\frac{5X}{5} = \frac{50}{5}$

$X = 10\text{ min}$

$\frac{D}{H} \times Q = \frac{\overset{5}{\cancel{50}}\ \cancel{\text{mg}}}{\underset{1}{\cancel{10}}\ \cancel{\text{mg}}} \times 1\text{ mL} = 5\text{ mL}$

Give 50 mg/10 min or 5 mL/10 min; 0.5 mL/min

1 min = 60 sec

$10\text{ min} = 10 \times 60 = 600\text{ sec}$

$\frac{5\text{ mL}}{600\text{ sec}} \times \frac{X\text{ mL}}{15\text{ sec}}$

$600X = 75$

$\frac{600X}{600} = \frac{75}{600}$

$X = 0.13\text{ mL/15 sec}$

31) $\frac{\text{Total mL}}{\text{Total h}} = \frac{1000\text{ mL}}{12\text{ h}} = 83.3\text{ mL/h}$

$= 83\text{ mL/h}; \frac{V}{T} \times C$

$= \frac{83\ \cancel{\text{mL}}}{\underset{6}{\cancel{60}}\text{ min}} \times \overset{1}{\cancel{10}}\text{ gtt/}\cancel{\text{mL}} = \frac{83\text{ gtt}}{6\text{ min}} = 13.8\text{ gtt/min}$

$= 14\text{ gtt/min}$

32) $\frac{V}{T} \times C = \frac{83\ \cancel{\text{mL}}}{\underset{4}{\cancel{60}}\text{ min}} \times \overset{1}{\cancel{15}}\text{ gtt/}\cancel{\text{mL}} = \frac{83\text{ gtt}}{4\text{ min}}$

$= 20.7\text{ gtt/min} = 21\text{ gtt/min}$

33) $\frac{V}{T} \times C = \frac{83\ \cancel{\text{mL}}}{\underset{1}{\cancel{60}}\text{ min}} \times \overset{1}{\cancel{60}}\text{ gtt/}\cancel{\text{mL}} = 83\text{ gtt/min}$

Remember, if drop factor is 60 gtt/mL, then mL/ h = gtt/min; so 83 mL/h = 83 gtt/min

43) 60 mL/125mL/h = 0.48 h × 60 min/h = 29 min; therefore, the 60 mL left will infuse over the 30-min lunch break (the IV bag will be empty before the nurse returns from lunch).

44) 400 mL/75 mL/h = 5.3 h, or 5 h 18 min

0730 + 0518 = 1248

45) $\frac{V}{T} \times C = R$

$\frac{250 \text{ mL}}{T \text{ min}} \times 10 \text{ gtt/mL} = 15 \text{ gtt/min}$

$250 \times 10 = 15 \text{ T min}$

$\frac{2500}{15} \times \text{T min}$

$T = 166.7 \text{ min} = 2.8\text{h} = 2 \text{ h } 48 \text{ min}$

46) $\frac{\text{Total volume}}{\text{Total time}}$

$\frac{250 \text{ mL}}{6 \text{ h}} \times 41.5 \text{ mL/h} = 42 \text{ mL/h}$

$\frac{V}{T} \times C = \frac{442 \text{ mL}}{\cancel{60}_{4} \text{ min}} \times \cancel{15}^{1} \text{ gtt/mL} = 10.5 = 11 \text{ gtt/min}$

47) a) $\frac{V}{T} = \frac{800 \text{ mL}}{75 \text{ mL/h}} = 10.66 = 10.7 \text{ h}$

0.7h × 60 min = 42 minutes. The IV will run for 10 h and 42 min.

b) $\frac{V}{T} \times C = \frac{75 \text{ mL}}{60 \text{ min}} \times 60 \text{ gtt/min} = 75 \text{ gtt/min}$

for microtubing

c) $\frac{V}{T} \times C = \frac{75 \text{ mL}}{60 \text{ min}} \times 10 \text{ gtt/min} = 12.5 \text{ gtt/min}$

= 13 gtt/min for macrotubing

While either tubing could be correct, select the macrotubing, which is easier to count and provides sufficient flow in the vein.

48) a) $\frac{V}{T} \times C = \frac{30 \text{ mL}}{\cancel{60}_{1} \cancel{\text{min}}} \times \cancel{60}^{1} \text{ gtt/}\cancel{\text{min}} = 30 \text{ gtt/min}$

for microtubing

$\frac{V}{T} \times C = \frac{\cancel{30}^{1} \text{ mL}}{\cancel{60}_{2} \cancel{\text{min}}} \times 10 \text{ gtt/}\cancel{\text{min}} = 5 \text{ gtt/mL}$

for macrotubing

b) Select the 500-mL bag of NS IV solution. Although the 250-mL bag could be used, it will empty in approximately 8 h, whereas the 500-mL bag will empty in approximately 16 h (this timing will also depend on the disease process and the rationale for the IV rate).

Select the microdrip tubing. Recall that blood flow in the vein exerts a pressure against a gravity-infused IV solution. If the flow rate is too slow, the blood may back up into the tubing and clot, resulting in the infusion stopping. Therefore, the microdrip tubing at 30 gtt/min will provide a better and easier way to control flow rate than 5 gtt/min with the macrotubing.

49) a) $\frac{V}{T} \times C = \frac{125 \text{ mL}}{\cancel{60}_{1} \cancel{\text{min}}} \times \cancel{60}^{1} \text{ gtt/}\cancel{\text{min}} = 125 \text{ gtt/min}$

for microtubing

$\frac{V}{T} \times C = \frac{125 \text{ mL}}{\cancel{60}_{6} \cancel{\text{min}}} \times \cancel{10}^{1} \text{ gtt/}\cancel{\text{min}} = \frac{125}{6} = 20.8$

= 21 gtt/mL

b) Select the 1000-mL bag of NS IV solution because of the rapid flow rate of infusion. Select the macrodrip tubing. The microdrip tubing needs to be run at 125 gtt/min, which is too many to be counted; therefore, the macrodrip tubing at 21 gtt/min is more easily counted.

Answers to Practice Problems—Chapter 13

1) 1.16; 1.7–2.3; Yes; 2; 0.5 **2)** 0.52; 41.6; 0.83 **3)** 0.4; 100 **4)** 2 **5)** 0.7 **6)** 0.78; 1950 **7)** 2.6 **8)** No **9)** 1.3; 26 **10)** 13 **11)** 0.32 **12)** 1.92 **13)** 1.63 **14)** 0.69 **15)** 1.67 **16)** 0.52 **17)** 560 000 **18)** 1085; 1.09 **19)** 1.9–3.8 **20)** 8 **21)** 40 **22)** 45; 90; 4.2; 30 **23)** 58.8 **24)** 60; 60; 1.9; 45 **25)** 22.8 **26)** 2; 22 **27)** 40 **28)** 6.2; 44 **29)** 93 **30)** 1520; 63 **31)** 1810; 75 **32)** 1250; 52 **33)** 200; 8 **34)** 1500–1875; 250–312.5; Yes; 2.8 **35)** 35; 2.8; 35 **36)** 123; No; it is an underdose; ordered is 100 mg; recommended is 123 mg; contact the prescriber for clarification. **37)** The previous dose was *not* safe. Further calculations should not be done until the prescriber is contacted and the dosage changed. **38)** 330–495; 110–165; Yes; 1.7 **39)** 25; 1.7; 25 **40)** 1800–2700; 300–450; No; exceeds maximum dose; do *not* give dosage ordered. **41)** The previous dose was not safe. Further calculations should not be done until the prescriber is contacted and the dosage changed. **42)** 2 500 000; 6 250 000; 416 677; 1 041 667 **43)** Yes; 2.6 **44)** 20; 2.6; 20

Selected Solutions to Practice Problems—Chapter 13

1) $\text{BSA (m}^2) = \sqrt{\frac{\text{ht (in)} \times \text{wt (lb)}}{3131}} = \sqrt{\frac{85 \times 50}{3131}}$

$= 1.16 \text{ m}^2$

Recommended dosage range:

$1.5 \text{ mg}/\cancel{\text{m}^2} \times 1.16 \cancel{\text{m}^2} = 1.74 \text{ mg} = 1.7 \text{ mg}$

$2 \text{ mg}/\cancel{\text{m}^2} \times 1.16 \cancel{\text{m}^2} = 2.32 \text{ mg} = 2.3 \text{ mg}$

Ordered dosage is safe.

$\frac{D}{H} \times Q = \frac{2 \cancel{\text{mg}}}{1 \cancel{\text{mg}}} \times 1 \text{ mL} = 2 \text{ mL}$

Give 2 mL/min

$\frac{2 \text{ mL}}{60 \text{ sec}} \times \frac{X \text{ mL}}{15 \text{ sec}}$

$60X = 30$

$\frac{60X}{60} = \frac{30}{60}$

$X = 0.5 \text{ mL (per 15 sec)}$

2) $11.4 \text{ kg} \times 2.2 \text{ lb/kg} = 25 \text{ lb}$

$\text{BSA} = 0.52 \text{ m}^2$

$80 \text{ mg}/\cancel{\text{m}^2}/\text{day} \times 0.52 \cancel{\text{m}^2} = 41.6 \text{ mg}$

$41.6 \cancel{\text{mg}}/50 \cancel{\text{mg}} \times 1 \text{ mL} = 0.83 \text{ mL}$

3) $\text{BSA} = 0.40 \text{ m}^2$

$250 \text{ mcg}/\cancel{\text{m}^2}/\text{day} \times 0.40 \cancel{\text{m}^2} = 100 \text{ mcg/day}$

$= 100 \text{ mcg/day}$

4) $\frac{D}{H} \times Q = \frac{100 \cancel{\text{mcg}}}{500 \cancel{\text{mcg}}} \times 10 \text{ mL} = 2 \text{ mL}$

6) $\text{BSA} = 0.78 \text{ m}^2$

$2\,500 \text{ units}/\cancel{\text{m}^2} \times 0.78 \cancel{\text{m}^2} = 1950 \text{ units}$

7) $\frac{D}{H} \times Q = \frac{1950 \cancel{\text{units}}}{750 \cancel{\text{units}}} \times 1 \text{ mL} = 2.6 \text{ mL}$

9) Metric: $\text{BSA (m}^2) = \sqrt{\frac{\text{ht (cm)} \times \text{wt (kg)}}{3600}}$

$= \sqrt{\frac{140 \times 43.5}{3600}} =$

$\sqrt{\frac{6090}{3600}} = \sqrt{1.69} = 1.3 \text{ m}^2$

$20 \text{ mg}/\cancel{\text{m}^2} \times 1.3 \cancel{\text{m}^2} = 26 \text{ mg}$

10) $\frac{D}{H} \times Q = \frac{\overset{13}{\cancel{26}} \cancel{\text{mg}}}{\underset{1}{\cancel{2}} \cancel{\text{mg}}} \times 1 \text{ mL} = 13 \text{ mL}$

11) Metric:

$\text{BSA (m}^2) = \sqrt{\frac{\text{ht (cm)} \times \text{wt (kg)}}{3600}} = \sqrt{\frac{60 \times 6}{3600}} =$

$\sqrt{\frac{360}{3600}} = \sqrt{0.1} = 0.316 \text{ m}^2 = 0.32 \text{ m}^2$

15) Metric: $\text{BSA (m}^2) = \sqrt{\frac{\text{ht (cm)} \times \text{wt (kg)}}{3600}}$

$= \sqrt{\frac{160 \times 63}{3600}}$

$= \sqrt{\frac{10\,080}{3600}} = \sqrt{2.8} = 1.673 \text{ m}^2 = 1.67 \text{ m}^2$

18) $500 \text{ mg}/\cancel{\text{m}^2} \times 2.17 \cancel{\text{m}^2} = 1085 \text{ mg}$

$1085 \text{ mg} = 1085 \div 1000 = 1.085 \text{ g} = 1.09 \text{ g}$

20) $6 \text{ mg}/\cancel{\text{m}^2} \times 1.34 \cancel{\text{m}^2} = 8.04 = 8 \text{ mg}$

21) $8.04 \text{ mg}/\cancel{\text{day}} \times 5 \cancel{\text{days}} = 40.2 \text{ mg} = 40 \text{ mg}$

22) Total volume $= 30 \text{ mL} + 15 \text{ mL} = 45 \text{ mL}$

Flow rate: $\frac{45 \text{ mL}}{\underset{1}{\cancel{30}} \text{ min}} \times \frac{\overset{2}{\cancel{60}} \cancel{\text{min}}}{\text{h}} = 90 \text{ mL/h}$

$\frac{D}{H} \times Q = \frac{420 \cancel{\text{mg}}}{\underset{100}{\cancel{500}} \cancel{\text{mg}}} \times \overset{1}{\cancel{5}} \text{ mL} = \frac{420}{100} \text{ mL}$

$= 4.2 \text{ mL medication}$

Add 4.2 mL med. to chamber and fill with D_5NS to 30 mL.

23) $4.2 \text{ mL}/\cancel{\text{dose}} \times 2 \cancel{\text{doses}}/\text{day} = 8.4 \text{ mL/day}$

$8.4 \text{ mL}/\cancel{\text{day}} \times 7 \cancel{\text{days}} = 58.8 \text{ mL (total)}$

24) Total volume: $45 \text{ mL} + 15 \text{ mL} = 60 \text{ mL}$

Flow rate: $\frac{60 \text{ mL}}{60 \text{ min}} = 60 \text{ mL/h}$

$\frac{D}{H} \times Q = \frac{285 \cancel{\text{mg}}}{75 \cancel{\text{mg}}} \times 0.5 \text{ mL} = 1.9 \text{ mL (med)}$

Add 1.9 mL med. to chamber and fill with IV fluid to 45 mL.

25) $1.9 \text{ mL}/\cancel{\text{dose}} \times 3 \cancel{\text{doses}}/\text{day} = 5.7 \text{ mL/day}$

$5.7 \text{ mL}/\cancel{\text{day}} \times 4 \cancel{\text{days}} = 22.8 \text{ mL (total)}$

26) $\frac{D}{H} \times Q = \frac{\overset{2}{\cancel{500}} \cancel{\text{mg}}}{\underset{1}{\cancel{250}} \cancel{\text{mg}}} \times 1 \text{ mL} = 2 \text{ mL (med)}$

$\frac{65 \text{ mL}}{60 \text{ min}} \times \frac{X \text{ mL}}{20 \text{ min}}$

$60X = 1300$

$\frac{60X}{60} = \frac{1300}{60}$

$X = 21.6 \text{ mL} = 22 \text{ mL}$

Add 2 mL med. to chamber and fill with IV fluid to 22 mL.

27) $2 \text{ mL/dose} \times 4 \text{ doses/day}$

$8 \text{ mL/day} \times 5 \text{ days} = 40 \text{ mL}$

30) $100\ \text{mL}/\cancel{\text{kg}}/\text{day} \times 10\ \cancel{\text{kg}} = 1000\ \text{mL/day}$ for first 10 kg

$50\ \text{mL}/\cancel{\text{kg}}/\text{day} \times 10\ \cancel{\text{kg}} = 500\ \text{mL/day}$ for next 10 kg

$20\ \text{mL}/\cancel{\text{kg}}/\text{day} \times 1\ \cancel{\text{kg}}$

$= \dfrac{20\ \text{mL/day for remaining 1 kg}}{1520\ \text{mL/day or per 24 h}}$

$\dfrac{1520\ \text{mL}}{24\ \text{h}} = 63.3\ \text{mL/h} = 63\ \text{mL/h}$

31) $78\ \text{lb} = 78 \div 2.2 = 35.45 = 35.5\ \text{kg}$

$100\ \text{mL}/\cancel{\text{kg}}/\text{day} \times 10\ \cancel{\text{kg}} = 1000\ \text{mL/day}$ for first 10 kg

$50\ \text{mL}/\cancel{\text{kg}}/\text{day} \times 10\ \cancel{\text{kg}} = 500\ \text{mL/day}$ for next 10 kg

$20\ \text{mL}/\cancel{\text{kg}}/\text{day} \times 15.5\ \cancel{\text{kg}}$

$= \dfrac{310\ \text{mL/day for remaining 15.5 kg}}{1810\ \text{mL/day or per 24 h}}$

$\dfrac{1810\ \text{mL}}{24\ \text{h}} = 75.4\ \text{mL/h} = 75\ \text{mL/h}$

33) $100\ \text{mL}/\cancel{\text{kg}}/\text{day} \times 2\ \cancel{\text{kg}} = 200\ \text{mL}$

$200\ \text{mL}/24\ \text{h} = 8\ \text{mL/h}$

34) Safe daily dosage range:

$100\ \text{mg}/\cancel{\text{kg}} \times 15\ \cancel{\text{kg}} = 1500\ \text{mg}$

$125\ \text{mg}/\cancel{\text{kg}} \times 15\ \cancel{\text{kg}} = 1875\ \text{mg}$

Safe single dosage range:

$\dfrac{1500\ \text{mg}}{6\ \text{doses}} = 250\ \text{mg/dose}$

$\dfrac{1875\ \text{mg}}{6\ \text{doses}} = 312.5\ \text{mg/dose}$

Yes, the dosage is safe.

$1\ \text{g} = 1000\ \text{mg}$

$\dfrac{D}{H} \times Q = \dfrac{275\ \cancel{\text{mg}}}{1000\ \cancel{\text{mg}}} \times 10\ \text{mL} = 2.75\ \text{mL} = 2.8\ \text{mL}$

35) IV fluid volume:

$\dfrac{53\ \text{mL}}{60\ \text{min}} = \dfrac{X\ \text{mL}}{40\ \text{min}}$

$60X = 2120$

$\dfrac{60X}{60} = \dfrac{2120}{60}$

$X = 35.3\ \text{mL} = 35\ \text{mL}$

Add 2.8 mL med. and fill with IV fluid to 35 mL.

40) Safe daily dosage range:

$200\ \text{mg}/\cancel{\text{kg}} \times 9\ \cancel{\text{kg}} = 1800\ \text{mg}$

$300\ \text{mg}/\cancel{\text{kg}} \times 9\ \cancel{\text{kg}} = 2700\ \text{mg}$

Safe single dosage range:

$\dfrac{1800\ \text{mg}}{6\ \text{doses}} = 300\ \text{mg/dose}$

$\dfrac{2700\ \text{mg}}{6\ \text{doses}} = 450\ \text{mg/dose}$

Dosage is *not* safe; exceeds maximum safe dosage.

Do *not* give dosage ordered; consult with prescriber.

42) Safe daily dosage:

$100\ 000\ \text{units}/\cancel{\text{kg}} \times 25\ \cancel{\text{kg}} = 2\ 500\ 000\ \text{units}$

$250\ 000\ \text{units}/\cancel{\text{kg}} \times 25\ \cancel{\text{kg}} = 6\ 250\ 000\ \text{units}$

Safe single dosage:

$\dfrac{2\ 500\ 000\ \text{units}}{6\ \text{doses}} = 416\ 666.6 = 416\ 667\ \text{units/dose}$

$\dfrac{6\ 250\ 000\ \text{units}}{6\ \text{doses}} = 1\ 041\ 666.6$

$= 1\ 041\ 667\ \text{units/dose}$

43) Yes, dosage is safe.

$\dfrac{D}{H} \times Q = \dfrac{525\ \cancel{000\ \text{units}}}{200\ \cancel{000\ \text{units}}} \times 1\ \text{mL}$

$= 2.62\ \text{mL} = 2.6\ \text{mL}$

44) $\dfrac{60\ \text{mL}}{60\ \text{min}} \times \dfrac{X\ \text{mL}}{20\ \text{min}}$

$60X = 1200$

$\dfrac{60X}{60} = \dfrac{1200}{60}$

$X = 20\ \text{mL}$

Add 2.6 mL of med. and fill with IV fluid to 20 mL.

Answers to Practice Problems—Chapter 14

1) 60 **2)** 11 **3)** 14 **4)** 50 **5)** 1 **6)** 12 **7)** 50 **8)** 63 **9)** 35 **10)** 6; 15 **11)** 60 **12)** 45 **13)** 60 **14)** 24 **15)** Yes **16)** 17; 22 **17)** 100; 127 **18)** 102 **19)** 8 mEq **20)** 2 **21)** 5 **22)** 50 **23)** 25 **24)** 7.4 **25)** 12; 18 **26)** 150; 50 **27)** 2 **28)** 35 **29)** 8 **30)** 63 **31)** 80 **32)** 0.4 **33)** 4 **34)** 4 **35)** 100 **36)** 0.2; 200 **37)** 30 **38)** 200; 50 **39)** 5 **40)** 550 **41)** 2450 **42)** 19 **43)** 129 **44)** 13; 39 **45)** 102.3; 80 **46)** 8000; 1000; 8 **47)** 18; 1800; 100; 18 **48)** q6h; 4000; 4; 200; 2; 20

49) Decrease rate by 2 units/kg/h; 18

Answers to Application of Clinical Reasoning

14-1) The nurse who prepares any IV solution with an additive should *carefully* compare the order and medication 3 times: before beginning to prepare the dose, after the dosage is prepared, and just before it is administered to the patient. Further, the nurse should verify the safety of the dosage using the Three-Step Approach (convert, think, and calculate). It was clear that the nurse realized the error when a colleague questioned what was being prepared and the nurse verified the actual order. Also taking the time to do the calculation on paper helps the nurse to "see" the answer and avoid a potentially life-threatening patient safety incident.

Standard Weight-Based Heparin Protocol Worksheet

Round Client's Total Body Weight to Nearest 10 kg: *100* kg
DO NOT Change the Weight Based on Daily Measurements

FOUND ON THE ORDER FORM		
Initial Bolus (80 units/kg)	*8000* units	*8* mL
Initial Infusion Rate (18 units/kg/h)	*1800* units/h	*18* mL/h

Make adjustments to the heparin drip rate as directed by the order form.
ALL DOSES ARE ROUNDED TO THE NEAREST 100 UNITS

Date	Time	APTT	Bolus	Rate Change units/h	Rate Change mL/h	New Rate	RN 1	RN 2
10/05/XX	*1730*	*37 sec*	*4000 units (4 mL)*	*+200 units/h*	*+2 mL/h*	*20 mL/h*	*G.P.*	M.S.
10/05/XX	*2330*	*77 sec*		*−200 units/h*	*−2 mL/h*	*18 mL/h*	*G.P.*	*M.S.*

Signatures	Initials
B. Swart, RN	*B.S.*
M. Smith, RN	*M.S.*

Selected Solutions to Practice Problems—Chapter 14

3) $\frac{50 \text{ mL}}{60 \text{ min}} \times \frac{X \text{ mL}}{30 \text{ min}}$

$60X = 1500$

$\frac{60X}{60} = \frac{1500}{60}$

$X = 25 \text{ mL total volume}$

25 mL (total) − 11 mL of medication = 14 mL D_5W

4) $\frac{\text{mL/h}}{\text{drop factor constant}} = \frac{50 \text{ mL/h}}{1} = 50 \text{ gtt/min;}$

when drop factor is 60 gtt/mL, then mL/h = gtt/min

6) $\frac{D}{H} \times Q = \frac{1200 \cancel{\text{units}}/h}{\underset{100}{\cancel{25\,000}} \cancel{\text{units}}} \times \overset{1}{\cancel{250}} \text{ mL} = \frac{\overset{12}{\cancel{1200}}}{\underset{1}{\cancel{100}}} \text{ mL/h}$

$= 12 \text{ mL/h}$

7) $\frac{D}{H} \times Q = \frac{5 \cancel{\text{mg}}/h}{\underset{1}{\cancel{100}} \cancel{\text{mg}}} \times \overset{10}{\cancel{1000}} \text{ mL} = 50 \text{ mL/h}$

8) $\frac{D}{H} \times Q = \frac{500 \cancel{\text{mg}}/h}{\underset{8}{\cancel{4000}} \cancel{\text{mg}}} \times \overset{1}{\cancel{500}} \text{ mL} = \frac{500}{8} \text{ mL/h}$

$= 62.5 \text{ mL/h} = 63 \text{ mL/h}$

9) $\frac{D}{H} \times Q = \frac{1400 \cancel{\text{units}}/h}{\underset{40}{\cancel{20\,000}} \cancel{\text{units}}} \times \overset{1}{\cancel{500}} \text{ mL} = \frac{1400}{40} \text{ mL/h}$

$= 35 \text{ mL/h}$

10) $1.5\text{L} = 1.5 \times 1000 = 1500 \text{ mL}$

$\frac{1500 \cancel{\text{mL}}}{4 \cancel{\text{mL}}/\text{min}} = 375 \text{ min}$

$375 \cancel{\text{min}} \div 60 \cancel{\text{min}}/\text{h} = 6.25 = 6\frac{1}{4} \text{ h} = 6 \text{ h } 15 \text{ min}$

11) $\frac{D}{H} \times Q = \frac{4 \cancel{\text{mg}}/\text{min}}{\underset{4}{\cancel{2000}} \cancel{\text{mg}}} \times \overset{1}{\cancel{500}} \text{ mL} = \frac{4}{4} \text{ mL/min}$

$= 1 \text{ mL/min,}$

which is the same as 60 mL/60 min or 60 mL/h

12) $\frac{D}{H} \times Q = \frac{3 \cancel{\text{mg}}/\text{min}}{\underset{4}{\cancel{1000}} \cancel{\text{mg}}} \times \overset{1}{\cancel{250}} \text{ mL} = \frac{3}{4} \text{ mL/min}$

$= 0.75 \text{ mL/min}$

$0.75 \text{ mL}/\cancel{\text{min}} \times 60 \cancel{\text{min}}/\text{h} = 45 \text{ mL/h}$

13) $\frac{D}{H} \times Q = \frac{2 \cancel{\text{mg}}/\text{min}}{\underset{2}{\cancel{1000}} \cancel{\text{mg}}} \times \overset{1}{\cancel{500}} \text{ mL} = \frac{2}{2} \text{ mL/min}$

$= 1 \text{ mL/min,}$

which is the same as 60 mL/60 min or 60 mL/h

14) $5 \text{ mcg}/\cancel{\text{kg}}/\text{min} \times 80 \cancel{\text{kg}} = 400 \text{ mcg/min}$

$\frac{D}{H} \times Q = \frac{400 \cancel{\text{mcg}}/\text{min}}{\underset{1000}{\cancel{250\,000}} \cancel{\text{mcg}}} \times \overset{1}{\cancel{250}} \text{ mL} = 0.4 \text{ mL/min}$

$0.4 \text{ mL}/\cancel{\text{min}} \times 60 \cancel{\text{min}}/\text{h} = 24 \text{ mL/h}$

15) Dmg/h/2000mg × 1000 mL = 75 mL/h

$\frac{D}{2} \times \frac{75}{1}$

$D = 150 \text{ mg/h}$

$150 \text{ mg}/\cancel{\text{h}} \div 60 \text{ min}/\cancel{\text{h}} = 2.5 \text{ mg/min,}$

2.5 mg/min within normal range of 1–5 mg/min, so it is safe

16) IVPB flow rate: $\frac{\text{mL/h}}{\text{drop factor constant}} = \frac{100 \text{ mL/h}}{6}$

$= 16.7 \text{ gtt/min} = 17 \text{ gtt/min}$

Total IVPB time:q6h × 1 h = 4 × 1 h = 4 h

Total IVPB volume:4 × 100 mL = 400 mL

Total regular IV volume: 3000 mL − 400 mL

= 2600 mL

Total regular IV time: 24 h − 4 h = 20 h

Regular IV rate: $\text{mL/h} = \frac{2600 \text{ mL}}{20 \text{ h}} = 130 \text{ mL/h;}$

$\frac{\text{mL/h}}{\text{drop factor constant}} = \frac{130 \text{ mL/h}}{6} = 21.7 \text{ gtt/min}$

$= 22 \text{ gtt/min}$

17) IVPB rate:

$\frac{50 \text{ mL}}{30 \text{ min}} \times \frac{X \text{ mL}}{60 \text{ min}}$

$30X = 3000$

$\frac{30X}{30} = \frac{3000}{30}$

X = 100 mL; 100 mL/60 min = 100 mL/h

Total IVPB time: qid × 30 min = 4 × 30 min

= 120 min = 120 ÷ 60 = 2 h

Total IVPB volume:4 × 50 mL = 200 mL

Total regular IV volume: 3000 mL − 200 mL

= 2800 mL

Total regular IV time: 24 h − 2 h = 22 h

Regular IV rate: $\frac{2800 \text{ mL}}{22 \text{ h}} = 127.2 \text{ mL/h}$

$= 127 \text{ mL/h}$

18) $125 \text{ lb} = \frac{125}{2.2} = 56.81 \text{ kg} = 56.8 \text{ kg}$

$3 \text{ mcg}/\cancel{\text{kg}}/\text{min} \times 56.8 \cancel{\text{kg}} = 170.4 \text{ mcg/min}$

$\frac{D}{H} \times Q = \frac{170.4 \cancel{\text{mcg}}/\text{min}}{\underset{100}{\cancel{50\,000}} \cancel{\text{mcg}}} \times \overset{1}{\cancel{500}} \text{ mL} = 1.7 \text{ mL/min}$

$1.7 \text{ mL/min} \times 60 \text{ min/h} = 102 \text{ mL/h}$

19) 1000 mL − 800 mL = 200 mL infused

$\frac{D}{H} \times Q = \frac{200 \cancel{\text{mL}}}{\underset{5}{\cancel{1000}} \cancel{\text{mL}}} \times 40 \text{ mEq} = 8 \text{ mEq}$

$X = 8 \text{ mEq}$

20) $\frac{125 \text{ mL}}{60 \text{ min}} = 2.1 \text{ mL/min} = 2 \text{ mL/min}$

21) $\frac{500 \cancel{\text{mL}}}{100 \cancel{\text{mL}}/\text{h}} = 5 \text{ h}$

22) $\frac{D}{H} \times Q = \frac{2 \cancel{\text{mEq}}/\text{h}}{\underset{1}{\cancel{40}} \cancel{\text{mEq}}} \times \overset{25}{\cancel{1000}} \text{ mL} = 50 \text{ mL/h, or}$

50 gtt/min (because drop factor is 60 gtt/mL)

23) $\frac{D}{H} \times Q = \frac{1250 \cancel{\text{units}}/\text{h}}{\underset{50}{\cancel{50\,000}} \cancel{\text{units}}} \times \overset{1}{\cancel{1000}} \text{ mL} = \frac{1250}{50} \text{ mL/h}$

$= 25 \text{ mL/h};$

25 gtt/min (because drop factor is 60 gtt/mL)

24) $\frac{5 \text{ mg}}{1 \text{ mL}} \times \frac{37 \text{ mg}}{X \text{ mL}}$

$5X = 37$

$\frac{5X}{5} = \frac{37}{5}$

$X = 7.4 \text{ mL}$

25) $10 \text{ units} = 10 \times 1000 = 10\,000 \text{ milliunits}$

$\frac{D}{H} \times Q = \frac{4 \cancel{\text{milliunits}}/\text{min}}{\underset{20}{\cancel{10\,000}} \cancel{\text{milliunits}}} \times \overset{1}{\cancel{500}} \text{ mL}$

$= \frac{4}{20} \text{ mL/min} = 0.2 \text{ mL/min}$ (for first 20 min)

$0.2 \text{ mL/min} \times 60 \text{ min/h} = 12 \text{ mL/h}$

$\frac{D}{H} \times Q = \frac{6 \cancel{\text{milliunits}}/\text{min}}{\underset{20}{\cancel{10\,000}} \cancel{\text{milliunits}}} \times \overset{1}{\cancel{500}} \text{ mL}$

$= \frac{6}{20} \text{ mL/min} = 0.3 \text{ mL/min}$ (for next 20 min)

$0.3 \text{ mL}/\cancel{\text{min}} \times 60 \cancel{\text{min}}/\text{h} = 18 \text{ mL/h}$

26) Bolus:

$\frac{3 \text{ g}}{30 \text{ min}} \times \frac{X \text{ g}}{60 \text{ min}}$

$\frac{30X}{30} = \frac{180}{30}$

$X = 6 \text{ g}$

$6 \text{ g}/60 \text{ min} = 6 \text{ g/h}$

$\frac{D}{H} \times Q = \frac{6 \cancel{\text{g}}/\text{h}}{\underset{1}{\cancel{20}} \cancel{\text{g}}} \times \overset{25}{\cancel{500}} \text{ mL} = 150 \text{ mL/h}$

Continuous infusion:

$\frac{D}{H} \times Q = \frac{2 \cancel{\text{g}}/\text{h}}{\underset{1}{\cancel{20}} \cancel{\text{g}}} \times \overset{25}{\cancel{500}} \text{ mL} = 50 \text{ mL/h}$

29) $\frac{\overset{8}{\cancel{4000}} \text{ mg}}{\underset{1}{\cancel{500}} \text{ mL}} = 8 \text{ mg/mL}$

30) $\frac{D}{H} \times Q = \frac{500 \cancel{\text{mg}}/\text{h}}{\underset{8}{\cancel{4000}} \cancel{\text{mg}}} \times \overset{1}{\cancel{500}} \text{ mL} = \frac{500}{8} \text{ mL/h}$

$= 62.5 \text{ mL/h} = 63 \text{ mL/h}$

31) $80 \text{ units} = 80 \times 1000 = 80\,000 \text{ milliunits}$

$\frac{\overset{80}{\cancel{80\,000}} \text{ milliunits}}{\underset{1}{\cancel{1000}} \text{ mL}} = 80 \text{ milliunits/mL}$

32) $\frac{200 \text{ mg}}{500 \text{ mL}} = 0.4 \text{ mg/mL}$

33) $4 \text{ mg} = 4 \times 1000 = 4000 \text{ mcg}$

$\frac{\overset{4}{\cancel{4000}} \text{ mcg}}{\underset{1}{\cancel{1000}} \text{ mL}} = 4 \text{ mcg/mL}$

35) $220 \text{ lb}/2.2 \text{ lb/kg} = 100 \text{ kg}$

36) $\frac{\overset{2}{\cancel{20}} \text{ mg}}{\underset{10}{\cancel{100}} \text{ mL}} = \frac{2}{10} \text{ mg/mL} = 0.2 \text{ mg/mL}$

$0.2 \text{ mg/mL} = 0.2 \times 1000 = 200 \text{ mcg/mL}$

37) $1 \text{ mcg}/\cancel{\text{kg}}/\text{min} \times 100 \cancel{\text{kg}} = 100 \text{ mcg/min}$

$\frac{D}{H} \times Q = \frac{100 \cancel{\text{mcg}}/\text{min}}{\underset{200}{\cancel{20\,000}} \cancel{\text{mcg}}} \times \overset{1}{\cancel{100}} \text{ mL} = \frac{100}{200} \text{ mL/min}$

$= 0.5 \text{ mL/min}$

$0.5 \text{ mL}/\cancel{\text{min}} \times 60 \cancel{\text{min}}/\text{h} = 30 \text{ mL/h}$

38) IVPB rates:

$\frac{100 \text{ mL}}{30 \text{ min}} \times \frac{X \text{ mL}}{60 \text{ min}}$

$30X = 6000$

$\frac{30X}{30} = \frac{6000}{30}$

$X = 200 \text{ mL}$ (per 60 min)

200 mL/60 min = 200 mL/h (ampicillin sodium)

gentamicin sulfate: 50 mL/h

39) ampicillin sodium: q6h $\times$ 30 min = 4 $\times$ 30 min

= 120 min = 120 $\div$ 60 = 2 h

gentamicin sulfate: q8h $\times$ 1h = 3 $\times$ 1 h = 3 h

Total IVPB time: 2 h + 3 h = 5 h

40) ampicillin sodium:

4 $\cancel{\text{doses}} \times 100 \text{ mL}/\cancel{\text{dose}}$ = 400 mL

gentamicin sulfate: 3 $\cancel{\text{doses}} \times 50 \text{ mL}/\cancel{\text{dose}}$ = 150 mL

Total IVPB volume: 400 mL + 150 mL = 550 mL

41) 3000 mL − 500 mL = 2450 mL

42) 24 h − 5 h = 19 h

43) 2450 mL/19 h = 129 mL/h

44) $4 \text{ mcg}/\cancel{\text{kg}}/\text{min} \times 86.4 \cancel{\text{kg}} = 345.6 \text{ mcg/min}$

$345.6 \text{ mcg}/\cancel{\text{min}} \times 60 \cancel{\text{min}}/\text{h} = 20\,736 \text{ mcg/h} =$

$20\,736 \text{ mcg/h} = 20\,736 \div 1000 = 20.736 \text{ mg/h}$

$= 21 \text{ mg/h}$

$\frac{D}{H} \times Q = \frac{21 \text{ mg/h}}{800 \text{ mg}} \times 500 \text{ mL} = \frac{105}{8} \text{ mL/h} =$

13.1 mL/h = 13 mL/h (initial rate)

12 mcg/kg/min × 86.4 kg = 1036.8 mcg/min

1036.8 mcg/min × 60 min/h = 62 208

62 208 mcg/h = 62 208 ÷ 1000 = 62 mg/h

$\frac{D}{H} \times Q = \frac{62 \text{ mg/h}}{800 \text{ mg}} \times 500 \text{ mL} = \frac{310}{8} \text{ mL/h} =$

38.7 mL/h = 39 mL/h (after titration)

46) 80 units/kg × 100 kg = 8000 units

1000 units/mL

$\frac{D}{H} \times Q = \frac{8000 \text{ units}}{1000 \text{ units}} \times 1 \text{ mL} = 8 \text{ mL}$

47) 18 units/kg/h

18 units/kg/h × 100 kg = 1800 units/h

25 000 units/250 mL or 100 units/mL

$\frac{D}{H} \times Q = \frac{1800 \text{ units/h}}{100 \text{ units}} \times 1 \text{ mL} = 18 \text{ mL/h}$

48) q6h

40 units/kg × 100 kg = 4000 units

$\frac{4000 \text{ units}}{1000 \text{ units}} \times 1 \text{ mL} = 4 \text{ mL}$

Increase rate: 2 units/kg/h × 100 kg = 200 units/h

Increase rate: $\frac{200 \text{ units/h}}{100 \text{ units}} \times 1 \text{ mL} = 2 \text{ mL/h}$

18 mL/h + 2 mL/h = 20 mL/h (new infusion rate)

49) Decrease rate by 2 units/kg/h.

2 units/kg/h × 100 kg = 200 units/h

$\frac{200 \text{ units/h}}{100 \text{ units}} \times 1 \text{ mL} = 2 \text{ mL/h}$

20 mL/h −2 mL/h = 18 mL/h (new infusion rate)

Answers to Section 4—Self-Evaluation

1) 0.9% NaCl **2)** 0.9 g NaCl/100 mL **3)** 0.45 g NaCl/100 mL **4)** 50 **5)** 4.5 **6)** 2.25 **7)** 37.5 **8)** 6.75 **9)** mL/h **10)** 21 **11)** 83 **12)** 1940 **13)** 1536 **14)** Give a total of 3000 mL IV solution per day to include normal saline (0.9% NaCl) with 20 milliequivalents of potassium chloride added per litre (1000 mL) *and* a piggyback IV solution of 250 mg cefazolin added to 100 mL of normal saline (0.9% NaCl) every 8 hours. To administer the order each day, give 900 mL NS with KCl over $7\frac{1}{2}$ hours × 3 administrations and 100 mL NS with cefazolin over $\frac{1}{2}$ hour × 3 administrations, q8h **15)** 120 **16)** 200 **17)** Reset rate to 118 mL/min, if policy and patient's condition permit. **18)** 1410 **19)** 59 **20)** 120 **21)** 5 **22)** 0.48 **23)** 1.3 **24)** 0.47 **25)** 17.4–35.3 **26)** Yes **27)** 18.5 **28)** 37 mL **29)** 120 **30)** 18.5 **31)** 0.8 **32)** 1.6 **33)** Yes **34)** 1.6 **35)** 2; 20 **36)** 7.5 **37)** 7.5 **38)** 43 **39)** 200 **40)** 43 **41)** 200 **42)** 50 **43)** 12 **44)** 15 **45)** 0.13 **46)** 8 **47)** 80 **48)** 20 **49)** 61 **50)** 38

Selected Solutions to Section 4—Self-Evaluation

4) D_5 0.33% NaCl = 5% dextrose = 5 g dextrose/100 mL

$\frac{5 \text{ g}}{100 \text{ mL}} \times \frac{X \text{ g}}{1000 \text{ mL}}$

100X = 5000

$\frac{100X}{100} = \frac{5000}{100}$

X = 50 g

5) D_5 0.45% NaCl = 0.45 g/100 mL

$\frac{0.45 \text{ g}}{100 \text{ mL}} \times \frac{X \text{ g}}{1000 \text{ mL}}$

100X = 0.45 × 1000

X = 450/100 = 4.5 g

10) $\frac{2000 \text{ mL}}{24 \text{ h}} = 83.3 \text{ mL/h} = 83 \text{ mL/h}$

$\frac{\text{mL/h}}{\text{drop factor constant}} = \text{gtt/min}$

$\frac{83\text{mL/h}}{4} = 20.7 \text{ gtt/min} = 21 \text{ gtt/min}$

12) $\frac{V}{T} \times C = R$: $\frac{400 \text{ mL}}{T \text{ min}} \times 15 \text{ gtt/mL} = 24 \text{ gtt/min}$

$\frac{400}{T} \times 15 = 24$

$\frac{6000}{T} = \frac{24}{1}$

24T = 6000

$$\frac{\cancel{24}T}{\cancel{24}} \quad \frac{6\cancel{0}00}{\cancel{24}}$$

$$T = 250 \text{ min}$$

$$250 \text{ min} = 250 \div 60 = 4\tfrac{1}{6}\text{ h} = 4 \text{ h } 10 \text{ min}$$

$$\begin{array}{l} 1530 \text{ hours} \\ \underline{+410 \text{ hours}} \\ 1940 \text{ hours} \end{array}$$

13) $\frac{V}{T} \times C = R: \frac{V \text{ mL}}{60 \text{ min}} \times 10 \text{ gtt/mL} = 32 \text{ gtt/min}$

$$\frac{10V}{60} \quad \frac{32}{1}$$

$$10V = 1920$$

$$\frac{10V}{10} = \frac{1920}{10}$$

$$V = 192 \text{ mL/h}; 192 \text{ mL}/\cancel{h} \times 8 \cancel{h} = 1536 \text{ mL}$$

(administered during your 8-h shift)

15) $\frac{2700 \text{ mL}}{22.5 \text{ h}} = 120 \text{ mL/h}$

16) $\frac{100 \text{ mL}}{30 \text{ min}} \quad \frac{X \text{ mL}}{60 \text{ min}}$

$$30X = 6000$$

$$\frac{30X}{30} = \frac{6000}{30}$$

$$X = 200 \text{ mL}$$

$200 \text{ mL}/60 \text{ min} = 200 \text{ mL/h}$

17) $\frac{1200 \cancel{\text{mL}}}{100 \cancel{\text{mL}}/\text{h}}$ 12 h (total time ordered to infuse 1200 mL)

$$\begin{array}{l} 2200 \text{ hours (current time)} \\ \underline{-1530} \text{ hours (start time)} \\ 0630 = 6 \text{ h } 30 \text{ min (elapsed time)} \end{array}$$

IV has run for $6\frac{1}{2}$ h so $5\frac{1}{2}$ h remaining

$$\frac{\text{remaining volume}}{\text{remaining time}} = \frac{650 \text{ mL}}{5.5 \text{ h}} = 118 \text{ mL/h}$$

(adjusted rate)

$$\frac{\text{Adjusted gtt/min} - \text{Ordered gtt/min}}{\text{Ordered gtt/min}} = \% \text{ of variation;}$$

$$\frac{118 - 100}{100} = \frac{18}{100} = 0.18 = 18\% \text{(variance is safe)}$$

If policy and patient's condition permit, reset rate to 118 mL/h.

18) 1st 10 kg: $100 \text{ mL}/\cancel{\text{kg}}/\text{day} \times 10 \cancel{\text{kg}} = 1000 \text{ mL/day}$

Remaining 8.2 kg: $50\text{mL}/\cancel{\text{kg}}/\text{day} \times 8.2 \cancel{\text{kg}} = \underline{410 \text{ mL/day}}$

1410mL/day

19) $\frac{1410 \text{ mL}}{24 \text{ h}} = 58.7 \text{ mL/h} = 59 \text{ mL/h}$

20) $1185 \text{ g} = 1185 \div 1000 = 1.185 \text{ kg} = 1.2 \text{ kg}$

1st 10 kg: $100 \text{ mL}/\cancel{\text{kg}}/\text{day} \times 1.2 \cancel{\text{kg}} = 120 \text{ mL/day}$

21) $\frac{120 \text{ mL}}{24 \text{ h}} = 5 \text{ mL/h}$

22) $\text{BSA (m}^2) = \sqrt{\frac{\text{ht (cm)} \times \text{wt (kg)}}{3600}} = \sqrt{\frac{77 \times 11}{3600}} =$

$$\sqrt{\frac{847}{3600}} = \sqrt{0.235} = 0.48 \text{ m}^2$$

23) $\text{BSA (m}^2) = \sqrt{\frac{\text{ht (cm)} \times \text{wt (kg)}}{3600}} = \sqrt{\frac{155 \times 39}{3600}} =$

$$\sqrt{1.679} = 1.295 \text{ m}^2 = 1.30 \text{ m}^2$$

25) Minimum safe dosage: $37 \text{ mg}/\cancel{\text{m}^2} \times 0.47 \cancel{\text{m}^2} = 17.4 \text{ mg}$

Maximum safe dosage: $75\text{mg}/\cancel{\text{m}^2} \times 0.47 \cancel{\text{m}^2} = 35.3 \text{ mg}$

27) $\frac{D}{H} \times Q = \frac{18.5 \cancel{\text{mg}}}{1 \cancel{\text{mg}}} \times 1 \text{ mL} = 18.5 \text{ mL}$

28) $2 \text{ mL}/\cancel{\text{mg}} \times 18.5 \cancel{\text{mg}} = 37 \text{ mL}$

29) $\frac{D}{H} \times Q = \frac{1 \cancel{\text{mg}}/\text{min}}{18.5 \cancel{\text{mg}}} \times 37 \text{ mL} = 2 \text{ mL/min}$

$2 \text{ mL}/\cancel{\text{min}} \times 60 \cancel{\text{min}}/\text{h} = 120 \text{ mL/h}$

30) At 1 mg/min, 18.5 mg will infuse in 18.5 min.

$$\frac{1 \text{ mg}}{1 \text{ min}} \quad \frac{18.5 \text{ mg}}{X \text{ min}}$$

$$X = 18.5 \text{ min}$$

32) $2 \text{ mg}/\cancel{\text{m}^2} \times 0.8 \cancel{\text{m}^2} = 1.6 \text{ mg}$

35) $\frac{D}{H} \times Q = \frac{\cancel{250 \text{ mg}}}{\cancel{125 \text{ mg}}} \times 1 \text{ mL} = 2 \text{ mL (cefazolin)}$

$$\frac{40 \text{ mL}}{60 \text{ min}} \quad \frac{X \text{ mL}}{30 \text{ min}}$$

$$60X = 1200$$

$$\frac{60X}{60} = \frac{1200}{60}$$

$$X = 20 \text{ mL}$$

36) $300 \text{ mcg/kg} \times 25 \text{ kg} = 7500 \text{ mg}$

$7500 \text{ mcg} \div 1000 = 7.5 \text{ mg}$

38) Total IVPB volume: $100 \text{ mL} \times 6 = 600 \text{ mL}$

Regular IV volume: $1500 \text{ mL} - 600 \text{ mL} = 900 \text{ mL}$

Total IVPB time of q4h: 30 min: $6 \times 30 \text{ min} = 180 \text{ min} = 180 \div 60 = 3 \text{ h}$

Total regular IV time: $24 \text{ h} - 3 \text{ h} = 21 \text{ h}$

Regular IV rate: mL/h $= \frac{900 \text{ mL}}{21 \text{ h}} = 42.8$ mL/h $=$ 43 mL/h

or 43 gtt/min because mL/h = gtt/min when drop factor is 60 gtt/mL.

$$\frac{\text{mL/h}}{\text{drop factor constant}} = \text{gtt/min}; \frac{43 \text{ mL/h}}{1} = 43 \text{ gtt/min}$$

39) $\frac{100 \text{ mL}}{30 \text{ min}} \times \frac{X \text{ mL}}{60 \text{ min}}$

$30X = 6000$

$\frac{30X}{30} = \frac{6000}{30}$

X = 200 mL; 200 mL/60 min = 200 mL/h or 200 gtt/min (because drop factor is 60 gtt/mL)

40) See #38, regular IV rate calculated at 42.8 mL/h or 43 mL/h.

41) See #39, IVPB rate calculated at 200 mL/h.

42) $\frac{D}{H} \times Q = \frac{\overset{1}{\cancel{2}} \cancel{\text{mEq}}/\text{h}}{\underset{20}{\cancel{40}} \cancel{\text{mEq}}} \times 1000 \text{ mL} = 50 \text{ mL/h}$

43) $\frac{5 \text{ mcg/min}}{25\,000 \text{ mcg}} \times 1000 \text{ mL}$

$= 0.2 \text{ mL/min} \times 60 \text{ min/h} = 12 \text{ mL/h}$

44) $\frac{15 \text{ units}}{1 \text{ L}} = \frac{15.000.}{1.000.} = \frac{15\,\cancel{000} \ \cancel{\text{milliunits}}}{1\cancel{000} \text{ mL}} =$ 15 $\cancel{\text{milliunits}}$/mL

45) $\frac{D}{H} \times Q = \frac{2 \ \cancel{\text{milliunits}}/\text{min}}{15 \ \cancel{\text{milliunits}}} \times 1 \text{ mL} =$ $\frac{2}{15}$ mL/min = 0.13 mL/min

46) $0.13 \text{ mL}/\cancel{\text{min}} \times 60 \ \cancel{\text{min}}/\text{h} = 7.8 = 8 \text{ mL/h}$

47) $\frac{\overset{4}{\cancel{20}} \ \cancel{\text{milliunits}}/\text{min}}{\underset{3}{\cancel{15}} \ \cancel{\text{milliunits}}} \times 1 \text{ mL} = \frac{4}{3} \text{ mL/min} =$ 1.33 mL/min

$1.33 \text{ mL}/\cancel{\text{min}} \times 60 \ \cancel{\text{min}}/\text{h} = 80 \text{ mL/h}$

48) $4 \text{ mcg}/\cancel{\text{kg}}/\text{min} \times 68 \ \cancel{\text{kg}} = 272 = 272 \text{ mcg/min}$

$\frac{272 \text{ mcg/min}}{400\,000 \text{ mcg}} \times 500 \text{ mL}$

$= 0.34 \text{ mL/min} \times 60 \text{ min/h} = 20 \text{ mL/h}$

49) $12 \text{ mcg/kg/min} \times 68 \text{ kg} = 816 \text{ mcg/min}$

$\frac{816 \text{ mcg/min}}{400\,000 \text{ mcg}} \times 500 \text{ mL}$

$= 1.02 \text{ mL/min} \times 60 \text{ min/h} = 61 \text{ mL/h}$

50) $\frac{D}{H} \times Q = \frac{750 \ \cancel{\text{units}}/\text{h}}{\underset{20}{\cancel{10\,000}} \ \cancel{\text{units}}} \times \cancel{500} \text{ mL} = \frac{750}{20} \text{ mL/h} =$

37.5 mL/h = 38 mL/h

APPENDIX B

Systems of Measurement

The apothecary system was the first system of medication measurement used by pharmacists and physicians. It originated in Greece and made its way to England through Rome and France. The English used the apothecary system during the late 1600s, and the colonists brought it to North America. A modified system of measurement for everyday use evolved and is now recognized as the household system.

The Apothecary System

New learners consider apothecary notations complicated. Instead of using the Arabic number system with symbols called digits (e.g., 1, 2, 3, 4, 5), the apothecary system uses the Roman numeral system, and quantities are represented by symbols (e.g., i, v, x). The Roman numeral system uses seven basic symbols and their various combinations to represent all the numbers in the Arabic number system. The most common numeral symbols used in dosage calculations are i, v, and x.

For further information regarding the apothecary system of measurement and its use in medication dosages, see Appendix C.

The Household System

Household units are likely to be used by the patient at home where hospital measuring devices are not available. The healthcare provider who is familiar with the household system will be able to provide patient education in an understandable language. Even though there is no standardized system of notation, usually the quantity, in Arabic numbers and fractions, is expressed first. An abbreviation of the unit follows the quantity. For the purpose of medication dosages, common household units and International System of Units (SI) equivalent units are given below.

Household Unit	Equivalent SI Unit
1 teaspoon	5 mL
1 tablespoon	15 mL
1 fluid ounce	30 mL
1 cup	250 mL*
1 quart	1 L*

* These are not exact equivalents but are commonly used as such.

For further information regarding the household system of measurement and its use in medication dosages, see Appendix D.

The International System of Units[1]

BASE QUANTITIES AND BASE UNITS USED IN SI

Base Quantity	Base Unit	Symbol
Length	Metre	m
Mass	Kilogram	kg
Time, duration	Second	s
Electric current	Ampere	A
Thermodynamic temperature	Kelvin	K
Amount of substance	Mole	mol
Luminous intensity	Candela	cd

[1] Bureau International des Poids et Mesures. (2011). The international system of units (SI). Retrieved from www.bipm.org/en/si/.

SI PREFIXES

Factor	Prefix	Symbol	Factor	Prefix	Symbol
10^{1}	Deca	da	10^{-1}	Deci	d
10^{2}	Hecto	h	10^{-2}	Centi	c
10^{3}	Kilo	k	10^{-3}	Milli	m
10^{6}	Mega	M	10^{-6}	Micro	μ, mc*
10^{9}	Giga	G	10^{-9}	Nano	n
10^{12}	Tera	T	10^{-12}	Pico	p
10^{15}	Peta	P	10^{-15}	Femto	f
10^{18}	Exa	E	10^{-18}	Atto	a
10^{21}	Zeta	Z	10^{-21}	Zepto	z
10^{24}	Yotta	Y	10^{-24}	Yocto	y

* The official SI symbol of micro is μ but in the health sector, in order to reduce the incidence of transcribing errors, the preferred form is mc.

APPENDIX C

The Apothecary System of Measurement

COMMON ROMAN NUMERALS USED IN MEDICATION DOSAGES

Arabic Numeral	Roman Notation	Apothecary Number	Arabic Numeral	Roman Notation	Apothecary Number
1	I	i, $\overline{\text{i}}$	8	VIII	viii, $\overline{\text{viii}}$
2	II	ii, $\overline{\text{ii}}$	9	IX	ix, $\overline{\text{ix}}$
3	III	iii, $\overline{\text{iii}}$	10	X	x, $\overline{\text{x}}$
4	IV	iv, $\overline{\text{iv}}$	15	XV	xv, $\overline{\text{xv}}$
5	V	v, $\overline{\text{v}}$	20	XX	xx, $\overline{\text{xx}}$
6	VI	vi, $\overline{\text{vi}}$	25	XXV	xxv, $\overline{\text{xxv}}$
7	VII	vii, $\overline{\text{vii}}$	30	XXX	xxx, $\overline{\text{xxx}}$

MATH TIP

To reduce the number of errors interpreting medical notation, a line can be drawn over the lower case Roman numerals to distinguish them from other letters in a word or phrase. The lower case *i* is dotted above, not below, the line.

Example:

℥ iii or $\overline{\text{iii}}$ is the apothecary notation for 3 ounces.

Because Canada sometimes uses the same manufacturers as our southern neighbour, the United States, healthcare providers may occasionally encounter syringes and medicine cups that identify the minim and dram scales. Special care is needed to avoid confusing the markings for minims and drams with the medication doses required.

In the apothecary system, weight, length, and a couple of volume units have no readily used equivalents in medication calculations. The following table lists the apothecary units of measurement and essential equivalents of volume that may be encountered in reading drug dosages.

APOTHECARY UNITS, ABBREVIATIONS, AND THEIR EQUIVALENTS

Unit	Abbreviation	Equivalent
Grain	gr	
Quart	qt	qt i = pt ii
Pint	pt	pt i = ℥ 16
Ounce or fluid ounce	℥	qt i = ℥ 32
Dram	ʒ	
Minim	D	

Note: The minim (D) and fluid dram (ʒ) are given only so that you will be able to recognize them.

MATH TIP

The symbols for ounce and dram are very similar. To help remember which is which, remember this: The ounce (℥) is a larger unit than the dram, and its symbol has one more loop than the dram (ʒ), or there is "more bounce to the ounce."

CAUTION

Notice that the abbreviations for the apothecary grain (*gr*) and the metric gram (*g*) can be confusing. The rule of putting the abbreviation or symbol before the quantity in apothecary measurement further distinguishes it from a metric measurement. If you are ever doubtful about the meaning that is intended, be sure to ask the writer for clarification.

QUICK REVIEW

In the apothecary system,

- The common units for dosage calculation are grain (gr) and ounce (℥).
- The quantity is best expressed in lower case Roman numerals. Amounts greater than 10 may be expressed in Arabic numbers, *except* 15 (xv), 20 (xx), and 30 (xxx).
- Quantities less than 1 are expressed as fractions, *except* $\frac{1}{2}$. One-half $\left(\frac{1}{2}\right)$ is expressed by the symbol *ss*.
- The abbreviation or unit symbol is clearly written *before* the quantity.
- If you are unsure about the exact meaning of any medical notation, do not guess or assume. Ask the writer for clarification.

APPENDIX D

HOUSEHOLD UNITS, ABBREVIATIONS, AND THEIR EQUIVALENTS

Unit	Abbreviation	Equivalent
Drop	gtt	
Teaspoon	tsp (or t)	
Tablespoon	Tbs (or T)	1 Tbs = 3 tsp
Ounce (fluid)	oz (℥)	1 oz = 2 Tbs
Ounce (weight)	oz	1 pound (lb) = 16 oz
Cup	cup	1 cup = 8 oz
Pint	pt	1 pt = 2 cups
Quart	qt	1 qt = 4 cups = 2 pt

Note: Like the minim (♏) and dram (ʒ), the drop (gtt) unit is given only for the purpose of recognition. There are no standard equivalents for *drop* to learn. The amount of each drop varies according to the diameter of the utensil used for administration. (See Figure 5-2 Calibrated Dropper and Figure 12-14 Intravenous Drip Chambers.)

MATH TIP

The abbreviations for tablespoon and teaspoon are very similar. To help remember which is which, remember this: Tablespoon is larger than teaspoon, and the abbreviation is expressed with a capital *T*. Teaspoon is the smaller unit, and the abbreviation is expressed with a lower case or small *t*. To avoid confusion and to minimize errors, use *Tbs* for *tablespoon* and *tsp* for *teaspoon*.

CAUTION

There is wide variation in household measures and common household measuring devices, such as tableware teaspoons. Therefore, using the household system or household measures for dosage measurement can constitute a safety risk. Advise patients and their families to use the measuring devices packaged with the medication or provided by the pharmacy, rather than using common household measuring devices.

QUICK REVIEW

In the household system,

- The common units used in healthcare are teaspoon, tablespoon, ounce, cup, pint, quart, and pound.
- The quantity is expressed in Arabic numbers with the unit abbreviation following the amount. Example: 5 t
- Quantities less than 1 are preferably expressed as common fractions. Example: $\frac{1}{2}$ cup
- When in doubt about the exact amount or the abbreviation used, do not guess or assume. Ask the writer to clarify.

APPENDIX E

Units of Measurement for Temperature

Knowing and recognizing significant temperatures is important in the healthcare system for a number of reasons, for example, to

- Recognize healthy body temperatures;
- Diagnose some disease states;
- Ensure aseptic and sterilizing procedures; and
- Recognize the safe maintenance of a "cold chain" in transporting and storing some medications, such as vaccines.

Three temperature scales are available today: Fahrenheit, Celsius, and Kelvin. The oldest scale is Fahrenheit. In 1724, the Fahrenheit scale was proposed by and named after a German physicist who described water freezing at 32°F and boiling at 212°F at normal atmospheric pressure.

Less than 20 years later, Celsius, a Swedish astronomer, proposed a scale in which the difference between the freezing and boiling temperatures of pure water was divided into 100°. The Celsius scale is used most commonly throughout the world today.

The Kelvin scale is the newest scale, developed in the mid-1800s. The kelvin is a base unit in the SI. The Kelvin scale is based on *absolute zero*, which is the equivalent of −273.16°C. Its intervals are equivalent to the Celsius scale.

On April 1, 1975, weather reporters and forecasters started using the SI, with Celsius temperatures replacing Fahrenheit. By September of that year, Canadians had rain dropping in millimetres and snow falling in centimetres.

The United States is a notable world exception in its continued use of the Fahrenheit scale. Since the United States is one of Canada's largest trading partners, many of Canada's household tools and equipment still show temperature in Fahrenheit. In addition, a number of healthcare tools and instruments still use the Fahrenheit scale. Although it is hoped that all health tools and instruments used by today's Canadian healthcare providers offer the option of using the Celsius scale, the topic of temperature measurements is included here as a resource in case conversion is required.

One final note is regarding the term *centigrade,* which is sometimes used interchangeably with the Celsius scale. *Centigrade* means *divided into 100* and is based on the Latin words *centrum*, meaning hundred, and *gradus,* meaning degree.

Since the Kelvin scale is mainly used by scientists, conversion between temperature scales will focus on the Fahrenheit and Celsius scales. Simple formulas are used for conversions.

In Figure D-1, note the 180° difference between the freezing and boiling points on the Fahrenheit thermometer; the difference between freezing and boiling on the Celsius thermometer is 100°. The ratio of the difference between the Fahrenheit and Celsius scales can be expressed as 180:100 or 180/100. When reduced, this ratio is equivalent to 9/5, or 1.8. One or the other of these constants is used in temperature conversions. When converting between Fahrenheit and Celsius, if necessary, carry the math process to hundredths and round to tenths.

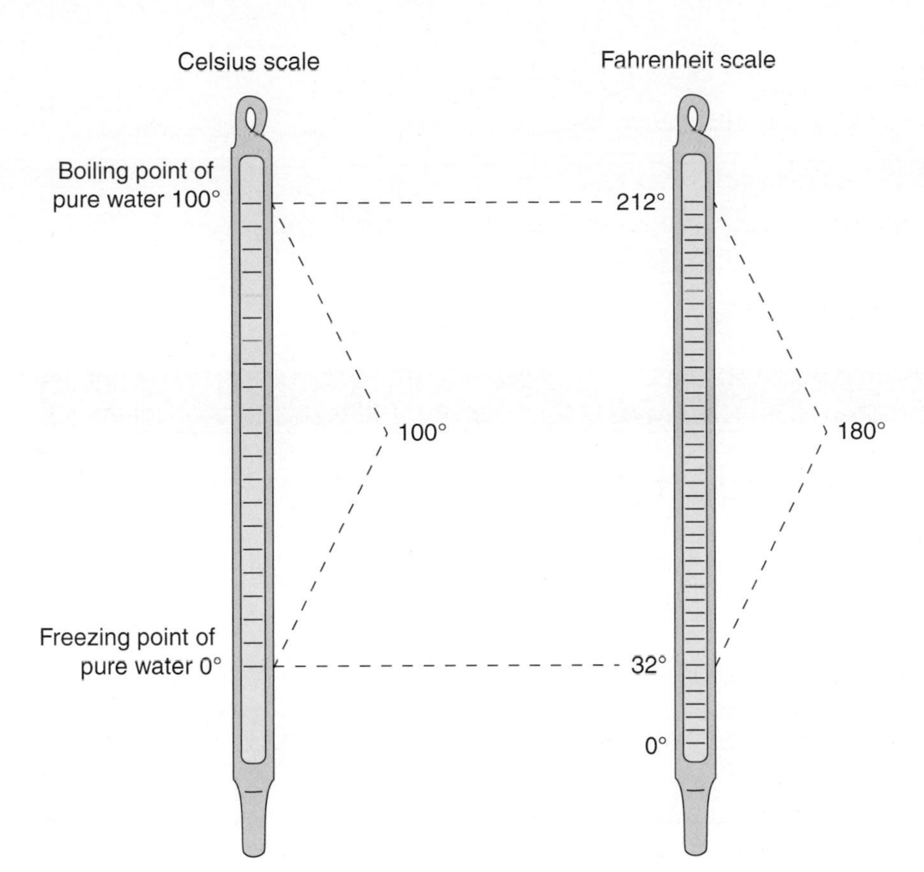

Note: Glass thermometers like those in Figure E-1 are for demonstration purposes. Electronic digital temperature devices are more commonly used in healthcare settings. Most electronic devices can instantly convert between the two scales, freeing the healthcare provider from doing the actual calculations. However, the healthcare provider's ability to understand the difference between Celsius and Fahrenheit remains important.

FIGURE E-1 Comparison of Celsius and Fahrenheit Temperature Scales

RULE

To convert Fahrenheit temperature to Celsius, subtract 32 and then divide the result by 1.8, or multiply by $\frac{5}{9}$.

$$°C = \frac{°F - 32}{1.8} \text{ or } °C = (°F - 32) \times \frac{5}{9}$$

Example:

Convert 98.6°F to °C.

$$°C = \frac{98.6 - 32}{1.8}$$

$$= \frac{66.6}{1.8}$$

$$°C = 37$$

RULE

To convert Celsius temperature to Fahrenheit, multiply by 1.8 or $\frac{9}{5}$ and add 32.

$$°F = 1.8 \times °C + 32 \text{ or } °F = \left(\frac{9}{5} \times °C\right) + 32$$

Note: One conversion is the reverse operation in the reverse order from the other.

Example:

Convert 35°C to °F.

$$°F = 1.8 \times 35 + 32$$
$$= 63 + 32$$
$$°F = 95$$

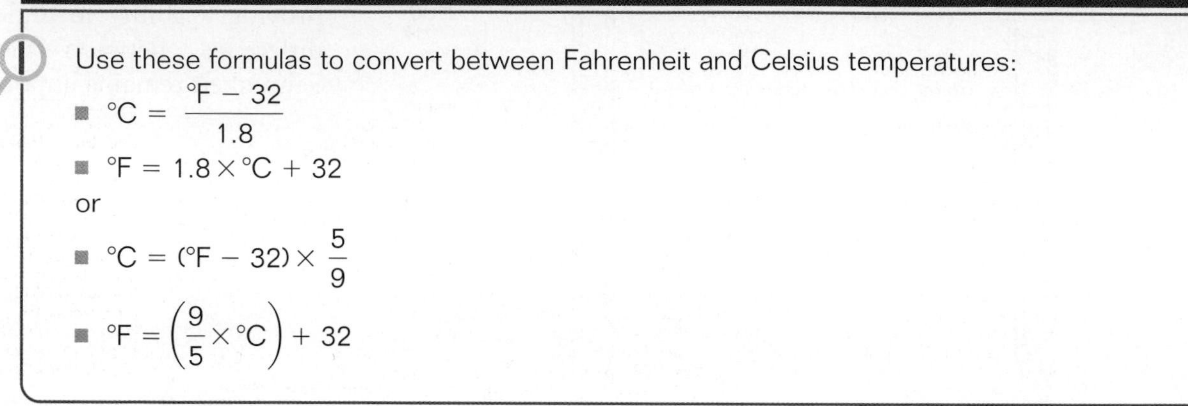

QUICK REVIEW

Use these formulas to convert between Fahrenheit and Celsius temperatures:

- $°C = \dfrac{°F - 32}{1.8}$
- $°F = 1.8 \times °C + 32$

or

- $°C = (°F - 32) \times \dfrac{5}{9}$
- $°F = \left(\dfrac{9}{5} \times °C\right) + 32$

INDEX